This book belongs to
Mr. & Mrs. R. Wayne Johnson

Nursing81
DRUG
HANDBOOK™

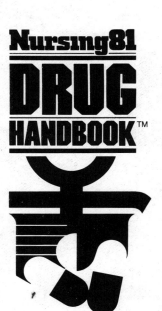

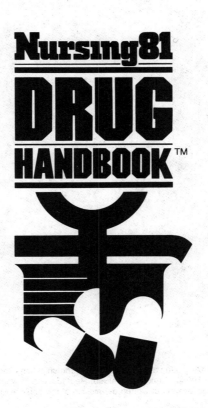

Nursing81
DRUG
HANDBOOK™

NURSING 81 BOOKS
INTERMED COMMUNICATIONS, INC.
HORSHAM, PENNSYLVANIA

NURSING81 DRUG HANDBOOK

ISSN 0273-320X

ISBN 0-916730-33-6

The clinical procedures described and recommended in this publication are based on research and consultation with medical and nursing authorities. To the best of our knowledge, these procedures reflect currently accepted clinical practice; nevertheless, they can't be considered absolute and universal recommendations. For individual application, treatment recommendations must be considered in light of the patient's clinical condition and, before administration of new or infrequently used drugs, in light of latest package-insert information. The authors and the publisher disclaim responsibility for any adverse effects resulting directly or indirectly from the suggested procedures, from any undetected errors, or from the reader's misunderstanding of the text.

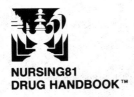

**NURSING81
DRUG HANDBOOK™**

PUBLISHER
Edward J. Quigley

EDITORIAL DIRECTOR
Helen Klusek Hamilton

CLINICAL DIRECTOR
Minnie Bowen Rose, RN, BSN, MEd

MANUFACTURING DIRECTOR
Bernard Haas

Intermed Communications Book Division

CHAIRMAN
Eugene W. Jackson

PRESIDENT
Daniel L. Cheney

RESEARCH DIRECTOR
Elizabeth O'Brien

PURCHASING DIRECTOR
Bacil Guiley

Staff for this volume

Clinical Pharmacy Editor: Larry Neil Gever, PharmD
Editors: June T. Norris, Jean Robinson, Avery Rome, Elaine Schott-Jones
Assistant Editors: Jean Axelrod, Saretta Berlin, Lisa Z. Cohen, Louise Lux-Sions, Laura Musmanno-Albert, Sanford Robinson, Norman Rudnick, Frank Wilson
Copy Editors: Barbara Hodgson, Linda Hewlings, Zena Sandler-Gordon
Indexer: Vonda Heller
Researchers: Carole Gan, June Gomez, Helen O'Connor, Sallie J. Rosenfeld
Designer: Kathaleen Motak Singel
Artists: Diane Fox, Sandra Simms
Typography Manager: David C. Kosten
Typography Assistants: Nancy Merz Ballner, Ethel Halle, Diane Paluba
Production Manager: Robert L. Dean

Clinical Consultants

Nancy Burns, RN, MSN, Assistant Professor, University of Texas School of Nursing, Arlington, Texas

Jeanne Dupont, RN, Head Nurse, Emergency Department, Massachusetts Eye and Ear Infirmary, Boston, Massachusetts

Margarethe Hawken, RN, MA, CNRN, Clinical Nurse Specialist in Neurology and Epilepsy, Seattle Veterans' Administration Medical Center, Seattle, Washington

Kathleen M. Hawkins, RN, Clinical Nurse Specialist in Dermatology, University of Colorado, Health Sciences Center, Denver, Colorado

Carolyn Holt, RN, BSEd, Coordinator, Nursing Staff Development, Columbus-Cuneo-Cabrini Medical Center, Chicago, Illinois

Gail D'Onofrio Long, RN, MS, Clinical Nurse Specialist in Medical Intensive Care and Coronary Care, University Hospital, Boston, Massachusetts

Elizabeth A. Phillips, RN, BA, Instructor in Nursing, St. Francis Medical Center School of Nursing, Trenton, New Jersey

Despina Seremelis, RN, BSN, Staff Nurse, Temple University Hospital, Philadelphia, Pennsylvania

Paula Brammer Vetter, RN, BSN, Clinical Instructor in Coronary Intensive Care, Cleveland Clinic Hospital, Cleveland, Ohio

Pharmacy Reviewers

Ron Ballentine, PharmD, Assistant Professor of Clinical Pharmacy, University of Houston; Drug Information Specialist, University of Texas System Cancer Center, M.D. Anderson Hospital and Tumor Institute, Houston, Texas

Peter W. Chan, PharmD, Clinical Pharmacist, Aurora, Colorado

Michael R. Cohen, BS, Assistant Director, Department of Pharmacy, Temple University Hospital; Clinical Assistant Professor, Temple University School of Pharmacy, Philadelphia, Pennsylvania

Lawrence J. Dwork, BS, Clinical Pharmacist, Grant Hospital, Columbus, Ohio

Matthew P. Fricker, BS, Clinical Pharmacist, Temple University Hospital, Philadelphia, Pennsylvania

Jay H. Hoffman, BS, Clinical Pharmacist, Thomas Jefferson University Hospital, Philadelphia, Pennsylvania

Alan W. Hopefl, PharmD, Assistant Professor of Clinical Pharmacy, St. Louis College of Pharmacy; Assistant Professor of Pharmacology in Medicine, St. Louis University School of Medicine, St. Louis, Missouri

Joseph A. Linkewich, PharmD, Associate Professor of Clinical Pharmacy, Philadelphia College of Pharmacy and Science, Philadelphia, Pennsylvania

Steven Meisel, PharmD, Deputy Chief Pharmacist, Keams Canyon Indian Hospital and Clinics, U.S. Public Health Service, Keams Canyon, Arizona

Linda Nelson, PharmD, Instructor in Clinical Pharmacy, Philadelphia College of Pharmacy and Science, Philadelphia, Pennsylvania

David R. Pipher, PharmD, Clinical Pharmacist, Medical College of Pennsylvania, Philadelphia, Pennsylvania

Susan Rogers, PharmD, Clinical Pharmacist, Thomas Jefferson University Hospital; Clinical Instructor, Philadelphia College of Pharmacy and Science, Philadelphia, Pennsylvania

Joel Shuster, PharmD, Director of Pharmacy Services, The Fairmount Institute; Clinical Assistant Professor, Philadelphia College of Pharmacy and Science, Philadelphia, Pennsylvania

William Simonson, PharmD, Associate Professor of Pharmacy, Oregon State University School of Pharmacy, Corvallis, Oregon

Joseph F. Steiner, PharmD, Assistant Professor of Family Practice, University of Wyoming, Family Practice Residency Center, Casper, Wyoming

Frank F. Williams, PharmD, Drug Information Pharmacist, Temple University Hospital, Philadelphia, Pennsylvania

EDITORIAL ADVISORY BOARD

Contents

Contributors

Richard Bailey, BS, Director of Pharmacy Service, Kensington Hospital, Philadelphia, Pennsylvania

Marquette L. Cannon, PharmD, Assistant Professor of Clinical Pharmacy, Temple University School of Pharmacy, Philadelphia, Pennsylvania

Peter W. Chan, PharmD, Clinical Pharmacist, Aurora, Colorado

Michael R. Cohen, BS, RPh, Assistant Director, Department of Pharmacy, Temple University Hospital, Philadelphia, Pennsylvania

Judith Hopfer Deglin, PharmD, Assistant Professor of Clinical Pharmacy, West Virginia University School of Pharmacy, Morgantown, West Virginia

Betty H. Dennis, MS, Assistant Professor of Clinical Pharmacy, University of North Carolina School of Pharmacy, Chapel Hill, North Carolina

Dina Dichek, BS, Pharmacist, Oakville-Trafalgar Memorial Hospital, Oakville, Ontario, Canada

Teresa P. Dowling, PharmD, Assistant Professor of Clinical Pharmacy, Philadelphia College of Pharmacy and Science, Philadelphia, Pennsylvania

Dan R. Ford, PharmD, Nuclear Pharmacist, National Radiopharmaceutical Company, Houston, Texas

Bruce M. Frey, PharmD, Clinical Pharmacist in Pediatrics, Thomas Jefferson University Hospital, Philadelphia, Pennsylvania

Lee Gardner, PharmD, Clinical Pharmacist, Kino Community Hospital, Tucson, Arizona

Marie Gardner, PharmD, Clinical Pharmacist, Tucson General Hospital, Tucson, Arizona

Philip P. Gerbino, PharmD, Associate Professor of Clinical Pharmacy, Philadelphia College of Pharmacy and Science, Philadelphia, Pennsylvania

Patricia J. Hedrick, PharmD, Clinical Pharmacist, University of Illinois Hospital, Chicago, Illinois

James R. Hildebrand, PharmD, Clinical Pharmacist, Thomas Jefferson University Hospital, Philadelphia, Pennsylvania

Arthur I. Jacknowitz, PharmD, Director, Drug Information Center, West Virginia University School of Pharmacy, Morgantown, West Virginia

Sandra G. Jue, PharmD, Clinical Pharmacist, Veterans Administration Medical Center, Boise, Idaho

Barbara H. Korberly, PharmD, Assistant Professor of Clinical Pharmacy, Philadelphia College of Pharmacy and Science, Philadelphia, Pennsylvania

Sheldon M. Leiman, BS, Assistant Director, Department of Pharmacy, Temple University Hospital, Philadelphia, Pennsylvania

Lauren F. McKaig, BS, Tutor in Clinical Pharmacy, Sunnybrook Medical Centre, University of Toronto, Toronto, Ontario, Canada

Kathryn Murphy, MSN, Instructor, Nursing of Children, University of Pennsylvania, Philadelphia, Pennsylvania

David W. Newton, PhD, Associate Professor of Pharmaceutics, Massachusetts College of Pharmacy and Allied Health Sciences, Boston, Massachusetts

Gerald N. Rotenberg, BS, FACA, Editor, Compendium of Pharmaceuticals and Specialties, Canadian Pharmaceutical Association, Toronto, Ontario, Canada

George David Rudd, MS, Assistant Professor of Clinical Pharmacy, University of North Carolina School of Pharmacy, Chapel Hill, North Carolina

Joel Shuster, PharmD, Director of Pharmacy Services, The Fairmount Institute, Philadelphia, Pennsylvania

Jamshid B. Tehrani, PhD, Pharmacist Manager, Skin and Cancer Pharmacy, Temple University Hospital, Philadelphia, Pennsylvania

C. Wayne Weart, PharmD, Associate Professor of Pharmacy and Family Practice, Medical University of South Carolina, Charleston, South Carolina

Frank F. Williams, PharmD, Drug Information Pharmacist, Temple University Hospital, Philadelphia, Pennsylvania

FOREWORD

In the adversary society that is developing in health care today, a dependable reference work on drug therapy is indispensable to every practicing nurse. Only a printed reference can validate the actions and side effects of the overwhelmingly complex array of drugs you may be asked to administer during ordinary duty. As the person who is responsible for administering most drugs, you need to be able to evaluate drug orders quickly—to check dosages with precision; to know the best route of administration; and to anticipate interactions, side effects, and possible toxicity.

The *Nursing81 Drug Handbook,* a handy pocket-sized drug reference, was compiled to give you all this information in an easily accessible form. Like the 1979 and 1980 editions of *Nurse's Guide to Drugs,* this edition summarizes all clinically relevant information on virtually all drugs currently used in the United States and Canada. It contains detailed information on more than 1,000 drugs—all of it completely reviewed, reevaluated, and updated by clinical pharmacists to assure the latest, most accurate information. You'll find newly approved drugs and newly approved indications for existing drugs. However, the information has been rearranged to fit a smaller, space-saving format. This book's comprehensive content is organized in a manner that makes the information easy to find. For example, the index makes each drug accessible by both generic and trade names. Drugs are grouped into 16 major sections, depending on their clinical use. Each drug entry is identified by both generic and trade names, and summarizes explicit dosage instruction for approved indications, side effects, clinically significant interactions, and nursing considerations. To help you focus quickly on significant side effects, this book italicizes the most hazardous and most common ones.

You will find the *Nursing81 Drug Handbook* a valuable daily resource. It's a dependable source of drug information that will help you meet your responsibility for administering drugs with confidence and skill.

LUTHER CHRISTMAN, *Ph.D., R.N.*
Vice President, Nursing Affairs and
Dean, College of Nursing, Rush University
Rush-Presbyterian-St. Luke's Medical Center
Chicago, Illinois

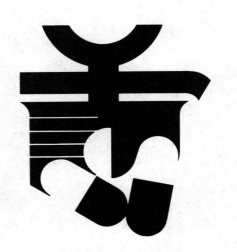

1

How to use Nursing81 Drug Handbook

Nursing81 Drug Handbook is meant to fill a very special need. It represents a joint effort by pharmacists and nurses to provide the nursing profession with drug information that focuses directly on what nurses need to know. With this in mind, it emphasizes clinical aspects, not pharmacology, and does not attempt to replace detailed pharmacology texts. For the same reason, the information is arranged in a format designed to make it readily accessible.

Introductory information
Following this chapter, Chapter 2 explains, in a general way, how drugs work. It also tells about side effects and adverse reactions, and gives general guidelines about drug use in pregnancy and the presence of drugs in breast milk. In the remaining chapters, all drugs are classified according to their common, therapeutic uses.

Drug information
Each chapter begins with an alphabetically arranged list of the generic names of drugs described in that chapter. Specific information on each drug is arranged under five headings: *Name; Indications and Dosage; Side Effects; Interactions;* and *Nursing Considerations.*

Each drug's generic name is immediately followed by an alphabetic list of its brand names. Brands available in both the United States and Canada are designated with a diamond (♦); those available *only* in Canada with a double diamond (♦♦). A brand name

with no symbol after it is available only in the United States. If a drug is a controlled substance, that too is clearly indicated (example: Controlled Substance Schedule II). Products listed, although generally available, may not be approved by the Food and Drug Administration. The mention of a brand name in no way implies endorsement of that product or guarantees its legality.

The section titled *Indications and Dosage* lists specific dosage instructions for adults and children, as applicable. Children's doses are usually indicated in terms of mg/Kg/day. Dosage instructions reflect current clinical trends in therapeutics and can't be considered an absolute and universal recommendation. For individual application, dosage instructions must be considered in context with the patient's clinical condition.

The section titled *Side Effects* lists each drug's commonly observed side effects (and selected rare ones if life-threatening). The most common and life-threatening side effects are italicized for easy reference. An exception to this rule is a side effect that, although it is normally considered quite hazardous, has been reported to be mild and reversible with the drug in question. For example, thrombocytopenia is considered a life-threatening side effect of mithramycin (a chemotherapeutic drug). On the other hand, the thrombocytopenia seen with methyldopa (Aldomet) is generally mild and reversible. Hence, thrombocytopenia listed as a side effect of mithramycin is italicized, whereas the same side effect under methyldopa is not. Side effects are grouped according to the body system in which they appear.

The next section, *Interactions,* lists each drug's confirmed, *clinically significant* interactions with other drugs, including additive effects, potentiated effects, and antagonistic effects. Also included are specific suggestions for dealing with dangerous drug interaction (for example, reducing doses or monitoring certain lab tests). Drug interactions are listed under the drug that is adversely affected. For example, magnesium trisilicate, an ingredient in antacids, interacts with tetracy-cline to cause decreased absorption of tetracycline. Therefore, this interaction is listed under tetracycline. To check on the possible effects of using two or more drugs simultaneously, refer to the interaction entry for *each* of the drugs in question.

The final section, *Nursing Considerations,* lists other useful information, starting with contraindications and precautions, followed by monitoring techniques and suggestions for prevention and treatment of side effects. Also included in this column are suggestions for promoting patient comfort, for patient teaching, and for preparing, administering, and storing each drug.

2

Drug actions, reactions, and interactions explained

Administration of any drug provokes a series of events within the body. The first event, when a drug combines with cell drug receptors, is known as the drug action. What follows as a result of this action of the drug is known as the drug effect. Depending upon the number of different cellular drug receptors affected by a given drug, a drug effect can be local or systemic, or both. For example, the antipeptic ulcer drug Tagamet (cimetidine) acts solely by blocking histamine receptor cells in the small intestine and the stomach. This is known as a local drug effect because the drug action is sharply limited to one area and does not spread to other parts of the body. On the other hand, Benadryl (diphenhydramine) produces a systemic effect in that it blocks histamine receptors in widespread areas of the body. In other words, local drug effects are specific to a limited number of organ systems, whereas systemic drug effects are generalized and affect different and diverse organ systems.

Three factors modify drug action

1. Absorption

Before a drug can act within the body, it must be absorbed into the bloodstream—usually after oral administration, the most frequently used route. Before a drug contained in a tablet or capsule can be absorbed, the dosage form must disintegrate, that is, break into smaller particles. Then, these smaller particles can dissolve in gastric juices. Only after so dissolving can a drug be absorbed into the blood-

stream. Once absorbed and circulating in the bloodstream, it is said to be bioavailable or ready to produce a drug effect. Of course, whether such absorption is complete or partial depends on several factors: the physiochemical effects of the drug, the formulation of the drug product, its interactions with other substances in the gastrointestinal tract, and various patient characteristics. These same factors also determine the speed of absorption. Thus, oral solutions and elixirs, which bypass the need for disintegration and dissolution, are usually absorbed more rapidly. Drugs administered intramuscularly must first be absorbed through the muscle into the bloodstream. Rectal suppositories must dissolve to be absorbed through the rectal mucosa. Of course, drugs administered intravenously are placed directly into the circulation and are completely and immediately bioavailable.

2. Distribution

After absorption, a drug moves from the bloodstream into various fluids and tissues within the body; this is distribution. Individual patient variations can greatly alter the amount of drug that is distributed throughout the body. For example, in an edematous patient, a given dose must be distributed to a larger volume than in a nonedematous patient; the amount of drug must sometimes be increased to account for this. Remember, the dosage should be decreased when the edema is corrected. Conversely, in an extremely dehydrated patient, the drug will be distributed to a much smaller volume, so the dose must then be decreased. The total area to which a drug is distributed is known as volume of distribution. Patients who are particularly obese may present another problem when considering drug distribution. Some drugs—such as digoxin, gentamicin, and tobramycin — are not well distributed to fatty tissue. Therefore, dosing based on actual body weight may lead to overdose and serious toxicity. In some cases, dosing must be based on lean body weight, which may be estimated from actuarial tables that give average weight range for height.

3. Metabolism and excretion (drug elimination)

Most drugs are metabolized in the liver and excreted by the kidneys. Hepatic diseases may affect one or more of the metabolic functions of the liver. Therefore, in patients with hepatic disease, the metabolism of a drug may be increased, decreased, or unchanged. Clearly, all patients with hepatic disease must be monitored closely for drug effect and toxicity. Some drugs (digoxin, gentamicin) are eliminated almost unchanged by the kidneys. For safe use of such drugs, renal function must be adequate or the drug will accumulate, producing toxic effects. Some drugs can alter the effect and excretion of other drugs. For example, they can stimulate hepatic metabolizing enzymes to speed up the rate of metabolism and change the drug effect. Or, they can block or promote renal excretion of other drugs, causing them to accumulate and enhance their effects, or causing them to be too rapidly excreted and so diminish their effects. Some slight elimination takes place by way of perspiration, saliva, breast milk, and so on. (Certain volatile anesthetics, however—halothane, for instance—are eliminated primarily by exhalation.)

The rate at which a drug is metabolized varies with the individual. In some patients, drugs are metabolized so quickly that their serum and tissue levels prove therapeutically inadequate. In others, the rate of metabolism is so slow that ordinary doses can produce toxic results.

Other modifying factors

An important factor that influences a drug's action and effect is its *binding to plasma proteins,* especially albumin, and other tissue components. Because only free, unbound drug can act in the body, such binding greatly influences effectiveness and duration of effect.

The *patient's age* is another important factor. Elderly patients usually have decreased hepatic function, less muscle mass, and diminished renal function. Consequently, lower doses and sometimes longer dosage intervals are needed to avoid toxicity in the elderly. With similar consequences, neonates have underdeveloped metabolic enzyme systems and inadequate renal function. They need highly individualized dosage and careful monitoring.

Underlying disease can also markedly affect drug action and effect. For example, acidosis may cause insulin resistance. Genetic diseases such as glucose-6-phosphate dehydrogenase (G-6-PD) deficiency and hepatic porphyria may turn drugs into toxins with serious consequences. Patients with G-6-PD deficiency may develop hemolytic anemia when given aspirin, sulfonamides, or any of a number of drugs. A genetically susceptible patient can develop an acute porphyria attack if given a barbiturate. Also, patients who have highly active hepatic enzyme systems (for example, rapid acetylators), when treated with isoniazid, can develop hepatitis from the rapid intrahepatic buildup of a toxic metabolite.

Things to consider about administration

1. Dosage forms do matter. Some tablets and capsules are too large to be readily swallowed by very ill patients. You may then request an oral solution or elixir of the same drug, but bear in mind that because a liquid is more easily and completely absorbed, it produces higher serum levels than a tablet. When a potentially toxic drug is given, the increased amount absorbed could cause toxicity. One example of this is digoxin tablets versus digoxin elixir. Sometimes a change in dosage form requires a change in dose.

2. Routes of administration are not therapeutically interchangeable. For example, phenytoin (Dilantin) is readily absorbed orally but is slowly and erratically absorbed intramuscularly. On the other hand, carbenicillin must be given parenterally because oral administration yields inadequate serum levels to treat systemic infections. However, it can be given orally to treat urinary tract infections because it concentrates in the urine.

3. The timing of drug administration can be important. Sometimes giving an oral drug during or shortly after mealtime decreases the amount of drug absorbed. This is not clinically significant with most drugs and may in fact be desirable with irritating drugs such as aspirin or phenylbutazone. But penicillins and tetracyclines should not be scheduled for administration at mealtimes because certain foods can inactivate them. If in doubt about the effect of food on a certain drug, check with a pharmacist.

4. Consider the patient's age, height, and weight. The doctor will need this information when calculating the dose for many drugs. It should be accurately recorded on the patient's chart. This chart should also include current laboratory data, especially kidney and liver function studies, so the doctor can consider them and adapt dosage as needed.

5. Watch for metabolic changes. Monitor for any physiologic change that might alter drug effect. Examples: depressed respiratory function and the development of acidosis or alkalosis.

6. Know the patient's history. Whenever possible, obtain a comprehensive family history from the patient or his family. Ask about past reactions to drugs, possible genetic traits that might alter drug response, and the current use of other drugs. Multiple drug therapy can dramatically change the effects of many drugs. These are known as drug interactions.

Drug interactions

When one drug administered in combination with or shortly after another drug alters the effect of one or both drugs, this is known as a drug interaction. Usually, the effect of one drug is increased or decreased. For instance, one drug may inhibit or stimulate the metabolism or excretion of the other; or it may release another from plasma protein-binding sites, freeing it for further action.

Combination therapy is based upon drug interaction. One drug, for example, may be given in order to potentiate another. Probenecid, which blocks the excretion of penicillin, is sometimes given with penicillin to maintain adequate serum levels of penicillin for a longer period. Often two drugs with similar action are given together precisely because of the additive effect that results. Aspirin and codeine, for instance, both analgesics, are often given in combination because together they provide greater relief from pain than either alone.

Drug interactions are sometimes used to prevent or antagonize certain side effects. Hydrochlorothiazide and spironolactone, both diuretics, are often administered in combination, because the former is potassium-depleting, while the latter is potassium-sparing.

But not all drug interactions are beneficial. Multiple drugs can interact to produce effects that are often undesirable and sometimes hazardous. Harmful drug interactions decrease efficiency or increase toxicity. A hypertensive patient well controlled with guanethidine may see his blood pressure rise to its former high level if he takes the antidepressant amitriptyline (Elavil) at the same time. Such a drug effect is known as antagonism. Drug combinations that produce these effects when used together should be avoided if possible. Another kind of inhibiting effect occurs when a tetracycline drug is administered concomitantly with calcium- or magnesium-containing drugs or foods (i.e., antacids or milk). These combine with tetracycline in the gastrointestinal tract and cause inadequate absorption of tetracycline.

Side effects

Any drug effect other than what is therapeutically intended can be called a side effect. It may be expected and benign, or unexpected and potentially harmful. For example, during hay fever season, a patient may have to contend with the drowsiness caused by chlorpheniramine to get relief from hay fever symptoms. In such a case, the dose may be adjusted up or down to balance therapeutic effect with side effect.

A side effect may be tolerated for a necessary therapeutic effect, or it may be hazardous and unacceptable and require discontinuation of the drug. Some side effects subside with continued use. As an example, the drowsiness associated with methyldopa (Aldomet) and the orthostatic hypotension associated with prazosin (Minipress) usually subside after several days, as the patient develops a tolerance to these effects. But many side effects are dose-related and lessen or disappear only if dosage is reduced. Although most side effects are not therapeutically desirable, an occasional one can be put to clinical use. An outstanding example of this is the drowsiness associated with diphenhydramine (Benadryl), which makes it clinically useful as a mild hypnotic.

Hypersensitivity, a term sometimes used interchangeably with drug allergy, is the result of an antigen-antibody immune reaction that occurs in the body when a drug is introduced into a susceptible patient. One of the most dangerous of all drug hypersensitivities is penicillin allergy. In its severest form, penicillin anaphylaxis can rapidly become fatal.

Rarely, idiosyncratic reactions occur. These are highly unpredictable, individual, and unusual. Probably the best known idiosyncratic drug reaction is the aplastic anemia caused by the antibiotic chloramphenicol (Chloromycetin). This reaction appears in only 1 out of 40,000 patients, but when it does, it is often fatal. A more common idiosyncratic reaction is extreme sensitivity to very low doses of a drug, or insensitivity to much higher than normally tolerated doses.

To deal with side effects correctly, you need to be alert to even minor changes in the patient's clinical status. Such minor changes may be an early warning of pending toxicity. Listen to the patient's complaints about his reactions to a drug, and consider each complaint objectively. You may be able to reduce undesirable side effects in several ways. Obviously, dosage reduction often helps. But often so does a simple rescheduling of the same dose. For example, Sudafed (pseudoephedrine) may produce stimulation that will be no problem if it's given early in the day; similarly, the drowsiness that occurs with antihistamines or tranquilizers can be totally harmless if the dose is given at bedtime.

Most important, your patient needs to be told what side effects to expect so he won't become worried or even stop taking the drug on his own. Of course, the patient should report any unusual or unexpected side effects to the doctor.

Recognizing drug allergies or serious idiosyncratic reactions can sometimes be lifesaving. Ask each patient about drugs he is taking or has taken in the past and what, if any, unusual effects he experienced from taking them. If a patient claims to be allergic to a drug, ask him to tell you exactly what happens when he takes it. He may be calling a harmless side effect such as upset stomach an allergic reaction, or he may have a true tendency to anaphylaxis. In either case, you and the doctor need to know this. Of course, you must record and report any clinical changes throughout the patient's hospital stay. If you suspect a hazardous side effect, withhold the drug until you can check with the pharmacist and the doctor.

Toxic reactions

Chronic drug toxicities are generally due to cumulative effect and the resulting buildup of the drug in the body. These effects may be extensions of the desired therapeutic effect. For example, guanethidine-induced norepinephrine depletion produces a desired antihypertensive effect, but in larger doses, this same biochemical action often produces orthostatic hypotension.

Drug toxicities usually occur when serum drug levels rise due to impaired metabolism or excretion. For example, blood levels of theophylline rise when hepatic dysfunction impairs metabolism of the drug. Similarly, digoxin toxicity can follow impaired renal function because digoxin is eliminated from the body almost exclusively by the kidneys (via glomerular filtration). Of course, toxic blood

levels also follow excessive dosage. Aspirin tinnitus (ringing in ears) is usually a sign that the safe dose has been exceeded.

Most drug toxicity is predictable and dose-related; fortunately, most drug toxicity is also readily reversible upon dosage adjustment. So it's essential to monitor patients carefully for physiological changes that might alter drug effect. Watch especially for impaired hepatic and renal function. Warn the patient about signs of pending toxicity, and tell him what to do if a toxic reaction occurs. Also, be sure to emphasize the importance of taking a drug exactly as prescribed. Warn the patient about serious problems that could arise if he changes the dose or the schedule for taking it.

Drugs and pregnancy

Ever since the thalidomide tragedy of the late 1950s—when thousands of malformed infants were born after their mothers used this mild sedative-hypnotic during pregnancy—use of drugs during pregnancy has been a source of serious medical concern and controversy. To identify drugs that may cause such teratogenic effects, preclinical drug studies always include tests on pregnant laboratory animals. These tests do point out gross teratogenicity but do not clearly establish safety. Because different species react to drugs in different ways, animal studies do not rule out possible teratogenic effects in humans. For example, the preliminary studies on thalidomide gave no warning of teratogenic effects, and it was subsequently released for general use in Europe.

To prevent such tragedies, just about every drug now carries a special warning on the official package insert. Such warnings state that safety in human pregnancy has not been established and use of the drug in pregnancy requires the expected therapeutic benefit be weighed against possible hazard to mother and child. With the exception of vitamins and minerals, no drug is approved caveat-free for use in pregnancy. Even Bendectin (a combination of the antihistamine doxylamine and the vitamin pyridoxine), for which nausea and vomiting of pregnancy is an official indication, carries a warning for cautious use during pregnancy.

What about the placental barrier? Once thought to protect the fetus from drug effects, the placenta isn't actually much of a barrier at all. Except for drugs with exceptionally large molecular structure, almost every drug administered to a pregnant woman crosses the placenta and enters the fetal circulation. An example of such large molecular size is heparin, the injectable anticoagulant. Theoretically, then, heparin could be used in a pregnant woman without fear of harming the fetus—but even heparin carries a warning for cautious use in pregnancy. Conversely, just because a drug crosses the placenta doesn't necessarily mean it's harmful to the fetus.

Actually, only one factor—stage of fetal development—seems clearly related to exaggerated risk during pregnancy. During two stages of pregnancy—the first and the third trimesters—the fetus is especially vulnerable to damage from maternal use of drugs. During these times, *all* drugs should be given with extreme caution. The most sensitive period for drug-induced fetal malformation is the first trimester, when fetal organs are differentiating (organogenesis). During this time, *all* drugs should be withheld unless doing so would jeopardize the mother's health. Theoretically, during this sensitive time, even aspirin could harm the fetus. So, strongly advise your patient to avoid *all* self-prescribed drugs during early pregnancy.

The other time of special fetal sensitivity to drugs is the last trimester.

The reason? At birth, when separated from his mother, the newborn must rely on his own metabolism to eliminate any remaining drug. Because his detoxifying systems are not fully developed, any residual drug may take a long time to be metabolized—and thus may induce prolonged toxic reactions. Consequently, drugs should be used only when absolutely necessary during the last 3 months of pregnancy.

Of course, in many circumstances, pregnant women must continue to take certain drugs. For example, an epileptic woman who is well controlled with an anticonvulsant should continue to take it even during pregnancy. Or a pregnant woman with a bacterial infection must receive antibiotics. In such cases, the potential risk to the fetus is overbalanced by the mother's need.

Following these general guidelines can prevent indiscriminate and potentially harmful use of drugs in pregnancy:
- Before a drug is prescribed for a woman of childbearing age, she should be asked the date of her last menstrual period and whether there is a possibility she is pregnant.
- Especially during the first and the third trimesters, a pregnant patient should avoid *all* drugs except those *essential* to maintain the pregnancy or maternal health.
- Topical drugs are not exempt from the warning against indiscriminate use during pregnancy. Many topically applied drugs can be absorbed in large enough amounts to be harmful to the fetus.
- When a pregnant patient needs *any* drug, the doctor should prescribe the *safest* possible drug in the *lowest* possible dose to minimize any harmful effect to the fetus.
- Every pregnant patient should check with her doctor before taking *any* drug.

Drugs and lactation

Most drugs a nursing mother takes do appear in breast milk. Drug levels in breast milk tend to be high when blood levels are high—generally, shortly after taking each dose. Therefore, the mother should be advised to breast-feed *before* taking medication, not *after*.

Nevertheless, with very few exceptions, a mother who wishes to breast-feed may continue to do so with her doctor's permission. The exceptions: Breast-feeding should be temporarily interrupted and replaced with bottle-feeding when the mother must take...

• tetracyclines
• chloramphenicol
• sulfonamides (during first 2 weeks postpartum)
• oral anticoagulants
• iodine-containing drugs
• antineoplastics.

To protect her infant, a nursing mother should avoid taking drugs indiscriminately. If she needs to take a drug to maintain her own health, she should first check with her doctor to be sure of taking the safest drug at the safest dose.

Amebicides and trichomonacides

carbarsone
chloroquine hydrochloride
chloroquine phosphate
diiodohydroxyquin
emetine hydrochloride
metronidazole
paromomycin sulfate

---

carbarsone

INDICATIONS & DOSAGE
Intestinal amebiasis—
Adults: 250 mg P.O. b.i.d. or t.i.d. for 10 days. Rectal (as retention enema): 2 g dissolved in 200 ml warm 2% sodium bicarbonate solution, every other night for 5 doses. Discontinue oral therapy when enema is given.
Children: average total dose is 75 mg/Kg P.O. daily in 3 divided doses over 10-day period. Recommended total varies according to age—2 to 4 years, 2 g total; 5 to 8 years, 3 g total; 9 to 12 years, 4 g total; and over 12, 5 g total.

SIDE EFFECTS
Blood: *agranulocytosis.*
CNS: neuritis, convulsions.
EENT: sore throat, retinal edema, visual disturbances.
GI: epigastric pain and burning, irritation, *nausea,* hepatitis, *vomiting,* diarrhea, anorexia, constipation, increased motility, abdominal cramps.
GU: polyuria, albuminuria.
Hepatic: hepatomegaly, jaundice.
Skin: eruptions, *exfoliative dermatitis,* pruritus.
Other: edema of wrists, ankles, and knees; weight loss; kidney damage; splenomegaly; *hemorrhagic encephalitis.*

INTERACTIONS
None significant.

NURSING CONSIDERATIONS
• Contraindicated as initial treatment in patients with hepatic or renal disease; in patients with contracted visual or color fields; and in patients with known hypersensitivity or intolerance to any arsenical treatment.
• Don't exceed recommended dose; toxicity may result. If second treatment is needed, allow at least 10 days between courses.
• Divide carbarsone capsule to obtain required dose. Give in ½ glass orange juice or milk, in small amount of 1% sodium bicarbonate solution, or in jelly or other food.
• Discontinue upon first sign of intolerance or toxicity. Fatal exfoliative dermatitis has been reported.
• Tell patient to report any unusual symptoms, even posttreatment.
• Liver function tests should precede therapy. Careful inspection of skin, vision testing, and palpation of liver and spleen should be repeated regularly.
• Monitor intake/output. Notify doctor of number, frequency, and character of stools.
• Give a cleansing enema before giving carbarsone enema.

• Deliver stool specimen to lab promptly; movements of parasites are seen only when stool is warm. Amebic cysts in stool indicate need for additional therapy. Stool specimen should be studied 1 week after stopping therapy and monthly for 1 year. To help prevent reinfestation, instruct patient in correct hygiene.

---

chloroquine hydrochloride
Aralen HCl
chloroquine phosphate
Aralen Phosphate♦, Chlorocon Roquine

INDICATIONS & DOSAGE
Extraintestinal amebiasis—
Adults: 160 to 200 mg chloroquine (hydrochloride) base I.M. daily for no more than 10 or 12 days. As soon as possible, substitute 1 g (600 mg base) chloroquine phosphate P.O. daily for 2 days; then 500 mg (300 mg base) daily for at least 2 to 3 weeks. Treatment is usually combined with an effective intestinal amebicide.
Rheumatoid arthritis—
250 mg chloroquine phosphate daily with evening meal.

SIDE EFFECTS
Blood: *agranulocytosis.*
CNS: mild and transient headache, neuromyopathy, psychic stimulation, fatigue, irritability, nightmares, convulsions, dizziness.
EENT: *visual disturbances* (blurred vision; difficulty in focusing; reversible corneal changes; generally irreversible, sometimes progressive or delayed retinal changes, e.g., narrowing of arterioles; macular lesions; pallor of optic disc; optic atrophy; patchy retinal pigmentation, often leading to blindness), ototoxicity, nerve deafness, vertigo, tinnitus.
GI: anorexia, abdominal cramps, diarrhea, nausea, vomiting.

Skin: pruritus, lichen planus-like eruptions, skin and mucosal pigmentary changes, pleomorphic skin eruptions.

INTERACTIONS
None significant.

NURSING CONSIDERATIONS
• Contraindicated in patients with retinal or visual field changes, porphyria. Use with extreme caution in presence of severe GI, neurologic, or blood disorders. Drug concentrates in liver; use cautiously in patients with hepatic disease or alcoholism. Use with caution in patients with G-6-PD deficiency or psoriasis; drug may exacerbate these conditions.
• Complete blood cell counts, including liver function studies, should be made periodically during prolonged therapy; if severe disorder appears which is not attributable to disease under treatment, drug may need to be discontinued.
• Overdosage can quickly lead to toxic symptoms: headache, drowsiness, visual disturbances, cardiovascular collapse, and convulsions, followed by sudden and early respiratory and cardiac arrest. Children are extremely susceptible to toxicity; avoid long-term treatment.
• Baseline and periodic ophthalmologic examinations needed. Report blurred vision, increased sensitivity to light, or muscle weakness. Check periodically for muscular weakness after long-term use. Audiometric exams recommended before, during, and after therapy, especially if long term.
• Give drug immediately before or after meals on same day each week.
• To avoid exacerbated drug-induced dermatoses, warn patient to avoid excessive exposure to sun.
• Each ml parenteral solution containing 50 mg dihydrochloride salt = 40 mg chloroquine base; each

---

500 mg tablet phosphate = 300 mg base.

diiodohydroxyquin
Gynovules♦♦, Inserfem, Yodoxin

INDICATIONS & DOSAGE
Intestinal amebiasis—
Adults: 630 to 650 mg P.O. t.i.d. for 20 days. Total daily dose should not exceed 2 g.
Children: usual dose: 30 to 40 mg/Kg of body weight daily in 2 to 3 divided doses for 20 days.
Additional courses of diiodohydroxyquin therapy should not be repeated before a resting interval of 2 to 3 weeks.

SIDE EFFECTS
Blood: *agranulocytosis.*
CNS: neurotoxicity, dysesthesia, weakness, vertigo, malaise, headache, agitation, retrograde amnesia, ataxia, peripheral neuropathy.
EENT: optic neuritis, optic atrophy, loss of vision.
GI: anorexia, nausea, vomiting, abdominal cramps, diarrhea, increased motility, constipation, epigastric burning and pain, gastritis, anal irritation and itching.
Skin: pruritus, hives, papular and pustular eruptions, urticaria, discoloration of hair and nails.
Other: thyroid enlargement, fever, chills, generalized furunculosis, hair loss.

INTERACTIONS
None significant.

NURSING CONSIDERATIONS
• Contraindicated in patients with known hypersensitivity to 8-hydroxyquinoline derivatives or iodine-containing preparations. Diiodohydroxyquin causes hepatic damage in such patients. Also contraindicated in patients with hepatic or renal disease, or preexisting optic neuropathy.
• Patient should have periodic ophthalmologic examinations during treatment.
• Give after meals. Crush tablets and mix with applesauce or chocolate syrup.
• Record intake/output and color and amount of stool. Send warm specimens to lab frequently.
• Watch for diarrhea during the first 2 to 3 days of treatment. Notify doctor if it continues past 3 days.
• Advise patient not to discontinue the medication prematurely. Tell him to notify doctor if skin rash occurs.

emetine hydrochloride

INDICATIONS & DOSAGE
Acute fulminating amebic dysentery—
Adults: 1 mg/Kg daily up to 65 mg daily (1 or 2 doses) deep S.C. or I.M. 3 to 5 days to control symptoms. Give another antiamebic drug simultaneously.
Children over 8 years: no more than 20 mg daily deep S.C. or I.M. for 3 to 5 days.
Children under 8 years: no more than 10 mg daily for 3 to 5 days.
Amebic hepatitis and abscess—
Adults: 65 mg daily (1 or 2 doses) deep S.C. or I.M. for 10 days.
Children over 8 years: no more than 20 mg daily for 10 days.
Children under 8 years: no more than 10 mg daily for 10 days.

SIDE EFFECTS
CNS: dizziness, headache, mild sensory disturbances, central or peripheral nerve function changes, neuromuscular symptoms (weakness, aching, stiffness, tenderness, pain, tremors).
CV: *acute toxicity*—can occur at any dose (hypotension, tachycardia,

precordial pain, dyspnea, *EKG abnormalities,* gallop rhythm, cardiac dilatation, severe acute degenerative myocarditis, pericarditis, congestive failure).
GI: *nausea, vomiting, diarrhea,* abdominal cramps, loss of sense of taste.
Metabolic: decreased serum potassium levels.
Skin: eczematous, urticarial purpuric lesions.
Local: skeletal muscle stiffness, aching, tenderness, muscle weakness at injection site.
Other: edema.

INTERACTIONS
None significant.

NURSING CONSIDERATIONS
• Contraindicated in patients with heart or kidney disease, except those with amebic abscess or hepatitis not controlled by chloroquine; patients who have received a course of emetine less than 6 to 8 weeks previously; children, except for severe dysentery unresponsive to other amebicides; and in those with polyneuropathy or muscle disease. Use with caution in aged or debilitated patients, patients with hypotension, or those about to undergo surgery.
• Record pulse rate and blood pressure 2 to 3 times daily. Discontinue use if drug produces tachycardia, precipitous fall in blood pressure, neuromuscular symptoms, marked gastrointestinal effects, or considerable weakness. Weakness and muscle symptoms usually precede more serious symptoms and serve as a guide for avoiding toxicity.
• Don't exceed recommended dose or extend therapy beyond 10 days. Patient confined to bed during treatment and for several days thereafter.
• Drug may alter EKG tracings for 6 weeks. EKG should be taken before therapy, after fifth dose, upon

completion, and 1 week after therapy. Patterns can resemble those of myocardial infarction. First and most consistent change is T wave inversion.
• Deep S.C. administration is preferred; I.M. acceptable, but I.V. route is dangerous and contraindicated. Injections cause necrosis and edema. Rotate sites and apply warm soaks.
• Record intake/output; odor and consistency of stools; and presence of mucus, blood, or other foreign matter. Send warm specimens to lab frequently. Repeat fecal examinations at 3-month intervals to assure elimination of amebae. Patients with acute amebic dysentery often become asymptomatic carriers. Check family members and suspected contacts.
• Suspect emetine-induced reaction if stools increase in number following initial relief of diarrhea.
• To help prevent reinfection, instruct patient in correct hygiene.
• Drug is very irritating. Avoid contact with eyes and mucous membranes.
• Restoration of body fluids and nutrients is an important adjunct to therapy.

---

metronidazole
Flagyl♦, Neo-Tric♦♦, Novonidazol♦♦, Trikacide♦♦

INDICATIONS & DOSAGE
Amebic hepatic abscess—
Adults: 500 to 750 mg P.O. t.i.d. for 5 to 10 days.
Children: 35 to 50 mg/Kg daily (in 3 doses) for 10 days.
Intestinal amebiasis—
Adults: 750 mg P.O. t.i.d. for 5 to 10 days.
Children: 35 to 50 mg/Kg daily (in 3 doses) for 10 days.
Follow this therapy with oral diiodohydroxyquin.
Trichomoniasis—

Adults (both male and female): 250 mg P.O. t.i.d. for 7 days or 2 g P.O. in single dose; 4 to 6 weeks should elapse between courses of therapy.
Refractory trichomoniasis—
Women: 250 mg P.O. b.i.d. for 10 days.

SIDE EFFECTS
Blood: leukopenia, neutropenia.
CNS: vertigo, headache, ataxia, incoordination, confusion, irritability, depression, restlessness, weakness, fatigue, drowsiness, insomnia, sensory neuropathy, paresthesias of the extremities, psychic stimulation, neuromyopathy.
CV: EKG change (flattened T wave).
EENT: blurred vision, difficulty in focusing, nasal congestion.
GI: abdominal cramping, stomatitis, *nausea, vomiting, anorexia,* diarrhea, constipation.
GU: darkened urine, polyuria, dysuria, pyuria, incontinence, cystitis, decreased libido, dyspareunia, dryness of vagina and vulva, sense of pelvic pressure.
Skin: pruritus, flushing.
Other: overgrowth of nonsusceptible organisms, especially *Candida* (glossitis, furry tongue), dry mouth, metallic taste, proctitis, fever.

INTERACTIONS
Alcohol: disulfiram-like reaction (nausea, vomiting, headache, cramps, flushing). Don't use together.
Disulfiram: acute psychoses and confusional states. Don't use together.

NURSING CONSIDERATIONS
Warning: This drug has been shown to be carcinogenic in mice and possibly rats. Unnecessary use should be avoided.
• Contraindicated in patients with a history of blood dyscrasia or CNS disorder, and in patients with retinal or visual field changes. Use with caution in patients with hepatic disease or alcoholism; in conjunction with known hepatotoxic drugs.
• Tell patients to avoid alcohol or alcohol-containing medications.
• Give with meals to minimize GI distress.
• Tell patients metallic taste and dark or reddish-brown urine are possible.
• Record number and character of stools when used in the treatment of amebiasis. Metronidazole should be used only after *Trichomonas vaginalis* has been confirmed by wet smear or culture or *Entamoeba histolytica* has been identified. Asymptomatic sexual partners of patients being treated for *Trichomonas vaginalis* infection should be treated simultaneously to avoid reinfection. Instruct patient in correct hygiene.
• Has been used to treat anaerobic infections.

---

paromomycin sulfate
Humatin

INDICATIONS & DOSAGE
Intestinal amebiasis, acute and chronic—
Adults and children: 25 to 35 mg/Kg daily P.O. in 3 doses for 5 to 10 days after meals.

SIDE EFFECTS
Blood: eosinophilia.
CNS: headache, vertigo.
EENT: ototoxicity.
GI: anorexia, nausea, vomiting, epigastric pain and burning, abdominal cramps, diarrhea, constipation, increased motility, steatorrhea, pruritus ani, malabsorption syndrome.
GU: hematuria, nephrotoxicity.
Skin: rash, exanthema, pruritus.
Other: overgrowth of nonsusceptible organisms.

INTERACTIONS
None significant.

Italicized side effects are common or life-threatening.

NURSING CONSIDERATIONS

• Contraindicated in impaired renal function or intestinal obstruction. Use with caution in ulcerative lesions of the bowel to avoid inadvertent absorption and resulting renal toxicity. Poorly absorbed orally but will accumulate with renal impairment or ulcerative lesions.

• Ask about history of sensitivity to this drug before giving first dose.

• Administer after meals.

• Emphasize personal hygiene, particularly handwashing before eating and after defecation.

• Criterion of cure is absence of amebae in stools examined weekly for 6 weeks after treatment and thereafter at monthly intervals for 2 years. Examine feces of family members or suspected contacts.

• Avoid high doses or prolonged therapy.

• Watch for signs of superinfection (continued fever and other signs of new infections, especially monilial infections).

4

Anthelmintics

antimony potassium tartrate
diethylcarbamazine citrate
gentian violet
mebendazole
piperazine adipate
piperazine citrate
piperazine phosphate
piperazine tartrate
pyrantel pamoate
pyrvinium pamoate
thiabendazole

antimony potassium tartrate
(not commercially available; must be
compounded)

INDICATIONS & DOSAGE
Schistosoma japonicum—
Adults: initially, 8 ml of 0.5% solution in sterile water for injection or
5% dextrose given slow I.V. Increase
each subsequent dose 4 ml until
11th day, when 28 ml are given. Give
28 ml on alternate days until a total of
360 ml (1.8 g).

SIDE EFFECTS
Blood: thrombocytopenia.
CV: hypotension, syncope, bradycar-
dia, EKG changes.
GI: nausea, vomiting, diarrhea,
colic, *hepatic necrosis.*
Other: dyspnea, severe arthralgia, al-
buminuria, fever, dermatitis.

INTERACTIONS
None significant.

NURSING CONSIDERATIONS
• Not for use in other worm infestations; toxicity with this agent is high.
• Solutions must be freshly prepared.
• Doses should be given 2 hours after
a light meal.
• Patient should lie down for 1 hour
after treatment.
• Antiemetics should not be given,
since they mask nausea and vomiting,
which are signs of hepatic toxicity.
• Extravasation may cause painful
cellulitis.
• Treatment of choice for *Schistosoma japonicum.*
• Avoid rapid injection. May lead to
severe cough, vomiting, or even fatal
reactions.

diethylcarbamazine citrate
Hetrazan

INDICATIONS & DOSAGE
Ascariasis (roundworm)—
Adults: 13 mg/Kg P.O. daily for
7 days.
Children: 6 to 10 mg/Kg P.O. t.i.d.
for 7 to 10 days.
*Loiasis, dipetalonemiasis, onchocer-
ciasis, Bancroftian or Malayan fila-
riasis*—
Adults and children:
2 mg/Kg P.O. t.i.d. for 3 to 4 weeks.
Repeat if necessary.
Tropical (pulmonary) eosinophilia—
Adults and children:
13 mg/Kg P.O. daily for 4 to 7 days.

SIDE EFFECTS

CNS: *headache, malaise, weakness,* lassitude, syncope.
CV: tachycardia, tachypnea, hypotension, leukocytosis, eosinophilia.
GI: anorexia, nausea, vomiting.
Skin: pruritus, dermatitis, bullous eruptions.
Other: arthralgia, myalgia, joint pain, swelling and edema of face and skin, severe pedal edema, fever, lymphadenitis, sweating, cough.

INTERACTIONS

None significant.

NURSING CONSIDERATIONS

• Use with caution in patients with hypertension; severe hepatic, renal, or cardiac disease; and in children under 1 year of age. Treat patients with recent history of malaria with an antimalarial agent first to prevent relapse in nonsymptomatic malarial infections.
• Administer carefully to avoid or control allergic or other untoward reactions. Minimize allergic reactions by giving with corticosteroids, antihistamines, or aspirin.
• Inform patient that side effects will usually be minor and transient.
• Instruct patient in good hygiene.
• Give immediately after meals. Drug has sweet but unpleasant taste.

---

gentian violet
Jayne's P-W Vermifuge

INDICATIONS & DOSAGE

Pinworms—
Adults: 60 mg P.O. t.i.d. 7 to 10 days.
Children: 2 mg/Kg P.O. daily in 2 to 3 doses for 8 to 10 days, not to exceed 90 mg/day. Discontinue treatment after 7 to 10 days. Resume if needed.

SIDE EFFECTS

CNS: headache, dizziness, lassitude.
GI: nausea, diarrhea, vomiting (purple), abdominal cramps.

INTERACTIONS

None significant.

NURSING CONSIDERATIONS

• Use with caution in patients with cardiac, hepatic, renal, or GI disease.
• Tablets must be taken whole with water. Give with meals.
• Patient should abstain from alcohol during treatment.
• If nausea and vomiting occur, stop treatment for 1 to 2 days; resume at reduced dosage and notify doctor. Warn that skin, clothing, vomitus, and feces will be stained purple.
• Instruct patient in good hygiene.

---

mebendazole
Vermox ♦

INDICATIONS & DOSAGE

Pinworm—
Adults, and children over 2 years: 100 mg P.O. as a single dose. If infestation persists 3 weeks later, repeat treatment.
Roundworm, whipworm, hookworm—
Adults, and children over 2 years: 100 mg P.O. b.i.d. for 3 days. If infestation persists 3 weeks later, repeat treatment.

SIDE EFFECTS

GI: occasional, transient abdominal pain and diarrhea in massive infestation and expulsion of worms.

INTERACTIONS

None significant.

NURSING CONSIDERATIONS

• Tablets may be chewed, swallowed, or crushed and mixed with food.

• No dietary restrictions, laxatives, or enemas necessary.
• To avoid reinfestation, wash peri-anal area daily. Change undergarments and bedclothes daily. Wash hands and clean fingernails after bowel movements and before meals. Treat all family members.

---

piperazine adipate
Entacyl♦♦
piperazine citrate
Antepar♦, Bryrel, Pin-Tega Tabs, Pipril, Ta-Verm, Vermazine
piperazine phosphate
Antepar Phosphate, Piperaval
piperazine tartrate
Razine Tartrate

INDICATIONS & DOSAGE
Pinworm—
Adults and children: 65 mg/Kg P.O. daily 7 to 8 days. Maximum daily dose is 2.5 g.
Roundworm—
Adults: 3.5 g P.O. in single doses for 2 consecutive days.
Children: 75 mg/Kg P.O. daily in single dose for 2 consecutive days. Maximum daily dose: 3.5 g.

SIDE EFFECTS
CNS: ataxia, tremors, choreiform movements, muscular weakness, myoclonus, hyporeflexia, paresthesias, convulsions, sense of detachment, EEG abnormalities, memory defect, headache, vertigo.
EENT: nystagmus, blurred vision, paralytic strabismus, cataracts with visual impairment, lacrimation, rhinorrhea, difficulty in focusing.
GI: *nausea, vomiting,* diarrhea, abdominal cramps.
Skin: urticaria, photodermatitis, *erythema multiforme,* purpura, eczematous skin reactions.

Other: arthralgia, fever, broncho-spasm.

INTERACTIONS
None significant.

NURSING CONSIDERATIONS
• Contraindicated in patients with hepatic and/or renal impairment, or convulsive disorders. Use with caution in patients with severe malnutrition or anemia.
• Discontinue if CNS or significant GI reactions occur.
• Because of potential neurotoxicity, avoid prolonged or repeated treatment, especially in children.
• No dietary restrictions, laxatives, or enemas necessary.
• May be taken with food.
• To avoid reinfestation, wash peri-anal area daily. Change undergarments and bedclothes daily. Wash hands and clean fingernails before meals and after bowel movements. Treat all family members.
• Protect from air, light, and moisture.

---

pyrantel pamoate
Antiminth, Combantrin♦♦

INDICATIONS & DOSAGE
Roundworm and pinworm—
Adults, and children over 2 years: single dose of 11 mg/Kg P.O. Maximum dose 1 g. For pinworm, dose should be repeated in 2 weeks.

SIDE EFFECTS
CNS: headache, dizziness, drowsiness, insomnia.
GI: anorexia, nausea, vomiting, gastralgia, cramps, diarrhea, tenesmus.
Skin: rashes.
Other: transient elevation of SGOT, fever, weakness.

Italicized side effects are common or life-threatening.

INTERACTIONS
None significant.

NURSING CONSIDERATIONS
• Use cautiously in severe malnutrition or anemia, or in hepatic dysfunction. Treat for anemia, dehydration, or malnutrition before giving drug.
• No dietary restrictions, laxatives, or enemas necessary.
• May be taken with food. Shake well before pouring.
• To avoid reinfestation, wash perianal area daily. Change undergarments and bedclothes daily. Wash hands and clean fingernails before meals and after bowel movements. Treat all family members.
• Protect from light. Store below 30° C. (86° F.).

---

pyrvinium pamoate
Pamovin♦♦, Povan, Pyr-Pam♦♦, Vanquin♦♦

INDICATIONS & DOSAGE
Pinworm—
Adults and children: 5 mg/Kg P.O. single dose (maximum 350 mg). Repeat in 2 weeks if needed.

SIDE EFFECTS
GI: nausea, vomiting, cramping, diarrhea (vomiting more common with suspension than with tablets).
Skin: photosensitivity, *erythema multiforme*.

INTERACTIONS
None significant.

NURSING CONSIDERATIONS
• Safe use with children who weigh less than 36 Kg not established.
• Swallow tablets whole to avoid staining teeth. May be taken with food.
• Warn that drug stains materials, skin, vomitus, and stools bright red.

• No dietary restrictions, laxatives, or enemas necessary.
• To avoid reinfestation, wash perianal area daily. Change undergarments and bedclothes daily. Wash hands and clean fingernails before meals and after bowel movements. Treat all family members.
• Protect from light.

---

thiabendazole
Mintezol♦

INDICATIONS & DOSAGE
Systemic infestation with pinworm, roundworm, threadworm, whipworm, cutaneous larva migrans, and trichinosis—
Adults or children over 70 Kg: 1.5 g P.O.
Adults or children under 70 Kg: 25 mg/Kg P.O. in 2 doses daily. Maximum dose is 3 g daily.
Cutaneous infestations—larva migrans (creeping eruption)—
Adults and children: dose depends on patient's weight. 70 Kg or over, 1.5 g P.O./dose; under 70 Kg, 4.6 mg/Kg/dose. 2 doses daily for 2 successive days. If active lesions still present 2 days after therapy, give second course.
*Pinworm—*2 doses daily for 1 day; repeat in 7 days.
*Roundworm, threadworm, whipworm—*2 doses daily for 2 successive days.
*Trichinosis—*2 doses daily for 2 to 4 successive days.

SIDE EFFECTS
CNS: impaired mental alertness, impaired physical coordination, *drowsiness, giddiness,* headache, dizziness.
GI: anorexia, nausea, vomiting, diarrhea, epigastric distress.
Skin: rash, pruritus, *erythema multiforme*.

Unmarked trade names available in the United States only.
♦ Also available in Canada   ♦♦ Available in Canada only.

Other: lymphadenopathy, fever, flush, chills.

INTERACTIONS
None significant.

NURSING CONSIDERATIONS
• Use with caution in patients with hepatic or renal dysfunction, severe malnutrition, anemia, and with patients who are vomiting. Supportive therapy indicated for anemic, dehydrated, or malnourished patients. In children under 15 Kg, weigh benefits against risks.
• Warn that medication may cause drowsiness and dizziness.
• Give after meals. Shake suspension before measuring; chew tablets before swallowing.
• Laxatives, enemas, and diet restrictions not needed.
• To avoid reinfestation, wash perianal area daily. Change undergarments and bedclothes daily. Wash hands and clean fingernails before meals and after bowel movements. Treat all family members.

5

Antifungals

amphotericin B
flucytosine
griseofulvin microsize
griseofulvin ultramicrosize
miconazole
nystatin

amphotericin B
Fungizone♦

INDICATIONS & DOSAGE
Systemic fungal infections (histoplasmosis, coccidioidomycosis, blastomycosis, cryptococcosis, disseminated moniliasis, aspergillosis, phycomycosis), meningitis—
Adults and children: initially, 1 mg in 250 ml of 5% dextrose infused over 2 to 4 hours; or 0.25 mg/Kg daily by slow infusion over 6 hours. Increase gradually as patient tolerance develops to maximum 1.0 mg/Kg daily. Therapy must not exceed 1.5 mg/Kg. If drug is discontinued for a week or more, administration must resume with initial dose and again increase gradually.
Topical (3% cream, lotion, ointment): apply liberally and rub well into affected area b.i.d. to q.i.d.
Intrathecal: 25 mcg/0.1 ml diluted with 10 to 20 ml of cerebrospinal fluid and administered by barbotage 2 or 3 times weekly. Initial dose should not exceed 50 mcg.
Coccidioidal arthritis—
Adults: 5 to 15 mg intra-articular into joint spaces.

SIDE EFFECTS
Blood: normochromic, normocytic anemia.
CNS: headache, peripheral neuropathy; with intrathecal administration—peripheral nerve pain, paresthesias.
GI: anorexia, weight loss, nausea, vomiting, dyspepsia, diarrhea, epigastric cramps.
GU: abnormal renal function with *hypokalemia, azotemia, hyposthenuria,* renal tubular acidosis, nephrocalcinosis; with large doses—permanent renal impairment, anuria, oliguria.
Local: burning, stinging, irritation, tissue damage with extravasation, *thrombophlebitis.*
Other: arthralgia, myalgia, muscle weakness secondary to hypokalemia, *fever, chills,* pain at site of injection, malaise, generalized pain.

INTERACTIONS
None significant.

NURSING CONSIDERATIONS
• Use cautiously in patients with impaired renal function.
• Use parenterally only in hospitalized patients, under close supervision, when diagnosis of potentially fatal fungal infection has been confirmed.
• Monitor vital signs; fever may appear 1 to 2 hours after start of I.V. infusion and should subside within 4 hours of discontinuation.
• Monitor intake/output; report change in appearance or volume. Renal damage usually reversible if drug is stopped with first sign of dysfunction.

• Perform liver and kidney function tests weekly. If BUN exceeds 40 mg/100 ml, or if serum creatinine exceeds 3 mg/100 ml, doctor may reduce or stop drug until kidney function improves. Monitor CBC weekly. Stop drug if elevated Bromsulphalein, alkaline phosphatase, or bilirubin.

• Monitor potassium levels closely. Report any signs of hypokalemia. Check calcium and magnesium levels periodically.

• In the dry state, store at 2° to 8° C. (35.6° to 46.4° F.). Protect from light. Expires 2 years after date of manufacture. Reconstitute with 10 ml sterile water only. Mixing with solutions containing sodium chloride, other electrolytes, or bacteriostatic agents such as benzyl alcohol causes precipitation. Do not use if solution contains precipitate or foreign matter. Use aseptic technique.

• Appears to be compatible with limited amounts of heparin sodium, hydrocortisone sodium succinate, and methylprednisolone sodium succinate.

• Reconstituted solution is stable for 1 week under refrigeration or 24 hours at room temperature. Protect from light. Wrap bottle in aluminum foil.

• Recommended infusion solution is 10 mg/100 ml of 5% dextrose in water.

• Severity of some side effects can be reduced by premedication with aspirin, antihistamines, antiemetics, or small doses of corticosteroids; addition of phosphate buffer and heparin to the solution; and alternate-day dose schedule. For severe reactions, drug may have to be stopped for varying periods.

• For I.V. infusion, an in-line membrane with mean pore diameter larger than 1 micron can be used. Infuse very slowly; rapid infusion may result in cardiovascular collapse. Warn of discomfort at infusion site.

• Antibiotics should be given separately; don't mix or piggyback with amphotericin.

• Advise patient that several months of therapy may be needed to assure adequate response.

• Topical preparations may stain clothing.

---

flucytosine
Ancobon, Ancotil♦ ♦

INDICATIONS & DOSAGE
For severe fungal infections caused by susceptible strains of Candida (including septicemia, endocarditis, urinary system and pulmonary infections) and Cryptococcus (meningitis, pulmonary infection, and possible urinary tract infections)—
Adults, and children weighing more than 50 Kg: 50 to 150 mg/Kg daily q 6 hours P.O.
Children weighing less than 50 Kg: 1.5 to 4.5 g/m²/day in 4 divided doses P.O.
Severe infections such as meningitis may require doses up to 250 mg/Kg.

SIDE EFFECTS
Blood: anemia, leukopenia, bone marrow depression, thrombocytopenia.
CNS: dizziness, drowsiness, confusion, headache.
GI: *nausea, vomiting, diarrhea,* abdominal bloating.
Metabolic: elevated serum alkaline phosphatase, SGOT, SGPT, BUN, serum creatinine.
Skin: occasional rash.

INTERACTIONS
None significant.

NURSING CONSIDERATIONS
• Use with extreme caution in pa-

Italicized side effects are common or life-threatening.

tients with impaired liver or kidney function, or bone marrow depression.
- Hematologic, and kidney and liver function studies should precede therapy and should be repeated at frequent intervals thereafter. Before treatment, susceptibility tests should establish that organism is flucytosine sensitive. Tests should be repeated weekly to monitor drug resistance.
- Flucytosine is well absorbed from the GI tract. Nausea, vomiting, stomach upset are reduced if capsules are given over a 15-minute period.
- Monitor intake and output; report any marked change.
- If possible, serum level assays of drug should be performed regularly to maintain flucytosine at therapeutic level (25 to 120 mcg/ml).
- Drug is often combined with amphotericin B; use may be synergistic, but may increase toxic effects.
- Store in light-resistant containers.
- Inform patient that adequate response may take weeks or months.

---

griseofulvin microsize
Fulvicin-U/F♦, Grifulvin V, Grisactin, Grisovin-FP♦♦, Grisowen
griseofulvin ultramicrosize
Fulvicin P/G, Gris-PEG

INDICATIONS & DOSAGE
Ringworm infections of skin, hair, nails (tinea corporis, tinea pedis, tinea cruris, tinea barbae, tinea capitis, and tinea unguium) when caused by Trichophyton, Microsporum, or Epidermophyton—
Adults: 500 mg (microsize) P.O. daily in single or divided doses. Severe infections may require up to 1 g daily.
Children over 22 Kg: 250 to 500 mg P.O. daily.
Children 13 to 22 Kg: 125 to 250 mg daily.
Adults: 125 mg tablet (ultramicro-

size), P.O. b.i.d. or 250 mg daily. Resistant fungal infections of tinea pedis and tinea unguium may require divided daily dose of 500 mg.
Children over 22 Kg: 125 mg to 250 mg daily, P.O.
Children 13 to 22 Kg: 62.5 mg to 125 mg daily, P.O.

SIDE EFFECTS
Blood: leukopenia, *granulocytopenia (requires discontinuation of drug)*.
CNS: headaches (in early stages of treatment), fatigue with large doses, occasional mental confusion, impaired performance of routine activities, psychotic symptoms.
GI: nausea, vomiting, excessive thirst, flatulence, diarrhea.
Metabolic: porphyria.
Skin: rash, urticaria, photosensitive reactions (may aggravate lupus erythematosus).
Other: estrogen-like effects in children, oral thrush.

INTERACTIONS
Barbiturates: decreased griseofulvin absorption. Divide into 3 doses of griseofulvin per day.

NURSING CONSIDERATIONS
- Contraindicated in patients with porphyria or hepatocellular failure. Since griseofulvin is a penicillin derivative, cross sensitivity is possible. Use cautiously in penicillin-sensitive patients. Use only when topical treatment fails to arrest mycotic disease.
- Blood studies should be repeated regularly.
- Advise patient that prolonged treatment may be needed to control infection and prevent relapse, even if symptoms abate in first few days of therapy. Tell patient to keep skin clean and dry and to maintain good hygiene. Caution him to avoid intense sunlight.
- Most effectively absorbed and causes least GI distress when given after high-fat meal.

• Effective treatment of tinea pedis may require concomitant use of topical agent.
• Diagnosis of infecting organism should be verified in lab. Continue drug until clinical and laboratory examinations confirm complete eradication.
• Because griseofulvin ultramicrosize is dispersed in polyethylene glycol (PEG), it is absorbed more rapidly and completely than microsize preparations and is effective at one half the usual griseofulvin dose.

miconazole
Monistat I.V.

INDICATIONS & DOSAGE
Treatment of systemic fungal infections (coccidioidomycosis, candidiasis, cryptococcosis, paracoccidioidomycosis), chronic mucocutaneous candidiasis—
Adults: 200 to 3,600 mg per day. Doses may vary with diagnosis and with infective agent. May divide daily dose over 3 infusions, 200 to 1,200 mg per infusion. Repeated courses may be needed due to relapse or reinfection.
Children: 20 to 40 mg/Kg per day. Do not exceed 15 mg/Kg per infusion.

SIDE EFFECTS
Blood: transient decreases in hematocrit, thrombocytopenia.
CNS: dizziness, drowsiness.
GI: *nausea, vomiting,* diarrhea.
Metabolic: *transient decrease in serum sodium.*
Skin: *pruritic rash.*
Local: *phlebitis at site of injection.*

INTERACTIONS
None significant.

NURSING CONSIDERATIONS
• Rapid injection of undiluted miconazole may produce arrhythmia.
• Premedication with antiemetic may lessen nausea and vomiting.
• Avoid administration at mealtime in order to lessen GI side effects.
• Lesser incidence and severity of side effects with this drug may offer a significant advantage over other antifungals.
• In treatment of fungal meningitis and urinary bladder infections, must be supplemented with intrathecal administration and bladder irrigation.
• Intravenous infusion should be given over 30 to 60 minutes.
• Inform patient that adequate response may take weeks or months.
• Transient elevations in serum cholesterol and triglycerides may be due to castor oil vehicle.

nystatin
Mycostatin♦, Nadostine♦♦, Nilstat♦, O-V Statin

INDICATIONS & DOSAGE
Gastrointestinal infections—
Adults: 500,000 to 1,000,000 units as oral tablets, t.i.d.
Treatment of oral, vaginal, and intestinal infections caused by Candida albicans (Monilia) and other Candida species—
Adults: 400,000 to 600,000 units oral suspension q.i.d. for oral candidiasis.
Children, and infants over 3 months: 250,000 to 500,000 units oral suspension q.i.d.
Newborn and premature infants: 100,000 units oral suspension q.i.d.
Vaginal infections—
Women: 100,000 units, as vaginal tablets, inserted high into vagina, daily or b.i.d. for 14 days.

SIDE EFFECTS
GI: transient nausea, vomiting, diarrhea (usually with large oral dosage).

INTERACTIONS
None significant.

NURSING CONSIDERATIONS
• Nystatin is virtually nontoxic and nonsensitizing when used orally, vaginally, topically; but advise patient to report redness, swelling, or irritation.
• Vaginal tablets can be used by pregnant women up to 6 weeks before term to prevent thrush in newborn. Continue therapy during menstruation. Instruct patient to wash applicator thoroughly after use.
• Explain that use of antibiotics, birth control pills, and corticosteroids; diabetes; reinfection by sexual partner; and tight-fitting panty hose are predisposing factors for vaginal infection and should be considered in management program.

• For treatment of oral candidiasis (thrush), tell patient to hold suspension in mouth for several minutes before swallowing. For treatment in infants, swab medication on oral mucosa. Patient should observe good mouth hygiene. Tell patient overuse of mouthwash or poorly fitting dentures, especially in older patients, may alter flora and promote infection.
• Advise patient to continue medication for 1 to 2 weeks after symptomatic improvement to ensure against reinfection. Consult doctor for exact length of therapy.
• Immunosuppressed patients sometimes take vaginal tablets (100,000 units) by mouth. Provides prolonged contact with oral mucosa.
• Instruct patient in careful hygiene for affected areas.
• Store in tightly closed, light-resistant containers in cool place. Check expiration date.
• Not effective against systemic infections.

Antimalarials

amodiaquine hydrochloride
chloroquine hydrochloride
chloroquine phosphate
hydroxychloroquine sulfate
primaquine phosphate
pyrimethamine
quinine sulfate

amodiaquine hydrochloride
Camoquin HCl

INDICATIONS & DOSAGE
Suppressive prophylaxis and treatment of acute attacks of malaria due to P. vivax, P. malariae, P. ovale, and susceptible strains of P. falciparum—
Adults: for suppression, single dose of 300 to 600 mg P.O. weekly, preferably on same day of week; for acute attacks, 600 mg P.O. initially, then 300 mg at 6, 24, and 48 hours.
Children: for suppression, 5 mg/Kg P.O. weekly, preferably on same day of week; for acute attacks, 10 mg/Kg P.O. divided into 3 doses at 12-hour intervals.

SIDE EFFECTS
Blood: *agranulocytosis, leukopenia, pancytopenia.*
CNS: mild and transient headache, neuromyopathy, polyneuritis, psychic stimulation, fatigue, irritability, nightmares, convulsions, dizziness, toxic psychosis.
EENT: visual disturbances (blurred vision; difficulty in focusing; reversible corneal changes; generally irreversible, sometimes progressive or de-layed, retinal changes, e.g., narrowing of arterioles; macular lesions; pallor of optic disc; optic atrophy; patchy retinal pigmentation, often leading to blindness); ototoxicity (nerve deafness, tinnitus, labyrinthitis).
GI: anorexia, abdominal cramps, diarrhea, nausea, vomiting.
Hepatic: toxic hepatitis.
Skin: pruritus, lichen planus-like eruptions, skin and mucosal pigmentary changes, pleomorphic skin eruptions.

INTERACTIONS
None significant.

NURSING CONSIDERATIONS
• Contraindicated in patients with retinal or visual field changes, porphyria, severe hepatic disease. Use with extreme caution in presence of severe GI, neurologic, or blood disorders. Use with caution in patients with G-6-PD deficiency or psoriasis; drug may exacerbate these conditions.
• Complete blood cell counts and liver function studies should be made periodically during prolonged therapy; if severe blood disorder appears which is not attributable to disease under treatment, drug may need to be discontinued.
• Overdosage can quickly lead to toxic symptoms: headache, drowsiness, visual disturbances, cardiovascular collapse and convulsions, followed by sudden and early respiratory and cardiac arrest. Children are extremely susceptible to toxicity; avoid long-term treatment.

- Baseline and periodic ophthalmologic examinations needed. Report blurred vision, increased sensitivity to light, or muscle weakness. Check periodically for muscular weakness after long-term use. Audiometric exams recommended before, during, and after therapy, especially if long term.
- Give immediately before or after meals on same day each week.
- To avoid exacerbated drug-induced dermatoses, warn patient to avoid excessive exposure to sun.

chloroquine hydrochloride
Aralen HCl, Roquine
chloroquine phosphate
Aralen Phosphate♦, Chlorocon

INDICATIONS & DOSAGE

Suppressive prophylaxis and treatment of acute attacks of malaria due to P. vivax, P. malariae, P. ovale, and susceptible strains of P. falciparum—
Adults: initially, 600 mg (base) P.O., then 300 mg P.O. at 6, 24, and 48 hours. Or 160 to 200 mg (base) I.M. initially; repeat in 6 hours if needed. Switch to oral therapy as soon as possible.
Children: initially, 10 mg (base)/Kg P.O., then 5 mg (base)/Kg dose P.O. at 6, 24, and 48 hours (do not exceed adult dose). Or 5 mg (base)/Kg I.M. initially; repeat in 6 hours if needed. Switch to oral therapy as soon as possible.
Malaria suppressive treatment—
Adults and children: 5 mg (base)/Kg P.O. (not to exceed 300 mg) weekly on same day of the week (begin 2 weeks before entering endemic area and continue for 8 weeks after leaving). If treatment begins after exposure, double the initial dose (600 mg for adults, 10 mg/Kg for children) in 2 divided doses, P.O. 6 hours apart.

SIDE EFFECTS

Blood: *agranulocytosis.*
CNS: mild and transient headache, neuromyopathy, psychic stimulation, fatigue, irritability, nightmares, convulsions, dizziness.
EENT: *visual disturbances* (blurred vision; difficulty in focusing; reversible corneal changes; generally irreversible, sometimes progressive or delayed, retinal changes, e.g., narrowing of arterioles; macular lesions; pallor of optic disc; optic atrophy; patchy retinal pigmentation, often leading to blindness); ototoxicity (nerve deafness, vertigo, tinnitus).
GI: anorexia, abdominal cramps, diarrhea, nausea, vomiting.
Skin: pruritus, lichen planus-like eruptions, skin and mucosal pigmentary changes, pleomorphic skin eruptions.

INTERACTIONS
None significant.

NURSING CONSIDERATIONS

- Contraindicated in patients with retinal or visual field changes, porphyria. Use with extreme caution in presence of severe GI, neurologic, or blood disorders. Drug concentrates in liver; use cautiously in patients with hepatic disease or alcoholism. Use with caution in patients with G-6-PD deficiency or psoriasis; drug may exacerbate these conditions.
- Complete blood cell counts and liver function studies should be made periodically during prolonged therapy; if severe blood disorder appears which is not attributable to disease under treatment, drug may need to be discontinued.
- Overdosage can quickly lead to toxic symptoms: headache, drowsiness, visual disturbances, cardiovascular collapse and convulsions, followed by sudden and early respiratory and cardiac arrest. Children are ex-

---

tremely susceptible to toxicity; avoid long-term treatment.
• Baseline and periodic ophthalmologic examinations needed. Report blurred vision, increased sensitivity to light, or muscle weakness. Check periodically for muscular weakness after long-term use. Audiometric exams recommended before, during, and after therapy, especially if long term.
• Give drug immediately before or after meals on same day each week.
• To avoid exacerbated drug-induced dermatoses, warn patient to avoid excessive exposure to sun.
• Each ml parenteral solution containing 50 mg dihydrochloride salt = 40 mg chloroquine base; each 500 mg tablet phosphate = 300 mg base.

---

hydroxychloroquine sulfate
Plaquenil Sulfate ♦

INDICATIONS & DOSAGE

Suppressive prophylaxis of attacks of malaria due to P. vivax, P. malariae, P. ovale, and susceptible strains of P. falciparum—
Adults and children: for suppression: 5 mg (base)/Kg body weight P.O. (not to exceed 310 mg) weekly on same day of the week (begin 2 weeks prior to entering and continue for 8 weeks after leaving endemic area). If not started prior to exposure, double initial dose (620 mg for adults, 10 mg/Kg for children) in 2 divided doses P.O. 6 hours apart.
Treatment of acute malarial attacks—
Adults, and children over 15 years: initially, 800 mg (sulfate) P.O., then 400 mg after 6 to 8 hours, then 400 mg daily for 2 days (total 2 g sulfate salt).
Children 11 to 15 years: 600 mg (sulfate) P.O. stat, then 200 mg

8 hours later, then 200 mg 24 hours later (total 1 g sulfate salt).
Children 6 to 10 years: 400 mg (sulfate) P.O. stat, then 2 doses of 200 mg at 8-hour intervals (total 800 mg sulfate salt).
Children 2 to 5 years: 400 mg (sulfate) P.O. stat, then 200 mg 8 hours later (total 600 mg sulfate salt).
Children under 1 year: 100 mg (sulfate) P.O. stat; then 3 doses of 100 mg 6 to 9 hours apart (total 400 mg sulfate salt).
Lupus erythematosus (chronic discoid and systemic)—
Adults: 400 mg P.O. daily or b.i.d., continued for several weeks or months, depending on response. Prolonged maintenance—200 to 400 mg P.O. daily.
Rheumatoid arthritis—
Adults: initially, 400 to 600 mg P.O. daily. When good response occurs (usually in 4 to 12 weeks), cut dosage in half.

SIDE EFFECTS

Blood: *agranulocytosis, leukopenia,* thrombocytopenia, *aplastic anemia.*
CNS: irritability, nightmares, ataxia, convulsions, psychic stimulation, toxic psychosis, vertigo, tinnitus, nystagmus, lassitude, fatigue, dizziness.
EENT: visual disturbances (blurred vision; difficulty in focusing; reversible corneal changes; generally irreversible, sometimes progressive or delayed, retinal changes, e.g., narrowing of arterioles; macular lesions; pallor of optic disc; optic atrophy; visual field defects; patchy retinal pigmentation, often leading to blindness); ototoxicity (irreversible nerve deafness, tinnitus, labyrinthitis).
GI: anorexia, abdominal cramps, diarrhea, nausea, vomiting.
Skin: pruritus, lichen planus-like eruptions, skin and mucosal pigmentary changes, pleomorphic skin eruptions, bleaching of hair.

Italicized side effects are common or life-threatening.

Other: weight loss, skeletal muscle weakness, hypoactive deep tendon reflexes.

INTERACTIONS
None significant.

NURSING CONSIDERATIONS
• Contraindicated in patients with retinal or visual field changes, porphyria. Use with extreme caution in presence of severe GI, neurologic, or blood disorders. Drug concentrates in the liver; use cautiously in patients with hepatic disease or alcoholism. Use with caution in patients with G-6-PD deficiency or psoriasis; drug may exacerbate these conditions.
• Complete blood cell counts and liver function studies should be made periodically during prolonged therapy; if severe blood disorder appears which is not attributable to disease under treatment, consider discontinuing.
• Overdosage can quickly lead to toxic symptoms: headache, drowsiness, visual disturbances, cardiovascular collapse and convulsions, followed by sudden and early respiratory and cardiac arrest. Children are extremely susceptible to toxicity; avoid long-term treatment.
• Baseline and periodic ophthalmologic examinations needed. Report blurred vision, increased sensitivity to light, or muscle weakness. Check periodically for muscular weakness after long-term use. Audiometric exams recommended before, during, and after therapy, especially if long term.
• Give drug immediately before or after meals on same day of each week.
• 100 mg sulfate salt = 77.5 mg hydroxychloroquine base.

---

primaquine phosphate

INDICATIONS & DOSAGE
Radical cure of relapsing vivax malaria, eliminating symptoms and infection completely; prevention of relapse—
Adults: 15 to 30 mg (base) P.O. daily for 14 days. (26.3 mg tablet = 15 mg of base).

SIDE EFFECTS
Blood: leukopenia, hemolytic anemia in G-6-PD deficiency, methemoglobinemia in NADH methemoglobin reductase deficiency, leukocytosis, acute intravascular hemolysis, mild anemia, *granulocytopenia, agranulocytosis.*
EENT: disturbances of visual accommodation.
GI: nausea, vomiting, epigastric distress, abdominal cramps.
Skin: urticaria.

INTERACTIONS
None significant.

NURSING CONSIDERATIONS
• Contraindicated in patients with lupus erythematosus and rheumatoid arthritis; in patients taking bone marrow depressants and potentially hemolytic drugs.
• Use with a fast-acting blood schizonticide, such as amodiaquine or chloroquine. Use full dose to reduce possibility of drug-resistant strains.
• Caucasians taking more than 30 mg daily, dark-skinned patients taking more than 15 mg (base) daily, and patients with severe anemia or suspected sensitivity should have frequent blood studies and urine examinations. Sudden fall in hemoglobin concentration, erythrocyte or leukocyte count, or marked darkening of the urine suggests impending hemolytic reactions.
• Observe closely for tolerance in pa-

Unmarked trade names available in the United States only.
♦ Also available in Canada   ♦ ♦ Available in Canada only.

tients with previous idiosyncrasy
(manifested by hemolytic anemia,
methemoglobinemia, or leukopenia);
family or personal history of favism;
erythrocytic G-6-PD deficiency or
NADH methemoglobin reductase
deficiency.
• Administer drug with meals or with
antacids.

pyrimethamine
Daraprim◆

INDICATIONS & DOSAGE
*Malaria prophylaxis and transmission
control—*
Adults, and children over 10: 25 mg
P.O. weekly.
Children 4 to 10 years old: 12.5 mg
P.O. weekly.
Children under 4: 6.25 mg P.O.
weekly.
Continue in all age groups at least
10 weeks after leaving endemic areas.
Acute attacks of malaria—
not recommended alone in nonim-
mune persons; use with faster-acting
antimalarials, as chloroquine, for
2 days to initiate transmission control
and suppressive cure.
Adults, and children over 15: 25 mg
P.O. daily for 2 days.
Children under 15: 12.5 mg P.O.
daily for 2 days.
Toxoplasmosis—
Adults: initially, 100 mg P.O., then
25 mg P.O. daily for 4 to 5 weeks;
during same time give 1 g sulfadiazine
P.O. q 6 hours.
Children: initially, 1 mg/Kg P.O.,
then 0.25 mg/Kg daily for 4 to
5 weeks, along with 100 mg sulfa-
diazine/Kg P.O. daily, divided
q 6 hours.

SIDE EFFECTS
Blood: megaloblastic anemia, bone
marrow depression, leukopenia,
thrombocytopenia, pancytopenia.

CNS: stimulation and convulsions
(acute toxicity).
GI: anorexia, vomiting, diarrhea,
atrophic glossitis.
Skin: rashes.

INTERACTIONS
*Folic acid and para-aminobenzoic
acid:* decreased antitoxoplasmic effects. May require dosage adjustment.

NURSING CONSIDERATIONS
• Contraindicated in chloroguanide-
resistant malaria. Use cautiously in
patients with convulsive disorders;
smaller doses may be needed. Also
use cautiously following treatment
with chloroguanide.
• Dosages required to treat toxoplasmosis approach toxic levels. Twice-
weekly blood counts, including platelets, are required. If signs of folic or
folinic acid deficiency develop, dosage should be reduced or discontinued while patient receives parenteral
folinic acid (leucovorin) until blood
counts become normal.
• Do not exceed recommended
dosage.
• Give with meals to minimize GI
distress.

quinine sulfate
Coco-Quinine

INDICATIONS & DOSAGE
*Malaria due to P. falciparum (chloro-
quine-resistant)—*
Adults: 650 mg P.O. q 8 hours for
10 days, with 25 mg pyrimethamine q
12 hours for 3 days, and with 500 mg
sulfadiazine q.i.d. for 5 days.

SIDE EFFECTS
Blood: hemolytic anemia, thrombocytopenia, agranulocytosis, hypoprothrombinemia.
CNS: severe headache, apprehension,
excitement, confusion, delirium, syn-

cope, hypothermia, convulsions (with toxic doses).
CV: decreased blood pressure, cardiovascular collapse with overdosage or rapid I.V. administration.
EENT: altered color perception, photophobia, blurred vision, night blindness, amblyopia, scotomata, diplopia, mydriasis, optic atrophy, tinnitus, impaired hearing.
GI: epigastric distress, diarrhea, nausea, vomiting.
GU: renal tubular damage, anuria.
Skin: rashes, pruritus.
Local: thrombosis at infusion site.
Other: asthma, flushing.

INTERACTIONS
Sodium bicarbonate: elevated quinine levels. Use together cautiously.

NURSING CONSIDERATIONS
• Contraindicated in patients with G-6-PD deficiency. Use with caution in patients with cardiovascular conditions.
• Discontinue if any signs of idiosyncrasy or toxicity occur.
• I.V. therapy must be used cautiously, as marked fall in blood pressure often follows. Monitor blood pressure frequently.
• I.V. route is preferred to I.M. route. Avoid extravasation.
• Has been used as a treatment for nocturnal leg cramps.
• Quinine is no longer used for acute attacks of malaria due to *Plasmodium vivax* or for suppression of malaria due to organism resistance.

7

Antituberculars and antileprotics

capreomycin sulfate
cycloserine
dapsone
ethambutol hydrochloride
ethionamide
isoniazid
para-aminosalicylic acid
sodium aminosalicylate
pyrazinamide
rifampin
streptomycin sulfate
sulfoxone sodium

---

capreomycin sulfate
Capastat Sulfate

INDICATIONS & DOSAGE
Adjunctive treatment in pulmonary tuberculosis—
Adults: 15 mg/Kg/day up to 1 g I.M. daily injected deeply into large muscle mass for 60 to 120 days; then 1 g 2 to 3 times weekly for a period of 18 to 24 months. Maximum dose should not exceed 20 mg/Kg daily. Must be given in conjunction with another antitubercular drug but *not* streptomycin sulfate.

SIDE EFFECTS
Blood: eosinophilia, leukocytosis, leukopenia.
CNS: headache.
EENT: *ototoxicity* (tinnitus, vertigo, hearing loss).
GU: *nephrotoxicity* (elevated BUN and nonprotein nitrogen, proteinuria, casts, red blood cells, leukocytes; tu-

bular necrosis, decreased creatinine clearance).
Local: pain, induration, excessive bleeding and sterile abscesses at injection site.

INTERACTIONS
None significant.

NURSING CONSIDERATIONS
• Contraindicated in patients receiving other ototoxic or nephrotoxic drugs. Use cautiously in patients with impaired renal function, history of allergies, or hearing impairment.
• Considered a "third-line" drug in the treatment of tuberculosis.
• Drug is never given I.V.; may cause neuromuscular blockade.
• Evaluate patient's hearing before and during therapy. Notify doctor if patient complains of tinnitus, vertigo, hearing impairment.
• Monitor renal function (output, specific gravity, blood urea nitrogen, urinalysis, serum creatinine) before and during therapy; notify doctor of decreasing kidney function. Dose must be reduced in renal impairment.
• Monitor serum potassium levels and liver function periodically.
• Reconstituted solutions can be stored for 48 hours at room temperature or 14 days if refrigerated. Straw- or dark-colored solution does not indicate a loss in potency.

cycloserine
Seromycin

INDICATIONS & DOSAGE
Adjunctive treatment in pulmonary or extrapulmonary tuberculosis—
Adults: initially, 250 mg P.O. every 12 hours for 2 weeks; then, if blood levels are below 25 to 30 mcg/ml and there are no clinical signs of toxicity, dose is increased to 250 mg P.O. q 8 hours for 2 weeks. If optimum blood levels are still not achieved, and there are no signs of clinical toxicity, then dose is increased to 250 mg P.O. q 6 hours. Maximum dose 1 g/day. If CNS toxicity occurs, drug is discontinued for 1 week, then resumed at 250 mg daily for 2 weeks. If no serious toxic effects occur, dose is increased by 250 mg increments every 10 days until blood level of 25 to 30 mcg/ml is obtained.

SIDE EFFECTS
CNS: drowsiness, headache, tremor, dysarthria, vertigo, confusion, loss of memory, *possible suicidal tendencies and other psychotic symptoms, nervousness,* hyperirritability, paresthesias, paresis, hyperreflexia.
Other: hypersensitivity (allergic dermatitis).

INTERACTIONS
Isoniazid: monitor for CNS toxicity (dizziness or drowsiness).

NURSING CONSIDERATIONS
• Contraindicated in patients with seizure disorders, depression or severe anxiety, severe renal insufficiency, or chronic alcoholism. Use cautiously in patients with impaired renal function; reduced dosage required.
• Considered a "third-line" drug in the treatment of tuberculosis.

• Obtain specimen for culture and sensitivity tests before therapy begins.
• Toxic reactions may occur with blood levels above 30 mcg/ml.
• Pyridoxine, anticonvulsants, tranquilizers, or sedatives may help to relieve side effects.
• Observe for personality changes.
• Monitor hematologic, kidney, and liver function studies.
• Instruct patient to take drug exactly as prescribed; warn against discontinuing use without doctor's advice.

dapsone
Avlosulfon♦

INDICATIONS & DOSAGE
Lepromatous leprosy—
Adults: weeks 1 to 4: 25 mg P.O. 2 times a week; weeks 5 to 8: 50 mg 2 times a week; weeks 9 to 12: 75 mg 2 times a week; weeks 13 to 16: 100 mg 2 times a week; weeks 17 to 20: 100 mg 3 times a week; weeks 21 to 24: 100 mg 4 times a week.
Children: reduced dosage, but not necessarily by body weight; usually approximately ½ of adult dose using same schedule.
Tuberculoid leprosy—
Adults: same as for *lepromatous leprosy* in adults but maximum dosage is 200 mg P.O. weekly (i.e., 100 mg 2 times a week).
Alternate dosage schedule—
Adults: 10 to 15 mg P.O. daily for 6 days a week slowly increased to 62.5 mg daily for 6 days a week over a 6-month period.

SIDE EFFECTS
Blood: anemia, especially hemolytic; methemoglobinemia; possible leukopenia.
CNS: psychosis, headache, dizziness, lethargy, severe malaise, paresthesias.
EENT: tinnitus, allergic rhinitis.

GI: anorexia, abdominal pain, nausea, vomiting.
Hepatic: hepatitis.
Skin: allergic dermatitis (generalized or fixed maculopapular rash).

INTERACTIONS
Probenecid: elevated levels of dapsone. Use together with extreme caution.

NURSING CONSIDERATIONS
• Contraindicated in renal amyloidosis. Use cautiously in chronic renal, hepatic, or cardiovascular disease; refractory types of anemia.
• Therapy should be interrupted if generalized, diffuse dermatitis occurs.
• Dapsone dosage should be reduced or temporarily discontinued if hemoglobin falls below 9 g/100 ml; if leukocyte count falls below 5,000; if erythrocyte count falls below 2.5 million or remains persistently low.
• Patient should receive hematinics during dapsone therapy.
• Antihistamines may help to combat dapsone-induced allergic dermatitis.
• Erythema nodosum type of "lepra reaction" may occur during therapy as a result of *Mycobacterium leprae* bacilli (malaise, fever, painful inflammatory induration in the skin and mucosa, iritis, neuritis). In severe cases, therapy should be stopped and glucocorticoids given cautiously.
• Twice-a-week dosage schedule reduces toxic effects.
• Monitor CBC frequently.

---

ethambutol hydrochloride
Etibi♦♦, Myambutol♦

INDICATIONS & DOSAGE
Adjunctive treatment in pulmonary tuberculosis—
Adults, and children over 13 years: initial treatment for patients who have not received previous antitubercular therapy 15 mg/Kg P.O. daily single dose.
Re-treatment: 25 mg/Kg P.O. daily single dose for 60 days with at least 1 other antitubercular drug; then decrease to 15 mg/Kg P.O. daily single dose.

SIDE EFFECTS
CNS: headache, dizziness, mental confusion, possible hallucinations, peripheral neuritis (numbness and tingling of extremities).
EENT: optic neuritis (vision loss and loss of color discrimination, especially red and green).
GI: anorexia, nausea, vomiting, abdominal pain.
Metabolic: elevated uric acid.
Skin: dermatitis, pruritus.
Other: anaphylactoid reactions, joint pain, fever, malaise, bloody sputum.

INTERACTIONS
None significant.

NURSING CONSIDERATIONS
• Contraindicated in patients with optic neuritis and children under 13. Use cautiously in patients with impaired renal function, cataracts, recurrent eye inflammations, gout, and diabetic retinopathy.
• Dose must be reduced in renal impairment.
• Perform visual acuity tests before and during therapy.
• Monitor renal, hematopoietic, and hepatic functions in long-term use.
• Observe patient for symptoms of gout.
• Instruct patient to take this drug exactly as prescribed; warn against discontinuing use without doctor's advice.
• Monitor serum uric acid.
• Peripheral neuritis may signal visual impairment. Question patient about paresthesias.

Italicized side effects are common or life-threatening.

ethionamide
Trecator SC

INDICATIONS & DOSAGE
Adjunctive treatment in pulmonary or extrapulmonary tuberculosis (when primary therapy with streptomycin, isoniazid, and aminosalicylic acid cannot be used or has failed)—
Adults: 500 mg to 1 g P.O. daily in divided doses. Concomitant administration of other effective anti-tubercular drugs and pyridoxine recommended.
Children: 12 to 15 mg/Kg P.O. daily in 3 to 4 doses. Maximum dose 750 mg.

SIDE EFFECTS
Blood: thrombocytopenia.
CNS: *peripheral neuritis,* psychic disturbances (especially mental depression).
CV: postural hypotension.
GI: *anorexia,* metallic taste in mouth, nausea, vomiting, sialorrhea, *epigastric distress,* diarrhea, stomatitis.
Skin: rash, *exfoliative dermatitis.*
Other: jaundice, hepatitis, elevated serum transaminase, weight loss.

INTERACTIONS
None significant.

NURSING CONSIDERATIONS
• Contraindicated in patients with severe hepatic damage. Use cautiously in patients with diabetes mellitus.
• Culture and sensitivity tests should be performed before starting therapy.
• Stop drug if skin rash occurs; may progress to exfoliative dermatitis.
• Monitor hepatic, hematopoietic, and renal function.
• Give with meals or antacids to minimize GI effects.
• Patient may require antiemetic.
• Pyridoxine may be ordered to prevent neuropathy.

• Instruct patient to take this drug exactly as prescribed; warn against discontinuing drug without doctor's advice.
• Patient should avoid excess alcohol ingestion because he may be more vulnerable to hepatic damage.

isoniazid (INH)
Hyzyd, Isotamine♦♦, Laniazid, Niconyl, Nydrazid, Rimifon♦♦, Rolazid, Teebaconin

INDICATIONS & DOSAGE
Primary treatment against actively growing tubercle bacilli—
Adults: 5 mg/Kg P.O. or I.M. daily single dose, up to 300 mg/day, continued for 18 months to 2 years.
Infants and children: 10 to 20 mg/Kg P.O. or I.M. daily single dose, up to 300 to 500 mg/day, continued for 18 months to 2 years. Concomitant administration of at least one other effective antitubercular drug is recommended.
Preventive therapy against tubercle bacilli of those closely exposed or those with positive skin test whose chest X-ray and bacteriological studies are consistent with nonprogressive tuberculous disease—
Adults: 300 mg P.O. daily single dose, continued for 1 year.
Infants and children: 10 mg/Kg P.O. daily single dose, up to 300 mg/day, continued for 1 year.

SIDE EFFECTS
Blood: *agranulocytosis,* hemolytic anemia, *aplastic anemia,* eosinophilia, leukopenia, neutropenia, thrombocytopenia, methemoglobinemia, pyridoxine-responsive hypochromic anemia.
CNS: *peripheral neuropathy* (especially in the malnourished, alcoholics, diabetics, and slow inactivators),

usually preceded by paresthesias of hands and feet.
GI: nausea, vomiting, epigastric distress, constipation, dryness of the mouth.
Hepatic: *hepatitis, occasionally severe and sometimes fatal, especially in the elderly.*
Metabolic: hyperglycemia, metabolic acidosis.
Local: irritation at the injection site.
Other: rheumatic and systemic lupus erythematosus-like syndromes; hypersensitivity (fever, rash, lymphadenopathy, vasculitis).

INTERACTIONS

Aluminum-containing antacids and laxatives: may decrease the rate and amount of isoniazid absorbed. Give isoniazid at least 1 hour before antacid or laxative.
Disulfiram: neurologic symptoms, including changes in behavior and coordination, may develop with concomitant isoniazid use. Avoid concomitant use.

NURSING CONSIDERATIONS

• Contraindicated in patients with acute hepatic disease, or isoniazid-associated hepatic damage. Use cautiously in patients with chronic non-isoniazid-associated hepatic disease, seizure disorders, severe renal impairment, chronic alcoholism; in elderly patients; in slow acetylator phenotypes (approximately 50% of Blacks and Caucasians).
• Monitor hepatic function if clinical signs of hepatic dysfunction occur during therapy. Tell patient to notify doctor immediately if symptoms of hepatic impairment occur (loss of appetite, fatigue, malaise, jaundice, dark urine).
• Alcohol may be associated with increased incidence of isoniazid-related hepatitis. Discourage use.
• Pyridoxine may be given to prevent peripheral neuropathy, especially in malnourished patients.
• Instruct patient to take this drug exactly as prescribed; warn against discontinuing drug without doctor's advice.
• Store drug at room temperature.
• Advise patient to avoid excessive laxative use.
• Advise patient to avoid cheese. May precipitate hypertensive crisis.
• Advise patient to take with food if gastrointestinal irritation occurs.

---

para-aminosalicylic acid
PAS, Nemasol Sodium♦♦
sodium aminosalicylate
Parasal Sodium, Pasdium, Teebacin

INDICATIONS & DOSAGE

Treatment of tuberculosis (para-aminosalicylic acid)—
Adults: 10 to 12 g P.O. daily, divided in 2 or 3 doses.
Children: 200 to 300 mg/Kg P.O. daily, divided in 3 or 4 doses.
Treatment of tuberculosis (sodium aminosalicylate)—
Adults: 14 to 16 g P.O. daily, divided in 3 or 4 doses.
Children: 200 to 300 mg/Kg P.O. daily, divided in 3 or 4 doses.

SIDE EFFECTS

Blood: *leukopenia, agranulocytosis,* eosinophilia, thrombocytopenia, hemolytic anemia.
CNS: encephalopathy.
CV: vasculitis.
GI: *nausea, vomiting,* diarrhea, abdominal pain.
GU: albuminuria, hematuria, crystalluria.
Hepatic: *jaundice, hepatitis.*
Metabolic: goiter, with or without myxedema; acidosis; hypokalemia.
Skin: rash.
Other: infectious mononucleosis-like syndrome, fever, lymphadenopathy.

Italicized side effects are common or life-threatening.

INTERACTIONS

Ascorbic acid, ammonium chloride: acidify urine and increase possibility of para-aminosalicylic acid crystalluria due to acidification. Avoid if possible.

Probenecid: may increase levels of para-aminosalicylic acid. Use together cautiously.

Rifampin: para-aminosalicylic acid may interfere with absorption of rifampin. Give these drugs 8 to 12 hours apart.

Diphenhydramine: inhibits PAS absorption. Monitor for decreased PAS effect.

NURSING CONSIDERATIONS

• Use cautiously in patients with impaired renal function, decreased hepatic function, and gastric ulcers.

• Sodium aminosalicylate should not be given to patients on sodium-restricted diets. A 15 g dose provides 1.6 g sodium.

• Give with meals or antacid to reduce gastrointestinal distress. Tell patient to swallow enteric-coated tablets whole and not with antacids.

• Monitor renal, hematopoietic, hepatic functions, and serum electrolytes.

• Tell patient to notify doctor at once if symptoms of hepatic impairment (loss of appetite, fatigue, malaise, jaundice, dark urine), fever, sore throat, or skin rash occur.

• Instruct patient to take any of these drugs exactly as prescribed; warn against discontinuing drug without doctor's advice.

• Protect from water, heat, sun. If drug turns brown or purple, don't use.

• Concomitant administration of at least one other effective antitubercular drug is recommended.

pyrazinamide
Tebrazid♦♦

INDICATIONS & DOSAGE

Hospitalized patients seriously ill with tuberculosis (when primary and secondary antitubercular drugs cannot be used or have failed)—

Adults: 20 to 35 mg/Kg P.O. daily, divided in 3 to 4 doses. Maximum dose 3 g daily.

SIDE EFFECTS

Blood: hemolytic anemia, hyperuricemia, possible bleeding tendency due to altered clotting mechanism or vascular integrity.

GI: anorexia, nausea, vomiting.

GU: dysuria.

Hepatic: *hepatitis.*

Metabolic: interference with control in diabetes mellitus, hyperuricemia.

Other: malaise, fever, arthralgia.

INTERACTIONS

None significant.

NURSING CONSIDERATIONS

• Contraindicated in patients with severe hepatic disease. Use cautiously in patients with diabetes mellitus or gout.

• Nearly 100% excreted in urine; reduced dose needed in renal impairment.

• Perform liver function studies and examination for jaundice, liver tenderness or enlargement before and frequently during therapy.

• Watch closely for signs of gout and of hepatic impairment (loss of appetite, fatigue, malaise, jaundice, dark urine, liver tenderness). Call doctor at once.

• Monitor hematopoietic studies and serum uric acid levels.

• Due to serious hepatotoxic effects, this drug is not recommended for initial therapy or long-term use.

• When used with surgical management of tuberculosis, start pyrazinamide 1 to 2 weeks preop and continue for 4 to 6 weeks postop.

rifampin
Rifadin♦, Rimactane♦

INDICATIONS & DOSAGE
Primary treatment in pulmonary tuberculosis—
Adults: 600 mg P.O. daily single dose 1 hour before or 2 hours after meals.
Children over 5 years: 10 to 20 mg/Kg P.O. daily single dose 1 hour before or 2 hours after meals. Maximum dose 600 mg daily.
Concomitant administration of other effective antitubercular drugs is recommended.
Meningococcal carriers—
Adults: 600 mg P.O. daily for 2 days.
Children over 5 years: 10 to 20 mg/Kg/day P.O., not to exceed 600 mg/day.

SIDE EFFECTS
Blood: eosinophilia, thrombocytopenia, transient leukopenia, hemolytic anemia, decreased hemoglobin.
CNS: headache, fatigue, *drowsiness,* ataxia, dizziness, mental confusion, generalized numbness.
EENT: visual disturbances, exudative conjunctivitis.
GI: epigastric distress, anorexia, nausea, vomiting, abdominal pain, diarrhea, flatulence, sore mouth and tongue.
GU: menstrual disturbances.
Metabolic: hyperuricemia.
Hepatic: *serious hepatotoxicity as well as transient abnormalities in liver function tests.*
Skin: pruritus, urticaria, rash.

INTERACTIONS
Aminosalicylic acid: may interfere

with absorption of rifampin. Give these drugs 8 to 12 hours apart.
Probenecid: may increase rifampin levels. Use cautiously.

NURSING CONSIDERATIONS
• Use cautiously in patients with hepatic disease or in those receiving other hepatotoxic drugs.
• Monitor hepatic function, hematopoietic studies, and serum uric acid levels.
• Warn patient about drowsiness and the possibility of red-orange discoloration of urine, feces, saliva, sweat, sputum, and tears. Soft contact lenses may be permanently stained.
• Tell patient to take this drug exactly as prescribed and to report side effects. Warn against discontinuing use without doctor's advice.
• Give 1 hour before or 2 hours after meals for optimal absorption.
• Increases enzyme activity of liver; may require increased doses of warfarin, corticosteroids, oral contraceptives, and oral hypoglycemics. See each drug entry for specific drug interactions.

streptomycin sulfate

INDICATIONS & DOSAGE
Primary treatment in tuberculosis—
Adults: with normal renal function, 1 g I.M. daily for 2 to 3 months, then 1 g 2 or 3 times a week. Inject deeply into upper outer quadrant of buttocks.
Children: with normal renal function, 20 mg/Kg daily in divided doses injected deeply into large muscle mass.
Give concurrently with other antitubercular agents, but not with capreomycin, and continue until sputum specimen becomes negative.

SIDE EFFECTS
Blood: eosinophilia, leukopenia, neu-

tropenia, pancytopenia, hemolytic anemia.
CNS: *transient paresthesias,* especially circumoral; lassitude.
CV: myocarditis.
EENT: *ototoxicity* (damage to vestibular and auditory portions of 8th cranial nerve, severe headache, *nausea, vomiting, vertigo,* ataxia, *tinnitus, roaring and sense of fullness in the ears,* hearing loss), optic nerve dysfunction (blurred vision, amblyopia).
GI: stomatitis.
GU: *nephrotoxicity* (transient proteinuria, increase in blood urea nitrogen and serum creatinine levels); nephrotoxicity less common than with other aminoglycosides.
Local: pain, irritation at injection site, *hypersensitivity* (rash, fever, urticaria, pruritus, angioneurotic edema).
Other: respiratory depression, muscle weakness, systemic lupus erythematosus syndrome.

INTERACTIONS
Other aminoglycosides, methoxyflurane: may increase streptomycin's ototoxic and nephrotoxic effects. Use cautiously.
Ethacrynic acid, furosemide: may increase streptomycin's ototoxic effects. Monitor carefully.
Dimenhydrinate: may mask symptoms of ototoxicity. Use together cautiously.

NURSING CONSIDERATIONS
• Contraindicated in patients with labyrinthine disease; those receiving other ototoxic or nephrotoxic drugs, neuromuscular blocking agents, and general anesthetics. Use cautiously in elderly patients and in those with impaired renal function.
• Monitor renal function studies. Reduce dose in renal impairment.
• Test patient's hearing before, during, and 6 months after therapy. No-

tify doctor if patient complains of tinnitus, roaring noises, fullness in ears.
• Observe patient for respiratory depression.
• To minimize renal damage, patient should be well hydrated.
• Watch for signs of superinfection (continued fever and other signs of new infections, especially of the upper respiratory tract).
• Very sensitizing topically. Protect hands when preparing drug.
• In primary treatment of tuberculosis, streptomycin is discontinued when sputum becomes negative.

---

sulfoxone sodium
Diasone Sodium♦

INDICATIONS & DOSAGE
Lepromatous and tuberculoid leprosy—
Adults: weeks 1 and 2: 330 mg P.O. 2 times a week; weeks 3 and 4: 330 mg 4 times a week; week 5 and following weeks: 330 mg daily for 6 days, skip a day and continue.
Children (4 years and older): give ½ the adult dose.

SIDE EFFECTS
Blood: possible leukopenia, *anemia, especially hemolytic;* methemoglobinemia.
CNS: psychosis, headache, dizziness, lethargy, severe malaise, paresthesias.
EENT: tinnitus, allergic rhinitis.
GI: anorexia, *abdominal pain,* nausea, vomiting.
Skin: allergic dermatitis (generalized or fixed maculopapular rash).
Other: hepatitis, drug fever, lepra reaction.

INTERACTIONS
None significant.

NURSING CONSIDERATIONS
• Contraindicated in renal amyloidosis. Use cautiously in chronic renal, hepatic, or cardiovascular disease, or refractory anemias.
• Therapy should be interrupted if generalized, diffuse dermatitis occurs.
• Sulfoxone sodium should be reduced or temporarily discontinued if hemoglobin falls below 9 g/100 ml; if leukocyte count falls below 5,000; if erythrocyte count falls below 2.5 million or remains persistently low.
• Patient should receive hematinics during sulfoxone sodium therapy.
• Antihistamines may help combat sulfoxone sodium-induced allergic dermatitis.

• Erythema nodosum type of "lepra reaction" may occur during sulfoxone sodium therapy as a result of circulating antigens caused by disintegrating *Mycobacterium leprae* bacilli (malaise, fever, painful areas of inflammatory induration in the skin and mucosa, iritis, neuritis). In severe cases, therapy should be interrupted and glucocorticoids given cautiously.
• Monitor CBC frequently.
• If drug fever is severe or frequent, interrupt therapy or reduce dosage.
• To minimize stomach upset, give drug with meals.
• Protect drug from light.

Aminoglycosides

amikacin sulfate
gentamicin sulfate
kanamycin sulfate
neomycin sulfate
streptomycin sulfate
tobramycin sulfate

---

amikacin sulfate
Amikin♦

INDICATIONS & DOSAGE
Serious infections caused by sensitive Pseudomonas aeruginosa, Escherichia coli, Proteus, Klebsiella, Serratia, Enterobacter, Acinetobacter, Providencia, Citrobacter, Staphylococcus—
Adults and children with normal renal function: 15 mg/Kg/day divided q 8 to 12 hours I.M. or I.V. infusion (in 100 to 200 ml dextrose 5% in water run in over 30 to 60 minutes). May be given by direct I.V. push if necessary.
Neonates with normal renal function: initially, 10 mg/Kg I.M. or I.V. infusion (in dextrose 5% in water run in over 1 to 2 hours), then 7.5 mg/Kg q 12 hours I.M. or I.V. infusion.
Meningitis—
Adults: systemic therapy as above; may also use up to 4 mg intrathecally or intraventricularly daily.
Children: systemic therapy as above; may also use 1 to 2 mg intrathecally daily.
Serious urinary tract infections—
Adults: 250 mg I.M. b.i.d.
Adults with impaired renal function: initially, 7.5 mg/Kg. Subsequent doses and frequency determined by serum amikacin levels and renal function studies.

SIDE EFFECTS
CNS: headache, lethargy, organic brain syndrome.
EENT: *ototoxicity (tinnitus, vertigo, hearing loss).*
GI: nausea, vomiting.
GU: *nephrotoxicity (cells or casts in urine, oliguria, proteinuria, decreased creatinine clearance, increased blood urea nitrogen and serum creatinine).*
Skin: rash, urticaria.

INTERACTIONS
I.V. ethacrynic acid, I.V. furosemide: increased ototoxicity. Use cautiously.
Dimenhydrinate: may mask symptoms of ototoxicity. Use with caution.
Carbenicillin: amikacin antagonism. Don't mix together in I.V. Schedule 1 hour apart.
Other aminoglycosides, methoxyflurane: increased ototoxicity and nephrotoxicity. Use together cautiously.

NURSING CONSIDERATIONS
• Use cautiously in patients with impaired renal function; in neonates and infants, elderly patients.
• Obtain specimen for culture and sensitivity before first dose. Therapy may begin pending test results.
• Weigh patient and obtain baseline renal function studies before therapy begins.
• Monitor renal function (output,

specific gravity, urinalysis, blood urea nitrogen, creatinine, and creatinine clearance). Notify doctor of decreasing renal function.
• Patient should be well hydrated while taking this drug.
• Evaluate patient's hearing before and during therapy. Notify doctor if patient complains of tinnitus, vertigo, hearing loss.
• Watch for superinfection (continued fever and other signs of new infections, especially of upper respiratory tract).
• Usual duration of therapy is 7 to 10 days. If no response after 3 to 5 days, therapy should be stopped and new specimens obtained for culture and sensitivity.
• Peak serum levels above 35 mcg/ml are associated with higher incidence of toxicity.
• After I.V. infusion, flush line with normal saline solution to clear all remaining drug.
• Amikacin is usually reserved for gentamicin-resistant organisms.

---

gentamicin sulfate
Cidomycin♦♦, Garamycin♦, U-Gencin

INDICATIONS & DOSAGE

Serious infections caused by sensitive Pseudomonas aeruginosa, Escherichia coli, Proteus, Klebsiella, Serratia, Enterobacter, Citrobacter, Staphylococcus—
Adults with normal renal function: 3 mg/Kg/day in divided dosage q 8 hours I.M. or I.V. infusion (in 50 to 200 ml of normal saline solution or dextrose 5% in water infused over 30 minutes to 2 hours). May be given by direct I.V. push if necessary. For life-threatening infections, patient may receive up to 5 mg/Kg/day in 3 to 4 divided dosages.
Children with normal renal func-

tion: 2 to 2.5 mg/Kg I.M. or I.V. infusion q 8 hours.
Infants and neonates over 1 week with normal renal function: 2.5 mg/Kg q 8 hours I.M. or I.V. infusion.
Neonates under 1 week: 2.5 mg/Kg I.V. q 12 hours. For I.V. infusion, dilute in normal saline solution or dextrose 5% in water and infuse over ½ to 2 hours.
Meningitis—
Adults: systemic therapy as above; may also use 4 to 8 mg intrathecally daily.
Children: systemic therapy as above; may also use 1 to 2 mg intrathecally daily.
Endocarditis prophylaxis for GI or GU procedure or surgery—
Adults: 1.5 mg/Kg I.M. or I.V. 30 to 60 minutes before procedure or surgery and q 8 hours after, for 2 doses. Given with aqueous penicillin G or ampicillin.
Children: 2 mg/Kg I.M. or I.V. 30 to 60 minutes before procedure or surgery and q 8 hours after, for 2 doses. Given with aqueous penicillin G or ampicillin.
Patients with impaired renal function: initial dose is same as for those with normal renal function. Subsequent doses and frequency determined by renal function tests.
Posthemodialysis to maintain therapeutic blood levels—
Adults: 1 to 1.7 mg/Kg I.M. or I.V. infusion after each dialysis.
Children: 2 mg/Kg I.M. or I.V. infusion after each dialysis.

SIDE EFFECTS

CNS: headache, lethargy, organic brain syndrome.
EENT: *ototoxicity (tinnitus, vertigo, hearing loss).*
GI: nausea, vomiting.
GU: *nephrotoxicity (casts or protein in the urine, oliguria, proteinuria, decreased creatinine clearance, in-*

creased blood urea nitrogen, nonpro-tein nitrogen, and serum creatinine levels).
Skin: rash, urticaria.

INTERACTIONS

I.V. ethacrynic acid, I.V. furosemide: increased ototoxicity. Use cautiously.
Dimenhydrinate: may mask symptoms of ototoxicity. Use with caution.
Carbenicillin: gentamicin antago-nism. Don't mix together in I.V. Schedule 1 hour apart.
Cephalosporins: increased nephrotox-icity. Use together cautiously.
Other aminoglycosides, methoxyflu-rane: increased ototoxicity and neph-rotoxicity. Use together cautiously.

NURSING CONSIDERATIONS

• Use cautiously in patients with im-paired renal function; in neonates and infants, elderly patients.
• Obtain specimen for culture and sensitivity before first dose. Therapy may begin pending test results.
• Weigh patient and obtain baseline renal function studies before therapy begins.
• Monitor renal function (output, specific gravity, urinalysis, blood urea nitrogen, creatinine, and creatinine clearance). Notify doctor of decreas-ing renal function.
• Patient should be well hydrated while taking this drug.
• After completing I.V. infusion, flush the line with normal saline solu-tion to clear all remaining drug.
• Evaluate patient's hearing before and during therapy. Notify doctor if patient complains of tinnitus, vertigo, hearing loss.
• Watch for superinfection (contin-ued fever and other signs of new in-fections, especially of upper respira-tory tract).
• Usual duration of therapy is 7 to 10 days. If no response in 3 to 5 days, therapy should be stopped and new

specimens obtained for culture and sensitivity.
• Peak serum levels above 12 mcg/ml and trough levels (those drawn just before next dose) above 2 mcg/ml are associated with higher incidence of toxicity.
• Draw blood for peak gentamicin level 1 hour after I.M. injection and 1 hour after I.V. infusion begins; trough levels, just before next dose.
• Hemodialysis (8 hours) removes up to 50% of drug from blood.
• Endocarditis prophylaxis is recom-mended for all patients with rheu-matic or congenital heart disease or prosthetic heart valve.
• After I.V. infusion, flush line with normal saline solution to clear all re-maining drug.
• Intrathecal form (without preserva-tives) should be used when intrathecal is indicated.

---

kanamycin sulfate
Kantrex♦, Klebcil

INDICATIONS & DOSAGE

Adjunctive treatment in hepatic coma—
Adults: 8 to 12 g/day P.O. in divided doses.
Preop bowel sterilization—
Adults: 1 g P.O. q 1 hour for 4 doses, then q 4 hours for 4 doses; or 1 g P.O. q 1 hour for 4 doses, then q 6 hours for 36 to 72 hours.
Intraperitoneal irrigation—
500 mg in 20 ml sterile distilled water instilled via catheter into wound after patient fully recovered from anes-thesia and neuromuscular blocking agent effects.
Serious infections caused by sensitive Escherichia coli, Proteus, Enterobac-ter aerogenes, Klebsiella pneumoniae, Serratia marcescens, Acinetobacter—
Adults and children with normal renal function: 15 mg/Kg/day di-

vided q 8 to 12 hours deep I.M. into upper outer quadrant of buttocks or I.V. infusion (diluted 500 mg/200 ml of normal saline solution or dextrose 5% in water infused at 60 to 80 drops/ minute). Maximum daily dose 1.5 g.
Neonates: 15 mg/Kg/day I.M. or I.V. divided q 12 hours.
Wound irrigation—up to 2.5 mg/ml in normal saline irrigation solution.

SIDE EFFECTS
CNS: headache, lethargy, organic brain syndrome.
EENT: *ototoxicity (tinnitus, vertigo, hearing loss).*
GI: nausea, vomiting.
GU: *nephrotoxicity (cells or casts in the urine, oliguria, proteinuria, decreased creatinine clearance, increased blood urea nitrogen and serum creatinine).*
Skin: rash, urticaria.

INTERACTIONS
Ethacrynic acid, furosemide: increased ototoxicity. Use cautiously.
Dimenhydrinate: may mask symptoms of ototoxicity. Use with caution.
Other aminoglycosides, methoxyflurane: increased ototoxicity and nephrotoxicity. Don't use together.

NURSING CONSIDERATIONS
• Oral use contraindicated in intestinal obstruction; in treatment of systemic infection. Use cautiously in impaired renal function, and the elderly.
• Obtain specimen for culture and sensitivity before first dose. Therapy may begin pending test results.
• Weigh patient and obtain baseline renal function studies before therapy begins.
• Monitor renal function (output, specific gravity, urinalysis, blood urea nitrogen, creatinine, and creatinine clearance). Notify doctor of decreasing renal function.
• Patient should be well hydrated while taking this drug.

• Evaluate patient's hearing before and during therapy. Notify doctor if patient complains of tinnitus, vertigo, hearing loss.
• Watch for superinfection (continued fever and other signs of new infection, especially of upper respiratory tract).
• If no response in 3 to 5 days, therapy should be stopped and new specimens obtained for culture and sensitivity.
• Peak serum levels over 30 mcg/ml are associated with increased incidence of toxicity.

neomycin sulfate
Mycifradin Sulfate♦, Neobiotic

INDICATIONS & DOSAGE
Adjunctive treatment in hepatic coma—
Adults: 1 to 3 g P.O. q.i.d. for 5 to 6 days; or 200 ml of 1% or 100 ml of 2% solution as enema retained for 20 to 60 minutes q 6 hours.
Infectious diarrhea caused by enteropathogenic Escherichia coli—
Adults: 50 mg/Kg/day P.O. in 4 divided doses for 2 to 3 days.
Children: 50 to 100 mg/Kg/day P.O. divided q 4 to 6 hours for 2 to 3 days.
Suppression of intestinal bacteria preoperatively—
Adults: 1 g P.O. q 1 hour for 4 doses, then 1 g q 4 hours for the balance of the 24 hours.
Children: 40 to 100 mg/Kg/day P.O. divided q 4 to 6 hours.
First dose should be preceded by saline cathartic.

SIDE EFFECTS
CNS: headache, lethargy, organic brain syndrome.
EENT: *ototoxicity (tinnitus, vertigo, hearing loss).*
GI: nausea, vomiting.
GU: *nephrotoxicity (cells or casts in*

the urine, oliguria, proteinuria, decreased creatinine clearance, increased blood urea nitrogen and serum creatinine).
Skin: rash, urticaria.

INTERACTIONS
Ethacrynic acid, furosemide: increased ototoxicity. Use cautiously.
Dimenhydrinate: may mask symptoms of ototoxicity. Use with caution.
Other aminoglycosides, methoxyflurane: increased ototoxicity and nephrotoxicity. Use together cautiously.

NURSING CONSIDERATIONS
• Contraindicated in intestinal obstruction. Use cautiously in patients with impaired renal function, ulcerative bowel lesions, and in elderly patients.
• Oral therapy not recommended for systemic infection; parenteral dosage form available for I.M. use but not recommended because of extreme ototoxicity and nephrotoxicity.
• Weigh patient and obtain baseline renal function studies before therapy begins.
• Monitor renal function (output, specific gravity, urinalysis, blood urea nitrogen, creatinine, and creatinine clearance). Notify doctor of decreasing renal function.
• Patient should be well hydrated while taking this drug.
• Watch for respiratory depression in renal disease, hypocalcemia, or neuromuscular diseases such as myasthenia gravis.
• Evaluate hearing of patient with hepatic or renal disease before and during prolonged therapy. Notify doctor if patient complains of tinnitus, vertigo, hearing loss. Onset of deafness may occur several weeks after drug is stopped.
• Watch for superinfection (continued fever and other signs of new infections, especially of upper respiratory tract).

• Sometimes used in the treatment of high blood cholesterol.
• Nonabsorbable at recommended dosage. However, more than 4 g of neomycin per day may be systemically absorbed and lead to nephrotoxicity.

---

streptomycin sulfate

INDICATIONS & DOSAGE
Nonhemolytic streptococcal endocarditis—
Adults: 1 g I.M. deep into upper outer quadrant of buttocks q 12 hours for 1 week, then 500 mg I.M. q 12 hours for 1 week with penicillin.
Treatment of tuberculosis—
Adults: initially, 0.75 to 1 g I.M. daily for 60 to 90 days, then 1 g 2 to 3 times weekly.
Endocarditis prophylaxis for dental and upper respiratory tract procedures—
Adults: 1 g I.M. 30 to 60 minutes before procedure. Used with penicillin.
Children: 20 mg/Kg I.M. 30 to 60 minutes before procedure. Used with penicillin.
Endocarditis prophylaxis for GI or GU procedures or surgery—
Adults: 1 g I.M. 30 to 60 minutes before procedure and q 12 hours for 2 doses after. Used with penicillin or ampicillin.
Children: 20 mg/Kg I.M. 30 to 60 minutes before procedure and q 12 hours for 2 doses after. Used with penicillin or ampicillin.
Patients with impaired renal function: initial dose is same as for those with normal renal function. Subsequent doses and frequency determined by renal function test results.
Enterococcal endocarditis—
Adults: 1 g I.M. q 12 hours for 2 weeks, then 500 mg I.M. q 12 hours for 4 weeks with penicillin.
Tularemia—
Adults: 1 to 2 g I.M. daily in divided

---

doses injected deep into upper outer quadrant of buttocks. Continue until patient is afebrile for 5 to 7 days.

SIDE EFFECTS
EENT: *ototoxicity (tinnitus, vertigo, hearing loss).*
GU: some nephrotoxicity (not nearly as frequent as with other aminoglycosides).
Skin: *exfoliative dermatitis.*
Local: pain, irritation, and sterile abscesses at injection site.
Other: *hypersensitivity* (rash, fever, urticaria, and angioneurotic edema).

INTERACTIONS
Dimenhydrinate: may mask symptoms of streptomycin-induced ototoxicity. Use together cautiously.
Ethacrynic acid, furosemide: increased ototoxicity. Use cautiously.
Other aminoglycosides, methoxyflurane: may increase streptomycin's ototoxic and nephrotoxic effects. Use cautiously.

NURSING CONSIDERATIONS
• Contraindicated in labyrinthine disease. Use cautiously in patients with impaired renal function and in the elderly.
• Obtain specimen for culture and sensitivity before first dose except when treating tuberculosis. Therapy may begin pending test results.
• Patient should be well hydrated while taking this drug.
• Evaluate patient's hearing before, during, and 6 months after therapy. Notify doctor if patient complains of tinnitus, roaring noises, or fullness in ears.
• Watch for superinfection (continued fever and other signs of new infections, especially of upper respiratory tract) and respiratory depression.
• Peak serum concentrations over 25 mcg/ml are associated with increased incidence of toxicity.
• Endocarditis prophylaxis is recom-

mended for all patients with rheumatic or congenital heart disease or with prosthetic heart valve. Patients should receive prophylactic antibiotics during GI or GU procedures or surgery, or during upper respiratory tract procedures.

---

tobramycin sulfate
Nebcin♦

INDICATIONS & DOSAGE
Serious infections caused by sensitive strains of Escherichia coli, Proteus, Klebsiella, Enterobacter, Serratia, Staphylococcus aureus, Pseudomonas, Citrobacter, Providencia—
Adults and children with normal renal function: 3 mg/Kg I.M. or I.V. daily divided q 8 hours. Up to 5 mg/Kg I.M. or I.V. daily divided q 6 to 8 hours for life-threatening infections.
Neonates under 1 week: up to 4 mg/Kg I.M. or I.V. daily divided q 12 hours. For I.V. use, dilute in 50 to 100 ml normal saline solution or dextrose 5% in water for adults and less volume for children. Infuse over 20 to 60 minutes.
Patients with impaired renal function: initial dose is same as for those with normal renal function. Subsequent doses and frequency determined by renal function study results.

SIDE EFFECTS
CNS: headache, lethargy, organic brain syndrome.
EENT: *ototoxicity (tinnitus, vertigo, hearing loss).*
GI: nausea, vomiting.
GU: *nephrotoxicity (cells or casts in the urine, oliguria, proteinuria, decreased creatinine clearance, increased blood urea nitrogen and serum creatinine).*
Skin: rash, urticaria.

Italicized side effects are common or life-threatening.

INTERACTIONS

I.V. ethacrynic acid, I.V. furosemide: increased ototoxicity. Use cautiously.
Dimenhydrinate: may mask symptoms of ototoxicity. Use with caution.
Carbenicillin: tobramycin antagonism. Don't mix together in I.V. Schedule 1 hour apart.
Cephalosporins: increased nephrotoxicity. Use together cautiously.
Other aminoglycosides, methoxyflurane: increased ototoxicity and nephrotoxicity. Use together cautiously.

NURSING CONSIDERATIONS

• Use cautiously in patients with impaired renal function and in the elderly.
• Obtain specimen for culture and sensitivity before first dose. Therapy may begin pending test results.
• Weigh patient and obtain baseline renal function studies before starting therapy.
• Usual duration of therapy is 7 to 10 days.
• Monitor renal function (output, specific gravity, urinalysis, blood urea nitrogen, creatinine, and creatinine clearance). Notify doctor of decreasing renal function.
• Patient should be well hydrated while taking this drug.
• Evaluate patient's hearing before and during therapy. Notify doctor if patient complains of tinnitus, vertigo, hearing loss.
• Watch for superinfection (continued fever and other signs of new infections, especially of upper respiratory tract).
• Peak serum levels over 12 mcg/ml are associated with increased incidence of toxicity.
• Draw blood for peak tobramycin level 1 hour after I.M. injection and 1 hour after I.V. infusion begins; draw blood for trough level just before next dose.
• After I.V. infusion, flush line with normal saline solution to clear all remaining drug.
• Recent studies indicate tobramycin is less nephrotoxic than gentamicin.

Penicillins

amoxicillin trihydrate
ampicillin
ampicillin sodium
carbenicillin disodium
carbenicillin indanyl sodium
cloxacillin sodium
cyclacillin
dicloxacillin sodium
hetacillin
hetacillin potassium
methicillin sodium
nafcillin sodium
oxacillin sodium
penicillin G benzathine
penicillin G potassium
penicillin G procaine
penicillin G sodium
penicillin V
penicillin V potassium
ticarcillin disodium

amoxicillin trihydrate
Amoxil♦, Larotid, Polymox♦,
Robamox, Sumox, Trimox, Utimox

INDICATIONS & DOSAGE
*Systemic infections caused by suscepti-
ble strains of gram-positive and gram-
negative organisms—*
Adults: 750 mg to 1.5 g P.O. daily,
divided into doses given q 8 hours.
Children: 20 to 40 mg/Kg P.O. daily,
divided into doses given q 8 hours.
Uncomplicated gonorrhea—
Adults: 3 g P.O. with 1 g probenecid
given as a single dose.

SIDE EFFECTS
Blood: anemia, thrombocytopenia,
thrombocytopenic purpura, eosinophilia, leukopenia.
GI: *nausea,* vomiting, *diarrhea.*
Other: *hypersensitivity (erythematous
maculopapular rash, urticaria, anaphylaxis),* overgrowth of nonsusceptible organisms.

INTERACTIONS
Probenecid: increased blood levels of
penicillin. Probenecid is often used
for this purpose.
*Chloramphenicol, erythromycin, tet-
racyclines:* antibiotic antagonism.
Give penicillins at least 1 hour before
bacteriostatic antibiotics.

NURSING CONSIDERATIONS
• Use cautiously in patients with
other drug allergies, especially to
cephalosporins (possible cross-allergenicity); in patients with mononucleosis, high incidence of maculopapular
rash in those receiving amoxicillin.
• Obtain cultures for sensitivity tests
before first dose. Unnecessary to wait
for results before beginning therapy.
• Before giving penicillin, ask patient
if he's had any previous allergic reactions to this drug. However, a negative
history of penicillin allergy is no
guarantee against a future allergic reaction.
• Tell patient to take medication exactly as prescribed, even after he feels
better. Entire quantity prescribed
should be taken.
• Give with food to prevent GI distress.
• Large doses may cause increased

yeast growths. Report symptoms to
doctor.
• With prolonged therapy, bacterial
and fungal superinfection may occur,
especially in the elderly, debilitated, or
those with low resistance to infection
due to immunosuppressors or irradiation. Close observation essential.
• Check expiration date. Warn patient
never to use leftover penicillin for a
new illness or to "share" penicillin
with family and friends.
• Tell patient to call the doctor if
rash, fever, or chills develop. A rash
is the most common allergic reaction.
• Amoxicillin and ampicillin have
similar clinical applications.

---

ampicillin
Amcill♦, Ampilean♦♦, Omnipen,
Penbritin♦, Pensyn, Pfizerpen A,
Roampicillin
ampicillin sodium
Amcill-S, Omnipen-N, Pen A/N, Pen-
britin-S, Polycillin-N, Principen/N,
Totacillin-N

INDICATIONS & DOSAGE
*Systemic infections caused by suscepti-
ble strains of gram-positive and gram-
negative organisms—*
Adults: 1 to 4 g P.O. daily, divided
into doses given q 6 hours; 2 to 12 g
I.M. or I.V. daily, divided into doses
given q 6 hours.
Children: 50 to 100 mg/Kg P.O.
daily, divided into doses given
q 6 hours; or 100 to 200 mg/Kg I.M.
or I.V. daily, divided into doses given
q 6 hours.
Meningitis—
Adults: 8 to 14 g I.V. daily for 3 days,
then I.M. divided q 3 to 4 hours.
Children: up to 300 mg/Kg I.V. daily
for 3 days, then I.M. divided
q 4 hours.
Uncomplicated gonorrhea—
Adults: 3.5 g P.O. with 1 g probenecid given as a single dose.

SIDE EFFECTS
Blood: anemia, thrombocytopenia,
thrombocytopenic purpura, eosinophilia, leukopenia.
GI: *nausea,* vomiting, *diarrhea,* glossitis, stomatitis.
Other: *hypersensitivity (erythematous
maculopapular rash, urticaria, anaphylaxis),* overgrowth of nonsusceptible organisms.

INTERACTIONS
Probenecid: increased blood levels of
penicillin. Probenecid is often used
for this purpose.
*Chloramphenicol, erythromycin, tet-
racyclines:* antibiotic antagonism.
Give penicillins at least 1 hour before
bacteriostatic antibiotics.

NURSING CONSIDERATIONS
• Use cautiously in patients with
other drug allergies, especially to
cephalosporins (possible cross-allergenicity); in patients with mononucleosis, high incidence of maculopapular
rash in those receiving ampicillin.
• Obtain cultures for sensitivity tests
before first dose. Unnecessary to wait
for results before beginning therapy.
• Before giving penicillin, ask patient
if he's had any previous allergic reactions to this drug. However, a negative
history of penicillin allergy is no
guarantee against a future allergic
reaction.
• Tell patient to take medication exactly as prescribed, even after he feels
better. Entire quantity prescribed
should be taken.
• Tell the patient to call the doctor if
rash, fever, or chills develop. A rash
is the most common allergic reaction.
• When given orally, drug may cause
GI disturbances. Food may interfere
with absorption, so give 1 to 2 hours
before meals or 2 to 3 hours after.
• Don't give I.M. or I.V. unless infection is severe or patient can't take oral
dose.
• Dosage should be altered in pa-

---

tients with impaired hepatic and renal functions.
• When giving I.V., mix with 5% dextrose in water or a saline solution. Don't mix with other drugs or solutions: they might be incompatible.
• Give I.V. intermittently to prevent vein irritation. Change site every 48 hours.
• Large doses may cause increased yeast growths. Report symptoms to doctor.
• With prolonged therapy, bacterial or fungal superinfection may occur, especially in the elderly, debilitated, or those with low resistance to infection due to immunosuppressors or irradiation. Close observation is essential.
• Check expiration date. Warn patient never to use leftover penicillin for a new illness or to "share" penicillin with family and friends.
• Initial dilution in vial is stable for 1 hour. Follow manufacturer's direction for stability data when ampicillin is further diluted for I.V. infusion.

---

carbenicillin disodium
Geopen, Pyopen♦

INDICATIONS & DOSAGE

Systemic infections caused by susceptible strains of gram-positive and especially gram-negative organisms (Proteus, Pseudomonas aeruginosa)—
Adults: 30 to 40 g daily I.V. infusion, divided into doses given q 4 to 6 hours.
Children: 300 to 500 mg/Kg daily I.V. infusion, divided into doses given q 4 to 6 hours.
Urinary tract infections—
Adults: 200 mg/Kg daily I.M. or I.V. infusion, divided into doses given q 4 to 6 hours.
Children: 50 to 200 mg/Kg daily I.M. or I.V. infusion, divided into doses given q 4 to 6 hours.

SIDE EFFECTS

Blood: *bleeding with high doses*, neutropenia, eosinophilia, leukopenia, *thrombocytopenia*.
CNS: *convulsions*, neuromuscular irritability.
GI: nausea.
Local: pain at injection site, vein irritation, phlebitis.
Metabolic: *hypokalemia*.
Other: *hypersensitivity (edema, fever, chills, rash, pruritus, urticaria, anaphylaxis)*, overgrowth of nonsusceptible organisms.

INTERACTIONS

Probenecid: increased blood levels of penicillin. Probenecid is often used for this purpose.
Gentamicin, tobramycin: chemically incompatible. Don't mix together in I.V. Give 1 hour apart.
Chloramphenicol, erythromycin, tetracyclines: antibiotic antagonism. Give penicillins at least 1 hour before bacteriostatic antibiotics.

NURSING CONSIDERATIONS

• Use cautiously in patients with other drug allergies, especially to cephalosporins (possible cross-allergenicity), those with bleeding tendencies, uremia, hypokalemia. Use cautiously in sodium-restricted patients; contains 4.7 mEq sodium/g.
• Obtain cultures for sensitivity tests before starting therapy. However, it's not necessary to wait for culture and sensitivity results before beginning therapy.
• Before giving penicillin, ask patient if he's had any previous allergic reactions to this drug. However, a negative history of penicillin allergy is no guarantee against a future allergic reaction.
• Dosage should be altered in patients with impaired hepatic and renal functions.
• Check CBC frequently. Drug may cause thrombocytopenia.

- Monitor serum potassium.
- If patient has high serum level of this drug, he may have convulsions. Be prepared by keeping side rails up on bed and tongue blade handy.
- When giving I.V., mix with 5% dextrose in water or other suitable I.V. fluids.
- Give I.V intermittently to prevent vein irritation. Change site every 48 hours.
- Large doses may cause increased yeast growths. Report symptoms to doctor.
- Almost always used with another antibiotic such as gentamicin.
- With prolonged therapy, other superinfections may occur, especially in the elderly, debilitated, or those with low resistance to infection due to immunosuppressors or irradiation. Close observation is essential.
- Check expiration date.

---

carbenicillin indanyl sodium
Geocillin, Geopen Oral♦♦

INDICATIONS & DOSAGE
Urinary tract infection and prostatitis caused by susceptible strains of gram-negative organisms—
Adults: 382 to 764 mg P.O. q.i.d. Not recommended for children.

SIDE EFFECTS
Blood: leukopenia, neutropenia, eosinophilia, anemia, thrombocytopenia.
GI: *nausea,* vomiting, *diarrhea, flatulence, abdominal cramps, unpleasant taste.*
Other: *hypersensitivity (rash, chills, fever, urticaria, pruritus, anaphylaxis),* overgrowth of nonsusceptible organisms.

INTERACTIONS
None significant.

NURSING CONSIDERATIONS
- Use cautiously in patients with other drug allergies, especially to cephalosporins (possible cross-allergenicity).
- Obtain cultures for sensitivity tests before starting therapy.
- Before giving penicillin, ask patient if he's had any previous allergic reactions to this drug. However, a negative history of penicillin allergy is no guarantee against a future allergic reaction.
- Tell patient to take medication exactly as prescribed, even after he feels better. Entire quantity prescribed should be taken.
- Tell patient to call the doctor if he develops rash, fever, or chills. A rash is the most common allergic reaction.
- When given orally, drug may cause GI disturbances. Food may interfere with absorption, so give 1 to 2 hours before meals or 2 to 3 hours after.
- Large doses may cause increased yeast growths. Report symptoms to doctor.
- With prolonged therapy, other superinfections may occur, especially in the elderly, debilitated, or those with low resistance to infection due to immunosuppressors or irradiation. Close observation is essential.
- Check expiration date. Warn patient never to use leftover penicillin for a new illness or to "share" penicillin with family and friends.
- Use only in patients whose creatinine clearance is 10 ml/minute or more.
- Excellent treatment for *Pseudomonas* urinary tract infections in ambulatory patients.
- May be useful in treatment of cystitis, but not pyelonephritis.
- Not effective for any systemic infection because blood levels are nil.

---

cloxacillin sodium
Bactopen♦♦, Cloxapen♦, Novo-
cloxin♦♦, Orbenin♦♦, Tegopen♦

INDICATIONS & DOSAGE
*Systemic infections caused by
penicillinase-producing staphylococci—*
Adults: 2 to 4 g P.O. daily, divided
into doses given q 6 hours.
Children: 50 to 100 mg/Kg P.O.
daily, divided into doses given
q 6 hours.

SIDE EFFECTS
Blood: eosinophilia.
GI: *nausea,* vomiting, *epigastric distress, diarrhea.*
Other: *hypersensitivity (rash, urticaria, chills, fever, sneezing, wheezing, anaphylaxis),* overgrowth of nonsusceptible organisms.

INTERACTIONS
Probenecid: increased blood levels of
penicillin. Probenecid is often used
for this purpose.
*Chloramphenicol, erythromycin, tet-
racyclines:* antibiotic antagonism.
Give penicillins at least 1 hour before
bacteriostatic antibiotics.

NURSING CONSIDERATIONS
• Use with caution in patients with
other drug allergies, especially to
cephalosporins (possible cross-allergenicity).
• Obtain cultures for sensitivity tests
before starting therapy.
• Before giving penicillin, ask patient
if he's had any previous allergic reactions to this drug. However, a negative
history of penicillin allergy is no
guarantee against a future allergic reaction.
• Tell patient to take medication exactly as prescribed, even if he feels
better. Entire quantity prescribed
should be taken.

• Tell patient to call the doctor if
rash, fever, or chills develop. A rash
is the most common allergic reaction.
• When given orally, drug may cause
GI disturbances. Food may interfere
with absorption, so give 1 to 2 hours
before meals or 2 to 3 hours after.
• Large doses may cause increased
yeast growths. Report symptoms to
doctor.
• With prolonged therapy, other superinfections may occur, especially in
the elderly, debilitated, or those with
low resistance to infection due to immunosuppressors or irradiation. Close
observation is essential.
• Check expiration date. Warn patient
never to use leftover penicillin for a
new illness or to "share" penicillin
with family and friends.

cyclacillin
Cyclapen

INDICATIONS & DOSAGE
*Systemic and urinary tract infections
caused by susceptible strains of gram-
positive and gram-negative organisms—*
Adults: 250 to 500 mg P.O. q.i.d. in
equally spaced doses.
Children: 50 to 100 mg/Kg/day in
equally divided doses.

SIDE EFFECTS
Blood: anemia, thrombocytopenia,
thrombocytopenic purpura, leukopenia, neutropenia, eosinophilia.
GI: *nausea,* vomiting, *diarrhea.*
Other: *hypersensitivity (edema, fever,
chills, rash, pruritus, urticaria, anaphylaxis),* overgrowth of nonsusceptible organisms.

INTERACTIONS
Probenecid: increased blood levels of
penicillin. Probenecid is often used
for this purpose.

Italicized side effects are common or life-threatening.

NURSING CONSIDERATIONS

- Contraindicated in patients allergic to other penicillins.
- Obtain cultures for sensitivity tests before starting therapy. However, it's not necessary to wait for culture and sensitivity results before beginning therapy.
- Before giving penicillin, ask patient if he's had any previous hypersensitive reactions to it. However, a negative history of penicillin allergy is no guarantee against a future allergic reaction.
- Tell patient he must take all medication exactly as prescribed, for as long as ordered, even after he feels better.
- Patients with renal insufficiency should receive less drug.
- Large doses of penicillin may cause increased yeast growths. Watch for signs and symptoms and report to doctor.
- With prolonged therapy, bacterial and fungal superinfection may occur, especially in the elderly, debilitated, or those with low resistance to infection due to immunosuppressors or irradiation. Close observation is essential.
- Check expiration date before giving this drug. Warn patient never to use leftover penicillin for a new illness or to "share" his penicillin with family and friends.
- Tell patient to call the doctor if he develops rash, fever, chills. A rash is the most common allergic reaction.

---

dicloxacillin sodium
Dycill, Dynapen♦, Pathocil, Veracillin

INDICATIONS & DOSAGE

Systemic infections caused by penicillinhase-producing staphylococci—

Adults: 1 to 2 g daily P.O. or I.M., divided into doses given q 6 hours.
Children: 25 to 50 mg/Kg P.O. or I.M. daily, divided into doses given q 6 hours.

SIDE EFFECTS

Blood: eosinophilia.
GI: *nausea,* vomiting, *epigastric distress,* flatulence, *diarrhea.*
Other: *hypersensitivity (pruritus, urticaria, rash, anaphylaxis),* overgrowth of nonsusceptible organisms.

INTERACTIONS

Chloramphenicol, erythromycin, tetracyclines: antibiotic antagonism. Give penicillins at least 1 hour before bacteriostatic antibiotics.
Probenecid: increased blood levels of penicillin. Probenecid is often used for this purpose.

NURSING CONSIDERATIONS

- Use cautiously in patients allergic to cephalosporins (possible cross-allergenicity).
- Obtain cultures for sensitivity tests before starting therapy.
- Before giving penicillin, ask patient if he's had any previous allergic reactions to this drug. However, a negative history of penicillin allergy is no guarantee against a future allergic reaction.
- Tell patient to take medication exactly as prescribed, even if he feels better. Entire quantity prescribed should be taken.
- Tell patient to call the doctor if rash, fever, or chills develop. A rash is the most common allergic reaction.
- When given orally, drug may cause GI disturbances. Food may interfere with absorption, so give 1 to 2 hours before meals or 2 to 3 hours after.
- Don't give I.M. unless infection is severe or patient can't take oral dose.
- Large doses may cause increased yeast growths. Report symptoms to doctor.

• With prolonged therapy, other superinfections may occur, especially in the elderly, debilitated, or those with low resistance to infection due to immunosuppressors or irradiation. Close observation is essential.

• Check expiration date. Warn patient never to use leftover penicillin for a new illness or to "share" penicillin with family and friends.

---

hetacillin
Versapen
hetacillin potassium
Versapen K

INDICATIONS & DOSAGE

Systemic infections caused by susceptible strains of gram-positive and gram-negative organisms—
Adults: 225 to 450 mg P.O. q.i.d.
Children: 22.5 to 45 mg/Kg P.O. daily, divided into doses given q 6 hours.
Hetacillin potassium may be given P.O., I.M., or I.V.

SIDE EFFECTS

Blood: thrombocytopenia, thrombocytopenic purpura, eosinophilia, leukopenia.
GI: vomiting, *nausea, epigastric distress, diarrhea,* glossitis, stomatitis.
Local: vein irritation, phlebitis.
Other: *hypersensitivity (chills, fever, anaphylaxis, maculopapular rash, urticaria),* overgrowth of nonsusceptible organisms.

INTERACTIONS

Chloramphenicol, erythromycin, tetracyclines: antibiotic antagonism. Give penicillins at least 1 hour before bacteriostatic antibiotics.
Probenecid: increased blood levels of penicillin. Probenecid is often used for this purpose.

NURSING CONSIDERATIONS

• Contraindicated in patients with mononucleosis. Use cautiously in patients with other drug allergies, especially to cephalosporins (possible cross-allergenicity), gastrointestinal disturbances.

• Obtain cultures for sensitivity tests before starting therapy. Unnecessary to wait for culture and sensitivity results before beginning therapy.

• Before giving penicillin, ask patient if he's had any previous allergic reactions to this drug. However, a negative history of penicillin allergy is no guarantee against a future allergic reaction.

• Tell patient to take medication exactly as prescribed, even if he feels better. Entire quantity prescribed should be taken.

• Tell patient to call the doctor if rash, fever, or chills develop. A rash is the most common allergic reaction.

• When given orally, drug may cause GI disturbances. Food may interfere with absorption, so give 1 to 2 hours before meals or 2 to 3 hours after.

• Don't give I.M. or I.V. unless infection is severe or patient can't take oral dose.

• When giving I.V., mix with appropriate I.V. solutions.

• Give I.V. intermittently to prevent vein irritation. Change site every 48 hours.

• Large doses may cause increased yeast growths. Report symptoms to doctor.

• With prolonged therapy, other superinfections may occur, especially in the elderly, debilitated, or those with low resistance to infection due to immunosuppressors or irradiation. Close observation is essential.

• Parenteral hetacillin potassium containing lidocaine is for I.M. injection only. Question patient about possible allergy to lidocaine.

• Check expiration date. Warn patient never to use leftover penicillin for a

---

Italicized side effects are common or life-threatening.

new illness or to "share" penicillin with family and friends.
• Very similar to ampicillin.

methicillin sodium
Azapen, Celbenin, Staphcillin♦

INDICATIONS & DOSAGE
Systemic infections caused by penicillinase-producing staphylo-cocci—
Adults: 4 to 12 g I.M. or I.V. daily, divided into doses given q 4 to 6 hours.
Children: 100 to 200 mg/Kg I.M. or I.V. daily, divided into doses given q 4 to 6 hours.

SIDE EFFECTS
Blood: *eosinophilia,* hemolytic anemia, transient neutropenia.
CNS: neuropathy, convulsions at high doses.
GI: glossitis, stomatitis.
GU: interstitial nephritis.
Local: *thrombophlebitis.*
Other: *hypersensitivity (chills, fever, edema, rash, urticaria, anaphylaxis),* overgrowth of nonsusceptible organisms.

INTERACTIONS
Chloramphenicol, erythromycin, tetracyclines: antibiotic antagonism. Give penicillins at least 1 hour before bacteriostatic antibiotics.
Probenecid: increased blood levels of penicillin. Probenecid is often used for this purpose.

NURSING CONSIDERATIONS
• Use cautiously in patients with other drug allergies, especially to cephalosporins (possible cross-allergenicity), and in infants.
• Obtain cultures for sensitivity tests before starting therapy.
• Before giving penicillin, ask patient if he's had any previous allergic reac-

tions to this drug. However, a negative history of penicillin allergy is no guarantee against a future allergic reaction.
• If ordered 4 times a day, be sure to give every 6 hours—even during the night.
• Urinalysis should be done frequently.
• If patient has high serum level of this drug, he may have convulsions. Be prepared by keeping side rails up on bed and tongue blade handy.
• Dosage should be altered in patients with impaired hepatic and renal functions.
• When giving I.V., mix with a normal saline solution. Don't mix with others because methicillin may be inactivated. Initial dilution must be made with sterile water for injection.
• Give I.V. intermittently to prevent vein irritation. Change site every 48 hours.
• Large doses may cause increased yeast growths. Report symptoms to doctor.
• With prolonged therapy, other superinfections may occur, especially in the elderly, debilitated, or those with low resistance to infection due to immunosuppressors or irradiation. Close observation is essential.
• Check expiration date.

nafcillin sodium
Nafcil, Unipen♦

INDICATIONS & DOSAGE
Systemic infections caused by penicillinase-producing staphylo-cocci—
Adults: 2 to 4 g P.O. daily, divided into doses given q 6 hours; 2 to 12 g I.M. or I.V. daily, divided into doses given q 4 to 6 hours.
Children: 50 to 100 mg/Kg P.O. daily, divided into doses given q 4 to 6 hours; or 100 to 200 mg/Kg I.M. or

I.V. daily, divided into doses given q
4 to 6 hours.

SIDE EFFECTS
Blood: transient leukopenia, neutropenia, granulocytopenia, thrombocytopenia with high doses.
GI: *nausea,* vomiting, diarrhea.
Local: *thrombophlebitis.*
Other: *hypersensitivity (chills, fever,
rash, pruritus, urticaria, anaphylaxis).*

INTERACTIONS
*Chloramphenicol, erythromycin, tet-
racyclines:* antibiotic antagonism.
Give penicillins at least 1 hour before
bacteriostatic antibiotics.
Probenecid: increased blood levels of
penicillin. Probenecid is often used
for this purpose.

NURSING CONSIDERATIONS
• Use cautiously in patients with
other drug allergies, especially to
cephalosporins (possible cross-allergenicity), and gastrointestinal distress.
• Obtain cultures for sensitivity tests
before starting therapy.
• Before giving penicillin, ask patient
if he's had any previous allergic reactions to this drug. However, a negative
history of penicillin allergy is no
guarantee against a future allergic reaction.
• Tell patient to take medication exactly as prescribed, even if he feels
better. Entire quantity prescribed
should be taken.
• Tell patient to call the doctor if
rash, fever, or chills develop. A rash
is the most common allergic reaction.
• When given orally, drug may cause
GI disturbances. Food may interfere
with absorption, so give 1 to 2 hours
before meals or 2 to 3 hours after.
• Don't give I.M. or I.V. unless infection is severe or patient can't take oral
dose.
• When giving I.V., mix with 5%

dextrose in water or a saline solution.
Don't mix with others; they might be
incompatible.
• Give I.V. intermittently to prevent
vein irritation. Change site every
48 hours.
• Large doses may cause increased
yeast growths. Report symptoms to
doctor.
• With prolonged therapy, other superinfections may occur, especially in
the elderly, debilitated, or those with
low resistance to infection due to immunosuppressors or irradiation. Close
observation is essential.
• Check expiration date. Warn patient
never to use leftover penicillin for a
new illness or to "share" penicillin
with family and friends.

oxacillin sodium
Bactocill, Prostaphilin♦

INDICATIONS & DOSAGE
*Systemic infections caused by
penicillinase-producing staphylococci—*
Adults: 2 to 4 g P.O. daily, divided
into doses given q 6 hours; 2 to 12 g
I.M. or I.V. daily, divided into doses
given q 4 to 6 hours.
Children: 50 to 100 mg/Kg P.O.
daily, divided into doses given
q 6 hours; 100 to 200 mg/Kg I.M. or
I.V. daily, divided into doses given
q 4 to 6 hours.

SIDE EFFECTS
Blood: granulocytopenia, thrombocy-
topenia, eosinophilia, hemolytic ane-
mia, transient neutropenia.
CNS: neuropathy.
GI: oral lesions.
GU: interstitial nephritis.
Hepatic: hepatitis.
Local: *thrombophlebitis.*
Other: *hypersensitivity (fever, chills,
rash, urticaria, anaphylaxis),* over-
growth of nonsusceptible organisms.

Italicized side effects are common or life-threatening.

INTERACTIONS

Probenecid: increased blood levels of penicillin. Probenecid is often used for this purpose.

Sulfamethoxypyridazine: decreased serum levels of oxacillin. Avoid if possible.

Chloramphenicol, erythromycin, tetracyclines: antibiotic antagonism. Give penicillins at least 1 hour before bacteriostatic antibiotics.

NURSING CONSIDERATIONS

• Use cautiously in patients with other drug allergies, especially to cephalosporins (possible cross-allergenicity), and in premature babies and infants.

• Obtain cultures for sensitivity tests before starting therapy.

• Before giving penicillin, ask patient if he's had any previous allergic reactions to this drug. However, a negative history of penicillin allergy is no guarantee against a future allergic reaction.

• Tell patient essential to take medication exactly as prescribed, even if he feels better. Entire quantity prescribed should be taken.

• Tell patient to call the doctor if rash, fever, or chills develop. A rash is the most common allergic reaction.

• When given orally, drug may cause GI disturbances. Food may interfere with absorption, so give 1 to 2 hours before meals or 2 to 3 hours after.

• Don't give I.M. or I.V. unless infection is severe or patient can't take oral dose.

• Check liver function levels frequently. Monitor for elevated SGOT and SGPT.

• When giving I.V., mix with 5% dextrose in water or a saline solution. Don't mix with others; they might be incompatible.

• Give I.V. intermittently to prevent vein irritation. Change site every 48 hours.

• Large doses may cause increased yeast growths. Report symptoms to doctor.

• With prolonged therapy, other superinfections may occur, especially in the elderly, debilitated, or those with low resistance to infection due to immunosuppressors or irradiation. Close observation is essential.

• Check expiration date. Warn patient never to use leftover penicillin for a new illness or to "share" penicillin with family and friends.

---

penicillin G benzathine
Bicillin L-A♦, Megacillin Suspension♦♦, Permanpen

INDICATIONS & DOSAGE

Congenital syphilis—
Children under age 2: 50,000 units/ Kg I.M. as a single dose.

Group A streptococcal upper respiratory infections—
Adults: 1.2 million units I.M. in a single injection.
Children over 27 Kg: 900,000 units I.M. in a single injection.
Children under 27 Kg: 300,000 to 600,000 units I.M. in a single injection.

Prophylaxis of poststreptococcal rheumatic fever or glomerulonephritis—
Adults and children: 1,200,000 units I.M. once a month or 600,000 units twice a month.

Syphilis less than 1 year in duration—
Adults: 2,400,000 units I.M. in a single dose.

Syphilis of more than 1 year duration—
Adults: 2,400,000 units I.M. weekly for 3 successive weeks.

SIDE EFFECTS

Blood: eosinophilia, hemolytic anemia, thrombocytopenia, leukopenia.
CNS: neuropathy, convulsions with high doses.

Local: pain and sterile abscess at injection site.
Other: *hypersensitivity (maculopapular and exfoliative dermatitis, chills, fever, edema, anaphylaxis).*

INTERACTIONS
Chloramphenicol, erythromycin, tetracyclines: antibiotic antagonism. Give penicillins at least 1 hour before bacteriostatic antibiotics.
Probenecid: increased blood levels of penicillin. Probenecid is often used for this purpose.

NURSING CONSIDERATIONS
• Use cautiously in patients with other drug allergies, especially to cephalosporins (possible cross-allergenicity).
• Obtain cultures for sensitivity tests before starting therapy. Unnecessary to wait for culture and sensitivity results before beginning therapy.
• Before giving penicillin, ask patient if he's had any previous allergic reactions to this drug. However, a negative history of penicillin allergy is no guarantee against a future allergic reaction.
• Tell patient to call the doctor if rash, fever, or chills develop. Fever and eosinophilia are the most common allergic reactions.
• Shake medication well before injection.
• Never give I.V. Inadvertent I.V. administration has caused cardiac arrest and death.
• Very slow absorption time makes allergic reactions difficult to treat.
• Inject deeply into upper outer quadrant of buttocks in adults; in midlateral thigh in infants and small children.
• Check expiration date.

penicillin G potassium
Arcocillin, Biotic-T, Burcillin-G, Cryspen, Deltapen, Falapen♦♦, G-Recillin-T, Hyasorb, Hylenta♦♦, K-Cillin, K-Pen, Ka-Pen♦♦, Lanacillin, Megacillin♦♦, Novopen-G♦, Palocillin, Parcillin, Pensorb, Pentids, P-50♦♦, Pfizerpen

INDICATIONS & DOSAGE
Moderate to severe systemic infections—
Adults: 1.6 to 3.2 million units P.O. daily, divided into doses given q 6 hours (1 mg = 1,600 units); 1.2 to 24 million units I.M. or I.V. daily, divided into doses given q 4 hours.
Children: 25,000 to 100,000 units/ Kg P.O. daily, divided into doses given q 6 hours; or 25,000 to 300,000 units/Kg I.M. or I.V. daily, divided into doses given q 4 hours.

SIDE EFFECTS
Blood: hemolytic anemia, leukopenia, thrombocytopenia.
CNS: neuropathy, convulsions with high doses.
Metabolic: possible severe potassium poisoning with high doses (hyperreflexia, convulsions, coma).
Local: *thrombophlebitis.*
Other: *hypersensitivity (rash, urticaria, maculopapular eruptions, exfoliative dermatitis, chills, fever, edema, anaphylaxis),* overgrowth of nonsusceptible organisms.

INTERACTIONS
Chloramphenicol, erythromycin, tetracyclines: antibiotic antagonism. Give penicillins at least 1 hour before bacteriostatic antibiotics.
Probenecid: increased blood levels of penicillin. Probenecid is often used for this purpose.

Italicized side effects are common or life-threatening.

NURSING CONSIDERATIONS

• Use cautiously in patients with other drug allergies, especially to cephalosporins (possible cross-aller-genicity).

• Obtain cultures for sensitivity tests before starting therapy. Unnecessary to wait for culture and sensitivity results before beginning therapy.

• Before giving penicillin, ask patient if he's had any previous allergic reactions to this drug. However, a negative history of penicillin allergy is no guarantee against a future allergic reaction.

• Tell patient to take medication exactly as prescribed, even if he feels better.

• Tell patient to call the doctor if rash, fever, or chills develop. A rash is the most common allergic reaction.

• When given orally, drug may cause GI disturbances. Food may interfere with absorption, so give 1 to 2 hours before meals or 2 to 3 hours after.

• Don't give I.M. or I.V. unless infection is severe or patient can't take oral dose. Extremely painful when given I.M.

• If patient has high serum level of this drug, he may have convulsions. Be prepared by keeping side rails up on bed and tongue blade handy.

• When giving I.V., mix with 5% dextrose in water or a saline solution. Don't mix with other solutions; they might be incompatible.

• Give I.V. intermittently to prevent vein irritation. Change site every 48 hours.

• Large doses may cause increased yeast growths. Report symptoms to doctor.

• With prolonged therapy, other superinfections may occur, especially in the elderly, debilitated, or those with low resistance to infection due to immunosuppressors or irradiation. Close observation is essential.

• Monitor serum potassium.

• Check expiration date. Warn patient never to use leftover penicillin for a new illness or to "share" penicillin with family and friends.

---

penicillin G procaine

Ayercillin♦♦, Crysticillin A.S., Duracillin A.S., Pfizerpen A.S., Tu-Cillin, Wycillin♦

INDICATIONS & DOSAGE

Moderate to severe systemic infections—
Adults: 600,000 to 1.2 million units I.M. daily given as a single dose.
Children: 300,000 units I.M. daily given as a single dose.
Uncomplicated gonorrhea—
Adults and children over 12: give 1 g probenecid; then 30 minutes later give 4.8 million units of penicillin G procaine I.M., divided into 2 injection sites.
Pneumococcal pneumonia—
Adults and children over 12: 300,000 to 600,000 units I.M. daily q 6 to 12 hours.

SIDE EFFECTS

Blood: thrombocytopenia, hemolytic anemia, leukopenia.
CNS: arthralgia, convulsions.
Other: *hypersensitivity (rash, urticaria, chills, fever, edema, prostration, anaphylaxis),* overgrowth of nonsusceptible organisms.

INTERACTIONS

Chloramphenicol, erythromycin, tetracyclines: antibiotic antagonism. Give penicillins at least 1 hour before bacteriostatic antibiotics.
Probenecid: increased blood levels of penicillin. Probenecid is often used for this purpose.

NURSING CONSIDERATIONS

• Contraindicated in patients with hypersensitivity to procaine. Use cautiously in patients with other drug al-

---

Unmarked trade names available in the United States only.
♦ Also available in Canada   ♦♦ Available in Canada only.

lergies, especially to cephalosporins (possible cross-allergenicity).
• Obtain cultures for sensitivity tests before starting therapy. Unnecessary to wait for culture and sensitivity results before beginning therapy.
• Before giving penicillin, ask patient if he's had any previous allergic reactions to this drug. However, a negative history of penicillin allergy is no guarantee against a future allergic reaction.
• Tell patient to call doctor if rash, fever, or chills develop. A rash is the most common allergic reaction.
• Give deep I.M. in upper outer quadrant of buttocks in adults; in mid-lateral thigh in small children.
• Never give I.V. Inadvertent I.V. administration has caused death due to CNS toxicity from procaine.
• Large doses may cause increased yeast growths. Report symptoms to doctor.
• Due to slow absorption rate, allergic reactions are hard to treat.
• With prolonged therapy, other superinfections may occur, especially in the elderly, debilitated, or those with low resistance to infection due to immunosuppressors or irradiation. Close observation is essential.
• Check expiration date.

---

penicillin G sodium
Crystapen♦ ♦

INDICATIONS & DOSAGE
Moderate to severe systemic infections—
Adults: 1.2 to 24 million units daily I.M. or I.V., divided into doses given q 4 hours.
Children: 25,000 to 300,000 units/Kg daily I.M. or I.V., divided into doses given q 4 hours.

SIDE EFFECTS
Blood: hemolytic anemia, leukopenia, thrombocytopenia.
CNS: arthralgia, neuropathy, convulsions.
CV: *congestive heart failure with high doses.*
Other: *hypersensitivity (chills, fever, edema, maculopapular rash, exfoliative dermatitis, urticaria, anaphylaxis),* overgrowth of nonsusceptible organisms.

INTERACTIONS
Chloramphenicol, erythromycin, tetracyclines: antibiotic antagonism. Give penicillins at least 1 hour before bacteriostatic antibiotics.
Probenecid: increased blood levels of penicillin. Probenecid is often used for this purpose.

NURSING CONSIDERATIONS
• Contraindicated in patients on sodium restriction. Use cautiously in patients with other drug allergies, especially to cephalosporins (possible cross-allergenicity).
• Obtain cultures for sensitivity tests before starting therapy. Unnecessary to wait for culture and sensitivity results before beginning therapy.
• Before giving penicillin, ask patient if he's had any previous allergic reactions to this drug. However, a negative history of penicillin allergy is no guarantee against a future allergic reaction.
• If patient has high serum level of this drug, he may have convulsions. Be prepared by keeping side rails up on bed and tongue blade handy.
• When giving I.V., mix with 5% dextrose in water or a saline solution. Don't mix with others; they might be incompatible.
• Give I.V. intermittently to prevent vein irritation. Change site every 48 hours.
• Large doses may cause increased

Italicized side effects are common or life-threatening.

yeast growths. Report symptoms to doctor.
• With prolonged therapy, other superinfections may occur, especially in the elderly, debilitated, or those with low resistance to infection due to immunosuppressors or irradiation. Close observation is essential.
• Monitor vital signs frequently.
• Monitor serum sodium.
• Check expiration date.

---

penicillin V
Biotic Powder, Compocillin-V, Ledercillin VK♦, Pfizerpen VK♦, Robicillin-VK, SK-Penicillin VK, Uticillin VK, V-Cillin Drops, V-Pen
penicillin V potassium
Betapen VK, Biotic-V-Powder, Bopen V-K, Cocillin V-K, Compocillin-VK, Dowpen VK, Lanacillin VK, Ledercillin VK♦, LV, Nadopen-V♦♦, Novopen-V♦♦, Penapar VK, Penbec-V♦♦, Pen-Vee-K♦, Pfizerpen VK, PVF K♦♦, Repen-VK, Uticillin VK, V-Cillin K♦

INDICATIONS & DOSAGE
Mild to moderate systemic infections—
Adults: 250 to 500 mg (400,000 to 800,000 units) P.O. q 6 hours.
Children: 15 to 50 mg/Kg (25,000 to 90,000 units/Kg) P.O. daily, divided into doses given q 6 to 8 hours.

SIDE EFFECTS
Blood: eosinophilia, hemolytic anemia, leukopenia, thrombocytopenia.
CNS: neuropathy.
GI: *epigastric distress,* vomiting, diarrhea, *nausea.*
Other: *hypersensitivity (rash, urticaria, chills, fever, edema, anaphylaxis),* overgrowth of nonsusceptible organisms.

INTERACTIONS
Chloramphenicol, erythromycin, tetracyclines: antibiotic antagonism.

Give penicillins at least 1 hour before bacteriostatic antibiotics.
Neomycin: decreased absorption of penicillin. Give penicillin by injection.
Probenecid: increased blood levels of penicillin. Probenecid is often used for this purpose.

NURSING CONSIDERATIONS
• Use cautiously in patients with other drug allergies, especially to cephalosporins (possible cross-allergenicity) and GI disturbances.
• Obtain cultures for sensitivity tests before starting therapy. Unnecessary to wait for culture and sensitivity results before beginning therapy.
• Before giving penicillin, ask patient if he's had any previous allergic reactions to this drug. However, a negative history of penicillin allergy is no guarantee against a future allergic reaction.
• Tell patient to take medication exactly as prescribed, even if he feels better. Entire quantity prescribed should be taken.
• Tell patient to call the doctor if rash, fever, or chills develop. A rash is the most common allergic reaction.
• When given orally, drug may cause GI disturbances. Food may interfere with absorption, so give 1 to 2 hours before meals or 2 to 3 hours after.
• Large doses may cause increased yeast growths. Report symptoms to doctor.
• With prolonged therapy, other superinfections may occur, especially in the elderly, debilitated, or those with low resistance to infection due to immunosuppressors or irradiation. Close observation is essential.
• Check expiration date. Warn patient never to use leftover penicillin for a new illness or to "share" penicillin with family and friends.

---

ticarcillin disodium
Ticar

INDICATIONS & DOSAGE
Severe systemic infections caused by susceptible strains of gram-positive and especially gram-negative organisms (Pseudomonas, Proteus)—
Adults: 18 g I.V. or I.M. daily, divided into doses given q 4 to 6 hours.
Children: 200 to 300 mg/Kg I.V. or I.M. daily, divided into doses given q 4 to 6 hours.

SIDE EFFECTS
Blood: leukopenia, neutropenia, eosinophilia, *thrombocytopenia,* hemolytic anemia.
CNS: convulsions, neuromuscular excitability.
GI: nausea.
Metabolic: *hypokalemia.*
Local: pain at injection site, vein irritation, phlebitis.
Other: *hypersensitivity (rash, pruritus, urticaria, chills, fever, edema, anaphylaxis),* overgrowth of nonsusceptible organisms.

INTERACTIONS
Chloramphenicol, erythromycin, tetracyclines: antibiotic antagonism. Give penicillins at least 1 hour before bacteriostatic antibiotics.
Probenecid: increased blood levels of penicillin. Probenecid is often used for this purpose.
Gentamicin, tobramycin: chemically incompatible. Don't mix together in I.V. Give 1 hour apart.

NURSING CONSIDERATIONS
• Use cautiously in patients with other drug allergies, especially to cephalosporins (possible cross-allergenicity); impaired renal function; hemorrhagic conditions; hypokalemia; in sodium-restricted patients (contains 5.2 mEq sodium/g).
• Obtain cultures for sensitivity tests before starting therapy. Unnecessary to wait for culture and sensitivity results before beginning therapy.
• Before giving penicillin, ask patient if he's had any previous allergic reactions to this drug. However, a negative history of penicillin allergy is no guarantee against a future allergic reaction.
• Dosage should be decreased in patients with impaired hepatic and renal functions.
• Check CBC frequently. Drug may cause thrombocytopenia.
• If patient has high serum level of this drug, he may develop convulsions. Be prepared by keeping side rails up on bed and tongue blade handy.
• When giving I.V., mix with 5% dextrose in water or other suitable I.V. fluids.
• Give I.V. intermittently to prevent vein irritation. Change site every 48 hours.
• Large doses may cause increased yeast growths. Report symptoms to doctor.
• Almost always used with another antibiotic such as gentamicin.
• With prolonged therapy, other superinfections may occur, especially in the elderly, debilitated, or those with low resistance to infection due to immunosuppressors or irradiation. Close observation is essential.
• Monitor serum potassium.
• Check expiration date.

Italicized side effects are common or life-threatening.

10

Cephalosporins

cefaclor
cefadroxil monohydrate
cefamandole naftate
cefazolin sodium
cefoxitin sodium
cephalexin monohydrate
cephaloglycin dihydrate
cephaloridine
cephalothin sodium
cephapirin sodium
cephradine

---

cefaclor
Ceclor

INDICATIONS & DOSAGE
Treatment of infections of respiratory or urinary tract, skin and soft tissue, and otitis media due to H. influenzae, Streptococcus pneumoniae and pyogenes, E. coli, P. mirabilis, Klebsiella species, and staphylococci—
Adults: 250 to 500 mg P.O. q 8 hours. Total daily dose should not exceed 4 g.
Children: 20 mg/Kg/day P.O. in divided doses q 8 hours. In more serious infections, 40 mg/Kg/day are recommended, not to exceed 1 g per day.

SIDE EFFECTS
Blood: transient leukopenia, lymphocytosis, anemia, eosinophilia.
CNS: dizziness, headache, somnolence.
GI: *nausea,* vomiting, diarrhea, anorexia.
GU: red and white cells in urine, vaginal moniliasis and vaginitis.

Skin: *maculopapular rash,* dermatitis.
Other: hypersensitivity, fever.

INTERACTIONS
Probenecid: may inhibit excretion and increase blood levels of cefaclor. Use together cautiously.

NURSING CONSIDERATIONS
• Contraindicated in hypersensitivity to other cephalosporins. Use cautiously in impaired renal status and in those with history of sensitivity to penicillin. Ask patient if he's had any reaction to previous cephalosporin or penicillin therapy before administering first dose.
• Prolonged use may result in overgrowth of nonsusceptible organisms. Careful observation of patient for superinfection is essential.
• Obtain cultures for sensitivity tests before therapy, but therapy may begin pending results of culture and sensitivity tests.
• Cefaclor is newest cephalosporin.
• Major clinical use appears to be in treating otitis media caused by *H. influenzae* when resistant to ampicillin or amoxicillin.
• Mostly used in ambulatory setting.
• Tell patient to take medication exactly as prescribed, even after he feels better.
• Call doctor if skin rash develops.
• Store reconstituted suspension in refrigerator. Stable for 14 days if refrigerated. Shake well before using.
• Drug may be taken with meals.
• Cefaclor is a relatively expensive

antibiotic and should be used only when the organism is resistant to other agents.

---

cefadroxil monohydrate
Duricef

INDICATIONS & DOSAGE
Treatment of urinary tract infections caused by E. coli, P. mirabilis, and Klebsiella species, infections of skin and soft tissue, and streptococcal pharyngitis—
Adults: 500 mg to 2 g P.O. per day, depending on the infection being treated. Usually given in once daily or b.i.d. dosage.
Children: 30 mg/Kg/day in 2 divided doses.

SIDE EFFECTS
Blood: transient neutropenia, eosinophilia, leukopenia, anemia.
CNS: dizziness, headache, malaise, paresthesias.
GI: *nausea,* anorexia, vomiting, *diarrhea,* glossitis, *dyspepsia,* abdominal cramps, anal pruritus, tenesmus, oral candidiasis (thrush).
GU: genital pruritus and moniliasis.
Skin: *maculopapular and erythematous rashes.*
Other: dyspnea.

INTERACTIONS
Probenecid: may inhibit excretion and increase blood levels of cefadroxil. Use together cautiously.

NURSING CONSIDERATIONS
• Contraindicated in hypersensitivity to other cephalosporins. Use cautiously in impaired renal status and in those with history of sensitivity to penicillin. Ask patient if he's had any reaction to previous cephalosporin or penicillin therapy before administering first dose.
• Prolonged use may result in over-growth of nonsusceptible organisms. Careful observation of patient for superinfection is essential.
• Obtain cultures for sensitivity tests before therapy, but therapy may begin pending results of cultures and sensitivity tests.
• If creatinine clearance is below 50 ml/min, dosage interval should be increased so drug doesn't accumulate.
• Tell patient to take medication exactly as prescribed, even after he feels better.
• Call doctor if skin rash develops.
• Absorption not delayed by presence of food.
• Longer half-life permits twice-daily dosing.

---

cefamandole naftate
Mandol

INDICATIONS & DOSAGE
Treatment of serious infections of respiratory and genitourinary tract, skin and soft tissue infections, bone and joint infections, bloodstream and peritonitis due to E. coli and other coliform bacteria, S. aureus, (penicillinase and nonpenicillinase producing), S. epidermidis, group A beta-hemolytic streptococci, Klebsiella, H. influenzae, P. mirabilis, and Enterobacter species—
Adults: 500 mg to 1 g q 4 to 8 hours. In life-threatening infections up to 2 g q 4 hours may be needed.
Infants and children: 50 to 100 mg/Kg/day in equally divided doses q 4 to 8 hours. May be increased to total daily dose of 150 mg/Kg (not to exceed maximum adult dose) for severe infections.

Total daily dosage is same for I.M. or I.V. administration and depends on susceptibility of organism and severity of infection. In patients with impaired renal function, doses or frequency of administration must be modified according to degree of renal impairment, severity of infection, susceptibility of organism, and serum levels of drug. Should be injected deep I.M. into a large muscle mass, such as gluteus or lateral aspect of thigh.

SIDE EFFECTS

Blood: transient neutropenia, eosinophilia, hemolytic anemia.
CNS: headache, malaise, paresthesias, dizziness.
GI: nausea, anorexia, vomiting, diarrhea, glossitis, dyspepsia, abdominal cramps, tenesmus, anal pruritus, oral candidiasis (thrush).
GU: nephrotoxicity, genital pruritus and moniliasis.
Skin: *maculopapular and erythematous rashes, urticaria.*
Local: *at injection site—pain, induration, sterile abscesses,* temperature elevation, tissue slough; *phlebitis and thrombophlebitis with I.V. injection.*
Other: *hypersensitivity,* dyspnea.

INTERACTIONS

Probenecid: may inhibit excretion and increase blood levels of cefamandole. Use together cautiously.

NURSING CONSIDERATIONS

• Contraindicated in hypersensitivity to other cephalosporins. Use cautiously in impaired renal status and in those with history of sensitivity to penicillin. Ask patient if he's had any reaction to previous cephalosporin or penicillin therapy before administering first dose.
• Prolonged use may result in overgrowth of nonsusceptible organisms. Careful observation of patient for superinfection is essential.
• Obtain cultures for sensitivity tests before therapy, but therapy may begin pending results of cultures and sensitivity tests.

• Cephalosporin of choice for treatment of *Enterobacter* sepsis.
• Not as effective as cefoxitin in treating anaerobic infections.
• For most cephalosporin-sensitive organisms, cefamandole offers little advantage over previously available agents.
• For I.V. use, reconstitute 1 g with 10 ml of sterile water for injection, 5% dextrose or 0.9% sodium chloride for injection. May be combined with the following intravenous fluids: 0.9% sodium chloride injection, 5% dextrose injection, 10% dextrose injection, 5% dextrose and 0.9% sodium chloride injection, 5% dextrose and 0.45% sodium chloride injection, 5% dextrose and 0.2% sodium chloride injection, or sodium lactate injection.
• I.M. cefamandole not as painful as cefoxitin. Does not require addition of lidocaine.
• After reconstitution, remains stable for 24 hours at room temperature or 96 hours under refrigeration.

---

cefazolin sodium
Ancef♦, Kefzol♦

INDICATIONS & DOSAGE

Treatment of serious infections of respiratory and genitourinary tracts, skin and soft tissue infections, bone and joint infections, septicemia, and endocarditis due to E. coli, Enterobacteriaceae, gonococci, H. influenzae, Klebsiella, P. mirabilis, S. aureus, S. pneumoniae, and group A beta-hemolytic streptococci; and perioperative prophylaxis—
Adults: 250 mg I.M. or I.V. q 8 hours to 1 g q 6 hours.
Children over 1 month: 8 to 16 mg/Kg I.M. or I.V. q 8 hours, or 6 to 12 mg/Kg q 6 hours.

Total daily dosage is same for I.M. or

I.V. administration and depends on susceptibility of organism and severity of infection. Initial I.V. loading dose (usually 500 mg) recommended. Maximum dose for severe infections: 33 mg/Kg q 8 hours or 25 mg/Kg q 8 hours.

In patients with impaired renal function, doses or frequency of administration must be modified according to degree of renal impairment, severity of infection, susceptibility of organism, and serum levels of drug. Should be injected deep I.M. into a large muscle mass, such as gluteus or lateral aspect of thigh.

SIDE EFFECTS

Blood: transient neutropenia, leukopenia, eosinophilia, anemia.
CNS: dizziness, headache, malaise, paresthesias.
GI: nausea, anorexia, vomiting, diarrhea, glossitis, dyspepsia, abdominal cramps, anal pruritus, tenesmus, oral candidiasis (thrush).
GU: nephrotoxicity, genital pruritus and moniliasis, vaginitis.
Skin: *maculopapular and erythematous rashes, urticaria.*
Local: *at injection site—pain, induration, sterile abscesses, tissue slough; phlebitis and thrombophlebitis with I.V. injection.*
Other: *hypersensitivity,* dyspnea.

INTERACTIONS

Probenecid: may increase blood levels of cephalosporins. Use together cautiously.

NURSING CONSIDERATIONS

• Use cautiously in impaired renal status and in those with history of sensitivity to penicillin. Ask patient if he's had any reaction to previous cephalosporin or penicillin therapy before administering first dose.
• Avoid doses greater than 4 g daily in severe renal impairment.
• Prolonged use may result in over-

growth of nonsusceptible organisms. Watch carefully for superinfection.
• Obtain cultures for sensitivity tests before therapy, but therapy may begin pending results of cultures and sensitivity tests.
• Because of long duration of effect, most infections can be treated with a single dose q 8 hours.
• For I.M. administration, reconstitute with sterile water, bacteriostatic water, or 0.9% sodium chloride solution as follows: 2 ml to 250 mg vial; 2 ml to 500 mg vial; 2.5 ml to 1 g vial. Shake well until dissolved. Resultant concentration: 125 mg/ml, 225 mg/ml, 330 mg/ml, respectively.
• Not as painful as other cephalosporins when given I.M.
• Alternate injection sites if I.V. therapy lasts longer than 3 days. Use of small I.V. needles in the larger available veins may be preferable.
• For I.V. administration, reconstituted cefazolin sodium is diluted in 50 to 100 ml of 0.9% sodium chloride injection, 5% or 10% dextrose injection, 5% dextrose in lactated Ringer's, 5% dextrose and 0.9% sodium chloride, 5% dextrose and 0.45% or 0.2% sodium chloride, lactated Ringer's injection, Normosol-M in 5% dextrose in water, Ionosol B with 5% dextrose, or Plasma-Lyte with 5% dextrose.
• Reconstituted cefazolin sodium is stable for 24 hours at room temperature, for 96 hours under refrigeration.
• About 40% to 75% of patients receiving cephalosporins show a false positive direct Coombs' test; only a few of these indicate hemolytic anemia.
• Urine glucose tests with Benedict's Qualitative Reagent, Clinitest, or Fehling's solution may cause false positive reaction during cephalosporin therapy. Clinistix, Diastix, and Tes-Tape are not affected.

Italicized side effects are common or life-threatening.

cefoxitin sodium
Mefoxin

INDICATIONS & DOSAGE

Treatment of serious infection of respiratory and genitourinary tract, skin and soft tissue infections, bone and joint infections, bloodstream and intra-abdominal infections due to E. coli and other coliform bacteria, S. aureus (penicillinase and non-penicillinase), S. epidermidis, streptococci, Klebsiella, H. influenzae, and Bacteroides species, including B. fragilis—
Adults: 1 to 2 g q 6 to 8 hours for uncomplicated forms of infection. Up to 12 g/day in life-threatening infections.
Children: 80 to 160 mg/Kg/day.

Total daily dosage is same for I.M. or I.V. administration and depends on susceptibility of organism and severity of infection. In patients with impaired renal function, doses or frequency of administration must be modified according to degree of renal impairment, severity of infection, susceptibility of organism, and serum levels of drug. Should be injected deep I.M. into a large muscle mass such as gluteus or lateral aspect of thigh.

SIDE EFFECTS

Blood: transient neutropenia, eosinophilia, hemolytic anemia.
CNS: headache, malaise, paresthesias, dizziness.
GI: nausea, anorexia, vomiting, diarrhea, glossitis, dyspepsia, abdominal cramps, tenesmus, anal pruritus, oral candidiasis (thrush).
GU: nephrotoxicity, genital pruritus and moniliasis.
Skin: *maculopapular and erythematous rashes, urticaria.*
Local: *at injection site—pain, induration, sterile abscesses, temperature elevation, tissue slough; phlebitis and thrombophlebitis with I.V. injection.*
Other: *hypersensitivity,* dyspnea.

INTERACTIONS

Probenecid: may inhibit excretion and increase blood levels of cefoxitin. Use together cautiously.

NURSING CONSIDERATIONS

• Contraindicated in hypersensitivity to other cephalosporins. Use cautiously in impaired renal status and in those with history of sensitivity to penicillin. Ask patient if he's had any reaction to previous cephalosporin or penicillin therapy before administering first dose.
• Prolonged use may result in overgrowth of nonsusceptible organisms. Observe patient for superinfection.
• Obtain cultures for sensitivity tests before therapy, but therapy may begin pending results of cultures and sensitivity tests.
• A very useful cephalosporin when anaerobic or mixed aerobic-anaerobic infection is suspected, especially *Bacteroides fragilis.*
• For most cephalosporin-sensitive organisms, cefoxitin offers little advantage over previously available agents.
• For I.V. use, reconstitute 1 g with at least 10 ml of sterile water for injection, and 2 g with 10 to 20 ml. 5% dextrose and 0.9% sodium chloride for injection can also be used. These primary solutions can be further diluted with the following solutions: Ringer's injection, lactated Ringer's injection, 5% dextrose in lactated Ringer's injection, 5% or 10% invert sugar in water, 10% invert sugar in saline, 5% sodium bicarbonate injection, Aminosol 5% solution, Normosol-M in 5% dextrose in water, Ionosol B with 5% dextrose, Polyonic M 56 in 5% dextrose.
• I.M. injection can be reconstituted with 0.5% or 1% lidocaine HCl

(without epinephrine) to minimize pain on injection.
• May cause false positive for urine glucose with Clinitest tablets.
• May be useful in the treatment of resistant gonorrhea.
• After reconstitution, remains stable for 24 hours at room temperature or 1 week under refrigeration.

cephalexin monohydrate
Ceporex♦♦, Keflex♦

INDICATIONS & DOSAGE
Treatment of infections of respiratory or genitourinary tract, skin and soft tissue infections, bone and joint infections, and otitis media due to E. coli and other coliform bacteria; group A beta-hemolytic streptococci, H. influenzae, Klebsiella, P. mirabilis, S. pneumoniae, and staphylococci—
Adults: 250 mg to 1 g P.O. q 6 hours.
Children: 6 to 12 mg/Kg P.O. q 6 hours. Maximum 25 mg/Kg q 6 hours.

SIDE EFFECTS
Blood: transient neutropenia, eosinophilia, anemia.
CNS: dizziness, headache, malaise, paresthesias.
GI: *nausea, anorexia,* vomiting, *diarrhea,* glossitis, dyspepsia, abdominal cramps, anal pruritus, tenesmus, oral candidiasis (thrush).
GU: genital pruritus and moniliasis, vaginitis.
Skin: *maculopapular and erythematous rashes, urticaria.*
Other: *hypersensitivity,* dyspnea.

INTERACTIONS
Probenecid: may increase blood levels of cephalosporins. Use together cautiously.

NURSING CONSIDERATIONS
• Use cautiously in impaired renal

status and in those with history of sensitivity to penicillin. Ask patient if he's had any reaction to previous cephalosporin or penicillin therapy before administering first dose.
• Prolonged use may result in overgrowth of nonsusceptible organisms. Watch closely for superinfection.
• Obtain cultures for sensitivity tests before therapy, but therapy may begin pending results of cultures and sensitivity tests.
• Tell patient to take medication exactly as prescribed, even after he feels better. Group A beta-hemolytic streptococci infections should be treated for a minimum of 10 days.
• Call doctor if skin rash develops.
• Preparation of oral suspension: add required amount of water to powder in two portions. Shake well after each addition. After mixing, store in refrigerator. Stable for 14 days without significant loss of potency. Keep tightly closed and shake well before using.
• About 40% to 75% of patients receiving cephalosporins show a false positive direct Coombs' test, but only a few of these indicate hemolytic anemia.
• Urine glucose tests with Benedict's Qualitative Reagent, Clinitest, or Fehling's solution may give false positive results during cephalosporin therapy. Clinistix, Diastix, and Tes-Tape are not affected.

cephaloglycin dihydrate
Kafocin

INDICATIONS & DOSAGE
Treatment of acute and chronic urinary tract infections, including cystitis, pyelitis, pyelonephritis, and "asymptomatic bacteriuria" when due to susceptible strains of E. coli, Klebsiella, Enterobacter, Proteus, staphylococci, and enterococci—

Italicized side effects are common or life-threatening.

Adults: 250 to 500 mg P.O. q 6 hours.

SIDE EFFECTS
Blood: transient neutropenia, eosinophilia, anemia.
CNS: dizziness, headache, malaise, paresthesias.
GI: *nausea, anorexia, vomiting, diarrhea,* glossitis, dyspepsia, abdominal cramps, anal pruritus, tenesmus, oral candidiasis (thrush).
GU: genital pruritus and moniliasis, vaginitis.
Skin: *maculopapular and erythematous rashes, urticaria.*
Other: *hypersensitivity,* dyspnea.

INTERACTIONS
Probenecid: may increase blood levels of cephalosporins. Use together cautiously.

NURSING CONSIDERATIONS
• Use cautiously in impaired renal function and in those with history of sensitivity to penicillin. Ask patient if he's had any reaction to previous cephalosporin or penicillin therapy before administering first dose.
• Cephaloglycin serum levels are low; used only for urinary tract infections.
• Prolonged use may result in overgrowth of nonsusceptible organisms. Watch for superinfection.
• Obtain cultures for sensitivity tests before beginning therapy, but therapy may begin pending results of cultures and sensitivity tests.
• Tell patient to take medication exactly as prescribed, even after he feels better.
• About 40% to 75% of patients receiving cephalosporins show a false positive direct Coombs' test, but only a few of these indicate hemolytic anemia.
• Urine glucose tests with Benedict's Qualitative Reagent, Clinitest, or Fehling's solution may give false positive results during cephalosporin ther-

apy. Clinistix, Diastix, and Tes-Tape are not affected.

---

cephaloridine
Ceporan♦♦, Loridine♦

INDICATIONS & DOSAGE
Treatment of serious infections of respiratory tract, central nervous system, genitourinary tract, bones and joints, bloodstream, skin, and soft tissue due to E. coli and other coliform bacteria, gonococci, H. influenzae, Klebsiella, P. mirabilis, pneumococci, staphylococci (coagulase positive and coagulase negative), beta-hemolytic and other streptococci; also, gonorrhea and early syphilis when penicillin is contraindicated—
Adults: 250 mg to 1 g I.M. or I.V. q 6 to 12 hours. Not to exceed 4 g daily.
Children: 7 to 12 mg/Kg I.M. or I.V. q 6 hours.
*Severe infections—*up to 25 mg/Kg q 6 hours. Not recommended for children under 1 month or for premature infants.

Total daily dosage is same for I.M. or I.V. administration and depends on susceptibility of organism and severity of infection. Initial loading dose (usually 500 mg) recommended. In patients with impaired renal function, doses and frequency of administration must be modified according to degree of renal impairment, severity of infection, susceptibility of causative organism, and serum levels of drug. Should be injected deep I.M. into large muscle mass, such as gluteus or lateral aspect of thigh. I.V. preferable in severe or life-threatening infections.

SIDE EFFECTS
Blood: transient neutropenia, eosinophilia, anemia.

CNS: headache, malaise, paresthesias.
GI: nausea, anorexia, vomiting, diarrhea, glossitis, dyspepsia, abdominal cramps, tenesmus, anal pruritus, oral candidiasis (thrush).
GU: *nephrotoxicity (especially in doses greater than 4 g daily or in patients with renal impairment),* genital pruritus and moniliasis.
Skin: *maculopapular and erythematous rashes, urticaria.*
Local: at injection site—pain, induration, sterile abscesses, tissue slough; phlebitis and thrombophlebitis with I.V. injection.
Other: *hypersensitivity,* dyspnea.

INTERACTIONS

Probenecid: may increase blood levels of cephalosporins. Use together cautiously.
Ethacrynic acid, furosemide: may enhance nephrotoxicity of cephaloridine. Use cautiously.

NURSING CONSIDERATIONS

• Contraindicated in renal impairment, since drug causes a relatively high incidence of dose-related nephrotoxicity. Use cautiously in patient with history of sensitivity to penicillin. Ask patient if he's had any reaction to previous cephalosporin or penicillin therapy before administering first dose. Safe use not established in patients with proteinuria, falling urinary output, rising BUN or serum creatinine, decreasing creatinine clearance, and those receiving other antibiotics with nephrotoxic potential.
• Prolonged use may result in overgrowth of nonsusceptible organisms. Watch for superinfection.
• Obtain cultures for sensitivity tests before beginning therapy, but therapy may begin pending results of cultures and sensitivity tests.
• Drug causes relatively little pain when given I.M.

• Good CNS penetration makes cephaloridine useful in treating meningitis.
• When giving this drug I.V., check frequently for vein irritation and phlebitis. Alternate injection sites if I.V. therapy lasts longer than 3 days. Use of small I.V. needles in the larger available veins may be preferable.
• Excreted in urine. Monitor renal function carefully. Watch for signs of impairment: casts in urine, proteinuria, decreased creatinine clearance of urine/plasma creatinine ratio. Avoid doses greater than 4 g daily.
• About 40% to 75% of patients receiving cephalosporins show a false positive direct Coombs' test, but only a few indicate hemolytic anemia.
• Urine glucose tests with Benedict's Qualitative Reagent, Clinitest, or Fehling's solution may give false positive results during cephalosporin therapy. Clinistix, Diastix, and Tes-Tape are not affected.

---

cephalothin sodium
Keflin Neutral♦

INDICATIONS & DOSAGE

Treatment of serious infections of respiratory, genitourinary, or gastrointestinal tract; skin and soft tissue infections (including peritonitis); bone and joint infections; septicemia; endocarditis; and meningitis due to E. coli and other coliform bacteria, Enterobacteriaceae, enterococci, gonococci, group A beta-hemolytic streptococci, H. influenzae, Klebsiella, P. mirabilis, Salmonella, S. aureus, Shigella, S. pneumoniae, staphylococci, and S. viridans—
Adults: 500 mg to 1 g I.M. or I.V. (or intraperitoneally) q 4 to 6 hours; in life-threatening infections, up to 2 g q 4 hours.
Children: 14 to 27 mg/Kg I.V. q 4 hours, or 20 to 40 mg/Kg q

Italicized side effects are common or life-threatening.

6 hours; dose should be proportionately less in accordance with age, weight, and severity of infection.

Dosage schedule is determined by degree of renal impairment, severity of infection, and susceptibility of causative organism. Should be injected deep I.M. into a large muscle mass, such as gluteus or lateral aspect of thigh. I.V. route is preferable in severe or life-threatening infections.

SIDE EFFECTS
Blood: transient neutropenia, eosinophilia, hemolytic anemia.
CNS: headache, malaise, paresthesias, dizziness.
GI: nausea, anorexia, vomiting, diarrhea, glossitis, dyspepsia, abdominal cramps, tenesmus, anal pruritus, oral candidiasis (thrush).
GU: nephrotoxicity, genital pruritus and moniliasis.
Skin: maculopapular and erythematous rashes, urticaria.
Local: *at injection site—pain, induration, sterile abscesses, temperature elevation, tissue slough; phlebitis and thrombophlebitis with I.V. injection.*
Other: *hypersensitivity,* dyspnea.

INTERACTIONS
Probenecid: may increase blood levels of cephalosporins. Use together cautiously.

NURSING CONSIDERATIONS
• Use cautiously in impaired renal functions and in those with history of sensitivity to penicillin. Ask patient if he's had any reaction to previous cephalosporin or penicillin therapy before administering first dose.
• Obtain cultures for sensitivity tests before beginning therapy, but therapy may begin pending results of cultures and sensitivity tests.
• Prolonged use may result in overgrowth of nonsusceptible organisms. Watch for superinfection.

• Drug causes severe pain when given I.M.; avoid this route if possible.
• When giving this drug I.V., check frequently for vein irritation and phlebitis. Alternate injection sites if I.V. therapy lasts longer than 3 days. Use of small I.V. needles in the larger available veins may be preferable. Addition of a small concentration of heparin (100 units) may reduce incidence of phlebitis.
• For I.M. administration, reconstitute each gram of cephalothin sodium with 4 ml of sterile water for injection, providing 500 mg in each 2.2 ml. If vial contents do not dissolve completely, add an additional 0.2 to 0.4 ml diluent, and warm contents slightly.
• For I.V. administration, dilute contents of 4 g vial with at least 20 ml of sterile water for injection, 5% dextrose injection, or 0.9% sodium chloride injection and add to one of following I.V. solutions: acetated Ringer's injection; 5% dextrose injection; 5% dextrose in lactated Ringer's injection; Ionosol B in 5% dextrose in water; lactated Ringer's injection; Normosol-N in 5% dextrose in water; Plasma-Lyte injection; Plasma-Lyte-N injection in 5% dextrose; Ringer's injection, or 0.9% sodium chloride injection. Choose solution and fluid volume according to patient's fluid and electrolyte status.
• About 40% to 75% of patients receiving cephalosporins show a false positive direct Coombs' test; only a few of these indicate hemolytic anemia.
• Urine glucose tests with Benedict's Qualitative Reagent, Clinitest, or Fehling's solution may give false positive results during cephalosporin therapy. Clinistix, Diastix, and Tes-Tape are not affected.

Unmarked trade names available in the United States only.
♦ Also available in Canada   ♦ ♦ Available in Canada only.

cephapirin sodium
Cefadyl♦

INDICATIONS & DOSAGE

Serious infections of respiratory, genitourinary, or gastrointestinal tract; skin and soft tissue infections; bone and joint infections (including osteomyelitis); septicemia; endocarditis due to S. pneumoniae, E. coli, group A beta-hemolytic streptococci, H. influenzae, Klebsiella, P. mirabilis, S. aureus, and S. viridans—
Adults: 500 mg to 1 g I.V. or I.M. q 4 to 6 hours up to 12 g daily.
Children over 3 months: 10 to 20 mg/Kg I.V. or I.M. q 6 hours; dose depends on age, weight, and severity of infection.

Should be injected deep I.M. into a large muscle mass, such as gluteus or lateral aspect of thigh. Depending upon causative organism and severity of infection, patients with reduced renal function may be treated adequately with a lower dose (7.5 to 15 mg/Kg q 12 hours). Patients with severely reduced renal function and who are to be dialyzed should receive same dose just before dialysis and q 12 hours thereafter.

SIDE EFFECTS

Blood: transient neutropenia, eosinophilia, anemia.
CNS: dizziness, headache, malaise, paresthesias.
GI: nausea, anorexia, vomiting, diarrhea, glossitis, dyspepsia, abdominal cramps, tenesmus, anal pruritus, oral candidiasis (thrush).
GU: nephrotoxicity, genital pruritus and moniliasis, vaginitis.
Skin: *maculopapular and erythematous rashes, urticaria.*
Local: *at injection site—pain, induration, sterile abscesses, tissue slough;*
phlebitis and thrombophlebitis with I.V. injection.
Other: *hypersensitivity,* dyspnea.

INTERACTIONS

Probenecid: may increase blood levels of cephalosporins. Use together cautiously.

NURSING CONSIDERATIONS

• Use cautiously in impaired renal function and in patients with a history of sensitivity to penicillin. Ask patient if he's had any reaction to previous cephalosporin or penicillin therapy before administering first dose.
• Prolonged use may result in overgrowth of nonsusceptible organisms. Watch for superinfection.
• Obtain cultures for sensitivity tests before beginning therapy, but therapy may begin pending results of cultures and sensitivity tests.
• For I.M. administration, reconstitute 1 g vial with 2 ml sterile water for injection or bacteriostatic water for injection so that 1.2 ml contains 500 mg of cephapirin. I.M. injection painful.
• When giving this drug I.V., check frequently for vein irritation and phlebitis. Alternate injection sites if I.V. therapy lasts longer than 3 days. Use of small I.V. needles in the larger available veins may be preferable.
• Prepare I.V. infusion using dextrose injection, sodium chloride injection, or bacteriostatic water for injection, as diluent: 20 ml yields 1 g per 10 ml; 50 ml yields 1 g per 25 ml; 100 ml yields 1 g per 50 ml.
• I.V. infusion with Y-tube: during infusion of cephapirin solution, it is desirable to stop other solution. Check volume of cephapirin solution carefully so that calculated dose is infused. When Y-tube is used, dilute 4 g vial with 40 ml of diluent.
• Compatible with following infusion solutions: sodium chloride injection; 5% dextrose in water; sodium lactate

injection; 5% dextrose in normal saline; 10% invert sugar in normal saline; 10% invert sugar in water; 5% dextrose and 0.2% sodium chloride injection; lactated Ringer's with 5% dextrose; 5% dextrose and 0.45% sodium chloride injection; Ringer's injection; lactated Ringer's; 10% dextrose injection; sterile water for injection; 20% dextrose injection; 5% sodium chloride in water; and 5% dextrose in Ringer's injection.

- Reconstituted cephapirin is stable and compatible for 10 days under refrigeration and for 24 hours at room temperature.
- About 40% to 75% of patients receiving cephalosporins show a false positive direct Coombs' test, but only a few indicate hemolytic anemia.
- Urine glucose tests with Benedict's Qualitative Reagent, Clinitest, or Fehling's solution may give false positive results during cephalosporin therapy. Clinistix, Diastix, and Tes-Tape are not affected.

---

cephradine
Anspor, Velosef♦

INDICATIONS & DOSAGE
Serious infection of respiratory, genitourinary, or gastrointestinal tract; skin and soft tissue infections; bone and joint infections; septicemia; endocarditis; and otitis media due to E. coli and other coliform bacteria, group A beta-hemolytic streptococci, H. influenzae, Klebsiella, P. mirabilis, S. aureus, S. pneumoniae, staphylococci, and S. viridans—
Adults: 500 mg to 1 g I.M. or I.V. 2 to 4 times daily; do not exceed 8 g daily. Or 250 to 500 mg P.O. q 6 hours. Severe or chronic infections may require larger and/or more frequent doses (up to 1 g P.O. q 6 hours).
Children over 1 year: 6 to 12 mg/Kg

P.O. q 6 hours. 12 to 25 mg/Kg I.M. or I.V. q 6 hours.
Otitis media— 19 to 25 mg/Kg P.O. q 6 hours. Do not exceed 4 g daily.
All patients, regardless of age and weight: larger doses (up to 1 g q.i.d.) may be given for severe or chronic infections. Parenteral therapy may be followed by oral. Injections should be given deep I.M. into a large muscle mass, such as gluteus or lateral aspect of thigh.

SIDE EFFECTS
Blood: transient neutropenia, eosinophilia.
CNS: dizziness, headache, malaise, paresthesias.
GI: *nausea, anorexia,* vomiting, heartburn, glossitis, dyspepsia, abdominal cramping, *diarrhea,* tenesmus, anal pruritus, oral candidiasis (thrush).
GU: genital pruritus and moniliasis, vaginitis.
Skin: *maculopapular and erythematous rashes, urticaria.*
Local: *at injection site—pain, induration, sterile abscesses, tissue slough; phlebitis and thrombophlebitis with I.V. injection.*
Other: *hypersensitivity,* dyspnea.

INTERACTIONS
Probenecid: may increase blood levels of cephalosporins. Use together cautiously.

NURSING CONSIDERATIONS
- Use cautiously in impaired renal function and in those with a history of sensitivity to penicillin. Ask patient if he's had any reaction to previous cephalosporin or penicillin therapy before administering first dose.
- Obtain cultures for sensitivity tests before beginning therapy, but therapy may begin pending results of cultures and sensitivity tests.
- Prolonged use may result in over-

---

growth of nonsusceptible organisms.
Watch for superinfection.
• When giving this drug I.V., check
frequently for vein irritation and phlebitis. Alternate injection sites if I.V.
therapy lasts longer than 3 days. Use
of small I.V. needles in the larger
available veins may be preferable.
• Tell patient to take medication exactly as prescribed, even after he feels
better. Group A beta-hemolytic streptococci infections should be treated
for a minimum of 10 days.
• I.M. injection painful
• For I.M. administration, reconstitute with sterile water for injection or
with bacteriostatic water for injection
as follows: 1.2 ml to 250 mg vial;
2 ml to 500 mg vial; 4 ml to 1 g vial.
I.M. solutions must be used within
2 hours if kept at room temperature
and within 24 hours if refrigerated.
Solutions may vary in color from light
straw to yellow without affecting
potency.
• When preparing cephradine for intravenous administration, when available, use preparation specifically supplied for infusion. Follow specific
product directions carefully when reconstituting.
• About 40% to 75% of patients receiving cephalosporins show a false
positive direct Coombs' test, but only
a few indicate hemolytic anemia.
• Urine glucose tests with Benedict's
Qualitative Reagent, Clinitest, or
Fehling's solution may give false positive results during cephalosporin therapy. Clinistix, Diastix, and Tes-Tape
are not affected.

11

Tetracyclines

demeclocycline hydrochloride
doxycycline hyclate
methacycline hydrochloride
minocycline hydrochloride
oxytetracycline hydrochloride
tetracycline hydrochloride
tetracycline phosphate complex

---

demeclocycline hydrochloride
Declomycin♦, Ledermycin

INDICATIONS & DOSAGE
Infections caused by susceptible gram-negative and gram-positive organisms, trachoma, amebiasis—
Adults: 150 mg P.O. q 6 hours or 300 mg P.O. q 12 hours.
Children over 8 years: 6 to 12 mg/Kg P.O. daily, divided q 6 to 12 hours.
Gonorrhea—
Adults: 600 mg P.O. initially, then 300 mg P.O. q 12 hours for 4 days (total 3 g).
Syndrome of Inappropriate ADH (a hypo-osmolar state)—
Adults: 600 to 1200 mg P.O. daily in divided doses.

SIDE EFFECTS
Blood: neutropenia, eosinophilia.
CV: pericarditis.
EENT: dysphagia, glossitis.
GI: anorexia, *nausea, vomiting, diarrhea,* enterocolitis, anogenital inflammation.
Metabolic: *increased BUN,* diabetes insipidus syndrome (polyuria, polydipsia, weakness).

Skin: *maculopapular and erythematous rashes, photosensitivity, increased pigmentation, urticaria.*
Other: hypersensitivity.

INTERACTIONS
Antacids (including NaHCO₃) and laxatives containing aluminum, calcium, and magnesium; food, milk, or other dairy products: decreased antibiotic absorption. Give antibiotic 1 hour before or 2 hours after any of the above.
Ferrous sulfate and other iron products, zinc: decreased antibiotic absorption. Give demeclocycline 3 hours after or 2 hours before iron administration.
Methoxyflurane: may cause nephrotoxicity with tetracyclines. Monitor carefully.

NURSING CONSIDERATIONS
• Use with extreme caution in impaired renal or hepatic function. Use of these drugs during last half of pregnancy and in children younger than age 8 may cause permanent discoloration of teeth, enamel defects, and retardation of bone growth.
• Obtain cultures before starting therapy.
• Check expiration date. Outdated or deteriorated demeclocycline may cause nephrotoxicity.
• Do not expose these drugs to light or heat; store in tight container.
• Watch for overgrowth of nonsensitive organisms. Check patient's tongue for monilia organisms. Stress

good oral hygiene. If superinfection occurs, drug should be discontinued.
• Observe patient for diarrhea.
• May cause false positive reading of Clinitest; false negative reading of Clinistix or Tes-Tape.
• Warn patient to avoid direct sunlight and ultraviolet light. A sunscreen may help avoid phototoxic reactions. Phototoxicity persists for some time after discontinuation of drug.
• Effectiveness is reduced when taken with milk or other dairy products, food, antacids, or iron products. Explain this to patient. Tell patient to take each dose with a full glass of water on an empty stomach, at least 1 hour before meals or 2 hours afterward. Give at least 1 hour before bedtime to prevent esophagitis.
• Instruct patient to take medication for as long as prescribed, exactly as prescribed, even after he feels better. Treat streptococcal infections for at least 10 days.

---

doxycycline hyclate
Doxychel, Vibramycin♦, Vibra Tabs

INDICATIONS & DOSAGE
Infections caused by sensitive gram-negative and gram-positive organisms, trachoma, amebiasis—
Adults: 100 mg P.O. q 12 hours on first day, then 100 mg P.O. daily; or 200 mg I.V. on first day in 1 or 2 infusions, then 100 to 200 mg I.V. daily.
Children over 8 years (under 45 Kg): 4.4 mg/Kg P.O. or I.V. daily, divided q 12 hours first day, then 2.2 to 4.4 mg/Kg daily. Over 45 Kg, same as adults.
Give I.V. infusion slowly (minimum time 1 hour). Infusion must be completed within 12 hours (within 6 hours in lactated Ringer's solution or 5% dextrose in lactated Ringer's).

Gonorrhea in patients allergic to penicillin—
Adults: 200 mg P.O. initially, followed by 100 mg P.O. at bedtime, and 100 mg P.O. b.i.d. for 3 days; or 300 mg P.O. initially and repeat dose in 1 hour.
Primary or secondary syphilis in patients allergic to penicillin—
Adults: 300 mg P.O. daily in divided doses for 10 days.

SIDE EFFECTS
Blood: neutropenia, eosinophilia.
CNS: benign intracranial hypertension.
CV: pericarditis.
EENT: sore throat, glossitis, dysphagia.
GI: anorexia, *epigastric distress, nausea,* vomiting, *diarrhea,* enterocolitis, anogenital inflammation.
Skin: *maculopapular and erythematous rashes, photosensitivity, increased pigmentation,* urticaria.
Local: thrombophlebitis.
Other: hypersensitivity.

INTERACTIONS
Antacids (including NaHCO$_3$) and laxatives containing aluminum, magnesium, or calcium: decreased antibiotic absorption. Give antibiotic 1 hour before or 2 hours after any of the above.
Ferrous sulfate and other iron products, zinc: decreased antibiotic absorption. Give doxycycline 3 hours after or 2 hours before iron administration.
Phenobarbital, carbamazepine, alcohol: decreased antibiotic effect. Avoid if possible.

NURSING CONSIDERATIONS
• Use of these drugs during last half of pregnancy and in children younger than age 8 may cause permanent discoloration of teeth, enamel defects, and retardation of bone growth.

- Patient may develop thrombophlebitis with I.V. administration.
- Obtain cultures before starting therapy.
- Check expiration date.
- Don't expose to light or heat. Protect from sunlight during infusion.
- Watch for overgrowth of nonsensitive organisms. Check patient's tongue for monilia organisms. Stress good oral hygiene. If superinfection occurs, drug should be discontinued.
- Observe patient for diarrhea.
- May be taken with milk or food if GI side effects develop.
- Do not give with antacids.
- Tell patient to take medication exactly as prescribed, even after he feels better. Treat streptococcal infections for at least 10 days.
- Reconstitute powder for injection with sterile water for injection. Use 10 ml for 100-mg vial and 20 ml in 200-mg vial. Dilute solution to 100 to 1,000 ml before giving. Do not infuse solutions more concentrated than 1 mg per ml.
- Reconstituted solution is stable for 72 hours refrigerated.
- Doxycycline may be used in patients with renal impairment; does not accumulate in or cause a significant rise in BUN.
- May cause false positive reading of Clinitest; false negative reading of Clinistix or Tes-Tape.
- Should not be taken within 1 hour of bedtime because of increased incidence of dysphagia.

---

methacycline hydrochloride
Rondomycin

INDICATIONS & DOSAGE

Infections caused by sensitive gram-negative and gram-positive organisms, trachoma, amebiasis—
Adults: 150 mg P.O. q 6 hours or 300 mg q 12 hours.

Children over 8 years: 6 to 12 mg/Kg P.O. daily, divided q 6 hours to q 12 hours.
Gonorrhea in patients sensitive to penicillin—
Adults: 900 mg P.O. initially, then 300 mg P.O. q.i.d. for total of 5.4 g.
Syphilis in patients sensitive to penicillin—
Adults: total dose of 18 to 24 g in equally divided doses over 10 to 15 days.

SIDE EFFECTS
Blood: neutropenia, eosinophilia.
CV: pericarditis.
EENT: dysphagia, glossitis.
GI: anorexia, *epigastric distress, nausea,* vomiting, *diarrhea,* enterocolitis, anogenital inflammation.
Metabolic: increased BUN.
Skin: *maculopapular and erythematous rashes, photosensitivity, urticaria.*
Other: hypersensitivity.

INTERACTIONS
Antacids (including NaHCO$_3$) and laxatives containing aluminum, magnesium, or calcium; food, milk, or other dairy products: decreased antibiotic absorption. Give antibiotic 1 hour before or 2 hours after any of the above.
Ferrous sulfate and other iron products, zinc: decreased antibiotic absorption. Give tetracyclines 3 hours after or 2 hours before iron administration.

NURSING CONSIDERATIONS
- Use with extreme caution in impaired renal or hepatic function. Use during last half of pregnancy and in children younger than age 8 may cause permanent discoloration of teeth, enamel defects, and retardation of bone growth.
- Obtain cultures before starting therapy.
- Check expiration date. Outdated or

deteriorated methacycline may cause nephrotoxicity.
- Do not expose these drugs to light or heat.
- Watch for overgrowth of nonsensitive organisms. Check patient's tongue for monilia organisms. Stress good oral hygiene. If superinfection occurs, drug should be discontinued.
- Observe patient for diarrhea.
- Warn patient to avoid direct sunlight and ultraviolet light. A sunscreen may help avoid phototoxic reactions. Phototoxicity persists for considerable time after discontinuation of drug.
- Effectiveness is reduced when taken with milk or other dairy products, food, antacids, or iron products. Explain this to patient. Tell patient to take each dose with a full glass of water on an empty stomach, at least 1 hour before meals or 2 hours afterward. Give at least 1 hour before bedtime to prevent esophagitis.
- Instruct patient to take medication exactly as prescribed, even after he feels better. Treat streptococcal infections for at least 10 days.
- May cause false positive reading of Clinitest; false negative reading of Clinistix or Tes-Tape.

---

minocycline hydrochloride
Minocin♦, Ultramycin♦♦, Vectrin

INDICATIONS & DOSAGE
Infections caused by sensitive gram-negative and gram-positive organisms, trachoma, amebiasis—
Adults: initially, 200 mg P.O., I.V.; then 100 mg q 12 hours or 50 mg P.O. q 6 hours.
Children over 8 years: initially, 4 mg/Kg P.O., I.V.; then 4 mg/Kg P.O. daily, divided q 12 hours. Give I.V. in 500 to 1,000 ml solution without calcium, over 6 hours.

Gonorrhea in patients sensitive to penicillin—
Adults: initially, 200 mg, then 100 mg q 12 hours for 4 days.
Syphilis in patients sensitive to penicillin—
Adults: initially, 200 mg, then 100 mg q 12 hours for 10 to 15 days.
Meningococcal carrier state—
100 mg P.O. q 12 hours for 5 days.

SIDE EFFECTS
Blood: neutropenia, eosinophilia.
CNS: *light-headedness.*
CV: pericarditis.
EENT: dysphagia, glossitis, *dizziness.*
GI: *anorexia,* epigastric distress, *nausea,* vomiting, *diarrhea,* enterocolitis, inflammatory lesions in anogenital region.
Metabolic: increased BUN.
Skin: maculopapular and erythematous rashes, photosensitivity, increased pigmentation, urticaria.
Local: *thrombophlebitis.*
Other: hypersensitivity.

INTERACTIONS
Antacids (including NaHCO₃) or laxatives containing aluminum, magnesium, or calcium: decreased antibiotic absorption. Give antibiotic 1 hour before or 2 hours after any of the above.
Ferrous sulfate or other iron products, zinc: decreased antibiotic absorption. Tetracyclines should be given 3 hours after or 2 hours before iron administration.
Methoxyflurane: may cause severe nephrotoxicity with tetracyclines. Monitor carefully.

NURSING CONSIDERATIONS
- Use with extreme caution in impaired renal or hepatic function. Use during last half of pregnancy and in children younger than age 8 may cause permanent discoloration of

---

teeth, enamel defects, and retardation of bone growth.
- Patient may develop thrombophlebitis with I.V. administration of this drug. Avoid extravasation.
- Obtain cultures before starting therapy.
- Check expiration date.
- Do not expose these drugs to light or heat. Keep cap tightly closed.
- Watch for overgrowth of nonsensitive organisms. Check patient's tongue for monilia organisms. Stress good oral hygiene. If superinfection occurs, drug should be discontinued.
- Observe patient for diarrhea.
- May be taken with food. Tell patient to take medication exactly as prescribed, even after he feels better. Treat streptococcal infections for at least 10 days, syphilis for 10 to 15 days, gonorrhea for at least 4 days, and meningococcal carriers for 5 days.
- Reconstitute 100 mg powder with 5 ml sterile water for injection, with further dilution of 500 to 1,000 ml for I.V. infusion. Stable for 24 hours at room temperature.
- May cause false positive reading of Clinitest; false negative reading of Clinistix or Tes-Tape.
- Vestibular toxicity resulting in dizziness can frequently occur with this drug.

---

oxytetracycline hydrochloride
Dalimycin, Oxlopar, Oxy-Kesso-Tetra, Oxytetrachlor, Terramycin♦, Uri-tet

INDICATIONS & DOSAGE
Infections caused by sensitive gram-negative and gram-positive organisms, trachoma, amebiasis—
Adults: 250 mg P.O. q 6 hours; 100 mg I.M. q 8 to 12 hours; 250 mg I.M. q 12 hours; or 250 to 500 mg I.V. q 6 to 12 hours.

Children over 8 years: 25 to 50 mg/Kg P.O. daily, divided q 6 hours; 15 to 25 mg/Kg I.M. daily, divided q 8 to 12 hours; or 10 to 20 mg/Kg I.V. daily, divided q 12 hours.
Brucellosis—
Adults: 500 mg P.O. q.i.d. for 3 weeks with streptomycin 1 g I.M. q 12 hours first week, once daily second week.
Syphilis in patients sensitive to penicillin—
Adults: 30 to 40 g total dose P.O., divided equally over 10 to 15 days.
Gonorrhea in patients sensitive to penicillin—
Adults: initially, 1.5 g P.O. followed by 0.5 g q.i.d. for a total of 9 g.

SIDE EFFECTS
Blood: neutropenia, eosinophilia.
CNS: benign intracranial hypertension.
CV: pericarditis.
EENT: dysphagia, glossitis.
GI: *anorexia, nausea,* vomiting, *diarrhea,* enterocolitis, anogenital inflammation.
Metabolic: *increased BUN.*
Skin: *maculopapular and erythematous rashes, urticaria, photosensitivity, increased pigmentation.*
Local: *irritation after I.M. injection, thrombophlebitis.*
Other: hypersensitivity.

INTERACTIONS
Antacids (including NaHCO₃) and laxatives containing aluminum, magnesium, or calcium; food, milk, or other dairy products: decreased antibiotic absorption. Give antibiotic 1 hour before or 2 hours after any of the above.
Ferrous sulfate and other iron products, zinc: decreased antibiotic absorption. Give tetracyclines 3 hours after or 2 hours before iron administration.
Methoxyflurane: may cause severe

---

nephrotoxicity with tetracyclines.
Monitor carefully.

NURSING CONSIDERATIONS

• Use with extreme caution in impaired renal or hepatic function. Use during last half of pregnancy and in children younger than age 8 may cause permanent discoloration of teeth, enamel defects, and retardation of bone growth.
• Patient may develop thrombophlebitis with I.V. administration. Avoid extravasation.
• Obtain cultures before starting therapy.
• Check expiration date. Outdated or deteriorated oxytetracycline may cause nephrotoxicity.
• Do not expose these drugs to light or heat.
• Inject I.M. dosage deeply. Warn that it may be painful. Rotate sites. I.M. preparations contain a local anesthetic; ask patient about hypersensitivity to local anesthetics.
• Watch for overgrowth of nonsensitive organisms. Check patient's tongue for monilia organisms. Stress good oral hygiene. If superinfection occurs, drug should be discontinued.
• Observe patient for diarrhea.
• Warn patient to avoid direct sunlight and ultraviolet light. A sunscreen may help avoid phototoxic reactions. Phototoxicity persists for considerable time after discontinuation of drug.
• Effectiveness is reduced when taken with milk or other dairy products, food, antacids, or iron products. Explain this to patient. Tell patient to take each dose with a full glass of water on an empty stomach, at least 1 hour before meals or 2 hours afterward. Give at least 1 hour before bedtime to prevent esophagitis.
• Tell patient to take medication exactly as prescribed, even after he feels better.
• For I.V. use, reconstitute 250 mg

and 500 mg powder for injection with 10 ml sterile water for injection.
• Dilute to at least 100 ml in 5% dextrose in water, normal saline, or Ringer's solution. Do not mix with any other drug.
• Store reconstituted solutions in refrigerator. Stable for 48 hours.
• May cause false positive reading of Clinitest; false negative reading of Clinistix or Tes-Tape.

---

tetracycline hydrochloride
Achromycin♦, Amer-Tet, Bicycline, Cefracycline♦♦, Centet-250, Cycline, Cyclopar, Maso-Cycline, Medicycline♦♦, Neo-Tetrine♦♦, Nor-Tet 500, Novotetra♦♦, Paltet 250, Panmycin, Partrex, Piracaps, Retet, Robitet, Sarocycline, Scotrex, SK-Tetracycline, Sumycin♦, T-125, T-250, Tet-Cy, Tetra-C, Tetrachel, Tetraclor, Tetra-Co, Tetracrine♦♦, Tetracyn♦, Tetralan, Tetralean♦♦, Tetram, Tetram S, Tetramax, Trexin, Triacycline♦♦
tetracycline phosphate complex
Tetrex♦

INDICATIONS & DOSAGE

Infections caused by sensitive gram-negative and gram-positive organisms, trachoma, amebiasis, Mycoplasma, Rickettsia, and Chlamydia—
Adults: 250 to 500 mg P.O. q 6 hours; 250 mg I.M. daily or 150 mg I.M. q 12 hours; or 250 to 500 mg I.V. q 8 to 12 hours (I.M. and I.V. hydrochloride salt only).
Children over 8 years: 25 to 50 mg/Kg P.O. daily, divided q 6 hours; 15 to 25 mg/Kg/day (maximum 250 mg) I.M. single dose or divided q 8 to 12 hours; or 10 to 20 mg/Kg I.V. daily, divided q 12 hours.
Brucellosis—
Adults: 500 mg P.O. q 6 hours for 3 weeks with streptomycin 1 g I.M. q 12 hours week 1 and daily week 2.

Italicized side effects are common or life-threatening.

*Gonorrhea in patients sensitive to pen-
icillin—*
Adults: initially,1.5 g P.O., then
500 mg q 6 hours for total of 9 g.
*Syphilis in patients sensitive to peni-
cillin—*
Adults: 30 to 40 g total in equally di-
vided doses over 10 to 15 days.
Acne—
Adults and adolescents: initially,
250 mg P.O. q 6 hours, then 125 to
500 mg P.O. daily or every other day.
Shigellosis—
Adults: 2.5 g P.O. in 1 dose.

SIDE EFFECTS
Blood: neutropenia, eosinophilia.
CNS: dizziness, headache.
CV: pericarditis.
EENT: sore throat, glossitis, dys-
phagia.
GI: anorexia, *epigastric distress, nau-
sea,* vomiting, *diarrhea,* stomatitis,
enterocolitis, inflammatory lesions in
anogenital region.
Hepatic: hepatotoxicity with doses
I.V.
Metabolic: *increased BUN.*
Skin: *maculopapular and erythema-
tous rashes, urticaria, photosensitiv-
ity, increased pigmentation.*
Local: *irritation after I.M. injection,
thrombophlebitis.*

INTERACTIONS
*Antacids (including NaHCO₃) and
laxatives containing aluminum,
magnesium, or calcium; food, milk,
or other dairy products:* decreased
antibiotic absorption. Give antibiotic
1 hour before or 2 hours after any of
the above.
*Ferrous sulfate and other iron prod-
ucts, zinc:* decreased antibiotic absorption. Give tetracyclines 3 hours
after or 2 hours before iron administration.
Methoxyflurane: may cause severe
nephrotoxicity with tetracyclines.
Monitor carefully.

NURSING CONSIDERATIONS
• Use with extreme caution in impaired renal or hepatic function. Use
during last half of pregnancy and in
children younger than age 8 may
cause permanent discoloration of
teeth, enamel defects, and retardation
of bone growth.
• Obtain cultures before starting
therapy.
• Effectiveness reduced when taken
with milk or other dairy products,
food, antacids, or iron products. Explain this to patient. Tell patient to
take each dose with a full glass of water on an empty stomach, at least 1
hour before meals or 2 hours afterward. Give at least 1 hour before bedtime to prevent esophagitis.
• Patient may develop thrombophlebitis with I.V. administration. Avoid
extravasation.
• Check expiration date. Outdated or
deteriorated tetracycline may cause
nephrotoxicity.
• Discard I.M. solutions after
24 hours because they deteriorate.
Exception: discard Achromycin solution in 12 hours.
• Do not expose these drugs to light
or heat.
• Inject I.M. dosage deeply. Warn
patient that it may be painful. Rotate
sites. I.M. preparations often contain
a local anesthetic; ask patient about
hypersensitivity to local anesthetics.
• Watch for overgrowth of nonsensitive organisms. Check patient's
tongue for monilia organisms. Stress
good oral hygiene. If superinfection
occurs, drug should be discontinued.
• Observe patient for diarrhea.
• Warn patient to avoid direct sunlight and ultraviolet light. A sunscreen may help avoid phototoxic reactions. Phototoxicity persists for
some time after discontinuation of
drug.
• Tell patient to take medication exactly as prescribed, even after he feels

better. Treat streptoccocal infections for at least 10 days.
• For I.V. use, reconstitute 100 mg and 250 mg powder for injection with 5 ml sterile water; with 10 ml for 500 mg. Dilute in 100 to 1,000 ml volume of 5% dextrose in 0.9% saline. Refrigerate dilute solution for I.V. use and use within 24 hours. Exception: use Achromycin solution immediately.
• Do not mix tetracycline solution with any other I.V. additive.
• For I.M. use, reconstitute 100 mg powder for injection with 2 ml sterile water for injection. Concentration will be 50 mg/ml. Amount of diluent for 250 mg injection varies according to brand. Check with pharmacy or follow manufacturer's instructions.
• May cause false positive readings of Clinitest; false negative reading of Clinistix or Tes-Tape.

12

Sulfonamides

co-trimoxazole
sulfachlorpyridazine
sulfacytine
sulfadiazine
sulfamerazine
sulfameter
sulfamethizole
sulfamethoxazole
sulfamethoxypyridazine
sulfapyridine
sulfasalazine
sulfisoxazole

co-trimoxazole
(sulfamethoxazole-trimethoprim)
Bactrim♦, Bactrim DS♦, Septra♦,
Septra DS♦

INDICATIONS & DOSAGE
*Urinary tract infections and shigello-
sis—*
Adults: 160 mg trimethoprim/800 mg
sulfa q 12 hours for 10 to 14 days in
urinary tract infections and 5 days in
shigellosis.
Children: 8 mg/Kg trimethoprim/
40 mg/Kg sulfa per 24 hours, in 2 divided doses q 12 hours (10 days for
urinary tract infections; 5 days in
shigellosis).
Otitis media—
Children: 8 mg/Kg trimethoprim/
40 mg/Kg sulfa per 24 hours, in 2 divided doses q 12 hours for 10 days.
Pneumocystis carinii pneumonitis—
Adults: 20 mg/Kg trimethoprim/ 100
mg/Kg sulfa per 24 hours, in equally
divided doses q 6 hours for 14 days.
Children (36 Kg/80 lb): 160 mg tri-
methoprim/800 mg sulfa q 6 hours for
14 days.
Chronic bronchitis—
Adults: 160 mg trimethoprim/800 mg
sulfa q 12 hours for 10 to 14 days.
Not recommended for infants less
than 2 months old.
Available as tablets or suspension
only.

SIDE EFFECTS
Blood: *agranulocytosis, aplastic anemia,* megaloblastic anemia, thrombocytopenia, leukopenia, hemolytic
anemia.
CNS: headache, mental depression,
convulsions, hallucinations.
GI: *nausea, vomiting, diarrhea,* abdominal pain, anorexia, stomatitis.
GU: toxic nephrosis with oliguria and
anuria, crystalluria, hematuria.
Skin: *erythema multiforme (Stevens-
Johnson syndrome), generalized skin
eruption, epidermal necrolysis, exfoliative dermatitis,* photosensitivity, urticaria, pruritus.
Other: *hypersensitivity, serum sickness, drug fever,* jaundice.

INTERACTIONS
*Ammonium chloride, ascorbic acid,
paraldehyde:* doses sufficient to acidify urine may cause precipitation of
sulfonamide and crystalluria. Don't
use together.
*PABA-containing local anesthetics
and other PABA drugs:* inhibited antibacterial action. Don't use together.

NURSING CONSIDERATIONS
• Contraindicated in porphyria. Use

cautiously and in reduced dosages in impaired hepatic or renal function and in severe allergy or bronchial asthma, G-6-PD deficiency, blood dyscrasias.
• Tell patient to drink a full glass of water with each dose and to drink plenty of water during the day to prevent crystalluria. Monitor fluid intake and urinary output.
• This combination is often used in extremely ill immunosuppressed patients when prescribed for treatment of *Pneumocystis* pneumonia.
• Oral suspension available for patients who cannot swallow large tablets.
• Note that the "DS" product means "double strength."
• Promptly report skin rash, sore throat, fever, or mouth sores.
• Tell patient to take 1 hour before or 2 hours after meals for best absorption.
• Used effectively for treatment of chronic bacterial prostatitis.
• Used prophylactically for recurrent urinary tract infections in women.
• Most side effects develop within 2 weeks of onset of therapy.

---

sulfachlorpyridazine
Cosulid, Sonilyn, Vetisulid

INDICATIONS & DOSAGE
Urinary tract infections and some systemic infections—
Adults: 2 to 4 g P.O. initially, then 500 mg to 1 g P.O. q 6 hours.
Children over 2 months: 75 mg/Kg P.O. initially, then 150 mg/Kg daily, divided into doses given q 6 hours. Maximum daily dose 6 g.

SIDE EFFECTS
Blood: *agranulocytosis, aplastic anemia,* megaloblastic anemia, thrombocytopenia, leukopenia, hemolytic anemia.

CNS: headache, mental depression, convulsions, hallucinations.
GI: *nausea, vomiting, diarrhea,* abdominal pain, anorexia, stomatitis.
GU: toxic nephrosis with oliguria and anuria, crystalluria, hematuria.
Skin: *erythema multiforme (Stevens-Johnson syndrome), generalized skin eruption, epidermal necrolysis, exfoliative dermatitis,* photosensitivity, urticaria, pruritus.
Other: *hypersensitivity, serum sickness, drug fever,* jaundice.

INTERACTIONS
Ammonium chloride, ascorbic acid, paraldehyde: doses sufficient to acidify urine may cause precipitation of sulfonamide and crystalluria. Don't use together.
PABA-containing local anesthetics and other PABA drugs: inhibited antibacterial action. Don't use together.

NURSING CONSIDERATIONS
• Contraindicated in porphyria. Use cautiously and in reduced dosages in impaired hepatic or renal function, asthma or blood dyscrasias, G-6-PD deficiency, history of multiple allergies.
• Tell patient to drink a full glass of water with each dose and to drink plenty of water throughout the day to prevent crystalluria. Monitor fluid intake and urinary output. Intake should be sufficient to produce output of 1,500 ml daily.
• To aid in prevention of crystalluria, sodium bicarbonate may be administered to alkalinize urine.
• Tell patient to take medication for as long as prescribed, even after he feels better.
• Monitor urine cultures, CBC, and urinalysis before and during therapy.
• Tell patient to report early signs of blood dyscrasias (sore throat, fever, pallor, or jaundice) immediately and to stop taking drug. Warn patient to

---

Italicized side effects are common or life-threatening.

avoid direct sunlight and ultraviolet light to prevent photosensitivity reaction.

---

sulfacytine
Renoquid

INDICATIONS & DOSAGE
Urinary tract infections—
Adults: initially, 500 mg P.O., then 250 mg P.O. q.i.d. for 10 days.

SIDE EFFECTS
Blood: *agranulocytosis, aplastic anemia*, megaloblastic anemia, thrombocytopenia, leukopenia, hemolytic anemia.
CNS: headache, mental depression, convulsions, hallucinations.
GI: *nausea, vomiting, diarrhea*, abdominal pain, anorexia, stomatitis.
GU: toxic nephrosis with oliguria and anuria, crystalluria, hematuria.
Skin: *erythema multiforme (Stevens-Johnson syndrome), generalized skin eruption, epidermal necrolysis, exfoliative dermatitis*, photosensitivity, urticaria, pruritus.
Other: *hypersensitivity, serum sickness, drug fever*, jaundice.

INTERACTIONS
Ammonium chloride, ascorbic acid, paraldehyde: doses sufficient to acidify urine may cause precipitation of sulfonamide and crystalluria. Don't use together.
PABA-containing local anesthetics and other PABA drugs: inhibited antibacterial action. Don't use together.

NURSING CONSIDERATIONS
• Contraindicated in porphyria. Use cautiously and in reduced dosages in impaired hepatic or renal function, bronchial asthma, history of multiple allergies, G-6-PD deficiency, blood dyscrasias.
• Tell patient to drink a full glass of

water with each dose and to drink plenty of water throughout the day to prevent crystalluria. Monitor fluid intake and urinary output. Intake should be sufficient to produce output of 1,500 ml daily.
• To aid in prevention of crystalluria, sodium bicarbonate may be administered to alkalinize urine.
• Tell patient to take medication for as long as prescribed, even after he feels better. Warn patient to avoid direct sunlight and ultraviolet light to prevent photosensitivity reaction.
• Monitor urine cultures, CBC, and urinalysis before and during therapy.
• Tell patient to report early signs of blood dyscrasias (sore throat, fever, pallor, or jaundice) immediately and to stop taking drug.

---

sulfadiazine
Microsulfon, Neo-Quinette

INDICATIONS & DOSAGE
Urinary tract infection—
Adults: initially, 2 to 4 g P.O., then 500 mg to 1 g P.O. q 6 hours.
Children: initially, 75 mg/Kg or 2 g/m² P.O., then 150 mg/Kg or 4 g/m² P.O. in 4 to 6 divided doses daily. Maximum daily dose 6 g.
Rheumatic fever prophylaxis, as an alternative to penicillin—
Children over 30 Kg: 1 g P.O. daily.
Children under 30 Kg: 500 mg P.O. daily.
Adjunctive treatment in toxoplasmosis—
Adults: 4 g P.O. in divided doses q 6 hours for 3 to 4 weeks, discontinued for 1 week, then repeated; given with pyrimethamine 75 mg P.O. daily for 1 to 3 days, then 25 mg P.O. daily for 3 to 4 weeks, discontinued for 1 week, then repeated using 25 mg P.O. daily.
Children: 100 mg/Kg P.O. in divided doses q 6 hours for 3 to 4 weeks, dis-

continued for 1 week, then repeated; given with pyrimethamine, 1 mg/Kg P.O. daily for 1 to 3 days, then 0.5 mg/Kg P.O. daily for 3 to 4 weeks, discontinued for 1 week, then repeated using 0.5 mg/Kg P.O. daily.

SIDE EFFECTS
Blood: *agranulocytosis, aplastic anemia,* megaloblastic anemia, thrombocytopenia, leukopenia, hemolytic anemia.
CNS: headache, mental depression, convulsions, hallucinations.
GI: *nausea, vomiting, diarrhea,* abdominal pain, anorexia, stomatitis.
GU: toxic nephrosis with oliguria and anuria, crystalluria, hematuria.
Skin: *erythema multiforme (Stevens-Johnson syndrome), generalized skin eruption, epidermal necrolysis, exfoliative dermatitis,* photosensitivity, urticaria, pruritus.
Local: irritation, extravasation.
Other: *hypersensitivity, serum sickness, drug fever,* jaundice.

INTERACTIONS
Ammonium chloride, ascorbic acid, paraldehyde: doses sufficient to acidify urine may cause precipitation of sulfonamide and crystalluria. Don't use together.
PABA-containing local anesthetics and other PABA drugs: inhibited antibacterial action. Don't use together.

NURSING CONSIDERATIONS
• Contraindicated in porphyria or in infants younger than 2 months (except in congenital toxoplasmosis). Use cautiously and in reduced dosages in impaired hepatic or renal function, bronchial asthma, history of multiple allergies, G-6-PD deficiency, blood dyscrasias.
• Tell patient to drink a full glass of water with each dose and to drink plenty of water throughout the day to prevent crystalluria. Monitor fluid intake and urinary output. Intake should be sufficient to produce output of 1,500 ml daily. To aid in prevention of crystalluria, sodium bicarbonate may be administered to alkalinize urine.
• Tell patient to take medication for as long as prescribed, even if he feels better. Warn patient to avoid direct sunlight and ultraviolet light to prevent photosensitivity reaction.
• Give drug on schedule to maintain constant blood level.
• Watch for signs of blood dyscrasias (purpura, ecchymosis, sore throat, fever, pallor, or jaundice). Report them immediately.
• When giving I.V., make sure drug is well diluted. Infuse I.V. dosages slowly. If extravasation occurs, stop infusion and notify the doctor.
• Monitor urine cultures, CBC, and urinalysis before and during therapy.
• Mix with dextrose 5% in normal saline or Ringer's solution for I.V. infusion; any acidic solution (especially with pH below 9) causes precipitation. Use diluent cautiously. Discard solution if precipitation occurs.
• Sulfadiazine with pyrimethamine for treatment of toxoplasmosis may be continued for life. Therapy controls but does not cure toxoplasmosis.
• Folic or folinic acid may be used during rest periods in toxoplasmosis therapy to reverse hematopoietic depression and/or anemia associated with pyrimethamine and sulfadiazine.
• Protect drug from light.

---

sulfamerazine

INDICATIONS & DOSAGE
Antibacterial (rarely used alone)—
Adults: initially, 2 to 4 g P.O., then 500 mg to 1 g P.O. q 6 hours.
Children over 2 months: initially, 75 mg/Kg or 2 g/m^2, then 150 mg/Kg or 4 g/m^2 P.O. daily in 4 to 6 equally divided doses. Maximum daily dose 6 g.

SIDE EFFECTS

Blood: *agranulocytosis, aplastic anemia,* megaloblastic anemia, thrombocytopenia, leukopenia, hemolytic anemia.
CNS: headache, mental depression, convulsions, hallucinations.
GI: *nausea, vomiting, diarrhea,* abdominal pain, anorexia, stomatitis.
GU: toxic nephrosis with oliguria and anuria, crystalluria, hematuria.
Skin: *erythema multiforme (Stevens-Johnson syndrome), generalized skin eruption, epidermal necrolysis, exfoliative dermatitis,* photosensitivity, urticaria, pruritus.
Other: *hypersensitivity, serum sickness, drug fever,* jaundice.

INTERACTIONS

Ammonium chloride, ascorbic acid, paraldehyde: doses sufficient to acidify urine may cause precipitation of sulfonamide and crystalluria. Don't use together.
PABA-containing local anesthetics and other PABA drugs: inhibited antibacterial action. Don't use together.

NURSING CONSIDERATIONS

• Contraindicated in infants younger than 2 months (except in congenital toxoplasmosis) and in porphyria. Use cautiously in impaired hepatic or renal function, asthma, blood dyscrasias, G-6-PD deficiency, history of multiple allergies.
• Although drug has low incidence of crystalluria, tell patient to drink a full glass of water with each dose and to drink plenty of water throughout the day to prevent crystalluria. Monitor fluid intake and urinary output. Intake should be sufficient to produce output of 1,500 ml daily. To aid in prevention of crystalluria, sodium bicarbonate may be administered to alkalinize urine.
• Tell patient to take medication for as long as prescribed, even after he feels better. Warn patient to avoid direct sunlight and ultraviolet light to prevent photosensitivity reaction. Instruct patient to report early signs of blood dyscrasias (sore throat, fever, pallor, or jaundice) immediately and to stop taking drug.
• Monitor urine cultures, CBC, and urinalysis before and during therapy.
• Used in combination sulfonamide preparations such as Triple Sulfa with pyrimethamine to treat toxoplasmosis.
• Watch for signs of GI superinfection during long-term therapy.
• When given preop, the patient should receive a low-residue diet and a minimum of enemas and cathartics.

sulfameter
Sulla♦

INDICATIONS & DOSAGE

Urinary tract infections only—
Adults, and children over 12: initially, 1.5 g P.O., then 500 mg daily.

SIDE EFFECTS

Blood: *agranulocytosis, aplastic anemia,* megaloblastic anemia, thrombocytopenia, leukopenia, hemolytic anemia.
CNS: headache, mental depression, convulsions, hallucinations.
GI: *nausea, vomiting, diarrhea,* abdominal pain, anorexia, stomatitis.
GU: toxic nephrosis with oliguria and anuria, crystalluria, hematuria.
Skin: *erythema multiforme (Stevens-Johnson syndrome), generalized skin eruption, epidermal necrolysis, exfoliative dermatitis,* photosensitivity, urticaria, pruritus.
Other: *hypersensitivity, serum sickness, drug fever,* jaundice.

INTERACTIONS

Ammonium chloride, ascorbic acid, paraldehyde: doses sufficient to acidify urine may cause precipitation of

sulfonamide and crystalluria. Don't use together.
PABA-containing local anesthetics and other PABA drugs: inhibited antibacterial action. Don't use together.

NURSING CONSIDERATIONS

• Contraindicated in patients weighing less than 45 Kg (100 pounds); porphyria. Use cautiously and in reduced dosages in impaired hepatic or renal function, those receiving oral hypoglycemic agents (sulfonylurea), in early pregnancy, blood dyscrasias, G-6-PD deficiency, asthma, and in patients with history of multiple allergies.
• Tell patient to drink a full glass of water with each dose and to drink plenty of water throughout the day to prevent crystalluria. Monitor fluid intake and urinary output. Intake should be sufficient to produce output of 2,000 to 2,500 ml daily. To aid in prevention of crystalluria, sodium bicarbonate may be administered to alkalinize urine.
• Tell patient to take medication for as long as prescribed, even after he feels better. Warn patient to avoid direct sunlight and ultraviolet light to prevent photosensitivity reaction. Instruct patient to report early signs of blood dyscrasias (sore throat, fever, pallor, or jaundice) immediately and to stop taking drug.
• Check patient's urine pH frequently. If it's very acidic, the doctor may want to order sodium bicarbonate to alkalinize it.
• Monitor urine cultures, CBC, and urinalysis before and during therapy.
• Long-acting sulfonamide; never use in place of short-acting sulfonamides to treat systemic infections.
• Associated with increased incidence of severe and fatal adverse reactions.

sulfamethizole
Bursul, Microsul, Proklar-M, Sulfasol, Sulfstat, Sulfurine, Thiosulfil♦, Unisul, Uri-Pak, Urifon, Utrasul

INDICATIONS & DOSAGE
Urinary tract infections only—
Adults: 500 mg to 1 g P.O. t.i.d. to q.i.d.
Children over 2 months: 30 to 45 mg/Kg P.O. daily, divided into doses given q 6 hours.

SIDE EFFECTS
Blood: *agranulocytosis, aplastic anemia,* megaloblastic anemia, thrombocytopenia, leukopenia, hemolytic anemia.
CNS: headache, mental depression, convulsions, hallucinations.
GI: *nausea, vomiting, diarrhea,* abdominal pain, anorexia, stomatitis.
GU: toxic nephrosis with oliguria and anuria, crystalluria, hematuria.
Skin: *erythema multiforme (Stevens-Johnson syndrome), generalized skin eruption, epidermal necrolysis, exfoliative dermatitis,* photosensitivity, urticaria, pruritus.
Other: *hypersensitivity, serum sickness, drug fever,* jaundice.

INTERACTIONS
Ammonium chloride, ascorbic acid, paraldehyde: doses sufficient to acidify urine may cause precipitation of sulfonamide and crystalluria. Don't use together.
PABA-containing local anesthetics and other PABA drugs: inhibited antibacterial action. Don't use together.

NURSING CONSIDERATIONS
• Contraindicated in porphyria. Use cautiously and in reduced dosages in impaired hepatic or renal function, blood dyscrasias, G-6-PD deficiency, asthma, history of multiple allergies.
• Tell patient to drink a full glass of

water with each dose and to drink plenty of water throughout the day to prevent crystalluria. Monitor fluid intake and urinary output. Intake should be sufficient to produce output of 1,500 ml daily. To aid in prevention of crystalluria, sodium bicarbonate may be administered to alkalinize urine.
• Tell patient to take medication for as long as prescribed, even after he feels better. Warn patient to avoid direct sunlight and ultraviolet light to prevent photosensitivity reaction. Instruct patient to report early signs of blood dyscrasias (sore throat, fever, pallor, or jaundice) immediately and to stop taking drug.
• Monitor urine cultures, CBC, and urinalysis before and during therapy.

sulfamethoxazole
Gantanol ♦

INDICATIONS & DOSAGE
Urinary tract and systemic infections—
Adults: initially, 2 g P.O., then 1 g P.O. b.i.d. up to t.i.d. for severe infections.
Children and infants over 2 months: initially, 50 to 60 mg/Kg P.O., then 25 to 30 mg/Kg b.i.d. Maximum dose should not exceed 75 mg/Kg daily.

SIDE EFFECTS
Blood: *agranulocytosis, aplastic anemia,* megaloblastic anemia, thrombocytopenia, leukopenia, hemolytic anemia.
CNS: headache, mental depression, convulsions, hallucinations.
GI: *nausea, vomiting, diarrhea,* abdominal pain, anorexia, stomatitis.
GU: toxic nephrosis with oliguria and anuria, crystalluria, hematuria.
Skin: *erythema multiforme (Stevens-Johnson syndrome),* generalized skin eruption, *epidermal necrolysis, exfo-*

liative dermatitis, photosensitivity, urticaria, pruritus.
Other: *hypersensitivity, serum sickness, drug fever,* jaundice.

INTERACTIONS
Ammonium chloride, ascorbic acid, paraldehyde: doses sufficient to acidify urine may cause precipitation of sulfonamide and crystalluria. Don't use together.
PABA-containing local anesthetics and other PABA drugs: inhibited antibacterial action. Don't use together.

NURSING CONSIDERATIONS
• Contraindicated in porphyria or in infants younger than 2 months (except in congenital toxoplasmosis). Use cautiously and in reduced dosages in impaired hepatic or renal function and in those with severe allergy or bronchial asthma, G-6-PD deficiency, blood dyscrasias.
• Tell patient to drink a full glass of water with each dose and to drink plenty of water during the day to prevent crystalluria. Monitor fluid intake/urinary output. Intake should be sufficient to produce output of 1,500 ml daily. To aid in prevention of crystalluria, sodium bicarbonate may be administered to alkalinize urine.
• Tell patient to take medication for as long as prescribed, even after he feels better. Warn patient to avoid direct sunlight and ultraviolet light to prevent photosensitivity reaction.
• Monitor urine cultures, CBC, and urinalysis before and during therapy.
• Sulfamethoxazole is also used in adjunctive therapy for treatment of toxoplasmosis following therapy with other first line agents.
• Instruct patient to report early signs of blood dyscrasias (sore throat, fever, pallor, or jaundice) immediately and to stop taking drug.

sulfamethoxypyridazine
Midicel

INDICATIONS & DOSAGE
Urinary and systemic infections—
Adults over 60 Kg: initially, 1 g P.O. followed by 500 mg daily or 1 g every other day. For severe infection, initially, 2 g P.O. followed by 500 mg daily.
Adults under 60 Kg: initially, 1 g P.O. followed by 250 mg P.O. daily.
Children over 2 months: initially, 30 mg/Kg P.O. followed by 15 mg/Kg P.O. daily. Maximum initial dose 1 g and 500 mg thereafter.

SIDE EFFECTS
Blood: *agranulocytosis, aplastic anemia,* megaloblastic anemia, thrombocytopenia, leukopenia, hemolytic anemia.
CNS: headache, mental depression, convulsions, hallucinations.
GI: *nausea, vomiting, diarrhea,* abdominal pain, anorexia, stomatitis.
GU: toxic nephrosis with oliguria and anuria, crystalluria, hematuria.
Skin: *erythema multiforme (Stevens-Johnson syndrome), generalized skin eruption, epidermal necrolysis, exfoliative dermatitis,* photosensitivity, urticaria, pruritus.
Other: *hypersensitivity, serum sickness, drug fever,* jaundice.

INTERACTIONS
Ammonium chloride, ascorbic acid, paraldehyde: doses sufficient to acidify urine may cause precipitation of sulfonamide and crystalluria. Don't use together.
PABA-containing local anesthetics and other PABA drugs: inhibited antibacterial action. Don't use together.

NURSING CONSIDERATIONS
• Contraindicated in porphyria. Use cautiously and in reduced dosages in impaired hepatic or renal function, asthma, blood dyscrasias, G-6-PD deficiency, history of multiple allergies.
• Administer immediately after meals.
• Watch for signs of Stevens-Johnson syndrome (high fever, rash, severe headache, stomatitis, conjunctivitis). Stop drug at once if these occur.
• Tell patient to drink a full glass of water with each dose and to drink plenty of water during the day to prevent crystalluria. Monitor fluid intake/urinary output. Intake should be sufficient to produce output of 1,500 ml daily. To aid in prevention of crystalluria, sodium bicarbonate may be administered to alkalinize urine.
• Tell patient to take medication for as long as prescribed, even after he feels better. Warn patient to avoid direct sunlight and ultraviolet light to prevent photosensitivity reaction.
• Monitor urine cultures, CBC, and urinalysis before and during therapy.
• Sulfamethoxypyridazine a long-acting sulfonamide and should not be used in place of short-acting sulfonamides to treat systemic infections.

sulfapyridine
Dagenan♦♦

INDICATIONS & DOSAGE
Dermatitis herpetiformis—
Adults: 500 mg P.O. q.i.d. until improvement noted, then decrease dose by 500 mg every 3 days until minimum effective maintenance dose achieved.

SIDE EFFECTS
Blood: *agranulocytosis, aplastic anemia,* megaloblastic anemia, thrombocytopenia, leukopenia, hemolytic anemia.
CNS: headache, mental depression, convulsions, hallucinations.

GI: *nausea, vomiting, diarrhea,* abdominal pain, anorexia, stomatitis.
GU: toxic nephrosis with oliguria and anuria, crystalluria, hematuria.
Skin: *erythema multiforme (Stevens-Johnson syndrome), generalized skin eruption, epidermal necrolysis, exfoliative dermatitis,* photosensitivity, urticaria, pruritus.
Other: *hypersensitivity, serum sickness, drug fever,* jaundice.

INTERACTIONS

Ammonium chloride, ascorbic acid, paraldehyde: doses sufficient to acidify urine may cause precipitation of sulfonamide and crystalluria. Don't use together.
PABA-containing local anesthetics and other PABA drugs: inhibited antibacterial action. Don't use together.

NURSING CONSIDERATIONS

• Contraindicated in porphyria. Use cautiously and in reduced dosages in impaired hepatic or renal function, G-6-PD deficiency, history of multiple allergies, asthma, blood dyscrasias.
• Tell patient to drink a full glass of water with each dose and to drink plenty of water during the day to prevent crystalluria. Monitor fluid intake/urinary output. Intake should be sufficient to produce output of 1,500 ml daily.
• Alkalinization of the urine may decrease the danger of crystalluria but may greatly increase renal tubular reabsorption of the drug, sustained blood levels, and risk of toxicity.
• Tell patient to take medication for as long as prescribed, even after he feels better. Warn patient to avoid direct sunlight and ultraviolet light to prevent photosensitivity reaction.
• Monitor urine cultures, CBC, and urinalysis before and during therapy.
• Sulfapyridine is an intermediate-acting sulfonamide with a high potential for toxicity; its use is restricted to treatment of dermatitis herpetiformis when sulfone therapy is contraindicated.
• Tell patient to report any side effects at once and to stop drug.

---

sulfasalazine
Azulfidine, Azulfidine En-Tabs, SAS-500

INDICATIONS & DOSAGE

Mild to moderate ulcerative colitis, adjunctive therapy in severe ulcerative colitis—
Adults: initially, 3 to 4 g P.O. daily in evenly divided doses; usual maintenance dose is 1.5 to 2 g P.O. daily in divided doses q 6 hours. May need to start with 1 to 2 g initially, with a gradual increase in dose to minimize side effects.
Children over 2 years: initially, 40 to 60 mg/Kg P.O. daily, divided into 3 to 6 doses; then 30 mg/Kg daily in 4 doses.
May need to start at lower dose if gastrointestinal intolerance occurs.

SIDE EFFECTS

Blood: *agranulocytosis, aplastic anemia,* megaloblastic anemia, thrombocytopenia, leukopenia, hemolytic anemia.
CNS: headache, mental depression, convulsions, hallucinations.
GI: *nausea, vomiting, diarrhea,* abdominal pain, anorexia, stomatitis.
GU: toxic nephrosis with oliguria and anuria, crystalluria, hematuria.
Skin: *erythema multiforme (Stevens-Johnson syndrome), generalized skin eruption, epidermal necrolysis, exfoliative dermatitis,* photosensitivity, urticaria, pruritus.
Other: *hypersensitivity, serum sickness, drug fever,* jaundice.

INTERACTIONS

Ammonium chloride, ascorbic acid,

paraldehyde: doses sufficient to acidify urine may cause precipitation of sulfonamide and crystalluria. Don't use together.
PABA-containing local anesthetics and other PABA drugs: inhibited antibacterial action. Don't use together.

NURSING CONSIDERATIONS
• Contraindicated in porphyria. Use cautiously and in reduced dosages in impaired hepatic or renal function and in those with severe allergy or bronchial asthma, G-6-PD deficiency.
• Tell patient to drink a full glass of water with each dose and to drink plenty of water during the day to prevent crystalluria. Monitor fluid intake/urinary output. Intake should be sufficient to produce output of 1,500 ml daily.
• Instruct patient to take medication for as long as prescribed, even after he feels better. Warn patient to avoid direct sunlight and ultraviolet light to prevent photosensitivity reaction.
• Monitor urine cultures, CBC, and urinalysis before and during therapy.
• Colors urine orange-yellow.
• Side effects are usually those affecting the GI tract. Minimize symptoms by spacing doses evenly.

sulfisoxazole
Barazole, Gantrisin♦, G-Sox, J-Sul, Lipo Gantrisin, Novosoxazole♦♦, Rosoxol, SK-Soxazole, Sosol, Soxa, Soxomide, Sulfagan, Sulfalar, Sulfizin, Sulfizole♦♦, Urisoxin, Urizole, Velmatrol

INDICATIONS & DOSAGE
Urinary tract and systemic infections—
Adults: initially, 2 to 4 g P.O., then 1 to 2 g P.O. q.i.d.; extended-release suspension 4 to 5 g P.O. q 12 hours.
Children over 2 months: initially, 75 mg/Kg P.O. daily or 2 g/m² P.O.

daily in divided doses q 6 hours, then 150 mg/Kg or 4 g/m² P.O. daily in divided doses q 6 hours; extended-release suspension 60 to 70 mg/Kg P.O. q 12 hours.
Adults, and children over 2 months: parenteral dosages (sulfisoxazole diolamine) initially, 50 mg/Kg or 1.125 g/m² by slow I.V. injection, then 100 mg/Kg daily or 2.25 g/m² daily in divided doses q 6 hours by slow I.V. injection. 40% solution must be diluted to a concentration of 5% for I.V. use.

SIDE EFFECTS
Blood: *agranulocytosis, aplastic anemia,* megaloblastic anemia, thrombocytopenia, leukopenia, hemolytic anemia.
CNS: headache, mental depression, convulsions, hallucinations.
GI: *nausea, vomiting, diarrhea,* abdominal pain, anorexia, stomatitis.
GU: toxic nephrosis with oliguria and anuria, crystalluria, hematuria.
Skin: *erythema multiforme (Stevens-Johnson syndrome), generalized skin eruption, epidermal necrolysis, exfoliative dermatitis,* photosensitivity, urticaria, pruritus.
Other: *hypersensitivity, serum sickness, drug fever,* jaundice.

INTERACTIONS
PABA-containing local anesthetics and other PABA drugs: inhibited antibacterial action. Don't use together.
Ammonium chloride, ascorbic acid, paraldehyde: doses sufficient to acidify urine may cause crystalluria and precipitation of sulfonamide. Don't use together.

NURSING CONSIDERATIONS
• Contraindicated in porphyria and in infants younger than 2 months (except in congenital toxoplasmosis). Use cautiously in impaired hepatic or renal function, severe allergy or bronchial asthma, G-6-PD deficiency.

• Tell patient to drink a full glass of water with each dose and to drink plenty of water throughout the day to prevent crystalluria. Monitor fluid intake and urinary output. Intake should be sufficient to produce output of 1,500 ml daily. To aid in prevention of crystalluria, sodium bicarbonate may be administered to alkalinize urine.

• Tell patient to take medication for as long as prescribed, even after he feels better. Warn patient to avoid direct sunlight and ultraviolet light to prevent photosensitivity reaction.

• Monitor urine cultures, CBC, and urinalysis before and during therapy.

• Parenteral form can be given I.M. or S.C., but these routes are discouraged. Administration of this form with parenteral fluids is not recommended.

• Diluents other than sterile distilled water may cause precipitation.

• Gantrisin suspension and Lipo Gantrisin suspension cannot be interchanged, since the latter is an extended-release preparation.

• Sulfisoxazole/pyrimethamine combination used to treat toxoplasmosis.

• Tell patient to report early signs of blood dyscrasias (sore throat, fever, pallor, or jaundice) immediately and to stop taking drug.

• Watch for signs of GI superinfection during long-term therapy.

• When given preop, the patient should receive a low-residue diet and a minimum of enemas and cathartics.

• Although often given, initial loading dose is not pharmacologically necessary.

13

Urinary tract germicides

methenamine hippurate
methenamine mandelate
methenamine sulfosalicylate
methylene blue
nalidixic acid
nitrofurantoin
nitrofurantoin macrocrystals
oxolinic acid

methenamine hippurate
Hiprex, Hip-Rex♦♦, Urex
methenamine mandelate
Mandacon, Mandelamine♦, Mande-
lets, Mandelurine♦♦, Methandine♦♦,
Prov-U-Sep, Renelate, Sterine♦♦
methenamine sulfosalicylate
Hexalet

INDICATIONS & DOSAGE
*Long-term prophylaxis or suppression
of chronic urinary tract infections
(hippurate)—*
Adults, and children over 12 years:
1 g P.O. q 12 hours.
Children 6 to 12 years: 500 mg to
1 g P.O. q 12 hours.
*Urinary tract infections, infected re-
sidual urine in patients with neurogenic bladder (mandelate)—*
Adults: 1 g P.O. q.i.d. after meals.
Children 6 to 12 years: 500 mg P.O.
q.i.d. after meals.
Children under 6 years: 50 mg/Kg
divided in 4 doses after meals.
*Long-term prophylaxis or suppression
of chronic urinary tract infections
(sulfosalicylate)—*
Adults, and children over 12: 1 g

P.O. q.i.d. after meals with ½ glass
of water.
Children 6 to 12 years: 500 mg P.O.
q.i.d. after meals with ½ glass water.

SIDE EFFECTS
GI: *nausea.*
GU: with high doses, urinary tract ir-
ritation, dysuria, frequency, albumin-
uria, hematuria.
Hepatic: elevated liver enzymes.
Skin: rashes.

INTERACTIONS
Alkalinizing agents: inhibited methenamine action. Don't use together.
Acetazolamide: antagonized methenamine effect. Use together cautiously.

NURSING CONSIDERATIONS
• Contraindicated in renal insufficiency, severe hepatic disease, or severe dehydration.
• Ineffective against *Candida*
infection.
• Oral suspension contains vegetable
oil. Administer cautiously to elderly
or debilitated patients because aspiration could cause lipid pneumonia.
• Monitor intake/output. Intake
should be at least 1,500 to 2,000 ml/
day.
• Obtain clean voided urine specimen
for culture and sensitivity before
starting therapy and repeat p.r.n.
• Limit intake of alkaline foods, such
as vegetables, milk, peanuts, fruits,
and fruit juices, except cranberry,
plum, and prune juices. These juices
or ascorbic acid may be used to acidify urine.

- Warn patient not to take antacids, including Alka-Seltzer and sodium bicarbonate.
- Maintain urine pH at 5.5 or less. Use Nitrazine paper to check pH.
- *Proteus* and *Pseudomonas* tend to raise urine pH; urinary acidifiers are usually necessary when treating these infections.
- Obtain liver function studies periodically during long-term therapy.
- Administer after meals to lessen GI upset.
- If rash appears, hold dose and contact doctor.

methylene blue
M-B Tabs, MG-Blue, Urolene Blue, Wright's Stain

INDICATIONS & DOSAGE
Cystitis, urethritis—
Adults: 65 mg P.O. b.i.d. or t.i.d. after meals with glass of water.
Methemoglobinemia and cyanide poisoning—
Adults and children: 1 to 2 mg/Kg of 1% sterile solution slow I.V.

SIDE EFFECTS
Blood: anemia (long-term use).
GI: nausea, vomiting, diarrhea.
GU: dysuria, bladder irritation.
Other: fever (large doses).

INTERACTIONS
None significant.

NURSING CONSIDERATIONS
- Contraindicated in patients with renal insufficiency.
- Monitor intake/output carefully. Intake should be at least 2,000 ml/day.
- Monitor hemoglobin; possibility of anemia from accelerated destruction of erythrocytes.
- Turns urine and stool blue-green.
- Seldom used as urinary antiseptic.

- I.V. form has been used to treat nitrite intoxication.

nalidixic acid
NegGram♦

INDICATIONS & DOSAGE
Acute and chronic urinary tract infections caused by susceptible gram-negative organisms (Proteus, Klebsiella, Enterobacter, and E. coli)—
Adults: 1 g P.O. q.i.d. for 7 to 14 days; 2 g daily for long-term use.
Children over 3 months: 55 mg/Kg P.O. daily divided q.i.d. for 7 to 14 days; 33 mg/Kg/day for long-term use.

SIDE EFFECTS
Blood: eosinophilia.
CNS: drowsiness, weakness, headache, dizziness, vertigo, convulsions in epileptics.
EENT: sensitivity to light, change in color perception, diplopia, blurred vision.
GI: *abdominal pain, nausea, vomiting,* diarrhea.
Skin: pruritus, photosensitivity, urticaria, rash.
Other: angioedema, fever, chills, increased intracranial pressure and bulging fontanels in infants and children.

INTERACTIONS
Nitrofurantoin: may antagonize nalidixic acid effect. Use together cautiously.

NURSING CONSIDERATIONS
- Contraindicated in convulsive disorders. Use with caution in impaired hepatic or renal function, epilepsy, or severe cerebral arteriosclerosis.
- Not effective against *Pseudomonas*.
- Report visual disturbances; usually disappear with reduced dose.
- Obtain clean voided urine specimen

for culture and sensitivity before starting therapy and repeat p.r.n.
• Obtain CBC, kidney and liver function studies during long-term therapy.
• Resistant bacteria may emerge within first 48 hours of therapy.
• May cause a false positive Clinitest reaction. Use Clinistix or Tes-Tape to monitor urine glucose. Also gives false elevations in urinary vanillylmandelic acid (VMA) and 17-ketosteroids. Repeat tests after therapy completed.
• Avoid undue exposure to sunlight due to photosensitivity. Patient may continue to be photosensitive up to 3 months after drug is discontinued.

nitrofurantoin
Cyantin, Furadantin, Furalan, Furatine♦♦, Furantoin, Ivadantin, J-Dantin, Nephronex♦♦, Nifuran♦♦, Nitrex, Novofuran♦♦, Parfuran, Sarodant
nitrofurantoin macrocrystals
Macrodantin♦

INDICATIONS & DOSAGE
Pyelonephritis, pyelitis, and cystitis due to susceptible E. coli, S. aureus, enterococci; certain strains of Klebsiella, Proteus, and Enterobacter—
Adults, and children over 12: 50 to 100 mg P.O. q.i.d. with meals. Or, 180 mg I.M. or I.V. b.i.d. in patients over 55 Kg; 5 to 7 mg/Kg daily I.M. or I.V. in patients under 55 Kg.
Children 1 month to 12 years: 5 to 7 mg/Kg P.O. daily, divided q.i.d.

SIDE EFFECTS
Blood: hemolysis in patients with G-6-PD deficiency (reversed after stopping drug).
CNS: peripheral neuropathy, headache, dizziness, drowsiness, ascending polyneuropathy with high doses or renal impairment.

GI: anorexia, *nausea, vomiting,* abdominal pain, *diarrhea.*
Hepatic: hepatitis.
Skin: maculopapular, erythematous, or eczematous eruption; pruritus; urticaria.
Other: asthmatic attacks in patients with history of asthma; *anaphylaxis;* drug fever; overgrowth of nonsusceptible organisms in the urinary tract; *pulmonary sensitivity reactions (cough, chest pains, fever, chills, dyspnea).*

INTERACTIONS
None significant.

NURSING CONSIDERATIONS
• Contraindicated in moderate to severe renal impairment, anuria, oliguria, creatinine clearance under 40 ml/min; in G-6-PD deficiency.
• Obtain clean voided urine specimen for culture and sensitivity before starting therapy and repeat p.r.n.
• Give with food or milk to minimize GI distress.
• I.M. route painful and should not be used for more than 5 days.
• Dilute I.V. nitrofurantoin to 500 ml of suitable I.V. solution before administering. Constitute in sterile water without preservatives.
• Monitor intake/output carefully. May turn urine brown or darker.
• Store in amber container. Keep away from metals other than stainless steel or aluminum to avoid precipitate formation. Warn patients not to use pillboxes made of these materials.
• Continue treatment for 3 days after sterile urine specimens obtained.
• Monitor pulmonary status.
• May cause false positive test results with urine sugar using copper sulfate reduction method (Clinitest) but not with glucose oxidase tests (Tes-Tape, Diastix, Clinistix).

Italicized side effects are common or life-threatening.

oxolinic acid
Utibid

INDICATIONS & DOSAGE
Cystitis, urethritis, pyelonephritis, pyelitis, caused by susceptible gram-negative organisms (Proteus, Klebsiella, E. coli, and Enterobacter)—
Adults: 1 tablet (750 mg) P.O. b.i.d. for 2 weeks.

SIDE EFFECTS
Blood: transient leukopenia.
CNS: *insomnia, dizziness, nervousness,* drowsiness, headache, impaired alertness, impaired physical coordination, weakness.
GI: *nausea,* abdominal cramps, anorexia, vomiting, diarrhea, constipation.

INTERACTIONS
Nitrofurantoin: decreased response to oxolinic acid. Avoid if possible.

NURSING CONSIDERATIONS
• Contraindicated in convulsive disorders. Use cautiously in impaired renal function; in older patients, as the drug may cause CNS stimulation.
• Safe use when taken concurrently with other CNS stimulants not established.
• Before and during therapy, monitor for development of resistant organisms by obtaining urine specimens for culture and sensitivity.
• Warn patient that drug may cause dizziness.
• Monitor intake/output.

14

Miscellaneous

amantadine hydrochloride
bacitracin
chloramphenicol
chloramphenicol palmitate
chloramphenicol sodium succinate
clindamycin hydrochloride
clindamycin palmitate
  hydrochloride
clindamycin phosphate
colistimethate sodium
erythromycin base
erythromycin estolate
erythromycin ethylsuccinate
erythromycin gluceptate
erythromycin lactobionate
erythromycin stearate
furazolidone
lincomycin hydrochloride
novobiocin calcium
novobiocin sodium
polymyxin B sulfate
spectinomycin dihydrochloride
trimethoprim
troleandomycin phosphate
vancomycin hydrochloride
vidarabine monohydrate

---

amantadine hydrochloride
Symmetrel♦

INDICATIONS & DOSAGE
Prophylaxis or symptomatic treatment of influenza type A virus, respiratory tract illnesses—
Adults, and children over 9 years:
200 mg P.O. daily in a single dose or divided b.i.d.
Children 1 to 9 years: 4.4 to
8.8 mg/Kg P.O. daily, divided b.i.d. or t.i.d. Don't exceed 150 mg daily. Symptomatic treatment should continue for 24 to 48 hours after symptoms disappear. Prophylaxis should start as soon as possible after initial exposure and continue for at least 10 days after exposure. May continue prophylactic treatment up to 90 days for repeated or suspected exposures if influenza vaccine unavailable. If used with influenza vaccine, continue dose for 2 to 3 weeks until protection from vaccine develops.

SIDE EFFECTS
CNS: depression, fatigue, confusion, dizziness, psychosis, hallucinations, anxiety, irritability, ataxia, insomnia, weakness, headache.
CV: peripheral edema, orthostatic hypotension, congestive heart failure.
GI: anorexia, nausea, constipation, vomiting, dry mouth.
GU: urinary retention.

INTERACTIONS
None significant.

NURSING CONSIDERATIONS
• Use cautiously in history of epilepsy, congestive heart failure, peripheral edema, hepatic disease, mental illness, eczematoid rash, renal impairment, orthostatic hypotension, cardiovascular disease, and in elderly patients.
• For best absorption, drug should be taken after meals.
• Instruct patient to report side effects to the doctor, especially dizzi-

ness, depression, anxiety, nausea, and urinary retention.
• Monitor electrolyte balance and urinary output.
• If orthostatic hypotension occurs, instruct patient not to stand or change positions too quickly.
• If insomnia occurs, dose should be taken several hours before bedtime.
• Prophylactic use recommended for patients who can't receive influenza virus vaccine.

bacitracin

INDICATIONS & DOSAGE
Pneumonia or empyema caused by susceptible staphylococci—
Infants over 2.5 Kg: 1,000 units/Kg I.M. daily, divided q 8 to 12 hours.
Infants under 2.5 Kg: 900 units/Kg I.M. daily, divided q 8 to 12 hours. Although the F.D.A. approves the use of bacitracin in infants only, adults with susceptible staphylococcal infections may receive 10,000 to 25,000 units I.M. q 6 hours (maximum 25,000 units/dose, 100,000 units/day).

SIDE EFFECTS
Blood: blood dyscrasias, eosinophilia.
GI: nausea, vomiting, anorexia, diarrhea, rectal itching or burning.
GU: nephrotoxicity *(albuminuria, cylindruria, oliguria, anuria, increased BUN, tubular and glomerular necrosis).*
Skin: urticaria, rash.
Local: *pain at injection site.*
Other: superinfection, fever, *anaphylaxis.*

INTERACTIONS
None significant.

NURSING CONSIDERATIONS
• Contraindicated in impaired renal

function. Use cautiously in superinfections or neuromuscular disease.
• Culture and sensitivity test should be done initially and p.r.n.
• For I.M. administration only. Give deeply I.M.; injection may be painful; often diluted with procaine hydrochloride. Do not give if patient sensitive to procaine or PABA derivatives.
• Maintain adequate fluid intake, and monitor urinary output closely.
• Obtain baseline renal function studies before starting therapy. Monitor renal function (BUN, serum creatinine, creatinine clearance) daily during therapy. Notify doctor of any change.
• Dilute in solution containing sodium chloride and 2% procaine hydrochloride. Concentration of bacitracin should be between 5,000 and 10,000 units/ml. Store in refrigerator. Drug is inactivated at room temperature.
• Report side effects to the doctor immediately.
• May be used with neomycin as a bowel prep, or in solution as a wound irrigant.
• Urine pH should be kept above 6.

chloramphenicol

chloramphenicol palmitate

chloramphenicol sodium succinate
Chloromycetin♦, Mychel, Novochlorocap♦♦

INDICATIONS & DOSAGE
Hemophilus influenzae, meningitis, acute S. typhi infection, severe infections caused by sensitive Salmonella species, Rickettsia, lymphogranuloma, psittacosis, various sensitive gram-negative organisms causing meningitis, bacteremia, or other serious infections—

Adults and children: 50 to
100 mg/Kg P.O. or I.V. daily, divided
q 6 hours. Maximum dose is 100 mg/
Kg/day.
**Prematures and neonates (2 weeks
or younger):** 25 mg/Kg P.O. or I.V.
daily, divided q 6 hours. I.V. route
must be used to treat meningitis.

SIDE EFFECTS
Blood: *aplastic anemia,* hypoplastic
anemia, *granulocytopenia,* thrombocytopenia.
CNS: headache, mild depression,
confusion, delirium, peripheral neuropathy with prolonged therapy.
EENT: optic neuritis (in cystic fibrosis patients), glossitis, decreased visual acuity.
GI: nausea, vomiting, stomatitis,
diarrhea, enterocolitis.
Other: infections by nonsusceptible
organisms, hypersensitivity reaction
(fever, rash, urticaria, *anaphylaxis),
"gray baby syndrome" (abdominal
distention, cyanosis, vasomotor collapse, death within a few hours of onset of symptoms).*

INTERACTIONS
Penicillins: antagonized antibacterial
effect. Give penicillin at least 1 hour
before.
Acetaminophen: elevated chloramphenicol levels. Monitor for chloramphenicol toxicity.

NURSING CONSIDERATIONS
• Use cautiously in impaired hepatic
or renal function, with other drugs
causing bone marrow depression or
blood disorders. Don't use for infections susceptible to other agents or for
trivial infections such as colds.
• Culture and sensitivity test should
be done initially and p.r.n.
• Monitor CBC, platelets, serum
iron, and reticulocytes before and every 2 days during therapy. Stop drug
immediately if anemia, reticulocyto-

penia, leukopenia, or thrombocytopenia develops.
• Give I.V. slowly over 1 minute.
Check injection site daily for phlebitis
and irritation.
• Instruct patient to report side effects to the doctor, especially nausea,
vomiting, diarrhea, fever, confusion,
sore throat, or mouth sores.
• Tell patient to take medication for
as long as prescribed, exactly as directed, even after he feels better.
• Reconstitute 1 g vial of powder for
injection with 10 ml sterile water for
injection. Concentration will be
100 mg/ml. Stable for 30 days at
room temperature, but refrigeration
recommended. Do not use cloudy
solutions.

clindamycin hydrochloride

**clindamycin palmitate
   hydrochloride**

clindamycin phosphate
Cleocin, Dalacin C♦♦

INDICATIONS & DOSAGE
*Infections caused by sensitive staphy-
lococci, streptococci, pneumococci,
Bacteroides, Fusobacterium, Clostridium perfringens, and other sensitive
aerobic and anaerobic organisms—*
Adults: 150 to 450 mg P.O. q 6
hours; or 300 mg I.M. or I.V. q 6, 8,
or 12 hours. Up to 2,700 mg I.M. or
I.V. daily, divided q 6, 8, or 12 hours.
May be used for severe infections.
Children over 1 month: 8 to 25 mg/
Kg P.O. daily, divided q 6 to 8 hours;
or 15 to 40 mg/Kg I.M. or I.V. daily,
divided q 6 hours.

SIDE EFFECTS
Blood: transient leukopenia, eosinophilia, thrombocytopenia.
GI: *nausea,* vomiting, abdominal
pain, *diarrhea, pseudomembranous*

enterocolitis, esophagitis, flatulence, anorexia, *bloody or tarry stools*.
Hepatic: elevated SGOT, alkaline phosphatase, bilirubin.
Skin: maculopapular rash, urticaria.
Local: *pain*, induration, *sterile abscess with I.M. injection;* thrombophlebitis, erythema, and pain following I.V. administration.
Other: unpleasant or bitter taste, *anaphylaxis*.

INTERACTIONS
Erythromycin: antagonist that may block access of clindamycin to its site of action; don't use together.

NURSING CONSIDERATIONS
• Contraindicated in known hypersensitivity to the antibiotic congener lincomycin; also in history of GI disease, especially colitis. Use cautiously in renal or hepatic disease, asthma, newborns, allergies.
• Culture and sensitivity test should be performed initially and p.r.n.
• Don't use in meningitis. Drug does not get into CSF.
• Don't refrigerate reconstituted oral solution, as it will thicken. Drug is stable for 2 weeks at room temperature.
• Instruct patient to report side effects to the doctor, especially diarrhea. Warn patient not to treat such diarrhea himself.
• Don't give diphenoxylate (Lomotil) to treat drug-induced diarrhea. May prolong and worsen diarrhea.
• Give deep I.M. Rotate sites. Warn that I.M. injection may be painful. Doses greater than 600 mg per injection are not recommended.
• When giving I.V., check site daily for phlebitis and irritation. For I.V. infusion, dilute each 300 mg in 50 ml solution, and give no faster than 30 mg/minute.
• Monitor renal and hepatic function during prolonged therapy.

• Topical form is now available to treat acne.

---

colistimethate sodium
Colistin Sulfate, Coly-Mycin M♦, Coly-Mycin S Oral

INDICATIONS & DOSAGE
Enterocolitis caused by sensitive E. coli, sensitive Shigella, gastroenteritis—
Infants and children: 5 to 15 mg/Kg P.O. daily, divided q 6 to 8 hours.
Severe infections, especially of urinary tract, caused by sensitive Pseudomonas, Enterobacteria, E. coli, and Klebsiella—
Adults and children: 2.5 to 5 mg/Kg I.M. or I.V. daily, divided q 6 to 12 hours. Maximum daily dose not to exceed 5 mg/Kg/day in patients with normal renal function.

SIDE EFFECTS
CNS: *circumoral and lingual paresthesias;* paresthesias of extremities; neuromuscular blockage with respiratory arrest, especially in patients with impaired renal function; dizziness; slurring of speech.
GI: nausea, vomiting, discomfort.
GU: *nephrotoxicity* (decreased urine output, increased blood urea nitrogen, increased serum creatinine).
Skin: pruritus, urticaria.
Local: pain at I.M. site.
Other: "drug fever," overgrowth of susceptible organisms.

INTERACTIONS
None significant.

NURSING CONSIDERATIONS
• Contraindicated in patients with known hypersensitivity to the antibiotic congener polymyxin B. Use cautiously in renal impairment.
• Give deep I.M. Rotate sites. Warn that I.M. injection may be painful.

• When giving I.V., check site daily for phlebitis and irritation. For direct intermittent I.V. administration, inject ½ daily dose over 3 to 5 minutes at 12-hour intervals.
• For continuous I.V. infusion, infuse ½ daily dose over 3 to 5 minutes; then infuse remainder 1 to 2 hours later at rate of 5 mg/hour.
• Monitor renal function (BUN, creatinine clearance, urinary output).
• Report side effects immediately, especially speech impairment or paresthesias. Watch for signs of superinfection.
• Store reconstituted oral suspension at 2° to 15° C. (35.6° to 59° F.), and use within 7 days.
• Use sterile water for injection to reconstitute. When mixing, swirl solution gently to avoid frothing. Always prepare I.V. infusion fresh. Use within 24 hours.

---

erythromycin base
E-Mycin♦, Erythromid♦♦, Ethril 500, Ilotycin♦, Novorythro♦♦, Robimycin♦, Staticin
erythromycin estolate
Ilosone♦, Novorythro♦♦
erythromycin ethylsuccinate
E.E.S., Erythrocin♦, Pediamycin, Wyamycin Liquid
erythromycin gluceptate
Ilotycin♦
erythromycin lactobionate
Erythrocin♦
erythromycin stearate
Bristamycin, E-Biotic, Ethril, Erypar, Erythrocin♦, Novorythro♦♦, Pfizer E, Romycin, SK-Erythromycin, Wintrocin, Wyamycin

---

INDICATIONS & DOSAGE
Acute pelvic inflammatory disease caused by N. gonorrhoeae—
Women: 500 mg I.V. (erythromycin gluceptate, lactobionate) q 6 hours for 3 days, then 250 mg (erythromycin base, estolate, stearate) or 400 mg (erythromycin ethylsuccinate) P.O. q 6 hours for 7 days.
Endocarditis prophylaxis for dental procedures—
Adults: 1 g (erythromycin base, estolate, stearate) P.O. before procedure, followed by 250 mg P.O. q 6 hours for 8 doses afterward; or 1,200 mg (erythromycin ethylsuccinate) P.O. before procedure, followed by 400 mg P.O. q 6 hours for 8 doses afterward.
Children: 20 mg/Kg (oral erythromycin salts) P.O.1½ to 2 hours before procedure, then 10 mg/Kg q 6 hours for 8 doses.
Intestinal amebiasis—
Adults: 250 mg (erythromycin base, estolate, stearate) P.O. q 6 hours for 10 to 14 days.
Children: 30 to 50 mg/Kg (erythromycin base, estolate, stearate) P.O. daily, divided q 6 hours for 10 to 14 days.
Mild-to-moderately severe respiratory tract, skin and soft tissue infections caused by sensitive group A beta-hemolytic streptococci, Diplococci pneumoniae, Mycoplasma pneumoniae, Corynebacterium diphtheriae, Bordetella pertussis, Listeria monocytogenes—
Adults: 250 to 500 mg (erythromycin base, estolate, stearate) P.O. q 6 hours; or 400 to 800 mg (erythromycin ethylsuccinate) P.O. q 6 hours; or 15 to 20 mg/Kg I.V. daily, as continuous infusion or divided q 6 hours.
Children: 30 mg/Kg to 50 mg/Kg (oral erythromycin salts) P.O. daily, divided q 6 hours; or 15 to 20 mg/Kg I.V. daily, divided q 4 to 6 hours.
Syphilis—
Adults: 500 mg (erythromycin base, estolate, stearate) P.O. q.i.d. for 15 days.

SIDE EFFECTS
EENT: hearing loss with high doses I.V.

Italicized side effects are common or life-threatening.

GI: *abdominal pain and cramping, nausea, vomiting, diarrhea.*
Hepatic: cholestatic hepatitis (with erythromycin estolate).
Skin: urticaria, rashes.
Local: *venous irritation, thrombophlebitis following I.V. injection.*
Other: overgrowth of nonsusceptible bacteria or fungi; *anaphylaxis;* fever.

INTERACTIONS
Clindamycin, lincomycin: may be antagonistic. Don't use together.
Penicillins: antagonized antibacterial effect. Give penicillin at least 1 hour before.

NURSING CONSIDERATIONS
• Erythromycin estolate contraindicated in hepatic disease. Use other erythromycin salts cautiously in impaired hepatic function.
• Culture and sensitivity test should be performed initially and p.r.n.
• For best absorption, instruct patient to take oral form of drug with a full glass of water 1 hour before or 2 hours after meals. If tablets are coated, they may be taken with meals. Don't drink fruit juice with medication. Chewable erythromycin tablets should not be swallowed whole.
• When dispensing or administering the suspension, be sure to note the concentration of a given product. Dispense by mg, not by ml.
• May cause overgrowth of nonsusceptible bacteria or fungi. Watch for signs and symptoms of superinfection.
• Tell patient to take medication for as long as prescribed, exactly as directed, even after he feels better. Treat streptococcal infections for 10 days.
• Report side effects, especially nausea, abdominal pain, or fever.
• Erythromycin estolate may cause serious hepatotoxicity in adults (reversible cholestatic hepatitis). Monitor hepatic function (bilirubin, SGOT,

SGPT, alkaline phosphatase). Other erythromycin salts cause hepatotoxicity to a lesser degree.
• I.V. dose should be administered over 20 to 60 minutes. Dilute each 250 mg in at least 100 ml 0.9% normal saline solution.
• Has been used successfully in the treatment of Legionnaire's disease.
• Topical form now available to treat acne.

---

furazolidone
Furoxone

INDICATIONS & DOSAGE
Gastroenteritis, adjunctive therapy in cholera—
Adults: 100 mg P.O. q.i.d.
Children 5 to 12 years: 25 to 50 mg P.O. q.i.d.
Children 1 to 4 years: 17 to 25 mg P.O. q.i.d.
Infants (1 month to 1 year): 8 to 17 mg P.O. q.i.d. Dosage based on 5 mg/Kg daily; maximum dose 8.8 mg/Kg daily.

SIDE EFFECTS
Blood: hemolytic anemia in infants under 1 month and G-6-PD deficiency; hypoglycemia; *agranulocytosis.*
CNS: headache, malaise.
GI: nausea, vomiting, abdominal pain, diarrhea.
Other: hypersensitivity reaction (arthralgia, fever, hypotension, rash, urticaria, angioedema).

INTERACTIONS
Sympathomimetics: hypertensive crisis. Don't use together.

NURSING CONSIDERATIONS
• Tell patient to take medication exactly as directed, even after he feels better.
• Report side effects to the doctor,

especially fever, rash, abdominal pain.
- Store medication in dark place at 2° to 15° C. (36.5° to 59° F.).
- Warn patient not to use over-the-counter nasal sprays or cold and hay fever products.
- Drug may turn urine brown. Flushing, nausea, sweating may occur following ethanol ingestion. Tell patient not to drink alcohol or use alcohol-containing medication.
- If patient is taking drug for more than 5 days, tell him not to eat broad beans, cheese, beer, wine, pickled herring, chicken livers, yeast extracts, or fermented products. Drug is similar to monoamine oxidase inhibitor.
- May cause false positive urine glucose with Benedict's Reagent.

---

lincomycin hydrochloride
Lincocin◆

INDICATIONS & DOSAGE
Respiratory tract, skin and soft tissue, and urinary tract infections; osteomyelitis, septicemia, caused by sensitive group A beta-hemolytic streptococci, pneumococci, and staphylococci—
Adults: 500 mg P.O. q 6 to 8 hours (not to exceed 8 g daily); or 600 mg I.M. daily or q 12 hours; or 600 mg to 1 g I.V. q 8 to 12 hours (not to exceed 8 g daily).
Children over 1 month: 30 to 60 mg/Kg P.O. daily, divided q 6 to 8 hours; or 10 mg/Kg I.M. daily or divided q 12 hours; or 10 to 20 mg/Kg I.V. daily, divided q 6 to 8 hours.
For I.V. infusion, dilute to 100 ml; infuse over 1 hour to avoid hypotension.

SIDE EFFECTS
Blood: *neutropenia, leukopenia,* thrombocytopenia, purpura.
CNS: dizziness, angioedema, headache.

CV: hypotension with rapid I.V. infusion.
EENT: glossitis, tinnitus.
GI: nausea, vomiting, *persistent diarrhea,* abdominal cramps, enterocolitis, stomatitis, pruritus ani.
GU: vaginitis.
Skin: rashes, urticaria.
Local: pain at injection site.
Other: hypersensitivity, cholestatic hepatitis.

INTERACTIONS
Antidiarrheal medication (kaolin, pectin, attapulgite): reduced oral absorption of lincomycin by as much as 90%. Antidiarrheals should be avoided or given at least 2 hours before lincomycin.

NURSING CONSIDERATIONS
- Contraindicated in known hypersensitivity to clindamycin. Use cautiously in history of GI disorders (especially colitis); asthma or other allergy; in hepatic or renal disease; and in endocrine or metabolic disorders.
- Culture and sensitivity tests should be done initially and p.r.n.
- For best absorption, instruct patient to take drug with a full glass of water 1 hour before or 2 hours after meals.
- Tell patient to take medication exactly as directed, even after he feels better.
- Tell patient to report side effects to doctor, especially diarrhea. Warn him not to treat diarrhea himself. Watch for signs of superinfection.
- Never treat drug-induced diarrhea with diphenoxylate (Lomotil); may prolong or worsen diarrhea.
- Monitor CBC and platelets. Stop drug immediately if neutropenia, leukopenia, or other blood disorders develop.
- Give deep I.M. Rotate sites. Warn that I.M. injection may be painful.
- When giving I.V., check site daily for phlebitis and irritation.
- Monitor hepatic function (alkaline

---

phosphatase, SGOT, SGPT, bilirubin).

novobiocin calcium

novobiocin sodium
Albamycin

INDICATIONS & DOSAGE
Serious infections from sensitive Staphylococcus aureus and Proteus when other antibiotics are contraindicated—
Adults: 250 to 500 mg P.O. q 6 hours, or 500 mg to 1 g q 12 hours (not to exceed 2 g daily).
Children: 15 to 45 mg/Kg P.O. daily, divided q 6 hours.

SIDE EFFECTS
Blood: pancytopenia, *leukopenia, agranulocytosis,* anemia, thrombocytopenia, eosinophilia.
GI: nausea, vomiting, anorexia, diarrhea, intestinal hemorrhage.
Hepatic: jaundice, hepatitis.
Skin: urticaria, *maculopapular dermatitis.*
Local: pain at injection site.
Other: *erythema multiforme,* fever in hypersensitivity reactions, swollen joints, overgrowth of nonsusceptible organisms.

INTERACTIONS
None significant.

NURSING CONSIDERATIONS
• Use cautiously in hepatic disease or blood disorders. Do not use in infants, as it may cause kernicterus.
• Culture and sensitivity tests should be done initially and p.r.n.
• For best absorption, instruct patient to take drug with a full glass of water 1 hour before or 2 hours after meals.
• Tell patient to take medication for as long as prescribed exactly as directed, even after he feels better.

• Report side effects, especially skin rash, fever, jaundice, or GI distress.
• Stop drug immediately if blood dyscrasia develops. Notify doctor.
• Monitor liver function (bilirubin, SGOT, SGPT, alkaline phosphatase).
• Monitor CBC, platelet, reticulocyte counts before and during therapy.

polymyxin B sulfate
Aerosporin♦

INDICATIONS & DOSAGE
Acute urinary tract infections or septicemia caused by sensitive P. aeruginosa, or when other antibiotics are ineffective or contraindicated; bacteremia caused by sensitive A. aerogenes and K. pneumoniae, or acute urinary tract infections caused by E. coli—
Adults and children: 15,000 to 25,000 units/Kg/day I.V. infusion, divided q 12 hours; or 25,000 to 30,000 units/Kg/day, divided q 4 to 8 hours. I.M. not advised due to severe pain at injection site.
Meningitis caused by sensitive P. aeruginosa or H. influenzae when other antibiotics ineffective or contraindicated—
Adults, and children over 2 years: 50,000 units intrathecally once daily for 3 to 4 days, then 50,000 units every other day for at least 2 weeks after cerebrospinal fluid tests are negative and cerebrospinal fluid sugar is normal.
Children under 2 years: 20,000 units intrathecally once daily for 3 to 4 days, then 25,000 units every other day for at least 2 weeks after cerebrospinal fluid tests are negative and cerebrospinal fluid sugar is normal.

SIDE EFFECTS
CNS: irritability, drowsiness, weakness, ataxia, respiratory paralysis, headache and meningeal irritation with intrathecal administration, pe-

ripheral and perioral paresthesias, convulsions, *coma*.
CV: facial flushing.
EENT: blurred vision.
GU: nephrotoxicity (albuminuria, cylindruria, hematuria, proteinuria, decreased urine output, increased BUN).
Skin: urticaria.
Local: *pain at I.M. injection site*.
Other: hypersensitivity reactions with fever, *anaphylaxis*.

INTERACTIONS
None significant.

NURSING CONSIDERATIONS
• Use cautiously in impaired renal function or myasthenia gravis.
• Give only to hospitalized patients under constant medical supervision.
• For meningitis, must give intrathecally to achieve adequate CSF levels.
• Give deep I.M. Warn that injection may be painful. If patient isn't allergic to procaine, use 1% procaine as diluent to decrease pain. Rotate sites.
• Don't give solution containing local anesthetics I.V. or intrathecally.
• When giving I.V., check site daily for phlebitis and irritation. Dilute each 500,000 units in 300 to 500 ml 5% dextrose in water; infuse over 60 to 90 minutes.
• Monitor renal function (BUN, serum creatinine, creatinine clearance, urinary output) before and during therapy. Intake should be sufficient to maintain output at 1,500 ml/day.
• Notify doctor immediately if patient develops fever, CNS side effects, rash, or symptoms of nephrotoxicity.

---

spectinomycin dihydrochloride
Trobicin♦

INDICATIONS & DOSAGE
Gonorrhea—

Adults: 2 to 4 g I.M. single dose injected deeply into the upper outer quadrant of the buttock.

SIDE EFFECTS
CNS: insomnia, dizziness.
GI: nausea.
GU: decreased urine output.
Skin: urticaria.
Local: pain at injection site.
Other: fever, chills (may mask or delay symptoms of incubating syphilis).

INTERACTIONS
None significant.

NURSING CONSIDERATIONS
• Not effective in the treatment of syphilis.
• Serologic test for syphilis should be done before treatment dose and 3 months after.
• Use 20-gauge needle to administer drug.
• Shake vial vigorously after reconstitution and before withdrawing dose. Store at room temperature after reconstitution and use within 24 hours.
• Should be reserved for penicillin-resistant strains of gonorrhea.

---

trimethoprim
Proloprim, Trimpex

INDICATIONS & DOSAGE
Treatment of uncomplicated urinary tract infections caused by susceptible strains of E. coli, P. mirabilis, Klebsiella, and Enterobacter species—
Adults: 100 mg P.O. every 12 hours for 10 days.
Not recommended for children under 12 years.

SIDE EFFECTS
Blood: thrombocytopenia, leukopenia, megaloblastic anemia, methemoglobinemia.

Italicized side effects are common or life-threatening.

GI: epigastric distress, nausea, vomiting, glossitis.
Skin: *rash, pruritus, exfoliative dermatitis.*
Other: fever.

INTERACTIONS
None significant.

NURSING CONSIDERATIONS
• Contraindicated in documented megaloblastic anemia due to folate deficiency.
• Clinical signs such as sore throat, fever, pallor, or purpura may be early indications of serious blood disorders. Complete blood counts should be done routinely. Prolonged use of trimethoprim at high doses may cause bone marrow depression.
• Dose should be decreased in patients with severely impaired renal function. Give cautiously to patients with impaired hepatic function.
• To be of benefit, full course of therapy should be completed.

troleandomycin phosphate
Tao

INDICATIONS & DOSAGE
Sensitive pneumococcal pneumonia or group A beta-hemolytic streptococcal respiratory tract infection—
Adults: 250 to 500 mg P.O. q 6 hours.
Children: 6.6 to 11 mg/Kg P.O. daily, q 6 hours.

SIDE EFFECTS
GI: *nausea,* vomiting, diarrhea.
Skin: urticaria and rashes in hypersensitivity reactions.
Other: cholestatic hepatitis (abdominal pain), jaundice, *anaphylaxis.*

INTERACTIONS
None significant.

NURSING CONSIDERATIONS
• Use cautiously in hepatic impairment.
• Drug is not recommended for routine use.
• For best absorption, instruct patient to take drug with a full glass of water 1 hour before or 2 hours after meals.
• Tell patient to take medication for as long as prescribed, exactly as directed, even after he feels better. Treat streptococcal infections at least 10 days.
• Monitor liver function (bilirubin, SGOT, SGPT, alkaline phosphatase).
• Report side effects, especially abdominal pain, nausea, or jaundice.

vancomycin hydrochloride
Vancocin♦

INDICATIONS & DOSAGE
Severe staphylococcal infections when other antibiotics ineffective or contraindicated—
Adults: 500 mg I.V. q 6 hours, or 1 g q 12 hours.
Children: 44 mg/Kg I.V. daily, divided q 6 hours.
Neonates: 10 mg/Kg I.V. daily, divided q 6 to 12 hours.
Antibiotic-associated pseudomembranous and staphylococcal enterocolitis—
Adults: 500 mg P.O. in 30 ml water q 6 hours.
Children: 44 mg/Kg P.O. daily, divided q 6 hours with 30 ml water.

SIDE EFFECTS
Blood: transient eosinophilia.
EENT: tinnitus, ototoxicity (deafness).
GI: nausea.
GU: nephrotoxicity (hyaline casts in urine, albuminuria, increased BUN).
Local: *pain or thrombophlebitis with I.V. administration. necrosis.*
Other: chills, fever, *anaphylaxis,*

overgrowth of nonsusceptible organisms.

INTERACTIONS
Oral contraceptives: cholestatic jaundice. Monitor bilirubin values.

NURSING CONSIDERATIONS
• Contraindicated in patients receiving other neurotoxic, nephrotoxic, or ototoxic drugs. Use cautiously in impaired liver, kidney function; also in preexisting hearing loss; in patients over 60 years; and in patients with allergies to other antibiotics.
• Tell patient to take medication exactly as directed, even after he feels better. Treat staphylococcal endocarditis for at least 4 weeks.
• Patients should receive auditory function tests before and during therapy.
• Tell patient to report side effects at once, especially dizziness, fullness or ringing in ears. Stop drug immediately.
• Do not give drug I.M.
• For I.V. infusion, dilute in 200 ml solution and infuse over 20 to 30 minutes. Check site daily for phlebitis and irritation. Report pain at infusion site. Avoid extravasation. Severe irritation and necrosis can result.
• Monitor kidney function (BUN, serum creatinine, urinalysis, creatinine clearance, urinary output) before and during therapy. Watch for signs of superinfection.
• Refrigerate I.V. solution after reconstitution and use within 96 hours.
• Oral preparation stable for 2 weeks if refrigerated.
• Has been used recently to treat pseudomembranous enterocolitis caused by clindamycin.

vidarabine monohydrate
Vira-A

INDICATIONS & DOSAGE
Herpes simplex virus encephalitis—
Adults: 15 mg/Kg/day for 10 days. Slowly infuse the total daily dose by I.V. infusion at a constant rate over 12 to 24 hour period. Avoid rapid or bolus injection.

SIDE EFFECTS
Blood: anemia, neutropenia, thrombocytopenia.
CNS: tremor, dizziness, hallucinations, confusion, psychosis, ataxia.
GI: *anorexia, nausea,* vomiting, diarrhea.
Hepatic: elevated SGOT, bilirubin.
Skin: pruritus, rash.
Local: pain at injection site.
Other: weight loss.

INTERACTIONS
None significant.

NURSING CONSIDERATIONS
• Will reduce mortality caused by herpes simplex virus encephalitis from 70% to 28%. No evidence that vidarabine is effective in encephalitis due to other viruses.
• Don't give I.M. or S.C. because of low solubility and poor absorption.
• Monitor hematologic tests such as hemoglobin, hematocrit, WBC, and platelets during therapy.
• Patient with impaired renal function may need dosage adjustment.
• Once in solution, vidarabine is stable at room temperature for at least 2 weeks.
• Use with an I.V. filter.
• Must be diluted to a concentration of less than 0.5 mg/ml.

Italicized side effects are common or life-threatening.

15

Cardiotonic glycosides

deslanoside
digitalis leaf
digitoxin
digoxin
gitalin
lanatoside C
ouabain

---

deslanoside
Cedilanid-D

INDICATIONS & DOSAGE
Congestive heart failure, paroxysmal atrial tachycardia, atrial fibrillation and flutter—
Adults: loading dose 1.2 to 1.6 mg I.M. or I.V. in 2 divided doses over 24 hours; for maintenance, use another glycoside.
Not recommended for children.

SIDE EFFECTS
The following are signs of toxicity that may occur with all cardiotonic glycosides:
CNS: *fatigue, generalized muscle weakness, agitation, hallucinations,* headache, malaise, dizziness, vertigo, stupor, paresthesias.
CV: *increased severity of congestive heart failure, arrhythmias (most commonly conduction disturbances with or without AV block, premature ventricular contractions, and supraventricular arrhythmias),* hypotension.
Toxic effects on heart may be life-threatening and require immediate attention.
EENT: *yellow-green halos around vi-sual images, blurred vision,* light flashes, photophobia, diplopia.
GI: *anorexia, nausea,* vomiting, diarrhea.

INTERACTIONS
Amphotericin B, carbenicillin, ticarcillin, corticosteroids, and diuretics, including chlorthalidone, ethacrynic acid, furosemide, metolazone, and thiazides: hypokalemia, predisposing patient to digitalis toxicity. Monitor serum potassium.
Parenteral calcium, thiazides: hypercalcemia and hypomagnesemia, predisposing patient to digitalis toxicity. Monitor serum calcium and serum magnesium.

NURSING CONSIDERATIONS
• Contraindicated in presence of any digitalis-induced toxicity; ventricular fibrillation; ventricular tachycardia unless caused by congestive heart failure. Administering calcium salts to digitalized patient is contraindicated. Calcium affects contractility and excitability of heart very much as glycosides do and may lead to serious arrhythmias in digitalized patient. Use with extreme caution with acute myocardial infarction, incomplete AV block, chronic constrictive pericarditis, idiopathic hypertrophic subaortic stenosis, renal insufficiency, severe pulmonary disease, hypothyroidism; and in the elderly.
• Hypothyroid patients are very sensitive to glycosides; hyperthyroid patients may need larger doses.
• Obtain baseline data (heart rate and

rhythm, blood pressure, electrolytes, BUN, serum creatinine) before giving first dose.
- Question patient about recent use of cardiotonic glycosides (within the previous 2 to 3 weeks) before administering a loading dose. Always divide loading dose over first 24 hours unless clinical situation indicates otherwise.
- Use only for rapid digitalization, not maintenance.
- Dose is adjusted to patient's clinical condition and is monitored by serum levels of cardiotonic glycoside, calcium, potassium, magnesium, and by EKG.
- Take apical-radial pulse for a full minute. Record and report to doctor any significant changes (sudden increase or decrease in rate, pulse deficit, irregular beats, and particularly regularization of a previously irregular rhythm). Check blood pressure and obtain 12-lead EKG with these changes.
- Observe eating pattern. Ask patient about nausea, vomiting, anorexia, visual disturbances, and other symptoms of toxicity.
- I.M. injection is painful; give I.V. if possible.
- Monitor serum potassium carefully. Take corrective action *before* hypokalemia occurs.

---

digitalis leaf
Digifortis, Pil-Digis

INDICATIONS & DOSAGE
Congestive heart failure, paroxysmal atrial tachycardia, atrial fibrillation and flutter—
Adults: loading dose 1.2 to 1.8 g P.O. in divided doses over 24 hours; usual maintenance 100 mg P.O. daily. Not recommended for children.

SIDE EFFECTS
The following are signs of toxicity that may occur with all cardiotonic glycosides:
CNS: *fatigue, generalized muscle weakness, agitation, hallucinations,* headache, malaise, dizziness, vertigo, stupor, paresthesias.
CV: *increased severity of congestive heart failure, arrhythmias (most commonly conduction disturbances with or without AV block, premature ventricular contractions, and supraventricular arrhythmias),* hypotension.
Toxic effects on heart may be life-threatening and require immediate attention.
EENT: *yellow-green halos around visual images, blurred vision,* light flashes, photophobia, diplopia.
GI: *anorexia, nausea,* vomiting, diarrhea.

INTERACTIONS
Aminosalicylic acid, antacids, cholestyramine, kaolin-pectin, neomycin, colestipol: decreased absorption of digitoxin, the main active component of the digitalis leaf. Schedule doses as far as possible from administration of digitalis leaf.
Amphotericin B, carbenicillin, ticarcillin, corticosteroids, and diuretics, including chlorthalidone, ethacrynic acid, furosemide, metolazone, and thiazides: hypokalemia, predisposing patient to digitalis toxicity. Monitor serum potassium.
Parenteral calcium, thiazides: hypercalcemia and hypomagnesemia, predisposing patient to digitalis toxicity. Monitor serum calcium and serum magnesium.
Phenylbutazone, phenobarbital, phenytoin, rifampin: faster metabolism and shorter duration of action of digitoxin. Observe for underdigitalization.

NURSING CONSIDERATIONS
- Contraindicated in presence of any digitalis-induced toxicity; ventricular fibrillation; ventricular tachycardia

---

Italicized side effects are common or life-threatening.

unless caused by congestive heart failure. Administering calcium salts to digitalized patient is contraindicated. Calcium affects contractility and excitability of heart very much as glycosides do and may lead to serious arrhythmias in digitalized patient. Use with extreme caution in acute myocardial infarction, incomplete AV block, chronic constrictive pericarditis, idiopathic hypertrophic subaortic stenosis, renal insufficiency, severe pulmonary disease, hypothyroidism; and in the elderly.

• Hypothyroid patients are very sensitive to glycosides; hyperthyroid patients may need larger doses.

• Obtain baseline data (heart rate and rhythm, blood pressure, electrolytes, BUN, serum creatinine) before giving first dose.

• Question patient about recent use of cardiotonic glycosides (within the previous 2 to 3 weeks) before administering a loading dose. Always divide loading dose over first 24 hours unless clinical situation indicates otherwise.

• Dose is adjusted to patient's clinical condition and is monitored by serum levels of cardiotonic glycoside, calcium, potassium, magnesium, and by EKG.

• Take apical-radial pulse for a full minute. Record and report to doctor any significant changes (sudden increase or decrease in rate, pulse deficit, irregular beats, and particularly regularization of a previously irregular rhythm). Check blood pressure and obtain 12-lead EKG with these changes.

• Observe eating pattern. Ask patient about nausea, vomiting, anorexia, visual disturbances, and other symptoms of toxicity.

• Monitor serum potassium carefully. Take corrective action *before* hypokalemia occurs.

• Digitalis leaf is a long-acting drug; watch for cumulative effects.

• Withhold for 1 to 2 days before

elective electrocardioversion. Adjust dosage after cardioversion.

• Instruct patient and responsible family member about drug action, dosage regimen, how to take pulse, reportable signs, and follow-up plans.

• Therapeutic blood levels of serum digitoxin (the active agent in the leaf) range from 25 to 35 ng/ml.

---

digitoxin
Crystodigin, De-Tone, Purodigin♦

INDICATIONS & DOSAGE
Congestive heart failure, paroxysmal atrial tachycardia, atrial fibrillation and flutter—

Adults: loading dose 1.2 to 1.6 mg I.V. or P.O. in divided doses over 24 hours; maintenance 0.1 mg daily.

Children 2 to 12 years: loading dose 0.03 mg/Kg or 0.75 mg/m² I.M., I.V., or P.O. in divided doses over 24 hours; maintenance $^1/_{10}$ loading dose or 0.003 mg/Kg or 0.075 mg/m² daily. Monitor closely for toxicity.

Children 1 to 2 years: loading dose 0.04 mg/Kg over 24 hours in divided doses; maintenance 0.004 mg/Kg daily. Monitor closely for toxicity.

Children 2 weeks to 1 year: loading dose 0.045 mg/Kg I.M., I.V., or P.O. in divided doses over 24 hours; maintenance 0.0045 mg/Kg daily. Monitor closely for toxicity.

Premature infants, neonates, severely ill older infants: loading dose 0.022 mg/Kg I.M., I.V., or P.O. in divided doses over 24 hours; maintenance 0.0022 mg/Kg daily. Monitor closely for toxicity.

SIDE EFFECTS
The following are signs of toxicity that may occur with all cardiotonic glycosides:

CNS: *fatigue, generalized muscle weakness, agitation, hallucinations,*

---

headache, malaise, dizziness, vertigo, stupor, paresthesias.

CV: *increased severity of congestive heart failure, arrhythmias (most commonly conduction disturbances with or without AV block, premature ventricular contractions, and supraventricular arrhythmias),* hypotension.
Toxic effects on heart may be life-threatening and require immediate attention.

EENT: *yellow-green halos around visual images, blurred vision,* light flashes, photophobia, diplopia.

GI: *anorexia, nausea,* vomiting, diarrhea.

INTERACTIONS

Aminosalicylic acid, antacids, cholestyramine, colestipol, kaolin-pectin, neomycin: decreased absorption of oral digitoxin. Schedule doses as far as possible from oral digitoxin administration.

Amphotericin B, carbenicillin, ticarcillin, corticosteroids, and diuretics, including chlorthalidone, ethacrynic acid, furosemide, metolazone, and thiazides: hypokalemia, predisposing patient to digitalis toxicity. Monitor serum potassium.

Parenteral calcium, thiazides: hypercalcemia and hypomagnesemia, predisposing patient to digitalis toxicity. Monitor serum calcium and serum magnesium.

Phenylbutazone, phenobarbital, phenytoin, rifampin: faster metabolism and shorter duration of digitoxin. Observe for underdigitalization.

NURSING CONSIDERATIONS

• Contraindicated in presence of any digitalis-induced toxicity; ventricular fibrillation; ventricular tachycardia unless caused by congestive heart failure. Administering calcium salts to digitalized patient is contraindicated. Calcium affects contractility and excitability of heart very much as glycosides do and may lead to serious arrhythmias in digitalized patient. Use with extreme caution in acute myocardial infarction, incomplete AV block, chronic constrictive pericarditis, idiopathic hypertrophic subaortic stenosis, renal insufficiency, severe pulmonary disease, hypothyroidism; and in the elderly.

• Hypothyroid patients are very sensitive to glycosides; hyperthyroid patients may need larger doses.

• Obtain baseline data (heart rate and rhythm, blood pressure, electrolytes, BUN, serum creatinine) before giving first dose.

• Question patient about recent use of cardiotonic glycosides (within the previous 2 to 3 weeks) before administering a loading dose. Always divide loading dose over first 24 hours unless clinical situation indicates otherwise.

• Dose is adjusted to patient's clinical condition and is monitored by serum levels of cardiotonic glycoside, calcium, potassium, magnesium, and by EKG.

• Take apical-radial pulse for a full minute. Record and report to doctor any significant changes (sudden increase or decrease in rate, pulse deficit, irregular beats, and particularly regularization of a previously irregular rhythm). Check blood pressure and obtain 12-lead EKG with these changes.

• Observe eating pattern. Ask patient about nausea, vomiting, anorexia, visual disturbances, and other symptoms of toxicity.

• Watch closely for signs of toxicity, especially in children and the elderly.

• Monitor serum potassium carefully. Take corrective action *before* hypokalemia occurs.

• I.M. injection is painful; give I.V. if parenteral route is necessary.

• Digitoxin is a long-acting drug; watch for cumulative effects.

• Withhold for 1 to 2 days before

Italicized side effects are common or life-threatening.

elective electrocardioversion. Adjust dose after cardioversion.
- Protect solution from light.
- Instruct patient and responsible family member about drug action, dosage regimen, how to take pulse, reportable signs, and follow-up plans.
- Do not substitute one brand for another.
- Therapeutic blood levels of digitoxin range from 25 to 35 ng/ml.

digoxin
Lanoxin♦, Masoxin, SK-Digoxin

INDICATIONS & DOSAGE
Congestive heart failure, atrial fibrillation and flutter, paroxysmal atrial tachycardia—
Adults: loading dose 0.5 to 1 mg I.V. or P.O. in divided doses over 24 hours; maintenance 0.125 to 0.5 mg I.V. or P.O. daily (average 0.25 mg). Larger doses are often needed for treatment of arrhythmias, depending on patient response.
Children over 2 years: loading dose 0.04 to 0.06 mg/Kg P.O. divided q 8 hours over 24 hours; I.V. loading dose 0.025 to 0.04 mg/Kg; maintenance 0.02 mg/Kg P.O. daily divided q 12 hours.
Children 1 month to 2 years: loading dose 0.06 to 0.075 mg/Kg P.O. divided into three doses over 24 hours; I.V. loading dose 0.035 to 0.05 mg/Kg; maintenance 0.02 to 0.025 mg/Kg P.O. daily divided q 12 hours.
Neonates under 1 month: loading dose 0.05 mg/Kg P.O. divided q 8 hours over 24 hours; I.V. loading dose 0.015 to 0.04 mg/kg; maintenance 0.0167 mg/Kg P.O. daily divided q 12 hours.
Premature infants: loading dose 0.04 mg/Kg I.V. divided into 3 doses over 24 hours; maintenance 0.0133 mg/Kg I.V. daily divided q 12 hours.

SIDE EFFECTS
The following are signs of toxicity that may occur with all cardiotonic glycosides:
CNS: *fatigue, generalized muscle weakness, agitation, hallucinations,* headache, malaise, dizziness, vertigo, stupor, paresthesias.
CV: *increased severity of congestive heart failure, arrhythmias (most commonly conduction disturbances with or without AV block, premature ventricular contractions, and supraventricular arrhythmias),* hypotension. *Toxic effects on heart may be life-threatening and require immediate attention.*
EENT: *yellow-green halos around visual images, blurred vision,* light flashes, photophobia, diplopia.
GI: *anorexia, nausea,* vomiting, diarrhea.

INTERACTIONS
Aminosalicylic acid, antacids, cholestyramine, colestipol, kaolin-pectin, neomycin: decreased absorption of oral digoxin. Schedule doses as far as possible from oral digoxin administration.
Quinidine: increased digoxin blood levels. Monitor for toxicity.
Amphotericin B, carbenicillin, ticarcillin, corticosteroids, and diuretics, including chlorthalidone, ethacrynic acid, furosemide, metolazone, and thiazides: hypokalemia, predisposing patient to digitalis toxicity. Monitor serum potassium.
Parenteral calcium, thiazides: hypercalcemia and hypomagnesemia, predisposing patient to digitalis toxicity. Monitor serum calcium and serum magnesium.

NURSING CONSIDERATIONS
- Contraindicated in presence of any digitalis-induced toxicity; ventricular fibrillation; ventricular tachycardia unless caused by congestive heart failure. Administering calcium salts to

digitalized patient is contraindicated. Calcium affects contractility and excitability of heart very much as glycosides do and may lead to serious arrhythmias in digitalized patient. Use with extreme caution in acute myocardial infarction, incomplete AV block, chronic constrictive pericarditis, idiopathic hypertrophic subaortic stenosis, renal insufficiency, severe pulmonary disease, hypothyroidism; and in the elderly. Dose must be reduced in renal impairment.

• Hypothyroid patients are very sensitive to glycosides; hyperthyroid patients may need larger doses.

• Obtain baseline data (heart rate and rhythm, blood pressure, electrolytes, BUN, serum creatinine) before giving first dose.

• Question patient about recent use of cardiotonic glycosides (within the previous 2 to 3 weeks) before administering a loading dose. Always divide loading dose over first 24 hours unless clinical situation indicates otherwise.

• Dose is adjusted to patient's clinical condition and is monitored by serum levels of cardiotonic glycoside, calcium, potassium, magnesium, and by EKG.

• Take apical-radial pulse for a full minute. Record and report to doctor any significant changes (sudden increase or decrease in rate, pulse deficit, irregular beats, and particularly regularization of a previously irregular rhythm). Check blood pressure and obtain 12-lead EKG with these changes.

• Observe eating pattern. Ask patient about nausea, vomiting, anorexia, visual disturbances, and other symptoms of toxicity.

• Monitor serum potassium carefully. Take corrective action *before* hypokalemia occurs.

• Withhold for 1 to 2 days before elective electrocardioversion. Adjust dose after cardioversion.

• Instruct patient and responsible family member about drug action, dosage regimen, how to take pulse, reportable signs, and follow-up plans.

• Don't substitute one brand for another.

• Therapeutic blood levels of digoxin range from 0.5 to 2.5 ng/ml.

gitalin
Gitaligin

INDICATIONS & DOSAGE
Congestive heart failure, atrial fibrillation and flutter, paroxysmal atrial tachycardia—
Adults: loading dose 2.5 mg P.O. initially, then 0.75 mg q 6 hours until therapeutic effect is attained (not to exceed 6 mg total in 24 hours); maintenance 0.25 to 1.25 mg daily.
Not recommended for children.

SIDE EFFECTS
The following are signs of toxicity that may occur with all cardiotonic glycosides:
CNS: *fatigue, generalized muscle weakness, agitation, hallucinations,* headache, malaise, dizziness, vertigo, stupor, paresthesias.
CV: *increased severity of congestive heart failure, arrhythmias (most commonly conduction disturbances with or without AV block, premature ventricular contractions, and supraventricular arrhythmias),* hypotension.
Toxic effects on heart may be life-threatening and require immediate attention.
EENT: *yellow-green halos around visual images, blurred vision,* light flashes, photophobia, diplopia.
GI: *anorexia, nausea,* vomiting, diarrhea.

INTERACTIONS
Aminosalicylic acid, antacids, cholestyramine, colestipol, kaolin-pectin, neomycin: decreased absorption of

---

oral gitalin. Schedule doses as far as possible from oral gitalin administration.

Amphotericin B, carbenicillin, ticarcillin, corticosteroids, and diuretics, including chlorthalidone, ethacrynic acid, furosemide, metolazone, and thiazides: hypokalemia, predisposing patient to digitalis toxicity. Monitor serum potassium.

Parenteral calcium, thiazides: hypercalcemia and hypomagnesemia, predisposing patient to digitalis toxicity. Monitor serum calcium and serum magnesium.

NURSING CONSIDERATIONS

• Contraindicated in presence of any digitalis-induced toxicity; ventricular fibrillation; ventricular tachycardia unless caused by congestive heart failure. Administering calcium salts to digitalized patient is contraindicated. Calcium affects contractility and excitability of heart very much as glycosides do and may lead to serious arrhythmias in digitalized patient. Use with extreme caution in acute myocardial infarction, incomplete AV block, chronic constrictive pericarditis, idiopathic hypertrophic subaortic stenosis, renal insufficiency, severe pulmonary disease, hypothyroidism; and in the elderly.

• Hypothyroid patients are very sensitive to glycosides; hyperthyroid patients may need larger doses.

• Obtain baseline data (heart rate and rhythm, blood pressure, electrolytes, BUN, serum creatinine) before giving first dose.

• Question patient about recent use of cardiotonic glycosides (within the previous 2 to 3 weeks) before administering a loading dose. Always divide loading dose over first 24 hours unless clinical situation indicates otherwise.

• Dose is adjusted to patient's clinical condition and is monitored by serum levels of cardiotonic glycoside, cal-

cium, potassium, magnesium, and by EKG.

• Take apical-radial pulse for a full minute. Record and report to doctor any significant changes (sudden increase or decrease in rate, pulse deficit, irregular beats, and particularly regularization of a previously irregular rhythm). Check blood pressure and obtain 12-lead EKG with these changes.

• Observe eating pattern. Ask patient about nausea, vomiting, anorexia, visual disturbances, and other symptoms of toxicity.

• Monitor serum potassium carefully. Take corrective action *before* hypokalemia occurs.

• Gitalin is a long-acting drug; watch for cumulative effects.

• Withhold for 1 to 2 days before elective cardioversion. Adjust dose after cardioversion.

• Instruct patient and responsible family member about drug action, dosage regimen, how to take pulse, reportable signs, and follow-up plans.

lanatoside C
Cedilanid♦

INDICATIONS & DOSAGE

Congestive heart failure, atrial fibrillation and flutter, paroxysmal atrial tachycardia—
Adults: average total dose for digitalization is 10 mg P.O. given as follows: loading dose. First day, 3.5 mg; second day, 2.5 mg; third day, 2 mg; thereafter 1.5 mg per day until digitalization obtained; maintenance 0.5 to 1.5 mg daily.
Not recommended for children.

SIDE EFFECTS

The following are signs of toxicity that may occur with all cardiotonic glycosides:
CNS: *fatigue, generalized muscle*

weakness, agitation, hallucinations, headache, malaise, dizziness, vertigo, stupor, paresthesias.
CV: *increased severity of congestive heart failure, arrhythmias (most commonly conduction disturbances with or without AV block, premature ventricular contractions, and supraventricular arrhythmias),* hypotension.
Toxic effects on heart may be life-threatening and require immediate attention.
EENT: *yellow-green halos around visual images, blurred vision,* light flashes, photophobia, diplopia.
GI: *anorexia, nausea,* vomiting, diarrhea.

INTERACTIONS

Aminosalicylic acid, antacids, cholestyramine, kaolin-pectin, neomycin, colestipol: decreased absorption of digoxin formed in stomach from lanatoside C. Schedule doses as far as possible from lanatoside C administration.
Amphotericin B, carbenicillin, ticarcillin, corticosteroids, and diuretics, including chlorthalidone, ethacrynic acid, furosemide, metolazone, and thiazides: hypokalemia, predisposing patient to digitalis toxicity. Monitor serum potassium.
Parenteral calcium, thiazides: hypercalcemia and hypomagnesemia, predisposing patient to digitalis toxicity. Monitor serum calcium and serum magnesium.

NURSING CONSIDERATIONS

• Contraindicated in presence of any digitalis-induced toxicity; ventricular fibrillation; ventricular tachycardia unless caused by congestive heart failure. Administering calcium salts to digitalized patient is contraindicated. Calcium affects contractility and excitability of heart very much as glycosides do and may lead to serious arrhythmias in digitalized patient. Use with extreme caution in acute myocardial infarction, incomplete AV block,

chronic constrictive pericarditis, idiopathic hypertrophic subaortic stenosis, renal insufficiency, severe pulmonary disease, hypothyroidism; and in the elderly. Dose should be reduced in renal impairment.
• Hypothyroid patients are very sensitive to glycosides; hyperthyroid patients may need larger doses.
• Obtain baseline data (heart rate and rhythm, blood pressure, electrolytes, BUN, serum creatinine) before giving first dose.
• Question patient about recent use of cardiotonic glycosides (within the previous 2 to 3 weeks) before administering a loading dose. Always divide loading dose over first 24 hours unless clinical situation indicates otherwise.
• Dose is adjusted to patient's clinical condition and is monitored by serum levels of cardiotonic glycoside, calcium, potassium, magnesium, and by EKG.
• Take apical-radial pulse for a full minute. Record and report to doctor any significant changes (sudden increase or decrease in rate, pulse deficit, irregular beats, and particularly regularization of a previously irregular rhythm). Check blood pressure and obtain 12-lead EKG with these changes.
• Observe eating pattern. Ask patient about nausea, vomiting, anorexia, visual disturbances, and other symptoms of toxicity.
• Monitor serum potassium carefully. Take corrective action *before* hypokalemia occurs.
• Withhold for 1 to 2 days before elective electrocardioversion. Adjust dose after cardioversion.
• Instruct patient and responsible family member about drug action, dosage regimen, how to take pulse, reportable signs, and follow-up plans.

Italicized side effects are common or life-threatening.

ouabain

posing patient to toxicity. Monitor serum calcium and serum magnesium.

INDICATIONS & DOSAGE
Congestive heart failure, atrial fibrillation and flutter, paroxysmal atrial tachycardia—
Adults: loading dose 0.25 to 0.5 mg by slow I.V. injection. Additional 0.1 mg doses may be given every hour until a therapeutic effect is achieved or a total of 1mg is given. For maintenance, use another glycoside.
Not recommended for children.

SIDE EFFECTS
The following are signs of toxicity that may occur with all cardiotonic glycosides:
CNS: *fatigue, generalized muscle weakness, agitation, hallucinations,* headache, malaise, dizziness, vertigo, stupor, paresthesias.
CV: *increased severity of congestive heart failure, arrhythmias (most commonly conduction disturbances with or without AV block, premature ventricular contractions, and supraventricular arrhythmias), hypotension.*
Toxic effects on heart may be life-threatening and require immediate attention.
EENT: *yellow-green halos around visual images, blurred vision,* light flashes, photophobia, diplopia.
GI: *anorexia, nausea,* vomiting, diarrhea.

INTERACTIONS
Amphotericin B, carbenicillin, ticarcillin, corticosteroids, and diuretics, including chlorthalidone, ethacrynic acid, furosemide, metolazone, and thiazides: hypokalemia, predisposing patient to toxicity. Monitor serum potassium.
Parenteral calcium, thiazides: hypercalcemia and hypomagnesemia, predis-

NURSING CONSIDERATIONS
• Contraindicated in presence of any digitalis-induced toxicity; ventricular fibrillation; ventricular tachycardia unless caused by congestive heart failure. Administering calcium salts to digitalized patient is contraindicated. Calcium affects contractility and excitability of heart very much as glycosides do and may lead to serious arrhythmias in digitalized patient. Use with extreme caution in acute myocardial infarction, incomplete AV block, chronic constrictive pericarditis, idiopathic hypertrophic subaortic stenosis, renal insufficiency, severe pulmonary disease, hypothyroidism; and in the elderly. Dose should be reduced in renal impairment.
• Hypothyroid patients are very sensitive to glycosides; hyperthyroid patients may need larger doses.
• Obtain baseline data (heart rate and rhythm, blood pressure, electrolytes, BUN, serum creatinine) before giving first dose.
• Question patient about recent use of cardiotonic glycosides (within the previous 2 to 3 weeks) before administering a loading dose. Always divide loading dose over first 24 hours unless clinical situation indicates otherwise.
• Use only for rapid digitalization, not maintenance.
• Dose is adjusted to patient's clinical condition and is monitored by serum levels of cardiotonic glycoside, calcium, potassium, magnesium, and by EKG.
• Take apical-radial pulse for a full minute. Record and report to doctor any significant changes (sudden increase or decrease in rate, pulse deficit, irregular beats, and particularly regularization of a previously irregular rhythm). Check blood pressure

and obtain 12-lead EKG with these changes.
• Observe eating pattern. Ask patient about nausea, vomiting, anorexia, visual disturbances, and other symptoms of toxicity.

• I.M. route is painful; absorption is unpredictable. Not recommended.
• Monitor serum potassium carefully. Take corrective action *before* hypokalemia occurs.

Italicized side effects are common or life-threatening.

16

Antiarrhythmics

atropine sulfate
bretylium tosylate
disopyramide
disopyramide phosphate
lidocaine hydrochloride
phenytoin
phenytoin sodium
procainamide hydrochloride
propranolol hydrochloride
quinidine bisulfate
quinidine gluconate
quinidine polygalacturonate
quinidine sulfate

atropine sulfate

INDICATIONS & DOSAGE
Bradycardia, bradyarrhythmia (junctional or escape rhythm)—
Adults: usually 0.5 to 1 mg I.V. push; repeat q 5 minutes, to maximum 2 mg. Lower doses (less than 0.5 mg) can cause bradycardia.
Children: 0.01 mg/Kg dose up to maximum 0.4 mg; or 0.3 mg/m² dose; may repeat q 4 to 6 hours.

SIDE EFFECTS
Blood: leukocytosis.
CNS: *with doses greater than 5 mg— headache, restlessness,* ataxia, disorientation, hallucinations, delirium, coma, *insomnia, dizziness.*
CV: *1 to 2 mg—tachycardia, palpitations; greater than 2 mg—extreme tachycardia, angina.*
EENT: *1 mg—slight mydriasis,* photophobia; *2 mg—blurred vision, mydriasis.*

GI: *dry mouth (common even at low doses),* thirst, *constipation,* nausea, vomiting.
GU: *urinary retention.*
Skin: 2 mg—flushed, dry skin; 5 mg or more—hot, dry, reddened skin.

INTERACTIONS
Methotrimeprazine: may produce extrapyramidal symptoms. Monitor patient carefully.

NURSING CONSIDERATIONS
• Side effects vary considerably with dose. Most common are dry mouth, which can be treated with pilocarpine syrup, and thirst. Recommend sucking sour hard candy.
• Watch for tachycardia in cardiac patients; report to doctor.
• Antidote for atropine overdose is physostigmine salicylate.
• Other anticholinergic drugs may increase vagal blockage.

bretylium tosylate
Bretylol

INDICATIONS & DOSAGE
Adults:
*Ventricular fibrillation—*5 mg/Kg by rapid I.V. injection. If necessary, increase dose to 10 mg/Kg and repeat q 15 to 30 minutes until 30 mg/Kg has been given.
*Other ventricular arrhythmias—*initially, 500 mg diluted to 50 ml with 5% dextrose or normal saline and infused I.V. over more than 8 minutes at

5 to 10 mg/Kg. Dose may be repeated in 1 to 2 hours. Thereafter, dose q 6 to 8 hours.
I.V. maintenance—infused in diluted solution of 500 ml 5% dextrose or normal saline at 1 to 2 mg/minute.
I.M. injection—5 to 10 mg/Kg undiluted. Repeat in 1 to 2 hours if needed. Thereafter, repeat q 6 to 8 hours.
Not recommended for children.

SIDE EFFECTS
CNS: *vertigo, dizziness, light-headedness, syncope* (usually secondary to hypotension).
CV: *severe hypotension (especially orthostatic), bradycardia,* anginal pain.
GI: severe nausea, vomiting (with rapid infusion).

INTERACTIONS
All antihypertensives: may potentiate hypotension. Monitor blood pressure.

NURSING CONSIDERATIONS
• Contraindicated in digitalis-induced arrhythmias. Use cautiously in fixed cardiac output, aortic stenosis, and pulmonary hypertension to avoid severe and sudden drop in blood pressure.
• Monitor blood pressure, heart rate, and rhythm frequently. Notify doctor immediately of any change. If supine systolic blood pressure falls below 75 mm Hg, notify doctor, who may order norepinephrine or dopamine, or volume expansion to raise blood pressure.
• Keep patient supine until tolerance to hypotension develops.
• Follow dosage directions carefully to avoid nausea and vomiting.
• Give I.V. injections for ventricular fibrillation as rapidly as possible. Do not dilute.
• Rotate I.M. injection sites, and don't exceed 5 ml volume.
• To be used with other cardioresuscitative measures.

• Avoid subtherapeutic doses (less than 5 mg/Kg), since such doses may cause hypotension.
• Ventricular tachycardia and other ventricular arrhythmias respond less rapidly to treatment than does ventricular fibrillation.
• Dosage should be decreased in renal impairment.
• Monitor carefully if pressor amines (sympathomimetics) are given to correct hypotension, as bretylium potentiates pressor amines.
• Not first-line therapy; used for refractory arrhythmias only. Ineffective treatment for atrial arrhythmias.
• Has been used investigationally to treat hypertension.
• Observe for increased anginal pain in susceptible patients.
• Observe patient for side effects and notify doctor.

---

disopyramide
Rythmodan♦
disopyramide phosphate
Norpace♦

INDICATIONS & DOSAGE
Premature ventricular contractions (unifocal, multifocal, or coupled); ventricular tachycardia not severe enough to require electric cardioversion—
Adults: Usual maintenance dose 150 to 200 mg P.O. q 6 hours; for patients who weigh less than 50 Kg or those with renal, hepatic, or cardiac impairment—100 mg P.O. q 6 hours. Recommended doses in advanced renal insufficiency: Creatinine clearance 15 to 40 ml/minute: 100 mg q 10 hours; creatinine clearance 5 to 15 ml/minute: 100 mg q 20 hours; creatinine clearance 1 to 5 ml/minute: 100 mg q 30 hours.

SIDE EFFECTS
CNS: dizziness, fatigue, muscle weakness, syncope.
CV: *hypotension, congestive heart failure, heart block.*
EENT: *blurred vision, dry eyes, dry nose.*
GI: nausea, vomiting, anorexia, bloating, abdominal pain, *constipation, dry mouth.*
GU: *urinary retention and hesitancy.*
Hepatic: cholestatic jaundice.
Skin: rash in 1% to 3% of patients.

INTERACTIONS
None significant.

NURSING CONSIDERATIONS
• Contraindicated in cardiogenic shock or second- or third-degree heart block with no pacemaker. Use cautiously in congestive heart failure, underlying conduction abnormalities, urinary tract diseases (especially prostatic hypertrophy), hepatic or renal impairment, myasthenia gravis, narrow-angle glaucoma. Adjust dosage in renal insufficiency.
• Discontinue if heart block develops, if QRS complex widens by more than 25%, or if Q-T interval lengthens by more than 25% above baseline.
• Correct any underlying electrolyte abnormalities before use.
• Watch for recurrence of arrhythmias; check for side effects; notify doctor.
• Check apical pulse before administering drug. Notify doctor if pulse rate is slower than 60 beats per minute or faster than 120 beats per minute.
• Teach patient the importance of taking drug on time, exactly as prescribed. To do this, he may have to use an alarm clock for night dosages.
• Relieve discomfort of dry mouth with chewing gum or hard candy.
• Manage constipation with proper diet or bulk laxatives.
• Use of disopyramide with other an-

tiarrhythmics may cause further myocardial depression.

---

lidocaine hydrochloride
Lido Pen Auto-Injector, Xylocaine♦

INDICATIONS & DOSAGE
Ventricular arrhythmias from myocardial infarction, cardiac manipulation, or cardiac glycosides, ventricular tachycardia—
Adults: 50 to 100 mg (1 to 1.5 mg/Kg) I.V. bolus at 25 to 50 mg/minute. Give half this amount to elderly or lightweight patients, and to those with congestive heart failure or hepatic disease. Repeat bolus q 3 to 5 minutes until arrhythmias subside or side effects develop. Don't exceed 300 mg total bolus during a 1-hour period. Simultaneously, begin constant infusion: 1 to 4 mg/minute. Use lower dose in elderly patients, those with congestive heart failure or hepatic disease, or patients who weigh less than 50 Kg. If single bolus has been given, repeat smaller bolus 15 to 20 minutes after start of infusion to maintain therapeutic serum level. After 24 hours continuous infusion, decrease rate by half.
I.M. administration: 200 to 300 mg in deltoid muscle only.

SIDE EFFECTS
CNS: *confusion, tremors,* lethargy, *stupor, restlessness,* slurred speech, euphoria, depression, *light-headedness,* muscle twitches, convulsions, coma.
CV: *hypotension,* bradycardia, further arrhythmias.
EENT: *tinnitus, blurred or double vision.*
Other: *anaphylaxis.*

INTERACTIONS
Barbiturates: may decrease patient's response to lidocaine. Adjust dose.

Phenytoin: additive cardiac depressant effects. Monitor carefully.
Procainamide: may increase neurologic side effects. Monitor carefully.

NURSING CONSIDERATIONS
• Contraindicated in complete or second-degree heart block. Use of lidocaine with epinephrine (for local anesthesia) to treat arrhythmias contraindicated. Use with caution in elderly patients, those with congestive heart failure, renal or hepatic disease, or patients who weigh less than 50 Kg. Such patients will need a reduced dose.
• If toxic signs (dizziness) occur, stop drug at once and notify doctor. Continued infusion could lead to convulsions and coma. Give O_2 via nasal cannula, if not contraindicated. Keep O_2 and CPR equipment handy.
• Patients receiving infusions must be *attended at all times*. Use an infusion pump or a microdropper and timer for monitoring infusion precisely. Never exceed an infusion rate of 4 mg/minute, if possible. A faster rate greatly increases risk of toxicity.
• Monitor patient's response, especially blood pressure, serum electrolytes, BUN, and creatinine. Notify doctor promptly if abnormalities develop.
• A bolus dose not followed by infusion will have a short-lived effect.
• A patient who has received lidocaine I.M. will show a 7-fold increase in serum CPK level. Such CPK originates in the skeletal muscle, not the heart. Test isoenzymes if using I.M. route.
• Used investigationally to treat refractory status epilepticus.

phenytoin
Dilantin Infatab♦, Dilantin Pediatric
phenytoin sodium
Dantoin♦♦, Dihycon, Dilantin♦, Di-Phen, Diphenylan Sodium, EKKO, Toin Unicelles

INDICATIONS & DOSAGE
Ventricular arrhythmias unresponsive to lidocaine or procainamide; supraventricular and ventricular arrhythmias induced by cardiac glycosides—
Adults: loading dose 1 g P.O. divided over first 24 hours, followed by 500 mg daily for 2 days, then maintenance dose 300 mg P.O. daily; 250 mg I.V. over 5 minutes until arrhythmias subside, side effects develop, or 1 g has been given. Infusion rate should never exceed 50 mg/minute (slow I.V. push).
Alternate method: 100 mg I.V. q 15 minutes until side effects develop, arrhythmias are controlled, or 1 g has been given. I.M. dose not recommended because of pain and erratic absorption.
Children: 3 to 8 mg/Kg P.O. or slow I.V. daily or 250 mg/m² daily given as single dose or divided in 2 doses.

SIDE EFFECTS
Blood: thrombocytopenia, leukopenia, *agranulocytosis, pancytopenia, lymphadenopathy*, megaloblastic anemia.
CNS: *ataxia*, slurred speech, insomnia, headache, muscle twitching, *lethargy*.
CV: *severe hypotension, vascular collapse (with rapid I.V. infusions greater than 50 mg/minute)*, vasodilation, asystole, ventricular fibrillation, A-V block.
EENT: *nystagmus, diplopia*, blurred vision.
GI: *gingival hyperplasia, nausea, vomiting*, constipation.
Metabolic: hyperglycemia.

Italicized side effects are common or life-threatening.

Skin: rash (*morbilliform* most common), dermatitis (bullous, *exfoliative*, purpuric), lupus erythematosus, Stevens-Johnson syndrome.

INTERACTIONS

Alcohol, barbiturates, folic acid, Loxitane: monitor for decreased phenytoin activity.

Oral anticoagulants, antihistamines, chloramphenicol, diazepam, diazoxide, disulfiram, INH, phenylbutazone, phenyramidol, salicylates, sulfamethizole, valproate: monitor for increased phenytoin activity.

NURSING CONSIDERATIONS

• Contraindicated in heart block, sinus bradycardia, Stokes-Adams attacks. Use cautiously in congestive heart failure, hepatic or renal dysfunction, elderly or debilitated patients, hypotension, myocardial insufficiency, respiratory depression. Cardiac patients on thyroid replacement therapy should be given I.V. phenytoin cautiously to prevent supraventricular tachycardia.
• Administer drug slow I.V. push, not to exceed 50 mg/minute in adults.
• Monitor blood pressure and EKG. Notify doctor if side effects occur.
• Don't mix with 5% dextrose I.V. fluids, as crystallization will occur. Flush I.V. line with saline before and after administration.
• Watch patients on phenytoin and other antiarrhythmics (disopyramide, quinidine, procainamide, propranolol) closely for signs of additive cardiac depression.
• Phenytoin can be diluted in normal saline and infused without precipitation. Such infusions should not take longer than 1 hour.
• Shake oral suspensions well to make dosage uniform. After giving suspension by nasogastric tube, flush tube with water to facilitate passage to stomach.
• Give drug with food or large glass of water to minimize gastric irritation.
• Avoid I.M. route of administration.
• Teach patient importance of taking drug on time, exactly as prescribed.
• Dose should be decreased in hepatic dysfunction.
• Serum levels greater than 20 mcg/ml may be toxic. The difference between therapeutic and toxic levels of phenytoin in the blood is very slight. If toxic symptoms occur, draw blood for serum level determination.
• Stress need for good oral hygiene to minimize gingival hyperplasia.
• Uremic patients may require dose adjustment for stabilization.
• Patients concurrently on phenytoin and barbiturates, prednisone, or isoniazid should have serum phenytoin levels checked frequently. Observe for phenytoin toxicity and for failure to respond adequately to phenytoin.
• Patients concurrently on digitoxin and phenytoin may need larger doses.
• Warn patient not to drink alcohol as he may lose control of previously stable antiarrhythmic effects.

---

procainamide hydrochloride
Procan SR, Pronestyl♦, Sub-Quin

INDICATIONS & DOSAGE
Adults:
Premature ventricular contractions, ventricular tachycardia, atrial arrhythmias unresponsive to quinidine, paroxysmal atrial tachycardia—
100 mg q 5 minutes slow I.V. push, no faster than 25 to 50 mg/minute until arrhythmias disappear, side effects develop, or 1 g has been given. Once arrhythmias disappear, give continuous infusion of 2 to 6 mg/minute. Usual effective dose 500 to 600 mg. If arrhythmias recur, repeat bolus as above and increase infusion rate; 0.5 to 1 g I.M. q 4 to 8 hours until oral therapy begins.

Loading dose for atrial fibrillation or paroxysmal atrial tachycardia—1 to 1.25 g P.O. If arrhythmias persist after 1 hour, give additional 750 mg. If no change occurs, give 500 mg to 1 g q 2 hours until arrhythmias disappear or side effects occur. Maintenance 0.5 to 1 g q 4 to 6 hours.

Loading dose for ventricular tachycardia—1 g P.O. Maintenance 50 mg/Kg daily given at 3-hour intervals; average 250 to 500 mg q 3 hours.

Note: Sustained-release tablet may be used for maintenance dosing when treating ventricular tachycardia, atrial fibrillation, and paroxysmal atrial tachycardia. Dose is 500 mg to 1 g q 6 hours.

SIDE EFFECTS
Blood: thrombocytopenia, *agranulocytosis,* hemolytic anemia, *increased ANA titer.*
CNS: hallucinations, confusion, convulsions, depression.
CV: *severe hypotension, bradycardia,* A-V block, ventricular fibrillation (after parenteral use).
GI: *nausea, vomiting, anorexia, diarrhea, bitter taste.*
Skin: *rash.*
Other: *fever, lupus erythematosus syndrome (especially after prolonged administration),* myalgia.

INTERACTIONS
None significant.

NURSING CONSIDERATIONS
• Contraindicated in hypersensitivity to procaine and related drugs; in those with complete, second-, or third-degree heart block unassisted by electric pacemaker, or with myasthenia gravis. Use with caution in congestive heart failure or other conduction disturbances, such as bundle branch block or cardiac glycoside intoxication, or with hepatic or renal insufficiency.

• Patients receiving infusions must be *attended at all times.* Use an infusion pump or a microdropper and timer to monitor the infusion precisely.
• Monitor blood pressure and EKG continuously during I.V. administration. Watch for prolonged Q-T and Q-R intervals, heart block, or increased arrhythmias. If these occur, withhold drug, obtain rhythm strip, and notify doctor immediately.
• Keep patient in supine position for I.V. administration.
• Watch closely for side effects and notify doctor if they occur. Instruct patient to report fever, rash, muscle pain, diarrhea, or pleuritic chest pain.
• Decrease dose in hepatic and renal dysfunction, and give over 6 hours. Half-life of procainamide is increased as much as threefold in these states.
• Patient with congestive heart failure has a lower volume of distribution and can be treated with lower doses.
• Positive antinuclear antibody titer common in about 60% of patients who don't have symptoms of lupus erythematosus syndrome. This response seems related to prolonged use, not dosage.
• After long-standing atrial fibrillation, restoration of normal rhythm may result in thromboembolism, due to dislodgement of thrombi from atrial wall. Anticoagulation usually advised before restoration of normal sinus rhythm.
• Stress importance of taking drug exactly as prescribed. Patient may have to set an alarm clock for night dosage.

propranolol hydrochloride
Inderal♦

INDICATIONS & DOSAGE
Supraventricular, ventricular, and atrial arrhythmias; tachyarrhythmias

due to excessive catecholamine action during anesthesia, hyperthyroidism, and pheochromocytoma; angina—
Adults: 1 to 3 mg I.V. diluted in 50 ml 5% dextrose in water or normal saline infused slowly, not to exceed 1 mg/minute. After 3 mg have been infused, another dose may be given in 2 minutes; subsequent doses no sooner than q 4 hours. Maintenance 10 to 80 mg P.O. t.i.d. or q.i.d.

SIDE EFFECTS

CNS: *fatigue, lethargy,* vivid dreams, hallucinations.
CV: *bradycardia, hypotension, congestive heart failure,* peripheral vascular disease.
GI: nausea, vomiting, diarrhea.
Metabolic: hypoglycemia without tachycardia.
Skin: rash.
Other: *increased airway resistance,* fever.

INTERACTIONS

Insulin, hypoglycemic drugs (oral): can alter requirements for these drugs in previously stabilized diabetics. Monitor for hypoglycemia.
Cardiac glycosides: cause excessive bradycardia and increased depressant effect on myocardium. Use together cautiously.
Aminophylline: antagonizes beta-blocking effects of propranolol. Use together cautiously.
Isoproterenol, glucagon: antagonized propranolol effect. May be used therapeutically and in emergencies.

NURSING CONSIDERATIONS

• Contraindicated in asthma or allergic rhinitis; during ethyl ether anesthesia; in sinus bradycardia and in heart block greater than first degree; in cardiogenic shock; in right ventricular failure secondary to pulmonary hypertension. Use with caution in congestive heart failure, diabetes mellitus, or respiratory disease.

• Always withdraw drug slowly. Abrupt withdrawal might precipitate myocardial infarction or aggravate angina, thyrotoxicosis, pheochromocytoma. Abrupt withdrawal in thyrotoxicosis may exacerbate hyperthyroidism or precipitate thyroid storm. In thyrotoxicosis, propranolol may mask clinical signs of hyperthyroidism.
• *Don't discontinue before surgery for pheochromocytoma.* Before any surgical procedure, notify anesthesiologist that patient is receiving propranolol.
• Double-check dose and route. I.V. doses much smaller than P.O.
• Check apical pulse rate and blood pressure before giving drug. If you detect extremes in pulse rate, withhold drug and notify doctor at once. Severe bradycardia may be treated with atropine 0.25 to 1 mg I.V.
• After long-standing atrial fibrillation, restoration of normal sinus rhythm may result in thromboembolism due to dislodgement of thrombi from atrial wall. Anticoagulation often advised before restoration of normal atrial rhythm.
• Monitor blood pressure, EKG, heart rate, and rhythm frequently, especially during I.V. administration. When propranolol is used with other antihypertensives, monitor blood pressure while patient is sitting and standing.
• Auscultate patient's lungs for rales and his heart for gallop rhythm or for third or fourth heart sounds. If these develop, notify doctor at once.

quinidine bisulfate
(66% quinidine base)
Biquin Durules♦♦
quinidine gluconate
(62% quinidine base)
Duraquin, Quinaglute Dura-Tabs♦,
Quinate♦♦
quinidine polygalacturonate
(60.5% quinidine base)
Cardioquin♦
quinidine sulfate
(83% quinidine base)
CinQuin, Quine, Quinidex
Extentabs♦, Quinora, SK-Quinidine
Sulfate

INDICATIONS & DOSAGE
Atrial flutter or fibrillation—
Adults: 200 mg quinidine sulfate or
equivalant base P.O. q 2 to 3 hours
for 5 to 8 doses with subsequent daily
increases until sinus rhythm is restored or toxic effects develop. Administer quinidine only after digitalization to avoid increasing A-V block.
Maximum 3 to 4 g daily.
*Paroxysmal supraventricular tachy-
cardia—*
Adults: 400 to 600 mg I.M. gluconate q 2 to 3 hours until toxic side effects develop or arrhythmia subsides.
*Premature atrial and ventricular con-
tractions; paroxysmal atrioventricular
junctional rhythm; paroxysmal atrial
tachycardia; paroxysmal ventricular
tachycardia; maintenance after cardioversion of atrial fibrillation or flutter—*
Adults: test dose 50 to 200 mg P.O.,
then monitor vital signs before beginning therapy.
Quinidine sulfate or equivalent base
200 to 400 mg P.O. q 4 to 6 hours; or
initially, quinidine gluconate 600 mg
I.M., then up to 400 mg q 2 hours,
p.r.n.; or quinidine gluconate 800 mg
I.V. diluted in 40 ml of 5% dextrose in
water, infused at 1 mg/minute.
Children: test dose 2 mg/Kg; 3 to

6 mg/Kg q 2 to 3 hours for 5 doses
P.O. daily.

SIDE EFFECTS
Blood: *hemolytic anemia, thrombocytopenia, agranulocytosis.*
CNS: *vertigo, headache,* confusion,
restlessness, cold sweat, pallor,
fainting.
CV: *premature ventricular contractions; severe hypotension; SA and A-V
block; ventricular fibrillation, tachycardia; aggravated congestive heart
failure; EKG changes (particularly
widening of QRS complex, notched P
waves, widened Q-T interval, ST segment depression).*
EENT: *tinnitus,* excessive salivation,
blurred vision.
GI: *diarrhea, nausea, vomiting,* anorexia, abdominal pains.
Skin: rash, petechial hemorrhage of
buccal mucosa, pruritus.
Other: angioedema, acute asthmatic
attack, respiratory arrest, *fever, cin-
chonism, light-headedness.*

INTERACTIONS
*Acetazolamide, antacids, sodium bi-
carbonate:* may increase quinidine
blood levels due to alkaline urine.
Monitor for increased effect.
Barbiturates, phenytoin: may antagonize quinidine activity. Monitor for
decreased quinidine effect.

NURSING CONSIDERATIONS
• Contraindicated in cardiac glycoside toxicity when A-V conduction is
grossly impaired; complete A-V block
with A-V nodal or idioventricular
pacemaker. Use with caution in myasthenia gravis. Anticholinergic drug
doses may have to be increased.
• May increase toxicity of digitalis
derivatives. Use with caution in patients previously digitalized. Follow
digoxin levels.
• Dosage varies—some patients may
require drug q 4 hours, others

Italicized side effects are common or life-threatening.

q 6 hours. Titrate dose by both clinical response and blood levels.
• When changing route of administration, alter dosage to compensate for variations in quinidine base content.
• Dose should be decreased in congestive heart failure and hepatic disease.
• Check apical pulse rate and blood pressure before starting therapy. If you detect extremes in pulse rate, withhold drug and notify doctor at once.
• Lidocaine may be effective in treating quinidine-induced arrhythmias, since it increases A-V conduction.
• GI side effects, especially diarrhea, are signs of toxicity. Notify doctor.

Check quinidine blood levels, which are toxic when greater than 8 mcg/ml. Decrease GI symptoms by giving with meals. Monitor drug response carefully.
• Instruct patient to notify doctor if skin rash, fever, unusual bleeding, bruising, ringing in ears, or visual disturbance occurs.
• After long-standing atrial fibrillation, restoration of normal sinus rhythm may result in thromboembolism due to dislodgement of thrombi from atrial wall. Anticoagulation often advised before restoration of normal atrial rhythm.
• Never use discolored (brownish) quinidine solution.

17

Antihypertensives

alkavervir
alseroxylon
clonidine hydrochloride
cryptenamine acetate
cryptenamine tannate
deserpidine
diazoxide
guanethidine sulfate
hydralazine hydrochloride
mecamylamine hydrochloride
methyldopa
metoprolol tartrate
minoxidil
nadolol
nitroprusside sodium
pargyline hydrochloride
phenoxybenzamine hydrochloride
phentolamine hydrochloride
phentolamine methanesulfonate
prazosin hydrochloride
propranolol hydrochloride
rauwolfia serpentina
rescinnamine
reserpine
trimethaphan camsylate

---

alkavervir
Veriloid

INDICATIONS & DOSAGE
Essential, renal or malignant hypertension; toxemia of pregnancy—
Adults: 3 to 5 mg P.O. daily, given in 3 to 4 divided doses not less than 4 hours apart. Give after meals. Initial recommended dose is 8 to 9 mg. No dosing recommendations for children.

SIDE EFFECTS
CNS: mental confusion.
CV: *orthostatic hypotension,* cardiac arrhythmias, *bradycardia.*
EENT: blurred vision, excessive salivation, unpleasant taste.
GI: *nausea, vomiting,* epigastric burning, hiccups.
Other: respiratory depression, bronchial constriction, sweating.

INTERACTIONS
Anesthetic agents: may cause additive hypotensive effect. Observe patient carefully.
Tricyclic antidepressants: may diminish hypotensive response. Avoid if possible.

NURSING CONSIDERATIONS
• Contraindicated in patients with pheochromocytoma. Use cautiously in patients with angina, cerebrovascular disease, bronchial asthma, or those receiving other antihypertensive drugs.
• Rarely used to treat hypertension because of unsatisfactory response and high incidence of side effects.
• The range between therapeutic and toxic doses of this drug is narrow. Call the doctor immediately if patient develops side effects.
• Monitor blood pressure and pulse rate closely. Keep phenylephrine or ephedrine handy in case severe hypotension develops. If patient develops bradycardia, he may require atropine.
• Teach patient about his disease and therapy. Explain why it's important to take this drug exactly as prescribed,

even when he's feeling well. Tell patient not to stop this drug suddenly, but to call the doctor if unpleasant side effects develop.
• Inform patient that orthostatic hypotension can be minimized by rising slowly and avoiding sudden position changes. Unpleasant taste can be relieved with sugarless chewing gum, hard sour candy, or ice chips; nausea and vomiting can be prevented by not eating for at least 4 hours after each dose.
• In very hot weather, patient may require smaller doses.
• Give this drug after meals.

---

alseroxylon
Raudolfin, Rauwiloid

INDICATIONS & DOSAGE
Mild, labile hypertension—
Adults: initially, 4 mg P.O. daily as a single dose or divided in 2 doses for 1 to 3 weeks. Maintenance dose: 2 mg or less daily.
No dosing recommendations for children.

SIDE EFFECTS
CNS: mental confusion, *depression, drowsiness, nervousness, anxiety,* insomnia, *nightmares,* sedation.
CV: *orthostatic hypotension, bradycardia.*
EENT: *mouth dryness, nasal stuffiness,* glaucoma.
GI: *hypersecretion of gastric acid, nausea, vomiting,* gastrointestinal bleeding.
Skin: pruritus, rash.
Other: *impotence, weight gain.*

INTERACTIONS
MAO inhibitors: may cause excitability and hypertension. Avoid if possible.

NURSING CONSIDERATIONS
• Use cautiously in patients with severe cardiac or cerebrovascular disease, peptic ulcer, ulcerative colitis, renal disease, gallstones, mental depressive disorders, or those undergoing surgery.
• Use cautiously in patients taking other antihypertensive drugs.
• Monitor patient's blood pressure and pulse rate frequently.
• Teach patient about his disease and therapy. Explain why it's important to take this drug exactly as prescribed, even when he's feeling well. Tell patient not to discontinue this drug suddenly, but to call the doctor if unpleasant side effects, such as mental depression, nightmares, or insomnia, develop. Watch patient closely for signs of mental depression.
• Effect of drug may last for 10 days after discontinuation.
• Warn patient that this drug can cause drowsiness.
• Warn female patient to notify doctor if she becomes pregnant.
• Inform patient that orthostatic hypotension can be minimized by rising slowly and avoiding sudden position changes. Mouth dryness can be relieved with sugarless chewing gum, hard sour candy, or ice chips.
• Tell patient to contact doctor if relief is needed for nasal stuffiness.
• Give this drug with meals.
• Patient should weigh himself daily and notify doctor of any weight gain.
• One mg of alseroxylon is approximately equal to 0.1 mg of reserpine.

---

clonidine hydrochloride
Catapres♦

INDICATIONS & DOSAGE
Essential, renal, and malignant hypertension—
Adults: initially, 0.1 mg P.O. b.i.d. Then increase by 0.1 to 0.2 mg daily

on a weekly basis. Usual dose range:
0.2 to 0.8 mg daily in divided doses.
Infrequently, doses as high as 2.4 mg
daily.
No dosing recommendations for
children.

SIDE EFFECTS
CNS: *drowsiness,* dizziness, fatigue,
sedation, nervousness, headache.
CV: orthostatic hypotension, brady-
cardia.
EENT: *mouth dryness.*
GI: *constipation.*
GU: urinary retention.
Other: impotence.

INTERACTIONS
*Tricyclic antidepressants and MAO in-
hibitors:* may decrease antihypertensive effect. Use together cautiously.

NURSING CONSIDERATIONS
• Use cautiously in patients with severe coronary insufficiency, myocardial infarction, cerebral vascular disease, chronic renal failure, history of
depression, or those taking other antihypertensives.
• Monitor blood pressure and pulse
rate frequently. Dosage is usually adjusted to patient's blood pressure and
tolerance.
• Reduce dose gradually over 2 to
4 days. If discontinued abruptly, this
drug may cause severe hypertension.
• Teach patient about his disease and
therapy. Explain why it's important to
take this drug exactly as prescribed,
even when he's feeling well. Tell patient not to discontinue this drug suddenly, but to call the doctor if unpleasant side effects develop. Warn
that this drug can cause drowsiness.
• Inform patient that orthostatic
hypotension can be minimized by rising slowly and avoiding sudden position changes. Mouth dryness can be
relieved with sugarless chewing gum,
hard sour candy, or ice chips.

• Last dose should be taken immediately before retiring.
• Has been used investigationally to
decrease the subjective symptoms of
opiate withdrawal, migraine headache
prophylaxis, and dysmenorrhea.

---

cryptenamine acetate
Unitensen Aqueous
cryptenamine tannate
Unitensen, Unitensyl♦ ♦

INDICATIONS & DOSAGE
*Mild to moderate hypertension, tox-
emia—*
Adults: initially, 2 mg P.O. b.i.d., increased at weekly intervals, depending on response. Total daily dose not
to exceed 12 mg daily.
I.V. (for hypertensive crises and convulsive toxemia)—0.5 ml (130 CSR
units) diluted to 20 ml with 5% dextrose in water. Administer at infusion
rate of 1 ml/min.
When giving this drug I.V., record
blood pressure every minute.

SIDE EFFECTS
CNS: mental confusion.
CV: *orthostatic hypotension,* cardiac
arrhythmias, *bradycardia.*
EENT: blurred vision, excessive sali-
vation, unpleasant taste.
GI: *nausea, vomiting,* epigastric
burning, hiccups.
Other: respiratory depression, bron-
chial constriction.

INTERACTIONS
Anesthetic agents: may cause additive
hypotensive effect. Observe patient
carefully.
Tricyclic antidepressants: may diminish hypotensive response. Avoid if
possible.

NURSING CONSIDERATIONS
• Contraindicated in patients with
pheochromocytoma. Use cautiously

Italicized side effects are common or life-threatening.

in patients with angina, cerebrovascular disease, bronchial asthma, renal insufficiency, or those taking other antihypertensives.
• Monitor blood pressure and pulse rate closely. If severe hypotension develops, stop infusion and notify doctor, as he may use phenylephrine or ephedrine to counteract effect. Hypotension should dissipate in 60 to 90 minutes. If patient develops bradycardia, he may require atropine. Notify doctor promptly.
• The range between therapeutic and toxic doses of this drug is narrow. Call doctor immediately if patient develops side effects.
• Teach patient about his disease and therapy. Explain why it's important to take this drug exactly as prescribed, even when he's feeling well. Tell patient not to discontinue this drug suddenly, but to call the doctor if unpleasant side effects develop.
• Inform patient that orthostatic hypotension can be minimized by rising slowly and avoiding sudden position changes. Unpleasant taste can be relieved with sugarless chewing gum, sour hard candy, or ice chips.

---

deserpidine
Harmonyl

INDICATIONS & DOSAGE
Mild essential hypertension—
Adults: 0.25 mg P.O. t.i.d. to q.i.d. for up to 2 weeks, then maintenance dose of 0.25 mg once daily may be adequate.
No dosing recommendations for children.

SIDE EFFECTS
CNS: mental confusion, *depression, drowsiness, nervousness,* anxiety, nightmares, sedation.
CV: bradycardia.

EENT: *mouth dryness, nasal stuffiness,* glaucoma.
GI: *hypersecretion of gastric acid, nausea, vomiting,* gastrointestinal bleeding.
Skin: pruritus, rash.
Other: *impotence, weight gain.*

INTERACTIONS
MAO inhibitors: may cause excitability and hypertension. Avoid if possible.

NURSING CONSIDERATIONS
• Contraindicated in patients with mental depression. Use cautiously in patients with severe cardiac or cerebrovascular disease, peptic ulcer, ulcerative colitis, gallstones, or mental depressive disorders; patients undergoing surgery; and in patients taking other antihypertensives or anticonvulsants.
• Monitor patient's blood pressure and pulse rate frequently.
• Teach patient about his disease and therapy. Explain why it's important to take this drug exactly as prescribed, even when he's feeling well. Tell patient not to discontinue this drug suddenly, but to call the doctor if unpleasant side effects, such as mental depression, insomnia, or loss of appetite, develop. Warn that drug can cause drowsiness.
• Watch patient closely for signs of mental depression. Warn him to notify doctor promptly if he starts having nightmares.
• Tell patient to avoid alcohol and to follow prescribed diet.
• Mouth dryness can be relieved with chewing gum, sour hard candy, or ice chips. Tell patient to contact doctor if relief is needed for nasal stuffiness.
• Give this drug with meals to increase absorption.
• Patient should weigh himself daily and notify doctor of any weight gain.
• The 0.1 mg dosage strength contains tartrazine dye which may pro-

duce allergic reactions in susceptible patients.

diazoxide
Hyperstat♦ (I.V. only)

INDICATIONS & DOSAGE
Hypertensive crisis—
Adults: 300 mg I.V. bolus push, administered in 30 seconds or less into peripheral vein. Repeat at intervals of 4 to 24 hours, p.r.n. Mini-boluses of 1 to 3 mg/Kg repeated at intervals of 5 to 15 minutes or infusions of 15 mg/minute are equally effective. Switch to therapy with oral antihypertensives as soon as possible.
Children: 5 mg/Kg I.V. rapid bolus push.

SIDE EFFECTS
CNS: sweating, flushing, warmth, *headaches,* dizziness, light-headedness, euphoria.
CV: *sodium and water retention, orthostatic hypotension,* angina, myocardial ischemia, arrhythmias, EKG changes.
GI: *nausea, vomiting,* abdominal discomfort.
Metabolic: *hyperglycemia,* hyperuricemia.
Local: inflammation and pain from extravasation.

INTERACTIONS
Hydralazine: may cause severe hypotension. Use together cautiously.
Thiazide diuretics: may increase the effects of diazoxide. Use together cautiously.

NURSING CONSIDERATIONS
• Use cautiously in patients with impaired cerebral or cardiac function, diabetes, uremia, or those taking other antihypertensives.
• Monitor blood pressure frequently. Notify doctor immediately if severe

hypotension develops. Keep levarterenol available.
• Monitor patient's intake and output carefully. If fluid or sodium retention develops, doctor may want to order furosemide.
• Take care to avoid extravasation.
• Weigh patients daily. Notify doctor of any weight increase.
• Watch diabetics closely for signs of severe hyperglycemia or hyperosmolar nonketotic coma. Insulin may be needed.
• Check patient's uric acid levels frequently. Report abnormalities to doctor.
• Inform patient that orthostatic hypotension can be minimized by rising slowly and avoiding sudden position changes.
• This drug may alter requirements for insulin, diet, or oral hypoglycemic drugs in previously controlled diabetics. Monitor blood glucose daily.
• Infusion of diazoxide has been shown to be as effective as a bolus in some patients.

guanethidine sulfate
Ismelin♦

INDICATIONS & DOSAGE
For moderate to severe hypertension; usually used in combination with other antihypertensives—
Adults: initially, 10 mg P.O. daily. Increase by 10 mg at weekly to monthly intervals, p.r.n. Usual dose is 25 to 50 mg daily. Some patients may require up to 300 mg.
Children: initially, 200 mcg/Kg P.O. daily. Increase gradually every 1 to 3 weeks to maximum of 8 times initial dose.

SIDE EFFECTS
CNS: *dizziness, weakness, syncope.*
CV: *orthostatic hypotension, brady-*

cardia, congestive heart failure, arrhythmias.
EENT: *nasal stuffiness*, mouth dryness.
GI: *diarrhea*.
GU: *inhibition of ejaculation*.
Other: *edema, weight gain*.

INTERACTIONS
Levodopa, alcohol: may increase hypotensive effect of guanethidine. Use together cautiously.
MAO inhibitors, ephedrine, levarterenol, methylphenidate, amphetamines, tricyclic antidepressants, phenothiazines: may inhibit the antihypertensive effect of guanethidine. Adjust dose accordingly.

NURSING CONSIDERATIONS
• Contraindicated in patients with pheochromocytoma. Use cautiously in patients with severe cardiac disease, recent MI, cerebrovascular disease, peptic ulcer, impaired renal function, bronchial asthma, or those taking other antihypertensives.
• Discontinue drug 2 to 3 weeks before elective surgery.
• Teach patient about his disease and therapy. Explain why it's important to take this drug exactly as prescribed, even when he's feeling well. Tell patient not to discontinue this drug suddenly, but to call the doctor if unpleasant side effects develop.
• Tell patient to avoid strenuous exercise.
• Inform patient that orthostatic hypotension can be minimized by rising slowly and avoiding sudden position changes. Mouth dryness can be relieved with sugarless chewing gum, hard sour candy, or ice chips.
• Give this drug with meals to increase absorption.
• If patient develops diarrhea, doctor may prescribe atropine or paregoric.

hydralazine hydrochloride
Apresoline♦, Dralzine, Hydralyn, Nor-Pres 25, Rolazine

INDICATIONS & DOSAGE
Essential hypertension—
(oral, alone or in combination with other antihypertensives); to reduce afterload in severe congestive heart failure (with nitrates); and severe essential hypertension (parenteral to lower blood pressure quickly).
Adults: initially, 10 mg P.O. q.i.d.; gradually increased to 50 mg q.i.d. Maximum recommended dosage is 200 mg daily, but some patients may require 300 to 400 mg daily.
I.V.—20 to 40 mg given slowly and repeated as necessary, generally q 4 to 6 hours. Switch to oral antihypertensives as soon as possible.
I.M.—20 to 40 mg repeated as necessary, generally q 4 to 6 hours. Switch to oral antihypertensives as soon as possible.
Children: initially, 0.75 mg/Kg P.O. daily in 4 divided doses (25 mg/m² daily). May increase gradually to 10 times this dose, if necessary.
I.V.—give slowly 1.7 to 3.5 mg/Kg daily or 50 to 100 mg/m² daily in 4 to 6 divided doses.
I.M.—1.7 to 3.5 mg/Kg daily or 50 to 100 mg/m² daily in 4 to 6 divided doses.

SIDE EFFECTS
CNS: peripheral neuritis, *headache, dizziness.*
CV: orthostatic hypotension, *tachycardia*, arrhythmias, *angina, palpitations, sodium retention.*
GI: *nausea, vomiting, diarrhea, anorexia.*
Skin: rash.
Other: *lupus erythematosus, weight gain.*

INTERACTIONS

Diazoxide: may cause severe hypotension. Use together cautiously.

NURSING CONSIDERATIONS

- Use cautiously in patients with cardiac disease or those taking other antihypertensives.
- Monitor patient's blood pressure and pulse rate frequently.
- Watch patient closely for sore throat, fever, muscle and joint aches, skin rash. Call doctor immediately if any of these develop.
- Teach patient about his disease and therapy. Explain why it's important to take this drug exactly as prescribed, even when he's feeling well. Tell patient not to discontinue this drug suddenly, but to call the doctor if unpleasant side effects develop.
- Inform patient that orthostatic hypotension can be minimized by rising slowly and avoiding sudden position changes.
- Give this drug with meals to increase absorption.
- Compliance may be improved by administering this drug b.i.d. Check with doctor.

---

mecamylamine hydrochloride
Inversine

INDICATIONS & DOSAGE

For moderate to severe essential hypertension and uncomplicated malignant hypertension—
Adults: initially, 2.5 mg P.O. b.i.d. Increase by 2.5 mg daily every 2 days. Average daily dose 25 mg given in 3 divided doses.
No dosing recommendations for children.

SIDE EFFECTS

CNS: dilated pupils, *blurred vision, paresthesias,* sedation, *fatigue, tremor, choreiform movements,* con-vulsions, psychic changes, dizziness, *weakness, headaches.*
CV: *orthostatic hypotension.*
EENT: *mouth dryness,* glossitis.
GI: *anorexia, nausea, vomiting, constipation, adynamic ileus, diarrhea.*
GU: urinary retention.
Other: decreased libido, impotence.

INTERACTIONS

Sodium bicarbonate and acetazolamide: may increase effect of mecamylamine. Use together cautiously. Watch for increased hypotensive effects and toxicity.

NURSING CONSIDERATIONS

- Contraindicated in patients with recent MI, uremia, chronic pylonephritis. Use cautiously in patients with lower urinary tract pathology, renal insufficiency, glaucoma, pyloric stenosis, coronary insufficiency, cerebral vascular insufficiency, or those taking other antihypertensives.
- Effects of this drug are increased by high environmental temperature, fever, stress, or severe illness.
- Don't withdraw this drug suddenly; rebound hypertension may occur. Tell patient to call the doctor if unpleasant side effects develop.
- Monitor patient's blood pressure frequently while he's standing.
- Give with meals for better absorption. Don't restrict sodium intake.
- If patient develops constipation from this drug, the doctor may want him to take milk of magnesia. Instruct patient to avoid bulk laxatives.
- Teach patient about his disease and therapy. Explain why it's important to take this drug exactly as prescribed, even when he's feeling well.
- Instruct patient that orthostatic hypotension can be minimized by rising slowly and avoiding sudden position changes. Mouth dryness can be relieved with sugarless chewing gum, sour hard candy, or ice chips.

Italicized side effects are common or life-threatening.

methyldopa
Aldomet♦, Dopamet♦♦, Medimet-250♦♦, Novomedopa♦♦

INDICATIONS & DOSAGE
For sustained mild to severe hypertension; should not be used for acute treatment of hypertensive emergencies—
Adults: initially, 250 mg P.O. b.i.d. to t.i.d. in first 48 hours. Then increase as needed every 2 days. Dosages may need adjustment if other antihypertensive drugs are added to or deleted from therapy.
Maintenance dosages—500 mg to 2 g daily in 2 to 4 divided doses. Maximum recommended daily dose is 3 g. I.V.—500 mg to 1 g q 6 hours, diluted in 5% dextrose in water, and administered over 30 to 60 minutes. Switch to oral antihypertensives as soon as possible.
Children: initially, 10 mg/Kg/day P.O. in 2 to 3 divided doses; or 20 to 40 mg/Kg/day I.V. in 4 divided doses. Increase dose daily until desired response. Maximum daily dose 65 mg/Kg.

SIDE EFFECTS
Blood: *hemolytic anemia,* reversible granulocytopenia, thrombocytopenia.
CNS: *sedation,* headache, asthenia, weakness, dizziness, *decreased mental acuity,* involuntary choreoathetotic movements, psychic disturbances, depression.
CV: bradycardia, *orthostatic hypotension,* aggravated angina, myocarditis, *edema and weight gain.*
EENT: *nasal stuffiness.*
GI: *dry mouth,* diarrhea.
Hepatic: *hepatic necrosis.*
Other: gynecomastia, lactation, skin rash, drug-induced fever, impotence.

INTERACTIONS
Norepinephrine, phenothiazines, tricyclic antidepressants, amphetamines: possible hypertensive effects. Monitor carefully.

NURSING CONSIDERATIONS
• Use cautiously in patients receiving other antihypertensives or MAO inhibitors. Monitor blood pressure and pulse rate frequently.
• Observe patient for side effects, particularly unexplained fever. Report side effects to doctor.
• If patient requires blood transfusion, make sure he gets direct and indirect Coombs' tests to avoid cross-matching problems.
• Monitor blood studies (complete blood count) before and during therapy.
• If patient has been on this drug for several months, positive reaction to direct Coombs' tests indicates hemolytic anemia.
• Weigh patient daily. Notify doctor of any weight increase. Salt and water retention may occur but can be relieved with diuretics.
• Tell patient that urine may turn dark in toilet bowls treated with bleach.
• Teach patient about his disease and therapy. Explain why it's important to take this drug exactly as prescribed, even when he's feeling well. Tell patient not to stop this drug suddenly, but to call the doctor if unpleasant side effects develop. Once-daily dosage given at bedtime will minimize drowsiness during daytime. Check with doctor.
• Inform patient that orthostatic hypotension can be minimized by rising slowly and avoiding position changes. Mouth dryness can be relieved with sugarless chewing gum, hard sour candy, or ice chips.

metoprolol tartrate
Betaloc♦♦, Lopresor♦♦, Lopressor

INDICATIONS & DOSAGE
For hypertension; may be used alone or in combination with other anti-hypertensives—
Adults: 50 mg b.i.d. P.O. initially. Up to 200 to 400 mg daily in 2 to 3 divided doses.
No dosage recommendations for children.

SIDE EFFECTS
CNS: *fatigue, lethargy,* vivid dreams, hallucinations.
CV: *bradycardia, hypotension, congestive heart failure,* peripheral vascular disease.
GI: nausea, vomiting, diarrhea.
Metabolic: hypoglycemia without tachycardia.
Skin: rash.
Other: *increased airway resistance,* fever.

INTERACTIONS
Insulin, hypoglycemic drugs (oral): can alter dosage requirements in previously stabilized diabetics. Observe patient carefully.
Cardiac glycosides: excessive bradycardia and increased depressant effect on myocardium. Use together cautiously.

NURSING CONSIDERATIONS
• Use cautiously in patients with heart block, congestive heart failure, diabetes, respiratory disease, or those taking other antihypertensives. Always check patient's apical pulse rate before giving this drug. If it's slower than 60 beats/minute, hold drug and call doctor immediately.
• Monitor blood pressure frequently. If patient develops severe hypotension, administer a vasopressor.
• Teach patient about his disease and therapy. Explain why it's important to take this drug, even when he's feeling well. Tell patient not to discontinue this drug suddenly; abrupt discontinuation can exacerbate angina and MI. Tell patient to call doctor if unpleasant side effects develop.
• Food may increase absorption of metoprolol. Give consistently with meals.

minoxidil
Loniten

INDICATIONS & DOSAGE
Treatment of severe hypertension—
Adults: 5 mg P.O. initially as a single dose. Effective dosage range is usually 10 to 40 mg/day. Maximum dose 100 mg/day.
Children (under 12): 0.2 mg/Kg as a single daily dose. Effective dosage range usually 0.25 to 1.0 mg/Kg/day. Maximum dose is 50 mg.

SIDE EFFECTS
CV: *edema, tachycardia, pericardial effusion and tamponade, congestive heart failure.*
Other: *hypertrichosis* (elongation, thickening, and enhanced pigmentation of fine body hair), breast tenderness, EKG changes.

INTERACTIONS
Guanethidine: severe orthostatic hypotension. Advise patient to stand up slowly.

NURSING CONSIDERATIONS
• Contraindicated in pheochromocytoma.
• Use only when other antihypertensives have failed. A potent vasodilator.
• About 8 out of 10 patients will experience hypertrichosis within 3 to 6 weeks of beginning treatment. Unwanted hair can be controlled with a

hair remover or shaving. Assure patient that extra hair will disappear within 1 to 6 months of stopping minoxidil. Advise patient, however, not to discontinue taking drug without first notifying doctor.
• Drug is usually prescribed with a beta-blocking drug to control tachycardia and a diuretic to counteract fluid retention. Make sure patient complies with total treatment regimen.
• A patient package insert (PPI) has been prepared by the manufacturer for minoxidil, describing in laytman's terms the drug and its side effects. Be sure your patient receives this insert and reads it thoroughly.
• Available as a 2.5 and 10 mg tablet.

---

nadolol
Corgard♦

INDICATIONS & DOSAGE
Treatment of hypertension—
Adults: 40 mg P.O. once daily, initially. Dosage may be increased in 40 to 80 mg increments until optimum response. Usual maintenance dosage range: 80 to 320 mg once daily. Doses of 640 mg may be necessary in rare cases.
Long-term management of angina pectoris—
Adults: 40 mg P.O. once daily, initially. Dosage may be increased in 40 to 80 mg increments until optimum response. Usual maintenance dosage range: 80 to 240 mg once daily.

SIDE EFFECTS
CNS: *fatigue, lethargy,* vivid dreams, hallucinations.
CV: *bradycardia, hypotension, congestive heart failure,* peripheral vascular disease.
GI: nausea, vomiting, diarrhea.
Metabolic: hypoglycemia without tachycardia.

Skin: rash.
Other: *increased airway resistance,* fever.

INTERACTIONS
Insulin, hypoglycemic drugs (oral): can alter dosage requirements in previously stabilized diabetics. Observe patient carefully.
Cardiac glycosides: excessive bradycardia and increased depressant effect on myocardium. Use together cautiously.

NURSING CONSIDERATIONS
• Contraindicated in bronchial asthma, sinus bradycardia and greater than first degree conduction block, and cardiogenic shock.
• Use cautiously in cardiac failure, chronic bronchitis, and emphysema.
• Always check patient's apical pulse before giving this drug. If slower than 60 beats/minute, hold drug and call doctor.
• Monitor blood pressure frequently. If patient develops severe hypotension, administer a vasopressor.
• Don't discontinue abruptly: can exacerbate angina and MI.
• Teach patient about his disease and therapy. Explain why it's important to take this drug, even when he's feeling well. Tell patient not to discontinue drug suddenly, but to call doctor if unpleasant side effects develop.
• This drug masks common signs of shock and hypoglycemia.
• Food may increase absorption of nadolol. Give consistently with meals.

---

nitroprusside sodium
Nipride♦

INDICATIONS & DOSAGE
To lower blood pressure quickly in hypertensive emergencies; to control hypotension during anesthesia; to re-

duce preload and afterload in cardiac pump failure or cardiogenic shock; may be used with or without dopamine—
Adults: 50-mg vial diluted with 2 to 3 ml of dextrose 5% in water I.V. and then added to 250, 500, or 1,000 ml dextrose 5% in water. Infuse at 0.5 to 10 mcg/Kg/min.
Average dose: 3 mcg/Kg/min. Maximum infusion rate: 10 mcg/Kg/min. Patients taking other antihypertensive drugs along with nitroprusside are very sensitive to this drug. Adjust dosage accordingly.

SIDE EFFECTS
The following effects generally indicate overdosage:
CNS: *headache, dizziness,* ataxia, loss of consciousness, coma, weak pulse, absent reflexes, widely dilated pupils, *restlessness, muscle twitching, diaphoresis.*
CV: distant heart sounds, dyspnea, palpitations, shallow breathing.
GI: *vomiting, nausea, abdominal pain.*
Metabolic: acidosis.
Skin: pink color.
Local: *tissue sloughing and necrosis with extravasation.*

INTERACTIONS
None significant.

NURSING CONSIDERATIONS
• Use cautiously in patients with hypothyroidism, hepatic or renal disease, or those receiving other antihypertensives.
• Due to light sensitivity, wrap I.V. solution in foil. It's not necessary to wrap the tubing in foil. Fresh solution should have faint brownish tint. Discard after 4 hours.
• Obtain baseline vital signs before giving this drug, and find out what parameters the doctor wants to achieve.
• Check blood pressure every 5 minutes at start of infusion and every

15 minutes thereafter. If severe hypotension occurs, turn off I.V. Nipride—effects of drug quickly reversed. Notify doctor. If possible, an arterial pressure line should be started. Regulate drug flow to specified level.
• Don't use bacteriostatic water for injection or sterile saline for reconstitution.
• Infuse with motorized infusion pump.
• This drug is best run piggyback through a peripheral line with no other medication. Don't adjust rate of main I.V. line while drug is running. Even small bolus of nitroprusside can cause severe hypotension.
• This drug can cause cyanide toxicity, so check serum thiocyanate levels every 72 hours. Watch for signs of thiocyanate toxicity: profound hypotension, metabolic acidosis, dyspnea, headache, loss of consciousness, ataxia, vomiting. If these occur, discontinue drug immediately and notify doctor.
• Extravasation can cause tissue irritation.

---

pargyline hydrochloride
Eutonyl

INDICATIONS & DOSAGE
For moderate to severe hypertension, usually given in combination with other drugs—
Adults: initially, 25 to 50 mg P.O. once daily, if not receiving any other antihypertensive drugs. Then increase dosage by 10 mg daily at weekly intervals. Maximum daily dosage 200 mg.
Usual daily dose for patients over age 65 or those who've had sympathectomy: 10 to 25 mg. When used in combination with other drugs, total daily dose pargyline should not exceed 25 mg.
No dosage recommendations for

children.

SIDE EFFECTS

CNS: *tremors,* convulsions, choreiform movements, psychic changes, *nightmares, hyperexcitability, sweating,* dizziness, fainting, drowsiness.
CV: palpitations, *orthostatic hypotension,* fluid retention.
EENT: *mouth dryness,* optic damage.
GI: *nausea, vomiting, increased appetite, constipation.*
Other: impotence.

INTERACTIONS

Amphetamines, ephedrine, levodopa, metaraminol, methotrimeprazine, methylphenidate, phenylephrine, phenylpropanolamine, pseudoephedrine: enhanced pressor effects. Use together cautiously.
Alcohol, barbiturates, and other sedatives; tranquilizers; narcotics; dextromethorphan; tricyclic antidepressants: unpredictable interactions. Should be used with caution and in reduced dosage.

NURSING CONSIDERATIONS

• Contraindicated in patients with advanced renal failure, pheochromocytoma, hyperthyroidism, or Parkinson's disease; in patients who are hyperactive and hyperexcitable. Use cautiously in patients receiving other antihypertensives, or who have hepatic disease.
• Discontinue this drug at least 2 weeks before elective surgery.
• Hypotensive effects of this drug are increased by high temperatures, fever, stress, or severe illness. If patient develops severe hypotension, counteract with ephedrine or phenylephrine.
• Monitor blood pressure and pulse rate frequently. Take blood pressure while patient is standing.
• Patient should have periodic ophthalmic evaluations during therapy.
• If patient is scheduled for surgery

and has been taking this drug, be sure narcotic dosages are reduced.
• This drug may require up to several weeks to reach optimal effect.
• Warn patient not to take any other medications, including over-the-counter cold remedies, without first asking doctor.
• This drug is an MAO inhibitor. Tell patient not to eat foods with high tyramine content: for example, aged cheese, chianti wine, sour cream, canned figs, raisins, chicken livers, yeast extract, chocolate, pickled herring, caffeine, cyclamates, cola drinks.
• Teach patient about his disease and therapy. Explain why it's important to take this drug exactly as prescribed, even when he's feeling well. Tell patient not to discontinue this drug suddenly, but to call the doctor if unpleasant side effects develop.
• Inform patient that orthostatic hypotension can be minimized by rising slowly and avoiding sudden position changes. Mouth dryness can be relieved with sugarless chewing gum, sour hard candy, or ice chips.

phenoxybenzamine hydrochloride
Dibenzyline

INDICATIONS & DOSAGE

To control hypertension and sweating secondary to pheochromocytoma; may be used in combination with propranolol to control excessive tachycardia—
Adults: initially, 10 mg P.O. daily. Increase by 10 mg daily every 4 days. Maintenance dose: 20 to 60 mg daily.
Children: initially, 0.2 mg/Kg or 6 mg/m^2 P.O. daily in a single dose. Maintenance dose: 12 to 36 mg/m^2 daily as a single dose or in divided doses.

SIDE EFFECTS
CNS: lethargy, drowsiness.
CV: *orthostatic hypotension, tachycardia,* shock.
EENT: *nasal stuffiness, miosis.*
GI: vomiting, abdominal distress.
Other: *impotence.*

INTERACTIONS
None significant.

NURSING CONSIDERATIONS
• Use cautiously in patients with cerebrovascular or coronary insufficiency, advanced renal disease, respiratory disease.
• Watch patient closely for side effects, and call doctor promptly if they occur. If severe hypotension develops, patient may require levarterenol to counteract effect.
• Nasal congestion, miosis, and impotence usually decrease upon continued therapy.
• Patient with tachycardia may require concurrent propranolol therapy.
• Monitor patient's heart rate and blood pressure frequently.
• This drug may take several weeks to achieve optimal effect.
• Monitor respiratory status carefully. This drug may aggravate symptoms of pneumonia and asthma.
• Teach patient about his disease and therapy. Explain why it's important to take this drug exactly as prescribed, even when he's feeling well. Tell patient not to discontinue this drug suddenly, but to call the doctor if unpleasant side effects develop.
• Inform patient that orthostatic hypotension can be minimized by rising slowly and avoiding sudden position changes. Mouth dryness can be relieved with sugarless chewing gum, sour hard candy, or ice chips.
• Used investigationally to treat chronic urinary retention.

phentolamine hydrochloride
Regitine
phentolamine methanesulfonate
Regitine, Rogitine♦ ♦

INDICATIONS & DOSAGE
To aid in diagnosis of pheochromocytoma; to control or prevent hypertension before or during pheochromocytomectomy—
Adults: P.O. therapeutic dose: 50 mg q.i.d.
I.V. diagnostic dose: 5 mg, with close monitoring of blood pressure.
Before surgical removal of tumor, give 2 to 5 mg I.M. or I.V. During surgery, patient may need small I.V. doses (1 mg) or small I.M. doses (3 mg).
Children: P.O. therapeutic dose: 5 mg/Kg daily or 150 mg/m^2 daily in 4 to 6 divided doses.
I.V. diagnostic dose: 0.1 mg/Kg or 3 mg/m^2 as single dose, with close monitoring of blood pressure.
Before surgical removal of tumor give 1 mg I.V. or 3 mg I.M. During surgery, patient may need small I.V. doses (1 mg).

SIDE EFFECTS
CNS: *dizziness, weakness, flushing.*
CV: *hypotension,* shock, *arrhythmias,* palpitations, *tachycardia,* angina pectoris.
GI: *diarrhea,* abdominal pain, *nausea, vomiting,* hyperperistalsis.
Other: *nasal stuffiness,* hypoglycemia.

INTERACTIONS
None significant.

NURSING CONSIDERATIONS
• Contraindicated in angina, coronary artery disease, and history of MI. Use cautiously in patients with gastritis or peptic ulcer and in those receiving other antihypertensives.

Italicized side effects are common or life-threatening.

• When this drug is given for diagnostic test, check patient's blood pressure first. Make frequent blood pressure checks during administration.
• Diagnosis positive for pheochromocytoma if severe hypotension results from I.V. test dose.
• Administer levarterenol to counteract severe hypotensive effect of this drug. Don't administer epinephrine to raise blood pressure, as this may cause further drop.
• Don't give sedatives or narcotics 24 hours before diagnostic test.

prazosin hydrochloride
Minipress♦

INDICATIONS & DOSAGE
For mild to moderate hypertension; used alone or in combination with a diuretic or other antihypertensive drugs; also used to decrease afterload in severe chronic congestive heart failure—
Adults: P.O. test dose: 1 mg given before bedtime to prevent "first-dose syncope." Initial dose: 1 mg t.i.d. Increase dosage slowly. Maximum daily dose 20 mg. Maintenance dose: 3 to 20 mg daily in 3 divided doses. A few patients have required dosages larger than this (up to 40 mg daily).
If other antihypertensive drugs or diuretics are added to this drug, decrease prazosin dosage to 1 to 2 mg t.i.d. and retitrate.

SIDE EFFECTS
CNS: *dizziness,* headache, drowsiness, weakness, *"first-dose syncope,"* depression.
CV: orthostatic hypotension, *palpitations.*
EENT: blurred vision.
GI: vomiting, diarrhea, abdominal cramps, dry mouth, constipation, *nausea.*
GU: priapism.

INTERACTIONS
None significant.

NURSING CONSIDERATIONS
• Use cautiously in patients receiving other antihypertensive drugs.
• Monitor patient's blood pressure and pulse rate frequently.
• If initial dose is greater than 1 mg, patient may develop severe syncope with loss of consciousness (first-dose syncope). Increase dosage slowly. Instruct patient to sit or lie down if he experiences dizziness.
• Teach patient about his disease and therapy. Explain why it's important to take this drug exactly as prescribed, even when he's feeling well. Tell patient not to discontinue this drug suddenly, but to call the doctor if unpleasant side effects develop.
• Inform patient that orthostatic hypotension can be minimized by rising slowly and avoiding sudden position changes. Mouth dryness can be relieved with sugarless chewing gum, sour hard candy, or ice chips.
• Investigationally, compliance may be improved by giving this drug once a day. Check with doctor.

propranolol hydrochloride
Inderal♦

INDICATIONS & DOSAGE
Hypertension (usually used with thiazide diuretics)—
Adults: initial treatment of hypertension: 80 mg P.O. daily in 2 to 4 divided doses. Increase at 3- to 7-day intervals to maximum daily dose of 640 mg. Usual maintenance dose for hypertension: 160 to 480 mg daily. No dosing recommendations for children.

SIDE EFFECTS
CNS: *fatigue, lethargy,* vivid dreams, hallucinations.

CV: *bradycardia, hypotension, congestive heart failure*, peripheral vascular disease.
GI: nausea, vomiting, diarrhea.
Metabolic: hypoglycemia without tachycardia.
Skin: rash.
Other: *increased airway resistance*, fever.

INTERACTIONS
Insulin, hypoglycemic drugs (oral): can alter requirements for these drugs in previously stabilized diabetics. Monitor for hypoglycemia.
Cardiac glycosides: excessive bradycardia and increased depressant effect on myocardium. Use together cautiously.
Aminophylline: antagonized beta-blocking effects of propranolol. Use together cautiously.
Isoproterenol, glucagon: antagonized propranolol effect. May be used therapeutically and in emergencies.

NURSING CONSIDERATIONS
• Contraindicated in diabetes mellitus, asthma, allergic rhinitis; during ethyl ether anesthesia; in sinus bradycardia and heart block greater than first degree; in cardiogenic shock; in right ventricular failure secondary to pulmonary hypertension. Use with caution in congestive heart failure, respiratory disease, and patients taking other antihypertensive drugs.
• Always check patient's apical pulse rate before giving this drug. If you detect extremes in pulse rates, hold medication and call the doctor immediately.
• Monitor blood pressure frequently. If patient develops severe hypotension, notify doctor. He may prescribe a vasopressor.
• Teach patient about his disease and therapy. Explain why it's important to take this drug exactly as prescribed, even when he's feeling well. Tell patient not to discontinue this drug sud-

denly; abrupt discontinuation can exacerbate angina and MI. Tell patient to call doctor if unpleasant side effects develop.
• This drug masks common signs of shock and hypoglycemia.
• Food may increase the absorption of propranolol. Give consistently with meals.
• Compliance may be improved by administering this drug on a twice-daily basis. Check with doctor.

rauwolfia serpentina
HBP, Hiwolfia, Hyper-Rauw, Hywolfia, Rau, Raudixin♦, Rauja, Raumason, Rauneed, Raupoid, Rauserpa, Rauserpin, Rausertina, Rauval, Rauwoldin, Rawfola, Ru-Hy-T, Serfia, Serfolia, T-Rau, Wolfina

INDICATIONS & DOSAGE
Mild to moderate hypertension—
Adults: initially and for 1 to 3 weeks thereafter, 200 to 400 mg P.O. daily as a single dose or in 2 divided doses. Maintenance dose: 50 to 300 mg/day. No dosing recommendations for children.

SIDE EFFECTS
CNS: mental confusion, *depression, drowsiness, nervousness*, anxiety, nightmares, sedation, headache.
CV: *orthostatic hypotension, bradycardia, syncope*.
EENT: *mouth dryness, nasal stuffiness*, glaucoma.
GI: *hypersecretion of gastric acid, nausea, vomiting*, gastrointestinal bleeding.
Skin: pruritus, rash.
Other: *impotence, weight gain*.

INTERACTIONS
MAO inhibitors: may cause excitability and hypertension. Use together cautiously.

Italicized side effects are common or life-threatening.

NURSING CONSIDERATIONS
- Contraindicated in patients with depression. Use cautiously in patients with severe cardiac or cerebrovascular disease, impaired renal function, peptic ulcer, ulcerative colitis, gallstones; those undergoing surgery; or taking other antihypertensives or tricyclic antidepressants.
- Monitor patient's blood pressure and pulse rate frequently.
- Teach patient about his disease and therapy. Explain why it's important to take this drug exactly as prescribed, even when he's feeling well. Tell patient not to discontinue this drug suddenly, but to call the doctor if unpleasant side effects develop. Warn that this drug can cause drowsiness.
- Watch patient closely for signs of mental depression. Warn him to notify doctor promptly if he starts having nightmares.
- Inform patient that orthostatic hypotension can be minimized by rising slowly and avoiding sudden position changes. Mouth dryness can be relieved with sugarless chewing gum, sour hard candy, or ice chips. Tell patient to contact doctor if relief is needed for nasal stuffiness.
- Give this drug with meals.
- Patient should weigh himself daily and notify doctor of any weight gain.
- Effects of this drug may last for 10 days after it's been discontinued.

---

rescinnamine
Anaprel, Cinnasil, Moderil

INDICATIONS & DOSAGE
For mild to moderate hypertension; may be used alone or in combination with other antihypertensives—
Adults: initially, 0.5 mg b.i.d. Maintenance dose: 0.25 to 0.5 mg daily.
No dosing recommendations for children.

SIDE EFFECTS
CNS: mental confusion, *depression, drowsiness, nervousness, anxiety, nightmares,* sedation, parkinsonism.
CV: *orthostatic hypotension, bradycardia, syncope.*
EENT: *mouth dryness, nasal stuffiness,* glaucoma.
GI: *hypersecretion of gastric acid, nausea, vomiting,* gastrointestinal bleeding.
Skin: pruritus, rash.
Other: *impotence, weight gain.*

INTERACTIONS
MAO inhibitors: may cause excitability and hypertension. Use together cautiously.

NURSING CONSIDERATIONS
- Contraindicated in patients with depression. Use cautiously in patients with severe cardiac or cerebrovascular disease, peptic ulcer, ulcerative colitis, gallstones, or those undergoing surgery. Also use cautiously in patients taking other antihypertensives.
- Monitor patient's blood pressure and pulse rate frequently.
- Teach patient about his disease and therapy. Explain why it's important to take this drug exactly as prescribed, even when he's feeling well. Tell patient not to discontinue this drug suddenly, but to call the doctor if unpleasant side effects develop. Warn that this drug can cause drowsiness.
- Watch patient closely for signs of mental depression. Warn him to notify doctor promptly if he starts having nightmares.
- Inform patient that orthostatic hypotension can be minimized by rising slowly and avoiding sudden position changes. Mouth dryness can be relieved with sugarless chewing gum, sour hard candy, or ice chips. Tell patient to contact doctor if relief is needed for nasal stuffiness.
- Give this drug with meals.

- Patient should weigh himself daily and notify doctor of any weight gain.
- Effects of this drug may last for 10 days after it's been discontinued.

---

reserpine
Alkarau, Arcum R-S, Bonapene, Broserpine, De Serpa, Elserpine, Geneserp #2, Hiserpia, Hyperine, Lemiserp, Maso-Serpine, Neo-Serp♦♦, Rauloydin, Raurine, Rau-Sed, Rauserpin, Releserp-5, Reserjen, Reserfia♦♦, Reserpanca♦♦, Reserpaneed, Reserpoid, Rolserp, Sandril, Serp, Serpalan, Serpena, Serpanray, Serpasil♦, Serpate, Sertabs, Sertina, Tensin, T-Serp, Tri-Serp, Vio-Serpine, Zepine

INDICATIONS & DOSAGE
Mild to moderate essential hypertension (oral); hypertensive emergencies (parenteral)—
Adults: initially, 0.5 mg P.O. daily for 1 to 2 weeks. Maintenance dose: 0.1 to 0.5 mg daily.
I.M—initially, 0.5 to 1 mg, followed by doses of 2 to 4 mg at 2-hour intervals. Maximum recommended dose 4 mg.
Children: 0.07 mg/Kg or 2 mg/m² with hydralazine I.M. every 12 to 24 hours.

SIDE EFFECTS
CNS: mental confusion, *depression, drowsiness, nervousness, anxiety, nightmares,* sedation.
CV: *orthostatic hypotension, bradycardia, syncope.*
EENT: *mouth dryness, nasal stuffiness,* glaucoma.
GI: *hyperacidity, nausea, vomiting,* gastrointestinal bleeding.
Skin: pruritus, rash.
Other: *impotence, weight gain.*

INTERACTIONS
MAO inhibitors: may cause excitabil-ity and hypertension. Use together cautiously.

NURSING CONSIDERATIONS
- Contraindicated in patients with depression. Use cautiously in patients with severe cardiac or cerebrovascular disease, peptic ulcer, ulcerative colitis, gallstones, mental depressive disorders; those undergoing surgery; and those taking other antihypertensive drugs.
- Monitor patient's blood pressure and pulse rate frequently.
- Teach patient about his disease and therapy. Explain why it's important to take this drug exactly as prescribed, even when he's feeling well. Tell patient not to discontinue this drug suddenly, but to call doctor if unpleasant side effects develop. Warn that this drug can cause drowsiness.
- Warn female patient to notify doctor if she becomes pregnant.
- Watch patient closely for signs of mental depression. Warn him to notify doctor promptly if he starts having nightmares.
- Inform patient that orthostatic hypotension can be minimized by rising slowly and avoiding sudden position changes. Mouth dryness can be relieved with sugarless chewing gum, sour hard candy, or ice chips. Tell patient to contact doctor if relief is needed for nasal stuffiness.
- Give this drug with meals.
- Patient should weigh himself daily and notify doctor of any weight gain.
- Effects of this drug may last for 10 days after it's been discontinued.
- Parenteral form erratically absorbed; largely replaced by other antihypertensives for hypertensive emergencies.

Italicized side effects are common or life-threatening.

trimethaphan camsylate
Arfonad♦

INDICATIONS & DOSAGE
To lower blood pressure quickly in hypertensive emergencies; for controlled hypotension during surgery—
Adults: 500 mg (10 ml) diluted in 500 ml dextrose 5% in water to yield concentration of 1 mg/ml I.V. Start I.V. drip at 1 to 2 mg/min and titrate to achieve desired hypotensive response. Range: 0.3 mg to 6 mg/min.

SIDE EFFECTS
CNS: dilated pupils.
CV: *severe orthostatic hypotension, tachycardia.*
GI: anorexia, *nausea, vomiting, dry mouth.*
GU: *urinary retention.*
Other: respiratory depression, *extreme weakness.*

INTERACTIONS
None significant.

NURSING CONSIDERATIONS
- Contraindicated in patients with anemia, respiratory insufficiency. Use cautiously in patients with arteriosclerosis; cardiac, hepatic, or renal disease; degenerative CNS disorders; Addison's disease; diabetes; those receiving glucocorticoids; or those receiving other antihypertensives.
- Monitor patient's blood pressure and vital signs frequently.
- If extreme hypotension occurs, discontinue drug and call doctor. Use phenylephrine or mephentermine to counteract hypotension.
- Watch closely for respiratory distress, especially if large doses are used.
- Use infusion pump to administer this drug slowly.
- Discontinue drug before wound closure in surgery to allow blood pressure to return to normal.
- Position patient to avoid cerebral anoxia.
- Patient should receive oxygen therapy during use of this agent.

18

Vasodilators

amyl nitrite
cyclandelate
dioxyline phosphate
dipyridamole
erythrityl tetranitrate
ethaverine hydrochloride
isosorbide dinitrate
isoxsuprine hydrochloride
mannitol hexanitrate
nicotinyl alcohol
nitroglycerin
nylidrin hydrochloride
papaverine hydrochloride
pentaerythritol tetranitrate
tolazoline hydrochloride

---

amyl nitrite

INDICATIONS & DOSAGE
Antidote for cyanide poisoning—
0.2 or 0.3 ml by inhalation for 30 to 60 seconds q 5 minutes until conscious.
Relief of angina pectoris, bronchospasm, biliary spasm—
Adults and children: 0.2 to 0.3 ml by inhalation (1 glass ampule inhaler), p.r.n.

SIDE EFFECTS
Blood: methemoglobinemia.
CNS: *headache, sometimes with throbbing;* dizziness; weakness.
CV: *orthostatic hypotension, tachycardia,* flushing, palpitations, fainting.
GI: nausea, vomiting.
Skin: cutaneous vasodilation.
Other: hypersensitivity reactions.

INTERACTIONS
None significant.

NURSING CONSIDERATIONS
• Contraindicated in hypersensitivity to nitrites. Use with caution in cerebral hemorrhage, hypotension, head injury, and glaucoma.
• Watch for orthostatic hypotension. Have patient sit down and avoid rapid position changes while inhaling drug.
• Extinguish all cigarettes before using or ampule may ignite.
• Wrap ampule in cloth and crush. Hold near patient's nose and mouth so vapor is inhaled.
• Effective within 30 seconds but has a short duration (4 to 8 minutes).
• Head-low position, deep breathing, and movement of extremities may help relieve dizziness, syncope, or weakness from postural hypotension.
• Drug is often abused. Claimed to have aphrodisiac benefits. Sometimes called "Amy."

---

cyclandelate
Cyclanfor, Cyclospasmol♦

INDICATIONS & DOSAGE
Adjunct in intermittent claudication, arteriosclerosis obliterans, vasospasm and muscular ischemia associated with thrombophlebitis, nocturnal leg cramps, Raynaud's phenomenon, selected cases of ischemic cerebral vascular disease—
Adults: initially, 200 mg P.O. q.i.d. (before meals and h.s.); maximum

400 mg P.O. q.i.d. When clinical response is noted, decrease dosage gradually until maintenance dosage is reached. Maintenance dose 400 to 800 mg daily in divided doses.

SIDE EFFECTS
CNS: *headache, tingling of the extremities, dizziness.*
CV: *mild flushing,* tachycardia.
GI: pyrosis, eructation, nausea, heartburn.
Other: *sweating.*

INTERACTIONS
None significant.

NURSING CONSIDERATIONS
• Use with extreme caution in severe obliterative coronary artery or cerebral vascular disease, since circulation to these diseased areas may be compromised by vasodilatory effects of the drug elsewhere (coronary steal syndrome). Use with caution in glaucoma, hypotension.
• Give with food or antacids to lessen GI distress.
• Use in conjunction with, not as a substitute for appropriate medical or surgical therapy of peripheral or cerebral vascular disease.
• Short-term therapy of little benefit. Instruct patient to expect long-term treatment and to continue to take medication.
• Side effects usually disappear after several weeks of therapy.

---

dioxyline phosphate
Paveril Phosphate♦

INDICATIONS & DOSAGE
Treatment of angina pectoris and conditions in which there is reflex spasm of blood vessels in arms, legs, or lungs; smooth-muscle spasm—
Adults: 100 to 400 mg 3 to 4 times daily, as required.

SIDE EFFECTS
CNS: dizziness, sedation.
CV: sweating, flushing, hypotension.
GI: nausea, abdominal cramps.

INTERACTIONS
None significant.

NURSING CONSIDERATIONS
• Alert patient to possible side effects.

---

dipyridamole
Persantine♦

INDICATIONS & DOSAGE
Long-term therapy of chronic angina pectoris, prevention of recurrent transient ischemic attack—
Adults: 50 mg P.O. t.i.d. at least 1 hour before meals, to maximum of 400 mg daily.
Inhibition of platelet adhesion in patients with prosthetic heart valves, in combination with warfarin—
Adults: 100 to 400 mg P.O. daily.
Transient ischemic attack—
Adults: 100 mg P.O. daily as a single dose.

SIDE EFFECTS
CNS: *headache, dizziness.*
CV: flushing, fainting, *hypotension.*
GI: *nausea,* vomiting, diarrhea.
Skin: rash.
Other: weakness.

INTERACTIONS
None significant.

NURSING CONSIDERATIONS
• Use with caution in hypotension, anticoagulant therapy.
• Observe for side effects, especially with large doses. Monitor blood pressure.
• Administer 1 hour before meals.
• Watch for signs of bleeding, pro-

longed bleeding time (large doses, long-term).
• Clinical response to antianginal therapy may not be evident before second or third month. Tell patient to continue drug despite lack of observable response.

erythrityl tetranitrate
Anginar, Cardilate♦

INDICATIONS & DOSAGE
Prophylaxis and long-term management of frequent or recurrent anginal pain, reduced exercise tolerance associated with angina pectoris—
Adults: 5 mg sublingually or bucally t.i.d. or 10 mg P.O., a.c. chewed t.i.d., increasing in 2 to 3 days if needed.

SIDE EFFECTS
CNS: *headache, sometimes with throbbing; dizziness;* weakness.
CV: *orthostatic hypotension, tachycardia, flushing, palpitations,* fainting.
GI: nausea, vomiting, sublingual burning.
Skin: cutaneous vasodilation.
Other: hypersensitivity reactions.

INTERACTIONS
None significant.

NURSING CONSIDERATIONS
• Contraindicated in hypersensitivity to nitrites, idiosyncrasy, head trauma, cerebral hemorrhage, severe anemia. Use with caution in hypotension.
• Monitor blood pressure, and intensity and duration of response to drug.
• May cause headaches, especially at first. Treat headache with aspirin or acetaminophen. Dosage may need to be reduced temporarily, but tolerance usually develops.
• Tell patient to take medication regularly, even long-term, if ordered, and

to keep it easily accessible at all times. Physiologically necessary but not habit-forming.
• Additional dose may be taken before anticipated stress or at bedtime if angina is nocturnal.
• Advise patient to avoid alcoholic beverages; they may produce unpleasant Antabuse-like side effects.
• May cause orthostatic hypotension. Patient should get out of bed, go up and down stairs, and change position slowly; he should lie down at first sign of dizziness.
• Teach patient to take sublingual tablet at first sign of attack. He should wet the tablet with saliva, place it under the tongue until completely absorbed, and sit down and rest. Burning sensation indicates potency. Dose may be repeated every 10 to 15 minutes for a maximum of 3 doses. If no relief, patient should call doctor or go to hospital emergency room. If patient complains of tingling, he may try holding tablet in buccal pouch.
• Teach patient to take oral tablet on empty stomach, either ½ hour before or 1 to 2 hours after meals; to swallow oral tablets whole; and chew chewable tablets thoroughly before swallowing.
• Drug should not be discontinued abruptly—coronary vasospasm may occur.
• Store medication in cool place, in tightly closed container, away from light. To assure freshness, replace supply every 3 months. Remove cotton from container, since it absorbs drug.

ethaverine hydrochloride
Cebral, Circubid, Etalent, Ethaquin, Ethatab, Ethavex, Isovex, Laverin, Myoquin, Neopavrin, Pavaspan, Roldiol, Spasodil

INDICATIONS & DOSAGE
Long-term treatment of peripheral and

cerebrovascular insufficiency associated with arterial spasm; spastic conditions of gastrointestinal and genitourinary tracts—

Adults: 100 to 200 mg P.O. t.i.d. or 150 mg of sustained-release preparation P.O. q 12 hours.

SIDE EFFECTS
CNS: *headache,* drowsiness.
CV: *hypotension, flushing,* sweating, vertigo, cardiac depression, arrhythmias.
GI: *nausea; anorexia; abdominal distress; dryness of throat;* constipation; diarrhea.
Hepatic: jaundice, altered liver function tests.
Skin: rash.
Other: respiratory depression, malaise, lassitude.

INTERACTIONS
None significant.

NURSING CONSIDERATIONS
• Contraindicated in complete A-V dissociation and in severe hepatic disease. Use with caution in women who are pregnant or of childbearing age; and in glaucoma or pulmonary embolus; may precipitate arrhythmias.
• Hold dose and call doctor if signs of hepatic hypersensitivity develop.
• Monitor and record vital signs during therapy.
• FDA has announced this drug may not be effective for disease states indicated.

---

isosorbide dinitrate
Angidil, Coronex♦♦, Iso-Bid, Iso-D, Isosorb, Isordil♦, Isotrate, Neo-Corovas-80, Onset, Sorate, Sorbitrate, Sorquad, Vasotrate

INDICATIONS & DOSAGE
*Treatment of acute anginal attacks (sublingual and chewable only); pro-*phylaxis in situations likely to cause attacks; treatment of chronic ischemic heart disease (by preload reduction); adjunct with other vasodilators, such as hydralazine and prazosin in treatment of severe chronic congestive heart failure—

Adults:
Sublingual form—2.5 to 10 mg under the tongue for prompt relief of anginal pain, repeated q 2 to 3 hours during acute phase, or q 4 to 6 hours for prophylaxis.
Chewable form—5 to 10 mg, p.r.n., for acute attack or q 2 to 3 hours for prophylaxis but only after initial test dose of 5 mg to determine risk of severe hypotension.
Oral form—5 to 30 mg P.O. q.i.d. for prophylaxis only (use smallest effective dose); sustained-release forms 40 mg P.O. q 6 to 12 hours.

SIDE EFFECTS
CNS: *headache, sometimes with throbbing; dizziness;* weakness.
CV: *orthostatic hypotension, tachycardia, palpitations,* fainting.
GI: nausea, vomiting, sublingual burning.
Skin: cutaneous vasodilation, *flushing.*
Other: hypersensitivity reactions.

INTERACTIONS
None significant.

NURSING CONSIDERATIONS
• Contraindicated in hypersensitivity to nitrites, idiosyncrasy, head trauma, cerebral hemorrhage, severe anemia. Use with caution in hypotension.
• Monitor blood pressure and intensity and duration of response to drug.
• May cause headaches, especially at first. Treat headache with aspirin or acetaminophen. Dosage may need to be reduced temporarily, but tolerance usually develops.
• Tell patient to take medication regularly, even long-term, if ordered, and

to keep it easily accessible at all times. Physiologically necessary but not habit-forming.

• Additional dose may be taken before anticipated stress or at bedtime if angina is nocturnal.

• Advise patient to avoid alcoholic beverages; they may produce unpleasant Antabuse-like side effects.

• May cause orthostatic hypotension. Patient should get out of bed, go up and down stairs, and change position slowly; he should lie down at first sign of dizziness.

• Teach patient to take sublingual tablet at first sign of attack. He should wet the tablet with saliva, place it under the tongue until completely absorbed, and sit down and rest. Burning sensation indicates potency. Dose may be repeated every 10 to 15 minutes for a maximum of 3 doses. If no relief, patient should call doctor or go to hospital emergency room. If patient complains of tingling, he may try holding tablet in buccal pouch.

• Warn patient not to confuse sublingual with oral form.

• Teach patient to take oral tablet on empty stomach, either ½ hour before or 1 to 2 hours after meals; to swallow oral tablets whole; and to chew chewable tablets thoroughly before swallowing.

• Drug should not be discontinued abruptly—coronary vasospasm may occur.

• Store in cool place, in tightly closed container, away from light.

• Has been used investigationally in treatment of congestive heart failure.

---

isoxsuprine hydrochloride
Rolisox, Vasodilan♦, Vasoprine

INDICATIONS & DOSAGE
Adjunct for relief of symptoms associated with cerebral vascular insufficiency, peripheral vascular diseases
(such as arteriosclerosis obliterans, thromboangitis obliterans, Raynaud's disease)—
Adults: 10 to 20 mg P.O. t.i.d. or q.i.d.; initially, 5 to 10 mg I.M. b.i.d. or t.i.d. in severe or acute conditions, to maximum of 10 mg. Intramuscular doses greater than 10 mg may be associated with hypotension and tachycardia and are not recommended.

SIDE EFFECTS
CNS: *dizziness,* nervousness, weakness, trembling, *light-headedness.*
CV: *hypotension, tachycardia, transient palpitations.*
GI: vomiting, abdominal distress, intestinal distention.
Skin: severe rash.

INTERACTIONS
None significant.

NURSING CONSIDERATIONS
• Contraindicated in immediate postpartum period, arterial bleeding; I.M. contraindicated in hypotension or tachycardia.

• Safe use in pregnancy and lactation not established, although drug has been used to inhibit contractions in premature labor.

• Do not give intravenously.

• Observe for hypotension with parenteral use.

• Discontinue if rash develops.

---

mannitol hexanitrate
Mannex, Vascunitol

INDICATIONS & DOSAGE
Chronic prophylaxis against attacks of angina pectoris—
Adults: 15 to 60 mg P.O. q 4 to 6 hours.

SIDE EFFECTS
CNS: *headache, sometimes with throbbing; dizziness;* weakness.

Italicized side effects are common or life-threatening.

CV: *orthostatic hypotension, tachycardia, flushing, palpitations,* fainting.
GI: nausea, vomiting, sublingual burning.
Skin: cutaneous vasodilation.
Other: hypersensitivity, rise in intraocular tension, increased intracranial pressure.

INTERACTIONS
None significant.

NURSING CONSIDERATIONS
• Contraindicated in idiosyncrasy, head trauma, cerebral hemorrhage, severe anemia. Use with caution in hypotension.
• Monitor blood pressure and intensity and duration of response to drug.
• Medication may cause headaches, especially at first. Treat headache with aspirin or acetaminophen. Dosage may need to be reduced temporarily, but tolerance usually develops.
• Tell patient to take medication regularly, even long-term, if ordered. Physiologically necessary but not habit-forming.
• Additional doses may be taken before anticipated stress or at bedtime if angina is nocturnal.
• Alcoholic beverages should be avoided, since they may produce unpleasant Antabuse-like side effects.
• Medication may cause orthostatic hypotension. Patient should get out of bed, go up and down stairs, or change position slowly; he should lie down at first sign of dizziness.
• Store medication in cool dark place in tightly covered container.
• Effective within 15 to 30 minutes; duration 4 to 6 hours.

nicotinyl alcohol
Roniacol♦

INDICATIONS & DOSAGE
Treatment of conditions of deficient circulation such as peripheral vascular disease, vascular spasm, varicose ulcers, decubital ulcers, Meniere's syndrome, vertigo—
Adults: 50 to 100 mg regular tablets P.O. b.i.d. or t.i.d. (may increase to 150 to 200 mg P.O. t.i.d. or q.i.d.); 150 to 300 mg sustained-release tablets P.O. b.i.d.; 5 to 10 ml of elixir P.O. t.i.d.

SIDE EFFECTS
CNS: paresthesias.
CV: *transient flushing.*
GI: *gastric irritation.*
Skin: minor rashes.
Other: allergic reactions.

INTERACTIONS
Clonidine: may inhibit vasodilation. Observe for lack of response.

NURSING CONSIDERATIONS
• Contraindicated in active peptic ulcer or gastritis.
• Tolerance to side effects develops with continued therapy.

nitroglycerin
Ang-O-Span, Cardabid, Corobid, Glyceryl Trinitrate, Gly-Trate, Nitrine, Nitrobid, Nitrocap, Nitrocels, Nitro-Dial, Nitroglyn, Nitrol♦, Nitro-Lyn, Nitrong♦, Nitrospan, Nitrostabilin♦♦, Nitrostat♦, Nitrotym, Nitro-TD, Nitrozem, Nyglycon, Trates, Vasoglyn

INDICATIONS & DOSAGE
Prophylaxis against chronic anginal attacks—
Adults: 1 sustained-release capsule q

8 to 12 hours; or 2% ointment: Start with ½ inch ointment, increasing with ½-inch increments until headache occurs, then decreasing to previous dose. Range of dosage with ointment 2 to 5 inches. Usual dose 1 to 2 inches.
Relief of acute angina pectoris, prophylaxis to prevent or minimize anginal attacks when taken immediately prior to stressful events—
Adults: 1 sublingual tablet (gr. $^1/_{400}$, $^1/_{200}$, $^1/_{150}$, $^1/_{100}$) dissolved under the tongue or in the buccal pouch immediately upon indication of anginal attack. May repeat q 5 minutes for 15 minutes.

SIDE EFFECTS
CNS: *headache, sometimes with throbbing; dizziness;* weakness; syncope.
CV: *orthostatic hypotension, tachycardia, flushing, palpitations,* fainting.
GI: nausea, vomiting.
Skin: cutaneous vasodilation.
Local: sublingual burning.
Other: hypersensitivity reactions.

INTERACTIONS
None significant.

NURSING CONSIDERATIONS
• Contraindicated in hypersensitivity to nitrites, idiosyncrasy, head trauma, cerebral hemorrhage, severe anemia. Use with caution in hypotension.
• Monitor blood pressure and intensity and duration of response to drug.
• May cause headaches, especially at first. Treat headache with aspirin or acetaminophen. Dosage may need to be reduced temporarily, but tolerance usually develops.
• Tell patient to take medication regularly, even long-term, if ordered, and to keep it easily accessible at all times. Physiologically necessary but not habit-forming.
• Additional dose may be taken be-

fore anticipated stress or at bedtime if angina is nocturnal.
• Advise patient to avoid alcoholic beverages; they may produce unpleasant Antabuse-like side effects.
• May cause orthostatic hypotension. Patient should get out of bed, go up and down stairs, and change position slowly; he should lie down at first sign of dizziness.
• Teach patient to take sublingual tablet at first sign of attack. He should wet the tablet with saliva; place it under the tongue until completely absorbed and sit down and rest. Burning sensation indicates potency. Dose may be repeated every 10 to 15 minutes for a maximum of 3 doses. If no relief, patient should call doctor or go to hospital emergency room. If patient complains of tingling, he may try holding tablet in buccal pouch.
• Teach patient to take oral tablet on empty stomach, either ½ hour before or 1 to 2 hours after meals; to swallow oral tablets whole; and chew chewable tablets thoroughly before swallowing.
• Store in cool dark place, in tightly closed container. To assure freshness, replace supply every 3 months. Remove cotton from container, since it absorbs drug.
• To apply ointment, spread in uniform thin layer on any nonhairy area. Do not rub in. Cover with plastic film to aid absorption and to protect clothing.
• Doctor may prescribe nitroglycerin by its chemical name, glyceryl trinitrate (GTN).

---

nylidrin hydrochloride
Arlidin♦, Pervadil♦♦, Rolidrin

INDICATIONS & DOSAGE
To increase blood supply in vasospastic disorders (arteriosclerosis obliterans, thromboangitis obliterans, diabetic vascular disease, night leg

cramps, Raynaud's phenomenon and disease, ischemic ulcer, frostbite, acrocyanosis, acroparasthesia, sequelae of thrombophlebitis); and in circulatory disturbances of the middle ear (primary cochlear ischemia, cochlear striae, vascular ischemia, macular or ampullar ischemia); other disturbances due to labyrinth artery spasm or obstruction—
Adults: 3 to 12 mg P.O. t.i.d. or q.i.d.

SIDE EFFECTS
CNS: trembling, *nervousness*, weakness, *dizziness*.
CV: *palpitations, hypotension,* flushing.
GI: *nausea, vomiting*.

INTERACTIONS
None significant.

NURSING CONSIDERATIONS
• Contraindicated in acute myocardial infarction, paroxysmal tachycardia, angina pectoris, thyrotoxicosis. Use with caution in uncompensated heart disease or peptic ulcer.

---

papaverine hydrochloride
Blupav, BP-Papaverine, Cerebid, Cerespan, Cirbed, Delapav, DiPav, J-Pav, Kavrin, Lapay, Myobid, Papacon, Papalease, Papital T.R., PapKaps-150, Meta-Kaps, P-A-V, Pavabid, Pavacap, Pavacen, Pavaclor, Pavacron, Pavadel, Pavadur, Pavadyl, Pavakey S.A., Pava-lyn, Pava-Par, Pava-Rx, Pavasule, Pavatime, Pavatran T.D., Pava-Wol, Paverolan, Pavex, PT-300, Ro-Papav, S.M.R.-Kaps, Sustaverine, Vasal, Vasocap, Vasospan, Vazosan

---

INDICATIONS & DOSAGE
Relief of cerebral and peripheral ischemia associated with arterial spasm and myocardial ischemia; treatment of smooth-muscle spasm (coronary occlusion, angina pectoris, sequelae of peripheral and pulmonary embolism, certain cerebral angiospastic states); and visceral spasms (biliary, ureteral, or gastrointestinal colic)—
Adults: 60 to 300 mg P.O. 1 to 5 times daily, or 150 to 300 mg sustained-release preparations q 8 to 12 hours; 30 to 120 mg I.M. or I.V. q 3 hours, as indicated.

SIDE EFFECTS
CNS: *headache*.
CV: *increased heart rate, increased blood pressure* (with parenteral use), depressed AV and intraventricular conduction, arrhythmias.
GI: constipation, *nausea*.
Other: *sweating, flushing*, malaise, increased depth of respiration.

INTERACTIONS
None significant.

NURSING CONSIDERATIONS
• Contraindicated for I.V. use in complete A-V block. Use with caution in glaucoma.
• Monitor blood pressure, heart rate and rhythm, especially in cardiac disease. Hold dose and notify doctor immediately if changes occur.
• Not often used parenterally, except when immediate effect is desired.
• Give I.V. slowly (over 1 to 2 minutes) to avoid side effects.
• Most effective when given early in the course of a disorder.
• Tell patient to take medication regularly; long-term therapy is required.
• Do not add lactated Ringer's injection to the injectable form; will precipitate.
• FDA has announced this drug may not be effective for disease states indicated.

Unmarked trade names available in the United States only.
♦ Also available in Canada ♦♦ Available in Canada only.

pentaerythritol tetranitrate
Angijen Green, Angitrate, Antora,
Arcotrate Nos. 1 & 2, Baritrate,
Blaintrate, Desatrate 30, Desatrate
50, Dilar, Dinate, Duotrate, El-
PETN, Kaytrate, Maso-Trol, Nap-
trate, Nitrin, Penta-Cap-No. 1, Penta-
E., Penta-E. S.A., Pentaforte-T,
Penta-Tal No. 1 & 2, Pentestan-80,
Pentetra, Pentrate T.D., Pentritol,
Pent-T-80, Pentylan, Peritrate♦,
PETN, Petro-20 mg, P-T♦♦, P-T-T,
Quintrate, Rate, Vasolate, Vasolate-
80

INDICATIONS & DOSAGE
Prophylaxis against angina pectoris—
Adults: 10 to 20 mg P.O. q.i.d.; may
be titrated upward to 40 mg P.O.
q.i.d. ½ hour before or 1 hour after
meals and h.s.; 80 mg sustained-release preparations P.O. b.i.d.

SIDE EFFECTS
CNS: *headache, sometimes with
throbbing; dizziness;* weakness.
CV: *orthostatic hypotension, tachy-
cardia, flushing, palpitations,*
fainting.
GI: nausea, vomiting.
Skin: cutaneous vasodilation.
Other: hypersensitivity reactions.

INTERACTIONS
None significant.

NURSING CONSIDERATIONS
• Contraindicated in idiosyncrasy,
head trauma, cerebral hemorrhage,
severe anemia. Use with caution in
hypotension and glaucoma.
• Monitor blood pressure and intensity and duration of response to drug.
• Medication may cause headaches,
especially at first. Treat with aspirin
or acetaminophen. Dosage may need
to be reduced temporarily, but tolerance usually develops.
• Medication should be taken regularly, even long-term, if ordered.
Physiologically necessary but not
habit-forming.
• Additional doses may be taken before anticipated stress or at bedtime
for nocturnal angina.
• Not to be used for relief of acute anginal attacks.
• Medication may cause orthostatic
hypotension. Patient should get out of
bed, go up and down stairs, or change
position slowly; he should lie down at
first sign of dizziness.
• Drug should not be discontinued
abruptly—coronary vasospasm may
occur.
• Store medication in cool place in
tightly covered, light-resistant
container.

tolazoline hydrochloride
Priscoline♦, Tazol, Toloxan, Tolzol

INDICATIONS & DOSAGE
*Spastic peripheral vascular disorders
associated with acrocyanosis, acro-
paresthesia, arteriosclerosis obliterans, Buerger's disease, causalgia,
diabetic arteriosclerosis, gangrene,
endarteritis, sequelae of frostbite,
post-thrombotic conditions, Raynaud's
disease, scleroderma—*
Adults:
Oral—25 mg 4 to 6 times daily, gradually increasing to maximum of
50 mg 6 times daily.
Parenteral—10 to 50 mg S.C., I.V., or
I.M. q.i.d. Start with low dose, increasing gradually until optimal response (as determined by appearance
of flushing) is reached.
Intra-arterial—50 to 75 mg/injection,
depending on response; 1 or 2 injections may be required initially, then
dose of 2 or 3 injections weekly to
maintain circulation, possibly coupled
with oral tolazoline between injections.

Italicized side effects are common or life-threatening.

SIDE EFFECTS

CV: *arrhythmias, anginal pain, hypertension, flushing,* burning sensation (following intra-arterial injection), transient postural vertigo, palpitations.
GI: *nausea, vomiting, diarrhea, epigastric discomfort, exacerbation of peptic ulcer.*
Other: weakness, paradoxical response in seriously damaged limbs, increased pilomotor activity, tingling, chilliness, apprehension.

INTERACTIONS

Ethyl alcohol: possible Antabuse reaction from accumulation of acetaldehyde. Use together cautiously.

NURSING CONSIDERATIONS

• Contraindicated in coronary artery disease, active peptic ulcer, or following cerebrovascular accident. Use with caution in history of peptic ulcer disease, gastritis, or known or suspected mitral stenosis.

• Keep patient warm during parenteral administration to increase response.
• Appearance of flushing usually indicates maximum tolerable dose.
• Monitor vital signs. Watch especially for blood pressure changes, arrhythmias.
• Instruct patient to avoid alcohol: chills and flushing may occur.
• Due to risks, technique, and precautions, intra-arterial injection should be done only by experienced personnel, in selected cases, and only after maximum benefit has been achieved with oral and parenteral therapy.
• Warn against exposure to cold, which can aggravate tissue damage.
• Often used to distinguish between functional (vasospastic) and organic (obstructive) forms of peripheral vascular disease.

19

Antilipemics

cholestyramine
clofibrate
colestipol hydrochloride
dextrothyroxine sodium
niacin
probucol
sitosterols

---

cholestyramine
Questran♦

INDICATIONS & DOSAGE
Primary hyperlipidemia, pruritus, and diarrhea due to excess bile acid—
Adults: 4 g before meals and h.s., not to exceed 32 g daily. Each scoop or packet of Questran contains 4 g cholestyramine.
Children: 240 mg/Kg/day P.O. in 3 divided doses with beverage or food. Safe dosage not established for children under 6.

SIDE EFFECTS
GI: *constipation,* fecal impaction, hemorrhoids, *abdominal discomfort,* flatulence, *nausea,* vomiting, steatorrhea.
Skin: *rashes,* irritation of skin, tongue, and perianal area.
Other: *vitamin deficiency A, D, and K from decreased absorption;* hyperchloremic acidosis with long-term use or very high dosage.

INTERACTIONS
None significant.

NURSING CONSIDERATIONS
• To mix, sprinkle powder on surface of preferred beverage or wet food. Let stand a few minutes, then stir to obtain uniform suspension.
• Mixing with carbonated beverages may result in excess foaming. To avoid, use large glass, mix slowly.
• Administer all other medications at least 1 hour before or 4 to 6 hours after cholestyramine to avoid blocking their absorption.
• Observe bowel habits; treat constipation as needed. If severe constipation develops, decrease dosage, add a stool softener, or discontinue drug.
• Monitor cardiac glycoside levels for patients receiving both medications concurrently. Should cholestyramine therapy be discontinued, cardiac glycoside toxicity may result unless dosage is adjusted.
• Watch for deficiencies of vitamins A, D, and K.
• May cause decreased absorption of many drugs due to binding. Check drug interaction list of individual drugs.

---

clofibrate
Atromid-S♦

INDICATIONS & DOSAGE
Hyperlipidemia and xanthoma tuberosum—
Adults: 2 g P.O. daily in 4 divided doses. Some patients may respond to lower doses as assessed by serum lipid monitoring.

Should not be used in children.

SIDE EFFECTS
Blood: leukopenia.
CNS: fatigue, weakness.
GI: *nausea, diarrhea, transient and reversible elevations of liver function tests, vomiting,* stomatitis, *dyspepsia,* flatulence.
GU: decreased libido.
Hepatic: gallstones.
Skin: rashes, urticaria, pruritus, dry skin and hair.
Other: *myalgias and arthralgias,* resembling a flu-like syndrome; *weight gain; polyphagia;* fever.

INTERACTIONS
Oral contraceptives: may antagonize clofibrate's lipid-lowering effect. Monitor serum lipid level.

NURSING CONSIDERATIONS
• Contraindicated in patients with severe renal or hepatic disease.
• Warn patient to report flu-like symptoms to doctor immediately.
• Monitor renal and hepatic function, blood counts, serum electrolyte, and blood sugar levels. If liver function tests show steady rise, clofibrate should be discontinued.
• Should not be used indiscriminately. May pose increased risk of gallstones and cancer.
• If significant lipid lowering is not achieved within 3 months, drug should be discontinued.

colestipol hydrochloride
Colestid

INDICATIONS & DOSAGE
Primary hypercholesterolemia and xanthomas—
Adults: 15 to 30 g P.O. daily in 2 to 4 divided doses.

SIDE EFFECTS
GI: *constipation (common, may require decreasing the dosage),* fecal impaction, hemorrhoids, abdominal discomfort, flatulence, nausea, vomiting, steatorrhea.
Skin: rashes, irritation of skin, tongue, and perianal area.
Other: vitamin deficiency A, D, and K from decreased absorption; hyperchloremic acidosis with long-term use or very high dosage.

INTERACTIONS
Oral hypoglycemics: may antagonize response to colestipol. Monitor serum lipid level.

NURSING CONSIDERATIONS
• Administer all other medications at least 1 hour before or 4 to 6 hours after colestipol to avoid blocking their absorption.
• Monitor cardiac glycoside levels for patients receiving both medications concurrently. Should colestipol therapy be discontinued, cardiac glycoside toxicity may result unless dosage is adjusted.
• Watch for vitamin A, D, and K deficiency.
• Lowering dosage or adding stool softener may relieve constipation.
• May cause decreased absorption of many drugs due to binding. Check drug interaction list of individual drugs.

dextrothyroxine sodium
Choloxin♦

INDICATIONS & DOSAGE
Hyperlipidemia in euthyroid patients, especially when cholesterol and triglyceride levels are elevated—
Adults: initial dose 1 to 2 mg daily, increased by 1 to 2 mg daily at monthly intervals to a total of 4 to 8 mg daily.

Children: initial dose 0.05 mg/Kg daily, increased by 0.05 mg/Kg daily at monthly intervals to a total of 4 mg daily.

SIDE EFFECTS
CV: palpitations, angina pectoris, arrhythmias, ischemic myocardial changes on EKG, myocardial infarction.
EENT: visual disturbances, ptosis.
GI: nausea, vomiting, diarrhea, constipation, decreased appetite.
Metabolic: *insomnia, weight loss, sweating,* flushing, hyperthermia, hair loss.
Other: menstrual irregularities.

INTERACTIONS
None significant.

NURSING CONSIDERATIONS
• Contraindicated for patients with hepatic or renal disease, or iodism. Patients with history of heart disease, including arrhythmias, hypertension, or angina pectoris, should receive very small doses.
• May increase need for insulin, diet therapy, or oral hypoglycemics in diabetics.
• If the use of anticoagulants is being considered, discontinue drug 2 weeks before surgery to avoid possible potentiation of anticoagulant effect.
• Observe patient for signs of hyperthyroidism, such as nervousness, insomnia, weight loss. If these occur, dosage should be decreased or drug discontinued.

niacin
Diacin, Efacin, Niac, Niacalex, Niacels, NICL, Nicobid, Nicocap, Nico-400, Nicolar, NiCord XL, Nico-Span, Nicotinex, Ni-Span, Tega-Span, Tinic, Wampocap

INDICATIONS & DOSAGE
Adjunctive treatment of hyperlipidemias, especially associated with hypercholesterolemia—
Adults: 1.5 to 3 g daily in 3 divided doses with or after meals, increased at intervals to 6 g daily.

SIDE EFFECTS
CV: *flushing* (which usually subsides in a few weeks).
GI: *nausea,* dyspepsia, vomiting, diarrhea, anorexia, flatulence, epigastric pain.
Metabolic: *glucose intolerance resulting in hyperglycemia in previously well-controlled diabetics, hyperuricemia,* liver function test abnormalities.
Skin: *pruritus,* sensation of burning or stinging.

INTERACTIONS
None significant.

NURSING CONSIDERATIONS
• Use cautiously in gout, diabetes, gallbladder or hepatic disease, peptic ulcer.
• Advise patient that pruritus and flushing noted in first few weeks of therapy usually lessen with continued use.
• Begin therapy with small doses; then increase gradually.
• Give with meals to minimize GI irritation. Cold water eases swallowing.

Italicized side effects are common or life-threatening.

probucol
Lorelco♦

INDICATIONS & DOSAGE
Primary hypercholesterolemia—
Adults: 2 tablets (500 mg total) P.O. b.i.d. with morning and evening meals.
Not recommended in children.

SIDE EFFECTS

GI: *diarrhea, flatulence, abdominal pain, nausea, vomiting.*
Other: *hyperhidrosis,* fetid sweat, angioneurotic edema.

INTERACTIONS
None significant.

NURSING CONSIDERATIONS
• Drug's effect is enhanced when taken with food.
• Contraindicated in arrhythmias. Drug should be stopped in any patient whose EKG shows prolonged Q-T interval.

sitosterols
Cytellin

INDICATIONS & DOSAGE
Adjunctive therapy for hypercholesterolemia or hyperbetalipoproteinemia—
Adults: 15 ml (3 g) P.O. before meals to a total of 45 ml (9 g) daily. May increase to 30 ml before large or high-fat meals; give fraction of usual dose before snacks.

SIDE EFFECTS
GI: anorexia; *diarrhea;* abdominal cramps; *bulky, light-colored stools;* nausea.

INTERACTIONS
None significant.

NURSING CONSIDERATIONS
• Administer other medications 1 hour before or 4 hours after sitosterols.
• Give sitosterols immediately before meals or snacks.
• Mix with milk, tea, coffee, or fruit juice for palatability.
• Maximum therapeutic effect during second and third month of therapy.

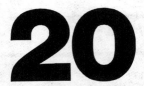

Nonnarcotic analgesics and antipyretics

acetaminophen
aspirin
butorphanol tartrate
choline magnesium trisalicylate
choline salicylate
ethoheptazine citrate
ethoxazene hydrochloride
fenoprofen calcium
ibuprofen
indomethacin
magnesium salicylate
meclofenamate
mefenamic acid
methotrimeprazine
nalbuphine hydrochloride
naproxen
oxyphenbutazone
phenacetin
phenazopyridine hydrochloride
phenylbutazone
salicylamide
salsalate
sodium salicylate
sodium thiosalicylate
sulindac
tolmetin sodium
zomepirac sodium

---

acetaminophen
Acephen, Atasol♦♦, Campain♦♦,
Datril, Dolanex, Liquiprin,
Paralgin♦♦, Phenaphen, Phendex,
Robigesic♦♦, Rounox♦♦, SK-Apap,
Tapar, Tempra♦, Tenlap, Tivrin♦♦,
Tylenol♦, Valadol

INDICATIONS & DOSAGE
Mild pain or fever—
Adults, and children over 10 years:
325 to 650 mg P.O. or rectally q 4
hours, p.r.n. Maximum 2.6 g daily.
Children under 1 year: 15 to
60 mg/dose
1 year: 60 mg/dose
2 years: 120 mg/dose
3 years: 180 mg/dose
4 years: 240 mg/dose
5 to 10 years: 325 mg/dose
May give P.O. or rectally q 4 to
6 hours. Maximum 1.2 g daily.

SIDE EFFECTS
Hepatic: severe liver toxicity with
large doses.
Skin: rash, urticaria.

INTERACTIONS
None significant.

NURSING CONSIDERATIONS
• Has no anti-inflammatory effect.
• Warn patient that high doses or unsupervised chronic use can cause liver
damage. Excessive ingestion of alcoholic beverages may hasten liver toxicity.
• Has little or no effect on prothrombin time.

aspirin

Acetal♦♦, Acetophen♦♦, Acetyl-Sal♦♦, Ancasal♦♦, A.S.A., Aspergum, Aspirjen Jr., Aspirin♦♦, Bayer Timed-Release, Buffinol, Decaprin, Ecotrin♦♦, Empirin, Entrophen♦♦, Measurin, Neopirine No. 25♦♦, Nova-Phase♦♦, Novasen♦♦, Rhonal♦♦, Sal-Adult♦♦, Sal-Infant♦♦, Supasa♦♦, Triaphen-10♦♦

INDICATIONS & DOSAGE

Adults:
Arthritis—2.6 to 5.2 g P.O. daily in divided doses.
Mild pain or fever— 325 to 650 mg P.O. or rectally q 4 hours, p.r.n.
Thromboembolic disorders—325 to 650 mg P.O. daily or b.i.d.
Transient ischemic attacks— 650 mg P.O. b.i.d. or 325 mg q.i.d.

Children:
Arthritis—90 to 130 mg/Kg P.O. daily divided q 4 to 6 hours.
Fever—40 to 80 mg/Kg P.O. or rectally daily divided q 6 hours, p.r.n.
Mild pain—65 to 100 mg/Kg P.O. or rectally daily divided q 4 to 6 hours, p.r.n.

SIDE EFFECTS

Blood: *prolonged bleeding time.*
EENT: *tinnitus and hearing loss (first signs of toxicity).*
GI: *nausea, vomiting, GI distress, occult bleeding.*
Hepatic: abnormal liver function studies.
Skin: *rash.*
Other: *hypersensitivity manifested by anaphylaxis.*

INTERACTIONS

Ammonium chloride (and other urine acidifiers): increased blood levels of aspirin products. Monitor for aspirin toxicity.
Antacids (and other urine alkalinizers): decreased levels of aspirin products. Monitor for decreased aspirin effect.
Oral anticoagulants: increased risk of bleeding. Avoid using together if possible.

NURSING CONSIDERATIONS

• Contraindicated in GI ulcer, GI bleeding, aspirin hypersensitivity. Use cautiously in hypoprothrombinemia, vitamin K deficiency, bleeding disorders, asthmatics with nasal polyps (may cause severe bronchospasm), and Hodgkin's disease (may cause profound hypothermia).
• Febrile, dehydrated children can develop toxicity rapidly.
• Give with food, milk, antacid, or large glass of water to reduce GI side effects.
• Warn patients to check with doctor or pharmacist before taking over-the-counter combinations containing aspirin.
• Therapeutic serum salicylate level in arthritis is 20 to 30 mg/100 ml.
• Alcohol may increase gastrointestinal blood loss.

butorphanol tartrate
Stadol

INDICATIONS & DOSAGE

Moderate to severe pain—
Adults: 1 to 4 mg I.M. q 3 to 4 hours, p.r.n.; or 0.5 to 2 mg I.V. q 3 to 4 hours, p.r.n.

SIDE EFFECTS

CNS: *sedation, headache, vertigo, floating sensation,* lethargy, confusion, nervousness, unusual dreams, agitation, euphoria, hallucinations, flushing.
CV: palpitations.
EENT: diplopia, blurred vision.
GI: *nausea,* vomiting, dry mouth.
Skin: rash, hives, *clamminess, excessive sweating.*

Other: *respiratory depression.*

INTERACTIONS
None significant.

NURSING CONSIDERATIONS
• Contraindicated in narcotic addiction; may precipitate narcotic abstinence syndrome. Use cautiously in head injury, increased intracranial pressure, acute MI, ventricular dysfunction, coronary insufficiency, respiratory diseases or depression, renal or hepatic dysfunction.
• Unlikely to cause dependence.
• Respiratory depression does not increase with increased dosage.
• Subcutaneous route not recommended.
• Also approved for use as a preoperative medication, as the analgesic component of balanced anesthesia, and in relief of postpartum pain.

---

choline magnesium trisalicylate
Trilisate

INDICATIONS & DOSAGE
Arthritis, mild—
Adults: 1 to 2 teaspoonfuls or tablets, each 500 mg salicylate, b.i.d.
Rheumatoid arthritis and osteoarthritis—
Adults: 2 to 3 teaspoonfuls or tablets b.i.d. Each tablet or teaspoonful equal in salicylate content to 650 mg aspirin.

SIDE EFFECTS
Blood: *prolonged bleeding time.*
EENT: *tinnitus and hearing loss (first signs of toxicity).*
GI: *nausea, vomiting, GI distress, occult bleeding.*
Hepatic: abnormal liver function studies.
Skin: *rash.*
Other: *hypersensitivity manifested by anaphylaxis.*

INTERACTIONS
Ammonium chloride (and other urine acidifiers): increased blood levels of salicylates. Monitor for salicylate toxicity.
Antacids (and other urine alkalinizers): decreased levels of salicylates. Monitor for decreased salicylate effect.
Oral anticoagulants: increased risk of bleeding. Avoid using together if possible.

NURSING CONSIDERATIONS
• Contraindicated in GI ulcer, GI bleeding, aspirin hypersensitivity. Use cautiously in hypoprothrombinemia, vitamin K deficiency, bleeding disorders, asthmatics with nasal polyps (may cause severe bronchospasm), and Hodgkin's disease (may cause profound hypothermia).
• May cause less GI distress than aspirin. If antacid needed, give 2 hours after meals and give choline magnesium trisalicylate before meals.
• May mix drug with water, fruit juice, or carbonated drinks.
• Febrile, dehydrated children can develop toxicity rapidly.
• Warn patient to check with doctor before taking over-the-counter combinations containing aspirin.
• Therapeutic serum salicylate level in arthritis is 20 to 30 mg/100 ml.
• Alcohol may increase gastrointestinal blood loss.

---

choline salicylate
Arthropan♦

INDICATIONS & DOSAGE
Arthritis—
Adults: 5 to 10 ml P.O. q.i.d.
Minor pain or fever—
Adults: 870 mg (5 ml) P.O. q 3 to 4 hours, p.r.n.
Children 3 to 6 years: 105 to 210 mg P.O. q 4 hours, p.r.n.

Italicized side effects are common or life-threatening.

Each 870 mg (5 ml) equals 650 mg aspirin.

SIDE EFFECTS
Blood: *prolonged bleeding time.*
EENT: *tinnitus and hearing loss (first signs of toxicity).*
GI: *nausea, vomiting, GI distress, occult bleeding.*
Hepatic: abnormal liver function studies.
Skin: *rash.*
Other: *hypersensitivity manifested by anaphylaxis.*

INTERACTIONS
Ammonium chloride (and other urine acidifiers): increased blood levels of salicylates. Monitor for salicylate toxicity.
Antacids (and other urine alkalinizers): decreased levels of salicylates Monitor for decreased salicylate effect.
Oral anticoagulants: increased risk of bleeding. Avoid using together if possible.

NURSING CONSIDERATIONS
• Contraindicated in GI ulcer, GI bleeding, aspirin hypersensitivity. Use cautiously in hypoprothrombinemia, vitamin K deficiency, bleeding disorders, asthmatics with nasal polyps (may cause severe bronchospasm), and Hodgkin's disease (may cause profound hypothermia).
• May cause less GI distress than aspirin. If antacid needed, give 2 hours after meals and give choline salicylate before meals.
• May mix drug with water, fruit juice, or carbonated drinks.
• Febrile, dehydrated children can develop toxicity rapidly.
• Warn patient to check with doctor before taking over-the-counter combinations containing aspirin.
• Therapeutic serum salicylate level in arthritis is 20 to 30 mg/100 ml.

• Alcohol may increase gastrointestinal blood loss.

---

ethoheptazine citrate
Zactane

INDICATIONS & DOSAGE
Mild pain—
Adults: 75 to 150 mg P.O. t.i.d. or q.i.d.

SIDE EFFECTS
CNS: dizziness, headache, syncope, nervousness.
EENT: visual disturbances.
GI: nausea, vomiting.
Skin: pruritus.

INTERACTIONS
None significant.

NURSING CONSIDERATIONS
• May use with aspirin for arthritic pain.
• Doesn't lower fever; may use alone when fever is valuable for diagnosis.
• Side effects other than GI distress and pruritus usually occur only when recommended dosage exceeded.

---

ethoxazene hydrochloride
Serenium

INDICATIONS & DOSAGE
Pain with urinary tract irritation or infection—
Adults: 100 mg a.c. P.O. t.i.d.

SIDE EFFECTS
GI: nausea, vomiting.

INTERACTIONS
None significant.

NURSING CONSIDERATIONS
• Contraindicated in hepatic and

Unmarked trade names available in the United States only.
♦ Also available in Canada   ♦ ♦ Available in Canada only.

renal disease. Use cautiously in GI disorders.
• Colors urine reddish-orange. May stain fabrics.
• Use only as analgesic. Use with antibiotic to treat urinary tract infection.

fenoprofen calcium
Nalfon♦

INDICATIONS & DOSAGE
Rheumatoid arthritis and osteoarthritis—
Adults: 300 to 600 mg P.O. q.i.d. Maximum 3.2 g daily.

SIDE EFFECTS
Blood: prolonged bleeding time.
CNS: headache, drowsiness, dizziness.
GI: *epigastric distress,* nausea, *occult blood loss.*
GU: reversible renal failure.
Skin: pruritus, rash, urticaria.

INTERACTIONS
None significant.

NURSING CONSIDERATIONS
• Contraindicated in renal disease and in asthmatics with nasal polyps. Use cautiously in GI disorders or allergy to other noncorticosteroid anti-inflammatory drugs, cardiac disease.
• Tell patient therapeutic effect may be delayed for 2 to 3 weeks.
• Check renal, hepatic, and auditory function periodically in long-term therapy. Stop drug if abnormalities occur.
• Give dose 30 minutes before or 2 hours after meals. If GI side effects occur, give with milk or meals.

ibuprofen
Motrin♦

INDICATIONS & DOSAGE
Arthritis, primary dysmenorrhea, postextraction dental pain—
Adults: 300 to 600 mg P.O. q.i.d.

SIDE EFFECTS
Blood: prolonged bleeding time.
CNS: headache, drowsiness, dizziness.
EENT: visual disturbances.
GI: *epigastric distress,* nausea, *occult blood loss.*
GU: reversible renal failure.
Skin: pruritus, rash, urticaria.
Other: aseptic meningitis, bronchospasm.

INTERACTIONS
None significant.

NURSING CONSIDERATIONS
• Contraindicated in asthmatics with nasal polyps. Use cautiously in GI disorders, allergy to other noncorticosteroid anti-inflammatory drugs, hepatic or renal disease, cardiac decompensation.
• Tell patient therapeutic effect may be delayed for 2 to 3 weeks.
• Check renal and hepatic function periodically in long-term therapy. Stop drug if abnormalities occur.
• Tell patient to report to doctor immediately any GI symptoms or signs of bleeding, visual disturbances, skin rashes, weight gain, or edema.
• Give with meals or milk to reduce GI side effects.

indomethacin
Indocid♦ ♦, Indocin

INDICATIONS & DOSAGE
Moderate to severe arthritis—

Italicized side effects are common or life-threatening.

Adults: 25 mg P.O. b.i.d. or t.i.d. with food or antacids; may increase dose by 25 mg daily q 7 days up to 200 mg daily.
Acute gouty arthritis—50 mg t.i.d. Reduce dose as soon as possible, then stop.

SIDE EFFECTS
Blood: *hemolytic anemia, aplastic anemia, agranulocytosis,* leukopenia, *thrombocytopenic purpura,* iron deficiency anemia.
CNS: *headache, dizziness,* depression, drowsiness, confusion, peripheral neuropathy, convulsions, psychic disturbances, syncope, *vertigo.*
CV: hypertension, edema.
EENT: blurred vision, corneal and retinal damage, hearing loss, tinnitus.
GI: *nausea, vomiting,* anorexia, *diarrhea, severe GI bleeding.*
GU: hematuria, acute renal failure.
Skin: pruritus, urticaria, angioedema.
Other: hypersensitivity (shock-like symptoms, rash, respiratory distress).

INTERACTIONS
Probenecid: decreased indomethacin excretion; watch for increased incidence of indomethacin side effects.
Furosemide: impaired response to both drugs. Avoid if possible.

NURSING CONSIDERATIONS
• Contraindicated in aspirin allergy, GI disorders. Use cautiously in epilepsy, parkinsonism, hepatic or renal disease, infection, history of mental illness, and in elderly patients.
• Severe headache may occur within 1 hour. Decrease dose if headache persists.
• Tell patient to notify doctor immediately if any visual changes occur. Patients taking drug long-term should have regular eye examinations.
• Very irritating to GI tract. Give with meals.

• Monitor for bleeding in patients receiving anticoagulants.
• Causes sodium retention; monitor for increased blood pressure in hypertensive patients.
• Used investigationally as prophylaxis for gout when colchicine is not well tolerated.

---

magnesium salicylate
Analate, Arthrin, Lorisal, Magan, Mobidin, MSG-600, Triact

INDICATIONS & DOSAGE
Adults:
Arthritis—up to 9.6 g daily in divided doses.
Mild pain or fever—600 mg P.O. t.i.d. or q.i.d.

SIDE EFFECTS
Blood: *prolonged bleeding time.*
EENT: *tinnitus and hearing loss (first signs of toxicity).*
GI: *nausea, vomiting, GI distress, occult bleeding.*
Hepatic: abnormal liver function studies.
Skin: *rash.*
Other: *hypersensitivity manifested by anaphylaxis.*

INTERACTIONS
Ammonium chloride (and other urine acidifiers): increased blood levels of aspirin products. Monitor for aspirin toxicity.
Antacids (and other urine alkalinizers): decreased levels of aspirin products. Monitor for decreased aspirin effect.
Oral anticoagulants: increased risk of bleeding. Avoid using together if possible.

NURSING CONSIDERATIONS
• Contraindicated in severe chronic renal insufficiency because of risk of magnesium toxicity; GI ulcer; GI

---

bleeding; aspirin hypersensitivity. Use cautiously in hypoprothrombinemia, vitamin K deficiency, bleeding disorders, and Hodgkin's disease (may cause profound hypothermia).
• Febrile, dehydrated children can develop toxicity rapidly.
• Give with food, milk, antacid, or large glass of water to reduce GI side effects.
• Warn patient to check with doctor before taking over-the-counter combinations containing aspirin.
• Therapeutic serum salicylate level in arthritis is 20 to 30 mg/100 ml.
• Alcohol may increase gastrointestinal blood loss.

meclofenamate
Meclomen

INDICATIONS & DOSAGE
Rheumatoid arthritis and osteoarthritis—
Adults: 200 to 400 mg/day P.O. in 3 or 4 equally divided doses.

SIDE EFFECTS
Blood: leukopenia, thrombocytopenia, *agranulocytosis, aplastic anemia.*
CNS: drowsiness, dizziness, nervousness, headache.
EENT: blurred vision, eye irritation.
GI: nausea, vomiting, *diarrhea,* hemorrhage.
GU: dysuria, hematuria, nephrotoxicity.
Skin: rash, urticaria.
Other: hepatotoxicity.

INTERACTIONS
None significant.

NURSING CONSIDERATIONS
• Contraindicated in GI ulceration or inflammation. Use cautiously in hepatic or renal disease, blood dyscra-

sias, diabetes mellitus, asthmatics with nasal polyps.
• Warn patient against activities that require alertness until response to drug is determined.
• Stop drug if rash or diarrhea develops.
• Should not be administered for more than 1 week at a time.
• Administer with food to minimize GI side effects.
• Almost identical in chemical structure to mefenamic acid.
• Available as 50 and 100 mg capsules.

mefenamic acid
Ponstan♦♦, Ponstel

INDICATIONS & DOSAGE
Mild to moderate pain, dysmenorrhea—
Adults, and children over 14 years: 500 mg P.O. initially, then 250 mg q 4 hours, p.r.n.
Maximum therapy 1 week.

SIDE EFFECTS
Blood: leukopenia, thrombocytopenia, *agranulocytosis, aplastic anemia.*
CNS: drowsiness, dizziness, nervousness, headache.
EENT: blurred vision, eye irritation.
GI: nausea, vomiting, *diarrhea,* hemorrhage.
GU: dysuria, hematuria, nephrotoxicity.
Skin: rash, urticaria.
Other: hepatotoxicity.

INTERACTIONS
None significant.

NURSING CONSIDERATIONS
• Contraindicated in GI ulceration or inflammation. Use cautiously in hepatic or renal disease, blood dyscra-

---

Italicized side effects are common or life-threatening.

sias, diabetes mellitus, asthmatics with nasal polyps.
- Warn patient against activities that require alertness until response to drug is determined.
- Severe hemolytic anemia may occur with prolonged use.
- Stop drug if rash or diarrhea develops.
- Should not be administered for more than 1 week at a time.
- Administer with food to minimize GI side effects.
- Can be used to treat menstrual pain.

methotrimeprazine
Levoprome, Nozinan♦♦

INDICATIONS & DOSAGE
Moderate to severe pain in nonambulatory patients—
Adults: 10 to 20 mg deep I.M. into large muscle mass, q 4 to 6 hours, p.r.n. Maximum dose 40 mg.

SIDE EFFECTS
Blood: *agranulocytosis.*
CNS: confusion, dizziness, *sedation,* weakness, amnesia.
CV: *orthostatic hypotension.*
EENT: nasal congestion.
GI: dry mouth, nausea, vomiting.
GU: difficult urination.
Local: pain, inflammation at injection site.
Other: chills, slurred speech.

INTERACTIONS
All antihypertensive agents and MAO inhibitors: increased orthostatic hypotension. Select other analgesic.

NURSING CONSIDERATIONS
- Contraindicated in phenothiazine hypersensitivity; cardiac, renal or hepatic disease; hypotension; coma; convulsive disorders. Use with extreme caution in elderly or debilitated patients with heart disease or any patients who may suffer severe consequences from a sudden drop in blood pressure.
- Used mainly in nonambulatory patients because of hypotension. Keep patient in bed or assist when out of bed for at least 6 hours after initial dose. Tolerance to this effect usually develops, but watch patient closely after each dose.
- May mix with atropine or scopolamine. Do not mix with other drugs.

nalbuphine hydrochloride
Nubain

INDICATIONS & DOSAGE
Moderate to severe pain—
S.C., I.M., or I.V.
Adults: 10 to 20 mg q 3 to 6 hours p.r.n. Maximum daily dose 160 mg.

SIDE EFFECTS
CNS: *sedation,* nervousness, depression, restlessness, crying, euphoria, hostility, unusual dreams, confusion, hallucinations, delusions.
GI: cramps, dyspepsia, bitter taste.
GU: urinary urgency.
Skin: itching, burning, urticaria.
Other: *respiratory depression,* physical and psychologic dependence.

INTERACTIONS
None significant.

NURSING CONSIDERATIONS
- Contraindicated in emotional instability, drug abuse, head injury, increased intracranial pressure. Use cautiously in hepatic and renal disease. These patients may overreact to customary doses.
- Causes respiratory depression which at 10 mg is equal to the respiratory depression produced by 10 mg of morphine.
- Psychologic and physiologic depen-

dence may occur, but it is less than that of pentazocine (Talwin).
• Respiratory depression can be reversed with naloxone.
• Also acts as a narcotic antagonist.
• Warn patient to avoid activities that require alertness until response to drug is determined.

naproxen
Naprosyn♦

INDICATIONS & DOSAGE
Arthritis—
Adults: 250 to 500 mg P.O. b.i.d. Maximum 1,000 mg daily.

SIDE EFFECTS
Blood: prolonged bleeding time.
CNS: headache, drowsiness, dizziness.
GI: *epigastric distress, occult blood loss,* nausea.
GU: reversible renal failure.
Skin: pruritus, rash, urticaria.

INTERACTIONS
None significant.

NURSING CONSIDERATIONS
• Use cautiously in renal disease, GI disorders, allergy to noncorticosteroid anti-inflammatory agents, and asthmatics with nasal polyps.
• Tell patient therapeutic effect may be delayed 2 to 3 weeks.
• Check renal and hepatic function periodically in long-term therapy. Stop drug if abnormalities occur.
• Dose can be given once daily very effectively. May increase patient compliance.

oxyphenbutazone
Oxalid, Tandearil

INDICATIONS & DOSAGE
Pain, inflammation in arthritis, bursitis, superficial venous thrombosis—
Adults: 100 to 200 mg P.O. with food or milk t.i.d. or q.i.d.
Acute gouty arthritis—
Adults: 400 mg initially as single dose, then 100 mg q 4 hours for 4 days or until relief is obtained.

SIDE EFFECTS
Blood: *bone marrow depression (fatal aplastic anemia, agranulocytosis, thrombocytopenia),* hemolytic anemia, leukopenia.
CNS: restlessness, confusion, lethargy.
CV: hypertension, *pericarditis, myocarditis, cardiac decompensation.*
EENT: optic neuritis, blurred vision, retinal hemorrhage or detachment, hearing loss.
GI: *nausea, vomiting, diarrhea,* ulcer, occult blood loss.
GU: proteinuria, hematuria, glomerulonephritis, nephrotic syndrome, *renal failure.*
Hepatic: *hepatitis.*
Metabolic: toxic and nontoxic goiter, respiratory alkalosis, and metabolic acidosis.
Skin: petechiae, pruritus, purpura, various dermatoses from rash to *toxic necrotizing epidermolysis.*

INTERACTIONS
Methandrostenolone: may increase oxyphenbutazone levels. Give together cautiously.

NURSING CONSIDERATIONS
• Contraindicated in senile patients; GI ulcer; blood dyscrasias; renal, hepatic, cardiac, and thyroid disease; polymyalgia rheumatica and temporal arteritis.

Italicized side effects are common or life-threatening.

- Tell patient to stop drug and notify doctor immediately if fever, sore throat, mouth ulcers, GI discomfort, black or tarry stools, bleeding, bruising, rash, or weight gain occurs.
- Give with food, milk, or antacids.
- Warn patient to remain under close medical supervision and to keep all doctor and lab appointments.
- Record patient's weight, intake, and output daily. May cause sodium retention and edema.
- Response should be seen in 2 or 3 days. Drug should be stopped if no response seen within 1 week.
- Monitor CBC every 2 weeks or weekly in elderly patients. Report any abnormality to doctor immediately.
- Patient over age 60 should not receive drug for longer than 1 week.

phenacetin

INDICATIONS & DOSAGE
Mild pain or fever—
Adults: 300 mg P.O. q 3 to 4 hours, p.r.n. Maximum 2.4 g daily.

SIDE EFFECTS
Blood: methemoglobinemia in toxic doses, hemolytic anemia in G-6-PD deficiency.
GI: nausea, vomiting.
GU: *papillary necrosis and chronic interstitial nephritis with long-term high doses.*
Skin: rash.

INTERACTIONS
None significant.

NURSING CONSIDERATIONS
- Repeated use contraindicated in anemia; cardiac, pulmonary, hepatic, or renal disease.
- Contained in many analgesic combinations. Warn patient to check ingredients of combination over-the-counter products.

phenazopyridine hydrochloride
Azodine, Azogesic, Azo-Pyridon, Azo-Standard, Azo-Sulfizin, Baridium, Di-Azo, Diridone, Phenazo♦♦, Phen-Azo, Phenazodine, Pyridiate, Pyridium♦, Urodine

INDICATIONS & DOSAGE
Pain with urinary tract irritation or infection—
Adults: 100 to 200 mg P.O. t.i.d.
Children: 100 mg P.O. t.i.d.

SIDE EFFECTS
CNS: headache.
GI: nausea.

INTERACTIONS
None significant.

NURSING CONSIDERATIONS
- Contraindicated in renal and hepatic insufficiency.
- Colors urine red or orange. May stain fabrics.
- Use only as analgesic. Use with antibiotic to treat urinary tract infection.
- Drug may be stopped in 3 days if pain relieved.
- May alter Clinistix or Tes-Tape results. Use Clinitest for accurate urinary glucose test results.
- Stop drug if skin or sclera becomes yellow-tinged. May indicate accumulation due to impaired renal excretion.

phenylbutazone
Algoverine♦♦, Anevral♦♦, Azolid, Butagesic♦♦, Butazolidin♦, Intrabutazone♦♦, Malgesic♦♦, Nadozone♦♦, Neo-Zoline♦♦, Phenbutazone♦♦, Phenylbetazone♦♦

INDICATIONS & DOSAGE
Pain, inflammation in arthritis, bursitis, acute superficial thrombophlebitis—

Adults: initially, 100 to 200 mg P.O.
t.i.d. or q.i.d. Maximum dose
600 mg per day. When improvement
is obtained, decrease dose to 100 mg
t.i.d. or q.i.d.
Acute, gouty arthritis—
Adults: 400 mg initially as single
dose, then 100 mg q 4 hours for
4 days or until relief is obtained.

SIDE EFFECTS
Blood: *bone marrow depression (fatal
aplastic anemia, agranulocytosis,
thrombocytopenia),* hemolytic anemia, leukopenia.
CNS: agitation, confusion, lethargy.
CV: hypertension, *pericarditis, myocarditis, cardiac decompensation.*
EENT: optic neuritis, blurred vision,
retinal hemorrhage or detachment,
hearing loss.
GI: *nausea, vomiting, diarrhea,* ulcer, occult blood loss.
GU: proteinuria, hematuria, glomerulonephritis, nephrotic syndrome,
renal failure.
Hepatic: *hepatitis.*
Metabolic: hyperglycemia, toxic and
nontoxic goiter, edema, respiratory
alkalosis, and metabolic acidosis.
Skin: petechiae, pruritus, purpura,
various dermatoses from rash to *toxic
necrotizing epidermolysis.*

INTERACTIONS
Barbiturates, antidepressants: may
impair phenylbutazone effect. Use together cautiously.
Cholestyramine: may alter phenylbutazone absorption. Give 1 hour before
cholestyramine.

NURSING CONSIDERATIONS
• Contraindicated in senility; GI ulcer; blood dyscrasias; renal, hepatic,
cardiac, and thyroid disease; polymyalgia rheumatica; temporal arteritis; and hypertension.
• Warn patient to stop drug and notify doctor immediately if fever, sore
throat, mouth ulcers, GI discomfort,
black or tarry stools, bleeding, bruising, rash, or weight gain occurs.
• Give with food, milk, or antacids.
• Patient should remain under close
medical supervision and keep all doctor and lab appointments.
• Record patient's weight, intake, and
output daily. May cause sodium retention and edema.
• Monitor CBC every 2 weeks or
weekly in elderly patients. Report any
abnormalities to doctor right away.
• Response should be seen in 3 to
4 days. Stop drug if no response
within 1 week.
• Patients over age 60 should not receive drug for longer than 1 week.

salicylamide
Amid-Sal, Doldram, Salamide

INDICATIONS & DOSAGE
Mild pain or fever—
Adults: 650 mg P.O. q.i.d., p.r.n.
Children: 65 mg/Kg/day divided into
6 doses.

SIDE EFFECTS
Blood: *prolonged bleeding time.*
EENT: *tinnitus and hearing loss (first
signs of toxicity).*
GI: *nausea, vomiting, GI distress, oc-
cult bleeding.*
Hepatic: abnormal liver function
studies.
Skin: *rash.*
Other: *hypersensitivity manifested by
anaphylaxis.*

INTERACTIONS
*Ammonium chloride (and other urine
acidifiers):* increased blood levels of
aspirin products. Monitor for aspirin
toxicity.
*Antacids (and other urine alkaliniz-
ers):* decreased levels of aspirin products. Monitor for decreased aspirin
effect.

Oral anticoagulants: increased risk of bleeding. Avoid using together if possible.

NURSING CONSIDERATIONS
• Contraindicated in GI ulcer, GI bleeding, aspirin hypersensitivity. Use cautiously in hypoprothrombinemia, vitamin K deficiency, bleeding disorders, and Hodgkin's disease (may cause profound hypothermia).
• Give with food, milk, antacid, or large glass of water to reduce GI side effects.
• Warn patient to check with doctor before taking over-the-counter combinations containing aspirin.
• Alcohol may increase gastrointestinal blood loss.

---

salsalate
Disalcid

INDICATIONS & DOSAGE
Minor pain or fever, arthritis—
Adults: 1 g P.O. b.i.d., t.i.d., or q.i.d., p.r.n.

SIDE EFFECTS
Blood: *prolonged bleeding time.*
EENT: *tinnitus and hearing loss (first signs of toxicity).*
GI: *nausea, vomiting, GI distress, occult bleeding.*
Hepatic: abnormal liver function studies.
Skin: *rash.*
Other: *hypersensitivity manifested by anaphylaxis.*

INTERACTIONS
Ammonium chloride (and other urine acidifiers): increased blood levels of aspirin products. Monitor for aspirin toxicity.
Antacids (and other urine alkalinizers): decreased levels of aspirin products. Monitor for decreased aspirin effect.

Oral anticoagulants: increased risk of bleeding. Avoid using together if possible.

NURSING CONSIDERATIONS
• Contraindicated in GI ulcer, GI bleeding, aspirin hypersensitivity. Use cautiously in hypoprothrombinemia, vitamin K deficiency, bleeding disorders, and Hodgkin's disease (may cause profound hypothermia).
• Give with food, milk, antacid, or large glass of water to reduce GI side effects.
• Warn patient to check with doctor before taking over-the-counter combinations containing aspirin.
• Therapeutic serum salicylate level in arthritis is 20 to 30 mg/100 ml.
• Alcohol may increase gastrointestinal blood loss.

---

sodium salicylate
Uracel

INDICATIONS & DOSAGE
Minor pain or fever—
Adults: 325 to 650 mg P.O. q 4 to 6 hours, p.r.n., or 500 mg slow I.V. infusion over 4 to 8 hours. Maximum dose 1 g daily.
Children: 40 to 100 mg/Kg P.O. q 4 to 6 hours, p.r.n.

SIDE EFFECTS
Blood: *prolonged bleeding time.*
EENT: *tinnitus and hearing loss (first signs of toxicity).*
GI: *nausea, vomiting, GI distress, occult bleeding.*
Hepatic: abnormal liver function studies.
Skin: *rash.*
Other: *hypersensitivity manifested by anaphylaxis.*

INTERACTIONS
Ammonium chloride (and other urine acidifiers): increased blood levels of

---

aspirin products. Monitor for aspirin toxicity.
Antacids (and other urine alkaliniz-ers): decreased levels of aspirin products. Monitor for decreased aspirin effect.
Oral anticoagulants: increased risk of bleeding. Avoid using together if possible.

NURSING CONSIDERATIONS

• Contraindicated in GI ulcer, GI bleeding, aspirin hypersensitivity. Use cautiously in hypoprothrombinemia, vitamin K deficiency, bleeding disorders, asthmatics with nasal polyps (may cause severe bronchospasm), and Hodgkin's disease (may cause profound hypothermia).
• Febrile, dehydrated children can develop toxicity rapidly.
• Give with food, milk, antacid, or large glass of water to reduce GI side effects.
• Enteric-coated or timed-release preparations are absorbed erratically and are ineffective for chronic therapy.
• Warn patient to check with doctor before taking over-the-counter combinations containing aspirin.
• Therapeutic serum salicylate level in arthritis is 20 to 30 mg/ml.
• Tinnitus, headache, dizziness, confusion, fever, sweating, thirst, drowsiness, dim vision, hyperventilation, and increased pulse rate are signs of mild toxicity.
• Alcohol may increase gastrointestinal blood loss.

---

sodium thiosalicylate
Arthrolate, Jecto Sal, Nalate, Osteolate, Thiodyne, Thiolate, Thiosal, TH Sal

---

INDICATIONS & DOSAGE
Adults:

Mild pain—50 to 100 mg I.M. daily or every other day.
Arthritis—100 mg I.M. daily.
Rheumatic fever—100 to 150 mg I.M. b.i.d. until asymptomatic.
Acute gout—100 mg I.M. q 3 to 4 hours for 2 days, then 100 mg I.M. daily until asymptomatic.

SIDE EFFECTS
Blood: *prolonged bleeding time.*
EENT: *tinnitus and hearing loss (first signs of toxicity).*
GI: *nausea, vomiting, GI distress, occult bleeding.*
Hepatic: abnormal liver function studies.
Skin: *rash.*
Other: *hypersensitivity manifested by anaphylaxis.*

INTERACTIONS
Ammonium chloride (and other urine acidifiers): increased blood levels of aspirin products. Monitor for aspirin toxicity.
Antacids (and other urine alkaliniz-ers): decreased levels of aspirin products. Monitor for decreased aspirin effect.
Oral anticoagulants: increased risk of bleeding. Avoid using together if possible.

NURSING CONSIDERATIONS
• Contraindicated in GI ulcer, GI bleeding, aspirin hypersensitivity. Use cautiously in hypoprothrombinemia, vitamin K deficiency, bleeding disorders, asthmatics with nasal polyps (may cause severe bronchospasm), and Hodgkin's disease (may cause profound hypothermia).
• Tinnitus, headache, dizziness, confusion, fever, sweating, thirst, drowsiness, dim vision, hyperventilation, and increased pulse rate are signs of mild toxicity.
• Alcohol may increase gastrointestinal blood loss.

---

sulindac
Clinoril

INDICATIONS & DOSAGE
Osteoarthritis, rheumatoid arthritis, ankylosing spondylitis—
Adults: 150 mg P.O. b.i.d. initially; may increase to 200 mg P.O. b.i.d.
Acute subacromial bursitis or supraspinatus tendinitis, acute gouty arthritis—
Adults: 200 mg P.O. b.i.d. for 7 to 14 days. Dose may be reduced as symptoms subside.

SIDE EFFECTS
Blood: prolonged bleeding time, *aplastic anemia.*
CNS: dizziness, headache, nervousness.
EENT: tinnitus.
GI: *epigastric distress, occult blood loss,* nausea.
Skin: rash, pruritus.
Other: edema.

INTERACTIONS
None significant.

NURSING CONSIDERATIONS
• Contraindicated in acute asthmatics whose condition is precipitated by aspirin or other nonsteroidal anti-inflammatory agents; in active ulcers and GI bleeding. Use cautiously in history of ulcers and GI bleeding, renal dysfunction, compromised cardiac function, hypertension.
• To reduce GI side effects, give with food, milk, or antacids.
• Patient should notify doctor and have complete visual exam if any visual disturbances occur.
• Tell patient to notify doctor immediately if prolonged bleeding occurs.
• Drug causes sodium retention.

tolmetin sodium
Tolectin♦, Tolectin DS

INDICATIONS & DOSAGE
Rheumatoid arthritis and osteoarthritis, juvenile rheumatoid arthritis—
Adults: 400 mg P.O. t.i.d. or q.i.d. Maximum 2 g daily.
Children: (2 yrs or older): 15 to 30 mg/Kg/day in divided doses.

SIDE EFFECTS
Blood: prolonged bleeding time. adequate. Don't exceed 600 mg per day.
Not recommended for children.
CNS: headache, dizziness, drowsiness.
GI: *epigastric distress, occult blood loss,* nausea.
GU: reversible renal failure.
Skin: rash, urticaria, pruritus.
Other: sodium retention, edema.

INTERACTIONS
None significant.

NURSING CONSIDERATIONS
• Contraindicated in asthmatics with nasal polyps. Use cautiously in cardiac and renal disease, and GI bleeding disorders.
• Give with food, milk, or antacids to reduce GI side effects.
• Tell patient therapeutic effect should begin within 1 week.
• Double strength capsule (400 mg) is available.

zomepirac sodium
Zomax

INDICATIONS & DOSAGE
Mild to moderately severe pain—
Adults: 100 mg P.O. q 4 to 6 hours as required p.r.n. In mild pain, 50 mg q

4 to 6 hours may be adequate. Don't exceed 600 mg per day.
Not recommended for children.

SIDE EFFECTS
EENT: tinnitus, taste change.
CNS: *drowsiness, dizziness, insomnia,* paresthesia, nervousness.
CV: *edema, hypertension,* cardiac irregularity, palpitations.
GI: *nausea, vomiting, diarrhea, dyspepsia,* constipation, flatulence, anorexia.
GU: urinary frequency, elevated BUN and creatinine, vaginitis, urinary tract infection.
Skin: rash, pruritus.
Other: chills.

INTERACTIONS
None significant.

NURSING CONSIDERATIONS
● Contraindicated in patients in whom aspirin and other nonsteroidal, anti-inflammatory drugs induce bronchospasm, rhinitis, urticaria, or other sensitivity reactions. Give cautiously to patients with a history of gastrointestinal bleeding, fluid retention, hypertension, and heart failure.
● A nonnarcotic analgesic with narcotic potency. In several studies has been shown to be as effective as morphine.
● No evidence of addiction with zomepirac.
● Give with food or antacids if gastrointestinal symptoms occur.

21

Narcotic analgesics

alphaprodine hydrochloride
anileridine hydrochloride
anileridine phosphate
Brompton's cocktail
codeine phosphate
codeine sulfate
fentanyl citrate
hydromorphone hydrochloride
levorphanol tartrate
meperidine hydrochloride
methadone hydrochloride
morphine sulfate
oxycodone hydrochloride
oxymorphone hydrochloride
pentazocine hydrochloride
pentazocine lactate
propoxyphene hydrochloride
propoxyphene napsylate

---

alphaprodine hydrochloride
Controlled Substance Schedule II
Nisentil♦

INDICATIONS & DOSAGE
Moderate to severe pain—
Adults: 0.4 to 0.6 mg/Kg I.V. or 0.4
to 1.2 mg/Kg S.C. q 2 hours, p.r.n.
Maximum 240 mg daily. Don't give
I.M.

SIDE EFFECTS
CNS: *sedation, clouded sensorium,
euphoria,* convulsions with large
doses.
CV: *hypotension,* bradycardia.
GI: *nausea, vomiting, constipation,*
ileus.
GU: *urinary retention.*

Other: *respiratory depression,* physical dependence.

INTERACTIONS
None significant.

NURSING CONSIDERATIONS
• Use with extreme caution in head
injury, increased intracranial pressure, shock, elderly or debilitated patients, increased cerebrospinal fluid
pressure, CNS depression, asthma,
COPD, respiratory depression, seizures, hepatic or renal disease, hypothyroidism, Addison's disease, alcoholism.
• Keep narcotic antagonist (naloxone) available when giving drug I.V.
• Monitor respirations of newborns
exposed to drug during labor.
• Rapid but short-lived effect makes
drug useful in minor surgery or in
urologic procedures; not useful for relief of chronic pain.
• Monitor respiratory and circulatory
status carefully.
• Related to meperidine.
• If used with other narcotic analgesics, general anesthetics, tranquilizers, sedatives, hypnotics, alcohol, tricyclic antidepressants, or MAO inhibitors, depressant effect is increased.
Reduce narcotic dose. Use together
with extreme caution.
• For better analgesic effect, give before patient has intense pain.
• When used postop, encourage turning, coughing, and deep breathing to
avoid atelectasis.

aniferidine hydrochloride

aniferidine phosphate
Controlled Substance Schedule II
Leritine♦

INDICATIONS & DOSAGE
Adjunct to anesthesia—
Adults: 50 to 100 mg added to 500 ml
5% dextrose in water for slow I.V. in-
fusion; initially, 5 to 10 mg followed
by slow infusion of 0.6 mg/min. Max-
imum dose 200 mg daily.
Moderate to severe pain—
Adults: 25 to 50 mg P.O., I.M., or
S.C. q 4 to 6 hours, p.r.n.
Preop—
Adults: 50 to 75 mg I.M. or S.C.

SIDE EFFECTS
CNS: *sedation, clouded sensorium,
euphoria,* convulsions with large
doses.
CV: *hypotension,* bradycardia.
GI: *nausea, vomiting, constipation,*
ileus.
GU: *urinary retention.*
Local: pain at injection site, local tis-
sue irritation, and induration after
S.C. injection; phlebitis after I.V. in-
jection.
Other: *respiratory depression,* physi-
cal dependence.

INTERACTIONS
None significant.

NURSING CONSIDERATIONS
• Use with extreme caution in increased intracranial pressure, increased cerebrospinal fluid pressure,
CNS depression, head injury, asthma,
COPD, respiratory depression, seizures, hepatic or renal disease, hypothyroidism, Addison's disease, elderly
or debilitated patients, alcoholism,
shock.
• Keep narcotic antagonist (naloxone) available when giving drug I.V.

• Warn ambulatory patient to avoid
activities that require alertness.
• Monitor respirations of newborns
exposed to drug during labor.
• S.C. injection more likely to cause
tissue irritation than I.M. route.
• Stopping drug after long-term use
may initiate withdrawal symptoms.
• Related to meperidine.
• Carefully aspirate before S.C. or
I.M. injection. Sudden I.V. injection
of more than 10 mg can cause cardiac
arrest.
• Monitor respiratory and circulatory
status carefully.
• If used with other narcotic analgesics, general anesthetics, tranquilizers, sedatives, hypnotics, alcohol, tricyclic antidepressants, or MAO inhibitors, depressant effect is increased.
Reduce narcotic dose. Use together
with extreme caution.

Brompton's cocktail
(Mixture containing varying amounts
of the following ingredients: morphine or methadone, cocaine or amphetamine, syrup or honey, alcohol
[90% to 98%] or gin, chloroform
water)
Controlled Substance Schedule II

INDICATIONS & DOSAGE
*Severe chronic pain of terminal
cancer—*
Adults: 10 to 20 ml of (standard phar-
macy-prepared mixture) q 3 to
4 hours (if morphine is used) or q 6 to
8 hours (if methadone is used). Must
be given around-the-clock. Dosage ti-
trations can be made at 48- to 72-hour
intervals. Maximum dose totally dependent on patient response.

SIDE EFFECTS
CNS: *sedation, clouded sensorium,
euphoria,* convulsions with large
doses.
CV: *hypotension,* bradycardia.

Italicized side effects are common or life-threatening.

GI: *nausea, vomiting, constipation,* ileus.
GU: *urinary retention.*
Other: *respiratory depression,* physical dependence.

INTERACTIONS
None significant

NURSING CONSIDERATIONS
• Use with extreme caution in head injury, increased intracranial pressure, shock, elderly or debilitated patients, increased cerebrospinal fluid pressure, CNS depression, asthma, COPD, respiratory depression, seizures, hepatic or renal disease, hypothyroidism, Addison's disease, alcoholism.
• Originated in Brompton Hospital in England to keep cancer patients in constant pain-free and euphoric state.
• Not commercially prepared—must be prepared by pharmacy.
• Has frequently proven to be effective when narcotic analgesics alone have failed to provide pain relief.
• Around-the-clock administration reduces patient's anticipation of pain and is major reason for effectiveness.
• If cocaine is ingredient in mixture—advise patient to swish mixture in mouth to aid absorption, as cocaine is absorbed only through oral mucosa.
• Phenothiazines are occasionally added to increase analgesic effect and prevent nausea.
• Most formulations are stable for up to 4 weeks at room temperature; storage in refrigerator may increase stability to 8 weeks.

codeine phosphate

codeine sulfate
Controlled Substance Schedule II

INDICATIONS & DOSAGE
Mild to moderate pain—
Adults: 15 to 60 mg P.O. or 15 to 60 mg (phosphate) S.C. or I.M. q 4 hours, p.r.n.
Children: 3 mg/Kg daily P.O. divided q 4 hours, p.r.n.

SIDE EFFECTS
CNS: *sedation, clouded sensorium, euphoria,* convulsions with large doses.
CV: *hypotension,* bradycardia.
GI: *nausea, vomiting, constipation,* ileus.
GU: *urinary retention.*
Other: *respiratory depression,* physical dependence.

INTERACTIONS
None significant.

NURSING CONSIDERATIONS
• Use with extreme caution in head injury, increased intracranial pressure, increased cerebrospinal fluid pressure, hepatic or renal disease, hypothyroidism, Addison's disease, acute alcoholism, seizures, severe CNS depression, bronchial asthma, COPD, respiratory depression, shock, elderly or debilitated patients.
• Warn ambulatory patient to avoid activities that require alertness.
• Monitor respiratory and circulatory status and bowel function.
• For full analgesic effect, give before patient has intense pain.
• Codeine and aspirin have additive effect. Give together for maximum pain relief.
• Do not administer discolored injection solution.
• If used with general anesthetics,

other narcotic analgesics, tranquilizers, sedatives, hypnotics, alcohol, tricyclic antidepressants, or MAO inhibitors, CNS depression is increased. Use together with extreme caution. Monitor patient's response.

fentanyl citrate
Controlled Substance Schedule II
Sublimaze♦

INDICATIONS & DOSAGE
Adjunct to general anesthesia—
Adults: 0.05 to 0.1 mg I.V. repeated q 2 to 3 minutes, p.r.n. Dose should be reduced in elderly and poor-risk patients.
Postop—
Adults: 0.05 to 0.1 mg I.M. q 1 to 2 hours, p.r.n.
Children 2 to 12 years: 0.02 to 0.03 mg per 9 Kg.
Preop—
Adults: 0.05 to 0.1 mg I.M. 30 to 60 minutes prior to surgery.

SIDE EFFECTS
CNS: *sedation, clouded sensorium, euphoria,* convulsions with large doses.
CV: *hypotension,* bradycardia.
GI: *nausea, vomiting, constipation,* ileus.
GU: *urinary retention.*
Other: *respiratory depression,* physical dependence.

INTERACTIONS
None significant.

NURSING CONSIDERATIONS
• Contraindicated in patients who have received MAO inhibitors within 14 days and with myasthenia gravis. Use cautiously in head injury, increased cerebrospinal fluid pressure, asthma, COPD, respiratory depression, seizures, hepatic or renal disease, hypothyroidism, Addison's disease, alcoholism, increased intracranial pressure, CNS depression, shock, elderly or debilitated patients.
• Keep narcotic antagonist (naloxone) and resuscitative equipment available when giving drug I.V.
• Monitor respirations of newborns exposed to drug during labor.
• Use as postop analgesic, only in recovery room. Make sure another analgesic is ordered for later use.
• Often used with droperidol (as Innovar) to produce neuroleptanalgesia.
• Monitor circulatory and respiratory status carefully.
• If used with other narcotic analgesics, general anesthetics, tranquilizers, alcohol, sedatives, hypnotics, tricyclic antidepressants, or MAO inhibitors, respiratory depression, hypotension, profound sedation, and coma may result. Fentanyl citrate dose should be reduced by ¼ to ⅓. Also give above drugs in reduced dosages.
• For better analgesic effect, give before patient has intense pain.
• When used postop, encourage turning, coughing, and deep breathing to avoid atelectasis.

hydromorphone hydrochloride
Controlled Substance Schedule II
Dilaudid♦

INDICATIONS & DOSAGE
Moderate to severe pain—
Adults: 2 to 4 mg P.O. q 4 to 6 hours, p.r.n.; or 2 to 4 mg I.M., S.C., or I.V. q 4 to 6 hours, p.r.n. (I.V. dose should be given over 3 to 5 minutes); or 3 mg rectal suppository at bedtime, p.r.n.

SIDE EFFECTS
CNS: *sedation, clouded sensorium, euphoria,* convulsions with large doses.
CV: *hypotension,* bradycardia.
GI: *nausea, vomiting, constipation,* ileus.

GU: *urinary retention.*
Local: induration with repeated S.C. injection.
Other: *respiratory depression,* physical dependence.

INTERACTIONS
None significant.

NURSING CONSIDERATIONS
• Contraindicated in increased intracranial pressure, status asthmaticus. Use with extreme caution in increased cerebrospinal fluid pressure, respiratory depression, hepatic or renal disease, hypothyroidism, shock, elderly or debilitated patients, Addison's disease, acute alcoholism, seizures, head injury, severe CNS depression, brain tumor, bronchial asthma, COPD.
• Warn ambulatory patient to avoid activities that require alertness.
• Monitor respiratory and circulatory status and bowel function.
• Keep narcotic antagonist (naloxone) available.
• Respiratory depression and hypotension can occur with I.V. administration. Give very slowly and monitor constantly.
• Rotate injection sites to avoid induration with S.C. injection.
• Commonly abused narcotic.
• If used with general anesthetics, other narcotic analgesics, tranquilizers, sedatives, hypnotics, alcohol, tricyclic antidepressants, or MAO inhibitors, CNS depression is increased. Hydromorphone dose should be reduced. Use together with extreme caution. Monitor patient's response.
• For better analgesic effect, give before patient has intense pain.
• When used postop, encourage turning, coughing, and deep breathing to avoid atelectasis.

levorphanol tartrate
Controlled Substance Schedule II
Levo-Dromoran♦

INDICATIONS & DOSAGE
Moderate to severe pain—
Adults: 2 to 3 mg P.O. or S.C. q 6 to 8 hours, p.r.n.

SIDE EFFECTS
CNS: *sedation, clouded sensorium, euphoria,* convulsions with large doses.
CV: *hypotension,* bradycardia.
GI: *nausea, vomiting, constipation,* ileus.
GU: *urinary retention.*
Other: *respiratory depression,* physical dependence.

INTERACTIONS
None significant.

NURSING CONSIDERATIONS
• Contraindicated in acute alcoholism, bronchial asthma, increased intracranial pressure, respiratory depression, and anoxia. Use with extreme caution in hepatic or renal disease, hypothyroidism, Addison's disease, seizures, head injury, severe CNS depression, brain tumor, COPD, shock, elderly or debilitated patients.
• Warn ambulatory patient to avoid activities that require alertness.
• Monitor circulatory and respiratory status and bowel function.
• Warn patient drug has bitter taste.
• Protect from light.
• Keep narcotic antagonist (naloxone) available.
• If used with general anesthetics, other narcotic analgesics, tranquilizers, sedatives, hypnotics, alcohol, tricyclic antidepressants, or MAO inhibitors, CNS depression is increased. Reduce levorphanol dose. Use together with extreme caution. Monitor patient's response.

- For better analgesic effect, give before patient has intense pain.
- When used postop, encourage turning, coughing, and deep breathing to avoid atelectasis.

---

meperidine hydrochloride
Controlled Substance Schedule II
Demer-Idine♦♦, Demerol♦, Pethidine HCl B.P.♦♦

INDICATIONS & DOSAGE
Moderate to severe pain—
Adults: 50 to 150 mg P.O., I.M., or S.C. q 3 to 4 hours, p.r.n.
Children: 1 mg/Kg P.O., I.M., or S.C. q 4 to 6 hours. Maximum— 100 mg q 4 hours, p.r.n.
Preop—
Adults: 50 to 100 mg I.M. or S.C. 30 to 90 minutes before surgery.
Children: 1 to 2.2 mg/Kg I.M. or S.C. 30 to 90 minutes before surgery.

SIDE EFFECTS
CNS: *sedation, clouded sensorium, euphoria,* convulsions with large doses.
CV: *hypotension,* bradycardia.
GI: *nausea, vomiting, constipation,* ileus.
GU: *urinary retention.*
Local: pain at injection site, local tissue irritation and induration after S.C. injection; phlebitis after I.V. injection.
Other: *respiratory depression,* physical dependence.

INTERACTIONS
MAO inhibitors, isoniazid: increased CNS excitation or depression can be severe or fatal. Don't use together.

NURSING CONSIDERATIONS
- Contraindicated if patient has used MAO inhibitors within 14 days. Use with extreme caution in increased intracranial pressure, increased cerebrospinal fluid pressure, shock, children under 12, CNS depression, head injury, asthma, COPD, respiratory depression, supraventricular tachycardias, seizures, acute abdominal conditions, hepatic or renal disease, hypothyroidism, Addison's disease, urethral stricture, prostatic hypertrophy, alcoholism, elderly or debilitated patients.
- Meperidine and active metabolite normeperidine accumulate in renal failure. Monitor for increased toxic effect in patients with poor renal function.
- Meperidine may be given slow I.V., preferably as a diluted solution. S.C. injection very painful.
- Keep narcotic antagonist (naloxone) available when giving drug I.V.
- Warn ambulatory patient to avoid activities that require alertness.
- Monitor respirations of newborns exposed to drug during labor. Have resuscitation equipment available.
- P.O. dose less than half as effective as parenteral dose. Give I.M. if possible. When changing from parenteral to P.O., dose should be increased.
- Syrup has local anesthetic effect. Give with full glass of water.
- Chemically incompatible with barbiturates. Don't mix together.
- Monitor respiratory and cardiovascular status carefully. Don't give if respirations below 12/minute or if change in pupils.
- Watch for withdrawal symptoms if stopped abruptly after long-term use.
- If used with other narcotic analgesics, general anesthetics, phenothiazines, sedatives, hypnotics, tricyclic antidepressants, or alcohol, respiratory depression, hypotension, profound sedation, or coma may occur. Reduce meperidine dose. Use together with extreme caution.
- For better analgesic effect, give before patient has intense pain.
- When used postop, encourage turn-

Italicized side effects are common or life-threatening.

ing, coughing, and deep breathing to avoid atelectasis.

methadone hydrochloride
Controlled Substance Schedule II
Dolophine, Westadone

INDICATIONS & DOSAGE
Severe pain—
Adults: 2.5 to 10 mg P.O., I.M., or S.C. q 3 to 4 hours, p.r.n.
Narcotic abstinence syndrome—
Adults: 15 to 40 mg P.O. daily (highly individualized).
Maintenance: 20 to 120 mg P.O. daily. Adjust dose as needed. Daily doses greater than 120 mg require special state and federal approval.

SIDE EFFECTS
CNS: *sedation, clouded sensorium, euphoria,* convulsions with large doses.
CV: *hypotension,* bradycardia.
GI: *nausea, vomiting, constipation,* ileus.
GU: *urinary retention.*
Local: pain at injection site, tissue irritation, induration following S.C. injection.
Other: *respiratory depression,* physical dependence.

INTERACTIONS
Rifampin: withdrawal symptoms; reduced blood levels of methadone. Use together cautiously.
Ammonium chloride and other urine acidifiers, phenytoin: may reduce methadone effect. Monitor for decreased pain control.

NURSING CONSIDERATIONS
• Contraindicated in obstetric analgesia. Give with extreme caution in acute abdominal conditions, elderly or debilitated patients, severe hepatic or renal impairment, hypothyroidism, Addison's disease, prostatic hypertrophy, urethral stricture, head injury, increased intracranial pressure, asthma, COPD, respiratory depression, CNS depression.
• Safe use in adolescents as maintenance drug not established.
• Oral dose is half as potent as injected dose.
• Rotate injection sites.
• Has cumulative effect; marked sedation can occur after repeated doses.
• Monitor circulatory and respiratory status and bowel function.
• Warn ambulatory patient to avoid activities that require alertness.
• One daily dose adequate for maintenance. No advantage to divide doses.
• Oral form legally required in maintenance programs.
• Give maintenance doses as oral liquid. Completely dissolve tablets in 120 ml of orange juice or powdered citrus drink.
• Constipation often severe with maintenance. Make sure stool softener or other laxative is ordered.
• Patient treated for narcotic abstinence syndrome will usually require an additional analgesic if pain control necessary.
• If used with general anesthetics, tranquilizers, sedatives, hypnotics, alcohol, tricyclic antidepressants or MAO inhibitors, respiratory depression, hypotension, profound sedation, or coma may occur. Use together with extreme caution. Monitor patient's response.

morphine sulfate♦
Controlled Substance Schedule II

INDICATIONS & DOSAGE
Severe pain—
Adults: 5 to 15 mg S.C. or I.M., or 30 to 60 mg P.O. q 4 hours, p.r.n. or around the clock. May be injected

---

Unmarked trade names available in the United States only.
♦ Also available in Canada   ♦♦ Available in Canada only.

slow I.V. (over 4 to 5 minutes) diluted in 4 to 5 ml water for injection.
Children: 0.1 to 0.2 mg/Kg dose S.C. Maximum 15 mg.

SIDE EFFECTS

CNS: *sedation, clouded sensorium, euphoria,* convulsions with large doses.
CV: *hypotension,* bradycardia.
GI: *nausea, vomiting, constipation,* ileus.
GU: *urinary retention.*
Other: *respiratory depression, physical dependence.*

INTERACTIONS

None significant.

NURSING CONSIDERATIONS

• Use with extreme caution in head injury, increased intracranial pressure, seizures, asthma, COPD, alcoholism, prostatic hypertrophy, severe hepatic or renal disease, acute abdominal conditions, hypothyroidism, Addison's disease, increased cerebrospinal fluid pressure, urethral stricture, cardiac arrhythmias, reduced blood volume, toxic psychosis, elderly or debilitated patients.
• Warn ambulatory patient to avoid activities that require alertness.
• Monitor circulatory and respiratory status and bowel function. Don't give if respirations below 12/minute.
• Drug of choice in relieving pain of myocardial infarction. May cause transient decrease in blood pressure.
• Keep narcotic antagonist (naloxone) and resuscitative equipment available.
• If used with general anesthetics, tranquilizers, sedatives, hypnotics, alcohol, tricyclic antidepressants, or MAO inhibitors, respiratory depression, hypotension, profound sedation, or coma may occur. Reduce morphine dose. Use together with extreme caution. Monitor patient's response.

• For better analgesic effect, give before patient has intense pain.
• When used postop, encourage turning, coughing, and deep breathing to avoid atelectasis.
• Newly available oral solution contains 10 mg/5 ml.

---

oxycodone hydrochloride
Controlled Substance Schedule II
Supeudol♦♦

Combinations:
Percocet♦♦, Percocet 5, Percocet-Demi♦♦, Percodan♦, Percodan-Demi♦, Tylox

---

INDICATIONS & DOSAGE

Moderate pain—
Adults: available in U.S. only in combination with other drugs, such as aspirin, phenacetin, and caffeine (Percodan, Percodan-Demi), or acetaminophen (Percocet 5, Tylox). 1 to 2 tablets P.O. q 6 hours, p.r.n. p.r.n.
Adults: (Supeudol) 1 to 3 suppositories rectally/day, p.r.n.
Children: (Percodan-Demi) ¼ to ½ tablet P.O. q 6 hours, p.r.n.

SIDE EFFECTS

CNS: *sedation, clouded sensorium, euphoria,* convulsions with large doses.
CV: *hypotension,* bradycardia.
GI: *nausea, vomiting, constipation,* ileus.
GU: *urinary retention.*
Other: *respiratory depression,* physical dependence.

INTERACTIONS

Anticoagulants: oxycodone hydrochloride products containing aspirin may increase anticoagulant effect. Monitor clotting times. Use together cautiously.

Italicized side effects are common or life-threatening.

NURSING CONSIDERATIONS

• Use with extreme caution in head injury, increased intracranial pressure, increased cerebrospinal fluid pressure, seizures, asthma, COPD, alcoholism, prostatic hypertrophy, severe hepatic or renal disease, acute abdominal conditions, urethral stricture, hypothyroidism, Addison's disease, cardiac arrhythmias, reduced blood volume, toxic psychosis, elderly or debilitated patients.

• Don't give to children, except for Percodan-Demi and Percocet-Demi.

• Warn ambulatory patient to avoid activities that require alertness.

• Monitor circulatory and respiratory status and bowel function. Do not give if respirations below 12/minute.

• For full analgesic effect, give before patient has intense pain.

• High level of analgesia when given P.O., but poor choice due to high risk of addiction and presence of phenacetin in some combinations.

• Give after meals or with milk.

• If used with general anesthetics, other narcotic analgesics, tranquilizers, sedatives, hypnotics, alcohol, tricyclic antidepressants, or MAO inhibitors, CNS depression is increased. Reduce oxycodone dose. Use together with extreme caution. Monitor patient's response.

---

oxymorphone hydrochloride
Controlled Substance Schedule II
Numorphan♦

INDICATIONS & DOSAGE
Moderate to severe pain—
Adults: 1 to 1.5 mg I.M. or S.C. q 4 to 6 hours, p.r.n., or 0.5 mg I.V. q 4 to 6 hours, p.r.n., or 2.5 to 5 mg rectally q 4 to 6 hours, p.r.n.

SIDE EFFECTS
CNS: *sedation, clouded sensorium,* *euphoria,* convulsions with large doses.
CV: *hypotension,* bradycardia.
GI: *nausea, vomiting, constipation,* ileus.
GU: *urinary retention.*
Other: *respiratory depression,* physical dependence.

INTERACTIONS
None significant.

NURSING CONSIDERATIONS
• Use with extreme caution in head injury, increased intracranial pressure, seizures, asthma, COPD, alcoholism, increased cerebrospinal fluid pressure, acute abdominal conditions, prostatic hypertrophy, severe hepatic or renal disease, urethral stricture, CNS depression, respiratory depression, hypothyroidism, Addison's disease, cardiac arrhythmias, reduced blood volume, toxic psychosis, elderly or debilitated patients.

• Warn ambulatory patient to avoid activities that require alertness.

• Monitor cardiovascular and respiratory status. Don't give if respirations below 12/minute.

• Well absorbed rectally. Alternative to narcotics with more limited dosage forms.

• Narcotic antagonists (naloxone) should be available.

• If used with general anesthetics, tranquilizers, sedatives, hypnotics, alcohol, tricyclic antidepressants, or MAO inhibitors, CNS depression is increased. Reduce oxymorphone dose. Use together with extreme caution. Monitor patient's response.

• For better analgesic effect, give before patient has intense pain.

• When used postop, encourage turning, coughing, and deep breathing to avoid atelectasis.

pentazocine hydrochloride

pentazocine lactate
Controlled Substance Schedule IV
Talwin♦

INDICATIONS & DOSAGE
Moderate to severe pain—
Adults: 50 to 100 mg P.O. q 3 to
4 hours, p.r.n. Maximum 600 mg
daily or 30 mg I.M., I.V., or S.C. q 3
to 4 hours, p.r.n. Maximum 360 mg
daily. Doses above 30 mg I.V. or 60
mg I.M. or S.C. not recommended.

SIDE EFFECTS
CNS: *sedation,* visual disturbances,
hallucinations, drowsiness, dizziness,
light-headedness, confusion, euphoria, headache.
GI: nausea, vomiting, dry mouth.
GU: urinary retention.
Local: induration, nodules, sloughing, and sclerosis of injection site.
Other: *respiratory depression,* physical and psychologic dependence.

INTERACTIONS
None significant.

NURSING CONSIDERATIONS
• Contraindicated in emotional instability, drug abuse, head injury, increased intracranial pressure. Use
cautiously in hepatic or renal disease,
myocardial infarction with nausea,
respiratory depression.
• Tablets not well absorbed.
• Possesses narcotic antagonist
properties.
• Psychologic and physiologic dependence may occur.
• Respiratory depression can be reversed with naloxone.
• Do not mix in same syringe with
soluble barbiturates.

• Warn ambulatory patient to avoid
activities that require alertness.

propoxyphene hydrochloride
Controlled Substance Schedule IV
Darvon, Depronal♦♦, Dolene, Dora-
phen, Harmar, Myospaz, Pargesic 65,
Pro-65♦♦, Pro-Pox 65, Proxagesic,
Ropoxy, Scrip-Dyne, SK-65, S-Pain-
65, 642♦♦

propoxyphene napsylate
Controlled Substance Schedule IV
Darvocet-N, Darvon-N♦

INDICATIONS & DOSAGE
Mild to moderate pain—
Adults: 65 mg (hydrochloride) P.O. q
4 hours, p.r.n.
Mild to moderate pain—
Adults: 100 mg (napsylate) P.O. q 4
hours, p.r.n.

SIDE EFFECTS
CNS: dizziness, headache, sedation,
euphoria, paradoxical excitement,
insomnia.
GI: nausea, vomiting, constipation.
Other: psychologic and physical
dependence.

INTERACTIONS
None significant.

NURSING CONSIDERATIONS
• Not to be prescribed in narcotic addiction.
• Warn ambulatory patient to avoid
activities that require alertness until
response to drug has been established.
• Warn patient not to exceed recommended dosage.
• Do not use caffeine or amphetamines to treat overdose: may cause
fatal convulsions. Use narcotic antagonist instead.

• May cause false decreases in urinary steroid excretion tests.
• 65 mg propoxyphene HCl equals 100 mg propoxyphene napsylate.

• Can be considered a mild narcotic analgesic.
• Advise patients to limit their intake of alcohol.

22

Narcotic antagonists

levallorphan tartrate
naloxone

---

levallorphan tartrate
Lorfan

INDICATIONS & DOSAGE
Severe narcotic-induced respiratory depression—
Adults: 1 mg I.V., then 1 to 2 doses of 0.5 mg at 10- to 15-minute intervals, p.r.n. Maximum total dose 3 mg.
Children: 0.02 mg/Kg I.V. May give 0.01 to 0.02 mg/Kg in 10 to 15 minutes.
Neonates (asphyxia neonatorum): 0.05 to 0.1 mg I.V. into umbilical vein immediately after delivery. May repeat in 5 to 10 minutes.

SIDE EFFECTS
CNS: lethargy, dizziness, drowsiness, restlessness, sense of heaviness in limbs; with high doses: psychic disturbances (hallucinations, disorientation, weird dreams); in neonates: irritability, increased crying.
CV: pallor.
EENT: miosis, pseudoptosis.
GI: nausea.
Other: sweating, respiratory depression.

INTERACTIONS
None significant.

NURSING CONSIDERATIONS
• Contraindicated in mild respiratory depression and in narcotic addiction.

(Violent withdrawal symptoms may occur.)
• Monitor respiratory depth and rate. Be prepared to give O_2, ventilation, and other resuscitative measures.
• May increase mild respiratory depression or that caused by nonnarcotic agents. Repeated doses may produce tolerance and increased respiratory depression.

---

naloxone
Narcan♦

INDICATIONS & DOSAGE
Pentazocine, propoxyphene, and narcotic-induced respiratory depression—
Adults: 0.4 mg I.V., S.C., or I.M. May repeat q 2 to 3 minutes, p.r.n., for 3 doses.
*Postop narcotic depression—*0.1 to 0.2 mg I.V. q 2 to 3 minutes, p.r.n. Adult concentration is 0.4 mg/ml.
Children: 0.01 mg/Kg dose I.M., I.V., S.C. May repeat q 2 to 3 minutes for 3 doses.
Note: If initial dose 0.01 mg/Kg does not result in clinical improvement, up to 10 times this dose (0.1 mg/Kg) may be needed to be effective.
Neonates (asphyxia neonatorum): 0.01 mg/Kg I.V. into umbilical vein. May repeat q 2 to 3 minutes for 3 doses. Neonatal concentration (for children also) is 0.02 mg/ml.

SIDE EFFECTS
With higher-than-recommended doses: nausea, vomiting.
In narcotic addicts: withdrawal symptoms.

INTERACTIONS
None significant.

NURSING CONSIDERATIONS
• Use cautiously in cardiac irritability and narcotic addiction.
• Safest drug to use when cause of respiratory depression uncertain.
• Monitor respiratory depth and rate. Be prepared to give O_2, ventilation, and other resuscitative measures.
• Ineffective in respiratory depression caused by nonnarcotics except pentazocine and propoxyphene.
• May dilute adult concentration (0.4 mg) by mixing 0.5 ml with 9.5 ml sterile water or saline for injection to make neonatal concentration (0.02 mg/ml).

23

Sedatives and hypnotics

amobarbital
amobarbital sodium
aprobarbital
barbital
butabarbital
butabarbital sodium
chloral hydrate
ethchlorvynol
ethinamate
flurazepam hydrochloride
glutethimide
hexobarbital
mephobarbital
methaqualone
methaqualone hydrochloride
methotrimeprazine hydrochloride
methyprylon
paraldehyde
pentobarbital
pentobarbital sodium
phenobarbital
phenobarbital sodium
propiomazine hydrochloride
secobarbital
secobarbital sodium
talbutal
triclofos sodium

---

amobarbital
Amytal♦, Isobec♦♦
amobarbital sodium
Controlled Substance Schedule II
Amytal Sodium♦

INDICATIONS & DOSAGE
Sedation—
Adults: usually 30 to 50 mg P.O.
b.i.d. or t.i.d. but may range from 15
to 120 mg b.i.d. to q.i.d.

Children: 3 to 6 mg/Kg/day P.O. divided into 4 equal doses.
Insomnia—
Adults: 65 to 200 mg P.O. or deep
I.M. at bedtime; I.M. injection not to
exceed 5 ml in any one site. Maximum dose 500 mg.
Children: 3 to 5 mg/Kg deep I.M. at
bedtime; I.M. injection not to exceed
5 ml in any one site.
Preanesthetic sedation—
Adults and children: 200 mg P.O. or
I.M. 1 to 2 hours before surgery.
Manic reactions; anticonvulsant—
Adults, and children over 6 years:
65 to 500 mg slow I.V.; rate not to exceed 100 mg/minute. Maximum dose
1 g.
Children under 6 years: 3 to
5 mg/Kg slow I.V. or I.M.

SIDE EFFECTS
CNS: *drowsiness, lethargy, hangover,*
paradoxical excitement in elderly
patients.
GI: nausea, vomiting.
Skin: rash, urticaria.
Local: pain, irritation, sterile abscess
at injection site.
Other: *Stevens-Johnson syndrome,*
angioedema.

INTERACTIONS
Alcohol or other CNS depressants, including other narcotic analgesics: excessive CNS and respiratory depression. Don't use together.
MAO inhibitors: inhibited metabolism
of barbiturates; may cause prolonged
CNS depression. Reduce barbiturate
dosage.

Rifampin: may decrease barbiturate levels. Monitor for decreased effect.

NURSING CONSIDERATIONS
• Contraindicated in uncontrolled severe pain, respiratory disease with dyspnea or obstruction, hypersensitivity to barbiturates, previous addiction to sedatives, porphyria. Use with caution in hepatic or renal impairment.
• Use injection solution within 30 minutes after opening container to minimize deterioration. Don't use cloudy or precipitated solution. Don't shake solution; mix with sterile water only.
• Reserve I.V. injection for emergency treatment. Give under close supervision. Be prepared to give artificial respiration. Administer slowly I.V.; not to exceed 100 mg/minute.
• Administer I.M. injection deeply. Superficial injection may cause pain, sterile abscess, and slough.
• Because barbiturates potentiate narcotics, reduce dose when giving during labor. Excessive dose may cause respiratory depression in neonate.
• Remove cigarettes of patient receiving hypnotic dose.
• Supervise walking; raise bed rails, especially for elderly patients.
• Long-term high dosage may cause drug dependence and severe withdrawal symptoms. Withdraw barbiturates gradually.
• Prevent hoarding or self-overdosing by patients who are depressed, suicidal, or drug-dependent, or who have a history of drug abuse. Warn patient about increased alcohol effects and against hazardous activity requiring alertness or skill.
• Watch for signs of barbiturate toxicity: coma, pupillary constriction, cyanosis, clammy skin, hypotension. Overdose can be fatal.
• Monitor prothrombin times carefully when patient on amobarbital starts or ends anticoagulant therapy.

Anticoagulant dose may need to be adjusted.

aprobarbital
Controlled Substance Schedule III
Alurate

INDICATIONS & DOSAGE
Sedation—
Adults: 15 to 40 mg P.O. t.i.d. or q.i.d.; usual dose 40 mg t.i.d.
Insomnia—
Adults: 40 to 160 mg P.O. at bedtime.

SIDE EFFECTS
CNS: *drowsiness, lethargy, hangover,* paradoxical excitement in elderly patients.
GI: nausea, vomiting.
Skin: rash, urticaria.
Other: *Stevens-Johnson syndrome,* angioedema.

INTERACTIONS
Alcohol or other CNS depressants, including narcotic analgesics: excessive CNS and respiratory depression. Don't use together.
MAO inhibitors: inhibited metabolism of barbiturates; may cause prolonged CNS depression. Reduce barbiturate dosage.
Rifampin: may decrease barbiturate levels. Monitor for decreased effect.

NURSING CONSIDERATIONS
• Contraindicated in uncontrolled severe pain, respiratory disease with dyspnea or obstruction, hypersensitivity to barbiturates, previous addiction to sedatives, porphyria. Use with caution in hepatic or renal impairment.
• Remove cigarettes of patient receiving hypnotic dose.
• Supervise walking; raise bed rails, especially for elderly patients.
• Long-term high dosage may cause drug dependence and severe with-

drawal symptoms. Withdraw barbiturates gradually.
- Prevent hoarding or self-overdosing by patients who are depressed, suicidal, or drug-dependent, or who have a history of drug abuse. Warn patient about increased alcohol effects and against hazardous activity requiring alertness or skill.
- Available as elixir only, with alcohol 20%.
- Monitor prothrombin times carefully when patient on aprobarbital starts or ends anticoagulant therapy. Anticoagulant dose may need to be adjusted.
- Watch for signs of barbiturate toxicity: coma, pupillary constriction, cyanosis, clammy skin, hypotension. Overdose can be fatal.

---

barbital
Controlled Substance Schedule IV
Barbital Sodium

INDICATIONS & DOSAGE
Insomnia—
Adults: 300 to 600 mg P.O. or I.M. 1 to 2 hours before bedtime.
Sedative—
Adults: 65 to 130 mg P.O. or I.M. b.i.d. or t.i.d.

SIDE EFFECTS
CNS: *drowsiness, lethargy, hangover,* paradoxical excitement in elderly patients.
GI: nausea, vomiting.
Skin: rash, urticaria.
Local: pain, swelling, thrombophlebitis.
Other: *Stevens-Johnson syndrome,* angioedema.

INTERACTIONS
Alcohol or other CNS depressants, including narcotic analgesics: excessive CNS and respiratory depression. Don't use together.

MAO inhibitors: inhibited metabolism of barbiturates; may cause prolonged CNS depression. Reduce barbiturate dosage.
Rifampin: may decrease barbiturate levels. Monitor for decreased effect.

NURSING CONSIDERATIONS
- Contraindicated in uncontrolled severe pain, respiratory disease with dyspnea or obstruction, hypersensitivity to barbiturates, previous addiction to sedatives, and porphyria. Use with caution in hepatic, renal, cardiac, or respiratory impairment.
- Use injection solution within 30 minutes after opening container to minimize deterioration. Don't use cloudy solution.
- Administer I.M. injection deeply. Superficial injection may cause pain, sterile abscess, and slough.
- Because barbiturates potentiate narcotics, reduce dose when giving during labor. Excessive dose may cause respiratory depression in neonate.
- Remove cigarettes of patient receiving hypnotic dose.
- Supervise walking; raise bed rails, especially for elderly patients.
- Long-term high dosage may cause drug dependence and severe withdrawal symptoms. Withdraw barbiturates gradually.
- Prevent hoarding or self-overdosing by patients who are depressed, suicidal, or drug-dependent, or who have a history of drug abuse. Warn about increased alcohol effects and against hazardous activity requiring alertness or skill.
- No analgesic action. May cause restlessness or delirium in presence of pain.
- Monitor prothrombin times carefully when patient on barbital starts or ends anticoagulant therapy. Anticoagulant dose may need to be adjusted.
- Watch for signs of barbiturate toxicity: coma, pupillary constriction,

---

Italicized side effects are common or life-threatening.

cyanosis, clammy skin, hypotension. Overdose can be fatal.

butabarbital
Buta-Barb♦♦, Butisol, Day-Barb♦♦, Medarsed, Neo-Barb♦♦
butabarbital sodium
Controlled Substance Schedule III
BBS, Butal, Butazem, Buticaps, Butisol Sodium♦, Sarisol No. 1, Soduben

INDICATIONS & DOSAGE
Sedation—
Adults: 15 to 30 mg P.O. t.i.d. or q.i.d.
Children: 6 mg/Kg P.O. divided t.i.d. Dosage range 7.5 to 30 mg P.O. t.i.d.
Preop—
Adults: 50 to 100 mg P.O. 60 to 90 minutes before surgery.
Insomnia—
Adults: 50 to 100 mg P.O. at bedtime.

SIDE EFFECTS
CNS: *drowsiness, lethargy, hangover,* paradoxical excitement in elderly patients.
GI: nausea, vomiting.
Skin: rash, urticaria.
Other: *Stevens-Johnson syndrome,* angioedema.

INTERACTIONS
Alcohol or other CNS depressants, including narcotic analgesics: excessive CNS and respiratory depression. Don't use together.
MAO inhibitors: inhibit the metabolism of barbiturates; may cause prolonged CNS depression. Reduce barbiturate dosage.
Rifampin: may decrease barbiturate levels. Monitor for decreased effect.

NURSING CONSIDERATIONS
• Contraindicated in uncontrolled severe pain, respiratory disease with dyspnea or obstruction, hypersensitiv-

ity to barbiturates, previous addiction to sedatives, porphyria. Use with caution in hepatic or renal impairment.
• Remove cigarettes of patient receiving hypnotic dose.
• Supervise walking; raise bed rails, especially for elderly patients.
• Long-term high dosage may cause drug dependence and severe withdrawal symptoms. Withdraw barbiturates gradually.
• Prevent hoarding or self-overdosing by patients who are depressed, suicidal, or drug-dependent, or who have a history of drug abuse. Warn patient about increased alcohol effects and against hazardous activity requiring alertness or skill.
• Butisol sodium elixir is sugar-free.
• Monitor prothrombin times carefully when patient on butabarbital starts or ends anticoagulant therapy. Anticoagulant dose may need to be adjusted.
• Watch for signs of barbiturate toxicity: coma, pupillary constriction, cyanosis, clammy skin, hypotension. Overdose can be fatal.
• Prolonged administration is not recommended: drug not shown to be effective after 14 days. A drug-free interval of at least 1 week is advised.

chloral hydrate
Controlled Substance Schedule IV
Aquachloral Supprettes, Chloralvan♦♦, Cohidrate, Noctec♦, Novochlorhydrate♦♦, Oradrate, S K Chloral Hydrate

INDICATIONS & DOSAGE
Sedation—
Adults: 250 mg P.O. or rectally t.i.d. after meals.
Children: 8 mg/Kg P.O. t.i.d. Maximum 500 mg t.i.d.
Insomnia—
Adults: 500 mg to 1 g P.O. or rectally 15 to 30 minutes before bedtime.

Children: 50 mg/Kg single dose.
Maximum dose 1 g.
Premedication for EEG—
Children: 25 mg/Kg single dose.
Maximum dose 1 g.

SIDE EFFECTS
CNS: *hangover, drowsiness,* night-
mares, dizziness, ataxia.
GI: *nausea,* vomiting, diarrhea, flat-
ulence.
Skin: hypersensitivity reactions.

INTERACTIONS
*Alcohol or other CNS depressants, in-
cluding narcotic analgesics:* excessive
CNS depression or vasodilation reaction. Use together cautiously.
Furosemide I.V.: sweating, flushes,
variable blood pressure, uneasiness.
Use together cautiously. Use a different hypnotic drug.

NURSING CONSIDERATIONS
• Contraindicated in marked hepatic
or renal impairment, hypersensitivity
to chloral hydrate or triclofos. Oral
administration contraindicated in gastric disorders. Use with caution in severe heart disease, mental depression,
suicidal tendencies.
• Dilute or administer with liquid to
minimize unpleasant taste and stomach irritation. Administer after meals.
• Prevent hoarding by patients who
are depressed, suicidal, or drug-dependent, or who have a history of
drug abuse. Warn about increased alcohol effects and against hazardous
activity requiring alertness or skill.
• Remove cigarettes of patient receiving hypnotic dose.
• Supervise walking; raise bed rails,
especially for elderly patients.
• Large dosage may raise BUN level.
• May cause false positives in glycosuria tests using cupric sulfate as Benedict's solution. Use Clinitest, Clinistix, or Tes-Tape.
• May interfere with fluorometric
tests for urine catecholamines and

Reddy, Jenkins, Thorn test for urinary
17-hydroxycorticosteroids. Do not
administer drug for 48 hours before
fluorometric test.
• Aqueous solutions incompatible
with alkaline substances.
• Store in dark container. Store suppositories in refrigerator.
• If patient is given anticoagulant,
monitor for increased prothrombin
times during the first several days of
therapy. Anticoagulant dose may need
to be adjusted.

---

ethchlorvynol
Controlled Substance Schedule IV
Placidyl♦

INDICATIONS & DOSAGE
Sedation—
Adults: 100 to 200 mg P.O. b.i.d. or
t.i.d.
Insomnia—
Adults: 500 mg to 1 g P.O. at bed-
time. May repeat 100 to 200 mg if
awakened in early a.m.

SIDE EFFECTS
Blood: thrombocytopenia.
CNS: facial numbness, drowsiness,
fatigue, nightmares, dizziness, resid-
ual sedation, muscular weakness, syn-
cope, ataxia.
CV: hypotension.
EENT: unpleasant aftertaste, blurred
vision.
GI: distress, nausea, vomiting.
Skin: rashes, urticaria.

INTERACTIONS
*Alcohol or other CNS depressants, in-
cluding narcotic analgesics; MAO inhibitors:* excessive CNS depression.
Use together cautiously.

NURSING CONSIDERATIONS
• Contraindicated in uncontrolled
pain and porphyria. Use cautiously in
hepatic or renal impairment; in el-

derly or debilitated patients; in mental depression with suicidal tendencies; if patient has previously overreacted to barbiturates or alcohol.
• Give with milk or food to minimize transient dizziness or ataxia caused by rapid absorption.
• May cause dependence and severe withdrawal symptoms. Withdraw gradually.
• Prevent hoarding or self-overdosing by patients who are depressed, suicidal, or drug-dependent, or who have a history of drug abuse. Overdosage very difficult to treat and has a high mortality rate. Warn about increased alcohol effects and against hazardous activity requiring alertness or skill.
• Watch for toxicity signs, such as poor muscle coordination, confusion, hypothermia, speech or vision disturbances, tremors, or weakness.
• 750 mg strength contains tartrazine dye. May cause allergic reactions in susceptible individuals.
• Remove cigarettes of patient receiving hypnotic dose.
• Supervise walking; raise bed rails, especially for elderly patients.
• Slight darkening of liquid from exposure to air and light doesn't affect safety or potency, but store in tight, light-resistant container to avoid possible deterioration.
• Monitor prothrombin times carefully when patient on ethchlorvynol starts or ends anticoagulant therapy. Anticoagulant dose may need to be adjusted.
• Drug is effective for short-term use only; treatment period should not exceed 1 week.

---

ethinamate
Controlled Substance Schedule IV
Valmid

INDICATIONS & DOSAGE
Insomnia—

Adults: 500 mg to 1 g P.O. 20 minutes before bedtime. Starting dose may be 250 mg for elderly or debilitated patients.
Preanesthetic—
Adults: 500 mg to 1 g P.O. 2½ hours preoperatively.

SIDE EFFECTS
Blood: thrombocytopenia.
GI: mild upset.
Skin: rashes, purpura.
Other: fever (allergic reaction).

INTERACTIONS
None significant.

NURSING CONSIDERATIONS
• Contraindicated for uncontrolled pain. Use cautiously in mental depression, suicidal tendencies, or history of drug abuse.
• Not usually given for daytime sedation due to short duration of effect.
• Long-term use may cause dependence and severe withdrawal symptoms. Withdraw gradually.
• Prevent hoarding or self-overdosing by patients who are depressed, suicidal, or drug-dependent, or who have a history of drug abuse. Warn about increased alcohol effects and against hazardous activity requiring alertness or skill.
• Abrupt withdrawal may cause blood pressure and pulse rate changes, sweating, and hallucinations.
• Remove cigarettes of patient receiving dose.
• Supervise walking; raise bed rails, especially for elderly patients.
• In overdosage, treat CNS and respiratory depression same as barbiturate intoxication; ethinamate is dialyzable.
• May cause falsely elevated urinary 17-ketosteroid (modified Zimmerman reaction) and 17-hydroxycorticosteroid levels (Porter-Silber test).
• Prolonged therapy not recommended; drug is not effective for more than 7 days.

---

flurazepam hydrochloride
Controlled Substance Schedule IV
Dalmane♦

INDICATIONS & DOSAGE
Insomnia—
Adults: 15 to 30 mg P.O. at bedtime.

SIDE EFFECTS
Blood: leukopenia, granulocytopenia.
CNS: *daytime sedation, dizziness, drowsiness, disturbed coordination,* lethargy, confusion, *headache.*

INTERACTIONS
Cimetidine: increased sedation. Monitor carefully.

NURSING CONSIDERATIONS
• Use cautiously in impaired hepatic or renal function, mental depression, suicidal tendencies, or history of drug abuse. Use caution and low end of dose range for elderly or debilitated patients.
• Prevent hoarding or self-overdosing by patients who are depressed, suicidal, or drug-dependent, or who have a history of drug abuse. Warn about increased alcohol effects and against hazardous activity requiring alertness or skill.
• Remove cigarettes of patient receiving dose.
• Supervise walking; raise bed rails, especially for elderly patients.

glutethimide
Controlled Substance Schedule III
Doriden♦, Rolathimide

INDICATIONS & DOSAGE
Insomnia—
Adults: 250 to 500 mg P.O. at bedtime. May be repeated, but not less than 4 hours before intended awaken-ing. Total daily dose should not exceed 1 g.
Preop—
Adults: 500 mg night before surgery; 500 mg to 1 g 1 hour before anesthesia.
First stage of labor—
500 mg at onset of labor; repeat once if necessary.
Sedative—
Adults: 125 to 250 mg t.i.d. after meals.

SIDE EFFECTS
CNS: *residual sedation,* paradoxical excitation, headache, vertigo.
EENT: dry mouth, blurred vision.
GI: irritation, nausea, diarrhea.
GU: bladder atony.
Skin: rashes, urticaria.

INTERACTIONS
Alcohol or other CNS depressants, including narcotic analgesics: excessive CNS depression. Use together cautiously.

NURSING CONSIDERATIONS
• Contraindicated in uncontrolled pain, severe renal impairment, porphyria. Use cautiously in mental depression, suicidal tendencies, history of drug abuse, prostatic hypertrophy, stenosing peptic ulcer, pyloroduodenal or bladder neck obstruction, narrow-angle glaucoma, cardiac arrhythmias.
• Drug is effective for short-term use only.
• Remove cigarettes of patient receiving dose.
• Supervise walking; raise bed rails, especially for elderly patients.
• Prevent hoarding or self-overdosing by patients who are depressed, suicidal, or drug-dependent, or who have a history of drug abuse. Warn about increased alcohol effects and against hazardous activity requiring alertness or skill for 7 to 8 hours after receiving this drug.

• Abrupt withdrawal may produce nausea, vomiting, nervousness, tremors, chills, fever, nightmares, insomnia, tachycardia, delirium, numbness of extremities, hallucinations, dysphagia, convulsions. Withdraw gradually.

• Monitor prothrombin times carefully when patient on glutethimide starts or ends anticoagulant therapy. Anticoagulant dose may need to be adjusted.

hexobarbital
Controlled Substance Schedule III
Sombulex

INDICATIONS & DOSAGE
Sedation—
Adults: 250 mg P.O., repeated as needed, q 2 to 3 hours.
Insomnia—
Adults: 250 to 500 mg P.O. at bedtime.

SIDE EFFECTS
CNS: *drowsiness, lethargy, hangover,* paradoxical excitement in elderly patients.
GI: nausea, vomiting.
Skin: rash, urticaria.
Other: *Stevens-Johnson syndrome,* angioedema.

INTERACTIONS
Alcohol or other CNS depressants, including narcotic analgesics: excessive CNS and respiratory depression. Do not use together.
MAO inhibitors: inhibit metabolism of barbiturates; may cause prolonged CNS depression. Reduce barbiturate dosage.
Rifampin: may decrease barbiturate levels. Monitor for decreased effect.

NURSING CONSIDERATIONS
• Contraindicated in uncontrolled severe pain, respiratory disease with dyspnea or obstruction, hypersensitivity to barbiturates, previous addiction to sedatives, porphyria. Use with caution in hepatic or renal impairment.

• May be used preop with atropine when morphine contraindicated.

• Because barbiturates potentiate narcotics, reduce dose when giving during labor. Excessive dose may cause respiratory depression in neonate.

• Remove cigarettes of patient receiving hypnotic dose.

• Supervise walking; raise bed rails, especially for elderly patients.

• Long-term high dosage may cause drug dependence and severe withdrawal symptoms. Withdraw barbiturates gradually.

• Prevent hoarding or self-overdosing by patients who are depressed, suicidal, or drug-dependent, or who have a history of drug abuse. Warn about increased alcohol effects and against hazardous activity requiring alertness or skill.

• Monitor prothrombin times carefully when patient on hexobarbital starts or ends anticoagulant therapy. Anticoagulant dose may need to be adjusted.

• Watch for signs of toxicity: coma, pupillary constriction (pupillary dilation with severe poisoning), clammy skin, hypotension. Overdose can be fatal.

mephobarbital
Controlled Substance Schedule IV
Mebaral♦

INDICATIONS & DOSAGE
Sedation—
Adults: 32 to 100 mg P.O. t.i.d. to q.i.d.
Children: 16 to 32 mg P.O. t.i.d. to q.i.d.
Incipient or active delirium tremens— 200 mg P.O. t.i.d.

SIDE EFFECTS

CNS: drowsiness, vertigo, headache, depression, residual sedation after hypnotic dose, paradoxical excitement.
GI: nausea, vomiting, diarrhea.
Skin: hypersensitivity reactions, jaundice.
Other: respiratory depression, apnea; discontinuance of hypnotic doses may induce nightmares or insomnia.

INTERACTIONS

Alcohol or other CNS depressants, including narcotic analgesics: excessive CNS and respiratory depression. Do not use together.
MAO inhibitors: inhibited metabolism of barbiturates; may cause prolonged CNS depression. Reduce barbiturate dosage.
Rifampin: may decrease barbiturate levels. Monitor for decreased effect.

NURSING CONSIDERATIONS

• Contraindicated in uncontrolled severe pain, respiratory disease with dyspnea or obstruction, hypersensitivity to barbiturates, previous addiction to sedatives, porphyria. Use with caution in hepatic or renal impairment, impaired cardiac or respiratory function.
• Remove cigarettes of patient receiving hypnotic dose.
• Supervise walking; raise bed rails, especially for elderly patients.
• Long-term high dosage may cause drug dependence and severe withdrawal symptoms. Withdraw barbiturates gradually.
• Prevent hoarding or self-overdosing by patients who are depressed, suicidal, or drug-dependent, or who have a history of drug abuse. Warn about increased alcohol effects and against hazardous activity requiring alertness or skill.
• Mephobarbital is metabolized to phenobarbital, the active agent.
• Monitor prothrombin times carefully when patient on mephobarbital starts or ends anticoagulant therapy. Anticoagulant dose may need adjustment.
• Watch for signs of toxicity.

---

methaqualone

Mequin, Quaalude, Sopor
methaqualone hydrochloride
Controlled Substance Schedule II
Parest, Parest 400, Rouqualone♦♦, Sedalone♦♦, Somnafac, Somnafac Forte, Triador♦♦, Tualone♦♦, Vitalone♦♦

INDICATIONS & DOSAGE

Sedation (methaqualone)—
Adults: 75 mg P.O. t.i.d. or q.i.d.
Insomnia (methaqualone)—
Adults: 150 to 300 P.O. at bedtime.
Insomnia (methaqualone hydrochloride)—
Adults: 200 to 400 mg P.O. at bedtime.

SIDE EFFECTS

CNS: headache, dizziness, fatigue, residual sedation, *transient paresthesias of extremities*, restlessness, anxiety.
EENT: dry mouth.
GI: anorexia, *nausea, vomiting*, epigastric discomfort.

INTERACTIONS

Alcohol or other CNS depressants, including narcotic analgesics: excessive CNS depression. Use together cautiously.

NURSING CONSIDERATIONS

• Contraindicated in history of drug abuse. Use cautiously in hepatic impairment, mental depression, suicidal tendencies.
• Remove cigarettes of patient receiving hypnotic dose.
• Supervise walking; raise bed rails, especially for elderly patients.

Italicized side effects are common or life-threatening.

- Warn about increased alcohol effects and against hazardous activity requiring alertness or skill.
- After switching from another hypnotic to methaqualone, onset of satisfactory hypnotic effect requires 5 to 7 consecutive nights of therapy.
- Prolonged administration of methaqualone is not recommended: drug not shown to be effective more than 14 days.
- One of major drugs of abuse "on the street." Because of high abuse potential, methaqualone is rarely clinically indicated.

---

methotrimeprazine hydrochloride
Levoprome, Nozinan♦♦

INDICATIONS & DOSAGE
Postop analgesia—
Adults, and children over 12 years: initially, 2.5 to 7.5 mg I.M. q 4 to 6 hours, then adjust dose.
Preanesthetic medication—
Adults, and children over 12 years: 2 to 20 mg I.M. 45 minutes to 3 hours prior to surgery.
Sedation, analgesia—
Adults, and children over 12 years: 10 to 20 mg deep I.M. q 4 to 6 hours as required.
Elderly: 5 to 10 mg I.M. q 4 to 6 hours.

SIDE EFFECTS
Blood: agranulocytosis and other dyscrasias after long-term high dosage.
CNS: *orthostatic hypotension, fainting, weakness, dizziness,* drowsiness, excessive sedation, amnesia, disorientation, euphoria, headache, slurred speech.
CV: *drop in blood pressure,* palpitations.
EENT: dry mouth, nasal congestion.
GI: nausea, vomiting, abdominal discomfort.

GU: difficulty urinating.
Local: *pain, inflammation, swelling at injection site.*

INTERACTIONS
All antihypertensive agents: increased orthostatic hypotension. Don't use together.

NURSING CONSIDERATIONS
- Contraindicated in concurrent antihypertensive drug therapy, including MAO inhibitors; also, in history of convulsive disorders; hypersensitivity to phenothiazines; severe cardiac, hepatic, or renal disease; previous overdose of CNS depressant; coma. Use with extreme caution in elderly or debilitated patient with heart disease or in any patient who may suffer serious consequences from a sudden drop in blood pressure.
- Use low initial dose in susceptible patient; increase gradually while frequently checking pulse, blood pressure, and circulation.
- Expect drop in blood pressure 10 to 20 minutes after I.M. injection.
- Keep patient in bed or closely supervised for 6 to 12 hours after initial doses because of orthostatic hypotension. If hypotension is severe, combat with phenylephrine, methoxamine, or levarterenol. Don't use epinephrine.
- Don't use for longer than 30 days except in terminal illness or when narcotics are contraindicated.
- In prolonged use, monitor liver function and blood studies periodically.
- Inject I.M. into large muscle masses. Rotate sites. Do not administer S.C., as local irritation results. I.V. injection not recommended.
- May be mixed in same syringe with reduced dose of atropine and scopolamine. Do not mix with other drugs. Protect solution from light.

methyprylon
Controlled Substance Schedule III
Noludar♦

INDICATIONS & DOSAGE
Insomnia—
Adults: 200 to 400 mg P.O. 15 minutes before bedtime.
Children over 3 months: 50 mg P.O. at bedtime, increased to 200 mg, if necessary. Maximum 400 mg/day.

SIDE EFFECTS
CNS: morning drowsiness, dizziness, headache, paradoxical excitation.
GI: nausea, vomiting, diarrhea, esophagitis.
Skin: rash.

INTERACTIONS
None significant.

NURSING CONSIDERATIONS
• Contraindicated in intermittent porphyria. Use cautiously in renal or hepatic impairment.
• Periodic blood counts are advisable during repeated or long-term use.
• Long-term high dosage may cause drug dependence and severe life-threatening withdrawal symptoms. Withdrawal should be gradual and closely monitored.
• Prevent hoarding or self-overdosing by patients who are depressed, suicidal, or drug-dependent, or who have a history of drug abuse. Warn about increased alcohol effect and against hazardous activity requiring alertness or skill.
• Remove cigarettes of patient receiving dose.
• Supervise walking; raise bed rails, especially for elderly patients.
• Value of this drug as a sedative has not been established.
• Overdosage symptoms include somnolence, confusion, constricted pupils, respiratory depression, hypotension, coma. Hemodialysis is useful in severe intoxication.

paraldehyde
Controlled Substance Schedule IV
Paral

INDICATIONS & DOSAGE
Sedation—
Adults: 4 to 10 ml P.O. or rectally; or 5 ml deep I.M. in upper outer quadrant of buttock. 3 to 5 ml I.V. (in emergency only).
Children: 0.15 ml/Kg P.O., rectally, or deep I.M.
Insomnia—
Adults: 10 to 30 ml P.O. or rectally; 10 ml I.M. or I.V.
Children: 0.3 ml/Kg P.O., rectally, or deep I.M.
Alcohol withdrawal syndrome—
Adults: 5 to 10 ml P.O. or rectally; or 5 ml deep I.M. q 4 to 6 hours for the first 24 hours, not to exceed a total of 60 ml P.O. or 30 ml I.M.; then q 6 hours on following days, not to exceed 40 ml P.O. or 20 ml I.M. per 24 hours.
Tetanus—
Adults: 4 to 5 ml I.V. (well diluted) or 12 ml (diluted 1:10) via gastric tube q 4 hours, p.r.n.; 5 to 10 ml I.M., p.r.n. to control seizures.

SIDE EFFECTS
CV: *I.V. administration may cause pulmonary edema or hemorrhage,* dilation of right side of heart, circulatory collapse.
GI: irritation, *foul breath odor.*
GU: nephrosis with prolonged use.
Skin: *erythematous rash.*
Local: *pain,* sterile abscesses, sloughing of skin, fat necrosis, muscular irritation, nerve damage at I.M. injection site (if injection is near nerve trunk).
Other: *respiratory depression.*

Italicized side effects are common or life-threatening.

INTERACTIONS

Alcohol: excessive CNS depression. Use with caution.

Disulfiram (Antabuse): increase in paraldehyde and acetaldehyde blood levels. Use together cautiously. May produce toxic disulfiram reaction.

NURSING CONSIDERATIONS

- Contraindicated in bronchopulmonary disease or gastroenteritis with ulceration. Use cautiously in hepatic impairment.
- Give rectal dose in olive oil or cottonseed oil as retention enema: 1 part paraldehyde, 2 parts oil, and 200 ml 0.9% sodium chloride solution.
- Dilute oral dose with iced juice or milk to mask taste and odor and to reduce GI distress.
- Use fresh supply; discard bottles opened more than 24 hours. Don't use if liquid has a brownish color, vinegary odor, or contains a precipitate.
- Drug reacts with plastic. Use glass syringe for parenteral dose, and don't put liquid in Styrofoam cup.
- Give I.M. injection deeply, away from nerve trunks, and massage injection site. Do not give more than 5 ml per injection site.
- Watch closely for respiratory depression, especially with repeated doses.
- Long-term high dosage may cause drug dependence and severe withdrawal symptoms. Withdraw gradually, with close monitoring.
- Remove cigarettes of patient receiving hypnotic dose.
- Supervise walking; raise bed rails, especially for elderly patients.
- Ventilate patient's room well to remove exhaled paraldehyde.
- No analgesic effect. May produce excitement or delirium in presence of pain.
- Oral or rectal administration of decomposed paraldehyde may cause severe corrosion of stomach or rectum.

pentobarbital
Controlled Substance Schedule II

pentobarbital sodium
Maso-Pent, Nembutal Sodium♦, Nova-Rectal♦♦, Penital, Pentogen♦♦

INDICATIONS & DOSAGE

Sedation—
Adults: 20 to 40 mg P.O. b.i.d., t.i.d., or q.i.d.
Children: 6 mg/Kg/day P.O. in divided doses.
Insomnia—
Adults: 100 to 200 mg P.O. at bedtime or 150 to 200 mg deep I.M.; 100 mg initially, I.V., then additional doses up to 500 mg; 120 to 200 mg rectally.
Children: 3 to 5 mg/Kg I.M. Maximum dose: 100 mg. Rectal dosages: 2 months to 1 year, 30 mg; 1 to 4 years, 30 to 60 mg; 5 to 12 years, 60 mg; 12 to 14 years, 60 to 120 mg.
Preanesthetic medication—
Adults: 150 to 200 mg I.M. or P.O. in 2 divided doses.

SIDE EFFECTS

CNS: *drowsiness, lethargy, hangover,* paradoxical excitement in elderly patients.
GI: nausea, vomiting.
Skin: rash, urticaria.
Other: *Stevens-Johnson syndrome,* angioedema.

INTERACTIONS

Alcohol or other CNS depressants, including narcotic analgesics: excessive CNS and respiratory depression. Do not use together.
MAO inhibitors: inhibited metabolism of barbiturates; may cause prolonged CNS depression. Reduce barbiturate dosage.
Rifampin: may decrease barbiturate levels. Monitor for decreased effect.

Unmarked trade names available in the United States only.
♦ Also available in Canada   ♦♦ Available in Canada only.

NURSING CONSIDERATIONS

• Contraindicated in uncontrolled severe pain, respiratory disease with dyspnea or obstruction, hypersensitivity to barbiturates, previous addiction to sedatives, porphyria. Use with caution in hepatic or renal impairment.
• Use injection solution within 30 minutes after opening container to minimize deterioration. Don't use cloudy solution.
• Parenteral solution alkaline. Avoid extravasation; may cause tissue necrosis.
• I.V. injection should be reserved for emergency treatment and should be given under close supervision. Be prepared to give artificial respiration.
• Administer I.M. injection deeply. Superficial injection may cause pain, sterile abscess, and slough.
• Do not mix with other medication.
• Because barbiturates potentiate narcotics, reduce dose when giving during labor. Excessive dose may cause respiratory depression in neonate.
• Remove cigarettes of patient receiving hypnotic dose.
• Supervise walking; raise bed rails, especially for elderly patients.
• Long-term high dosage may cause drug dependence and severe withdrawal symptoms. Withdraw barbiturates gradually.
• Prevent hoarding or self-overdosing by patients who are depressed, suicidal, or drug-dependent, or who have a history of drug abuse. Warn about increased alcohol effects and against hazardous activity requiring alertness or skill.
• No analgesic effect. May cause restlessness or delirium in presence of pain.
• Monitor prothrombin times carefully when patient on pentobarbital starts or ends anticoagulant therapy. Anticoagulant dose may need to be adjusted.
• Watch for signs of barbiturate tox-

icity: coma, pupillary constriction, cyanosis, clammy skin, hypotension. Overdose can be fatal.
• To insure accurate dosage, don't divide rectal suppositories.
• Nembutal sodium contains tartrazine dye; may cause allergic reactions in susceptible individuals.

---

phenobarbital
Barbipil, Barbita, Eskabarb♦, Gardenal♦, Henomint, Luminal♦, Orprine, PBR 12, Pheno-Squar, SK-Phenobarbital, Solfoton, Solu-barb, Stental
phenobarbital sodium
Controlled Substance Schedule IV
Luminal Sodium♦

INDICATIONS & DOSAGE
Sedation—
Adults: 30 to 120 mg P.O. daily in 2 or 3 divided doses.
Children: 6 mg/Kg P.O. divided t.i.d.
Insomnia—
Adults: 100 to 320 mg P.O. or I.M.
Children: 3 to 6 mg/Kg.
Preop sedation—
Adults: 100 to 200 mg I.M. 60 to 90 minutes before surgery.
Children: 16 to 100 mg I.M. 60 to 90 minutes before surgery.
Hyperbilirubinemia—
Neonates: 7 mg/Kg/day P.O. from first to fifth day of life, or 5 mg/Kg/day I.M. on first day, repeated P.O. on second to seventh days.
Chronic cholestasis—
Adults: 90 to 180 mg P.O. daily in 2 or 3 divided doses.
Children under 12 years: 3 to 12 mg/Kg/day P.O. in 2 or 3 divided doses.

SIDE EFFECTS
CNS: *drowsiness, lethargy, hangover* paradoxical excitement in elderly

---

Italicized side effects are common or life-threatening.

patients.
GI: nausea, vomiting.
Skin: rash, urticaria.
Local: pain, swelling, thrombophlebitis, necrosis, nerve injury.
Other: *Stevens-Johnson syndrome,* angioedema.

INTERACTIONS
Alcohol or other CNS depressants, including narcotic analgesics: excessive CNS and respiratory depression. Do not use together.
MAO inhibitors: inhibited metabolism of barbiturates; may cause prolonged CNS depression. Reduce barbiturate dosage.
Rifampin: may decrease barbiturate levels. Monitor for decreased effect.
Primidone: monitor for excessive phenobarbital blood levels.

NURSING CONSIDERATIONS
• Contraindicated in uncontrolled severe pain, respiratory disease with dyspnea or obstruction, hypersensitivity to barbiturates, previous addiction to sedatives, porphyria. Use with caution in impaired hepatic, renal, cardiac, or respiratory function; hyperthyroidism; diabetes mellitus; anemia; elderly or debilitated patients.
• Use injection solution within 30 minutes after opening container to minimize deterioration. Don't use cloudy solution.
• I.V. injection should be reserved for emergency treatment and should be given under close supervision. Be prepared to give artificial respiration.
• When given I.V., do not give more than 60 mg/minute.
• Give I.M. injection deeply. Superficial injection may cause pain, sterile abscess, and slough.
• Because barbiturates potentiate narcotics, reduce dose when giving during labor. Excessive dose may cause respiratory depression in neonate.

• Remove cigarettes of patient receiving hypnotic dose.
• Supervise walking; raise bed rails, especially for elderly patients.
• Long-term high dosage may cause drug dependence and severe withdrawal symptoms. Withdraw barbiturates gradually.
• Prevent hoarding or self-overdosing by patients who are depressed, suicidal, or drug-dependent, or who have a history of drug abuse. Warn about increased alcohol effects and against hazardous activity requiring alertness or skill.
• No analgesic action. May cause restlessness or delirium in presence of pain.
• Monitor prothrombin times carefully when patient on phenobarbital starts or ends anticoagulant therapy. Anticoagulant dose may need to be adjusted.
• Watch for signs of barbiturate toxicity: coma, pupillary constriction, cyanosis, clammy skin, hypotension. Overdose can be fatal.

---

propiomazine hydrochloride
Largon

INDICATIONS & DOSAGE
Sedation—
Adults: 20 to 40 mg I.M. or I.V.
Preop—
Adults: 10 to 20 mg I.M. or I.V.
During surgery; in conjunction with local, nerve block, or spinal anesthetic—
Adults: 20 to 40 mg I.M. or I.V. during early stages of labor, repeated q 3 hours, if necessary.
Sedation the night before surgery as a preanesthetic, or postop—
Children under 27 Kg: 0.55 to 1.1 mg/Kg I.M. or I.V.
Children 6 to 12 years: 25 I.M. or I.V. mg in a single dose.

Children 4 to 6 years: 15 mg I.M. or I.V. in a single dose.

SIDE EFFECTS
CNS: dizziness, confusion, amnesia (primarily in the elderly), restlessness.
CV: tachycardia, rise in blood pressure, transient hypotension with rapid I.V. infusion.
EENT: dry mouth.
GI: distress.
Skin: rashes.
Local: vein irritation and thrombophlebitis following I.V. injection.
Other: respiratory depression.

INTERACTIONS
None significant.

NURSING CONSIDERATIONS
• Contraindicated if patients have received large doses of other CNS depressants or are comatose. Use extreme caution with patients in hypertensive crisis.
• Give I.V. injection slowly to avoid transient fall in blood pressure.
• Inject in large, undamaged vein to minimize irritation. Avoid extravasation. Don't inject into artery; irritation may cause severe arteriospasm, impaired circulation, and gangrene.
• Do not give subcutaneously.
• Do not use solution for injection if it is cloudy or contains a precipitate.
• Antiemetic effect may mask signs of drug overdose or other disorders.
• Warn about increased effects of alcohol, tranquilizers, antihistamines, and other CNS depressants and against hazardous activity requiring alertness or skill.
• Supervise walking; raise bed rails, especially in elderly patients.
• Propiomazine reverses vasopressor effect of epinephrine. Use norepinephrine when vasopressor effect needed.

secobarbital
Seconal
secobarbital sodium
Controlled Substance Schedule II
Seco-8, Secogen Sodium♦♦, Seconal Sodium♦, Seral♦♦

INDICATIONS & DOSAGE
Sedation, preop—
Adults: 200 to 300 mg P.O. 1 to 2 hours before surgery.
Children: 50 to 100 mg P.O. or 4 to 5 mg/Kg rectally 1 to 2 hours before surgery.
Insomnia—
Adults: 100 to 200 mg P.O. or I.M.
Children: 3 to 5 mg/Kg I.M., not to exceed 100 mg, with no more than 5 ml injected in any one site. 4 to 5 mg/Kg rectally.
Acute tetanus convulsion—
Adults and children: 5.5 mg/Kg I.M. or slow I.V., repeated q 3 to 4 hours, if needed; I.V. injection rate not to exceed 50 mg per 15 seconds.
Acute psychotic agitation—
Adults: 50 mg/minute I.V. up to 250 mg I.V. initially, additional doses given cautiously after 5 minutes if desired response is not obtained. Not to exceed 500 mg total.
Status epilepticus—
Adults and children: 250 to 350 mg I.M. or I.V.

SIDE EFFECTS
CNS: *drowsiness, lethargy, hangover,* paradoxical excitement in elderly patients.
GI: nausea, vomiting.
Skin: rash, urticaria.
Other: *Stevens-Johnson syndrome,* angioedema.

INTERACTIONS
Alcohol or other CNS depressants, including narcotic analgesics: excessive CNS and respiratory depression. Do not use together.

MAO inhibitors: inhibited metabolism of barbiturates; may cause prolonged CNS depression. Reduce barbiturate dosage.
Rifampin: may decrease barbiturate levels. Monitor for decreased effect.

NURSING CONSIDERATIONS

• Contraindicated in uncontrolled severe pain, respiratory disease with dyspnea or obstruction, hypersensitivity to barbiturates, previous addiction to sedatives, porphyria. Use with caution in hepatic or renal impairment; also, in pregnant women with toxemia; or history of bleeding.
• Use injection solution within 30 minutes after opening container to minimize deterioration. Don't use cloudy solution.
• I.V. injection should be reserved for emergency treatment and should be given under close supervision. Be prepared to give artificial respiration.
• Give I.M. injection deeply. Superficial injection may cause pain, sterile abscess, and slough.
• Because barbiturates potentiate narcotics, reduce dose when giving during labor. Excessive dose may cause respiratory depression in neonate.
• Remove cigarettes of patient receiving hypnotic dose.
• Supervise walking; raise bed rails, especially for elderly patients.
• Long-term high dosage may cause drug dependence and severe withdrawal symptoms. Withdraw barbiturates gradually.
• Prevent hoarding or self-overdosing by patients who are depressed, suicidal, or drug-dependent, or who have a history of drug abuse. Warn about increased alcohol effects and against hazardous activity requiring alertness or skill.
• If patient has renal insufficiency, use sterile drug reconstituted with sterile water for injection. Avoid com-

mercial solution containing polyethylene glycol; may irritate kidneys.
• Secobarbital in polyethylene glycol must be refrigerated.
• Secobarbital sodium injection not compatible with lactated Ringer's solution.
• Sterile secobarbital sodium compatible with Ringer's injection and normal saline. Don't mix with acidic solutions.
• To reconstitute, rotate ampule. Do not shake.
• Monitor prothrombin times carefully when patient on secobarbital starts or ends anticoagulant therapy. Anticoagulant dose may need to be adjusted.
• Watch for signs of barbiturate toxicity: coma, pupillary construction, cyanosis, clammy skin, hypotension. Overdose can be fatal.

---

talbutal
Controlled Substance Schedule III
Lotusate

INDICATIONS & DOSAGE
Sedation—
Adults: 30 to 60 mg P.O. b.i.d. or t.i.d.
Insomnia—
Adults: 120 mg P.O. at bedtime.

SIDE EFFECTS
CNS: *drowsiness, lethargy, hangover,* paradoxical excitement in elderly patients.
GI: nausea, vomiting.
Skin: rash, urticaria.
Other: *Stevens-Johnson syndrome,* angioedema.

INTERACTIONS
Alcohol or other CNS depressants, including narcotic analgesics: excessive CNS and respiratory depression. Don't use together.
MAO inhibitors: inhibit the metabo-

lism of barbiturates; may cause prolonged CNS depression. Reduce barbiturate dosage.
Rifampin: may decrease barbiturate levels. Monitor for decreased effect.

NURSING CONSIDERATIONS
• Contraindicated in uncontrolled severe pain, respiratory disease with dyspnea obstruction, hypersensitivity to barbiturates, previous addiction to sedatives, porphyria. Use with caution in hepatic or renal impairment.
• Remove cigarettes of patient receiving hypnotic dose.
• Supervise walking; raise bed rails, especially for elderly patients.
• Long-term high dosage may cause drug dependence and severe withdrawal symptoms. Withdraw barbiturates gradually.
• Prevent hoarding or self-overdosing by patients who are depressed, suicidal, or drug-dependent, or who have a history of drug abuse. Warn about increased alcohol effects and against hazardous activity requiring alertness or skill.
• Monitor prothrombin times carefully when patient on talbutal starts or ends anticoagulant therapy. Anticoagulant dose may need to be adjusted.
• Watch for signs of barbiturate toxicity: coma, pupillary constriction, cyanosis, clammy skin, hypotension. Overdose can be fatal.

triclofos sodium
Triclos

INDICATIONS & DOSAGE
Insomnia—
Adults: 1.5 g P.O. 15 to 20 minutes before bedtime.
To induce sleep in EEG—
Children under 12 years: 22 mg/Kg P.O.

SIDE EFFECTS
CNS: light-headedness, dizziness, hangover, *drowsiness,* headache, ataxia.
GI: *nausea,* vomiting, flatulence, bad taste in mouth.
Skin: hypersensitivity reactions.

INTERACTIONS
Alcohol or other CNS depressants, including narcotic analgesics: excessive CNS depression or vasodilation. Use together cautiously.
Furosemide I.V.: possible sweating, flushes, variable blood pressure, uneasiness. Use together cautiously.

NURSING CONSIDERATIONS
• Contraindicated in hepatic or renal impairment, hypersensitivity to triclofos sodium or chloral hydrate, women in labor. Use with caution in cardiac arrhythmias, severe cardiac disease, mental depression, suicidal tendencies, or drug dependency.
• In prolonged use, monitor blood and hepatic function periodically.
• Withdraw slowly after prolonged use to avoid delirium, tremors, hallucinations.
• Prevent hoarding or self-overdosing by patients who are depressed, suicidal, or drug-dependent, or who have a history of drug abuse. Warn about increased alcohol effects and against hazardous activity requiring alertness or skill.
• Supervise walking; raise bed rails, especially for elderly patients.
• May cause false positives in glycosuria tests using cupric sulfate as Benedict's or Fehling's solution. Use Clinitest, Clinistix, or Tes-Tape.
• May interfere with fluorometric tests for urine catecholamines and Reddy, Jenkins, Thorn test for urinary 17-hydroxycorticosteroids. Don't administer drug for 48 hours before fluorometric test.

• Monitor prothrombin times carefully when patient on triclofos starts or ends anticoagulant therapy. Anticoagulant dose may need to be adjusted.

24

Anticonvulsants

acetazolamide
acetazolamide sodium
bromides
carbamazepine
clonazepam
diazepam
ethosuximide
ethotoin
magnesium sulfate
mephenytoin
mephobarbital
metharbital
methsuximide
paraldehyde
paramethadione
phenacemide
phenobarbital
phenobarbital sodium
phensuximide
phenytoin sodium (extended)
phenytoin sodium (prompt)
primidone
trimethadione
valproic acid
valproate sodium

---

acetazolamide
Acetazolam♦♦, Diamox♦, Hydrazol,
Roxolamide
acetazolamide sodium
Diamox♦

INDICATIONS & DOSAGE
*Myoclonic seizures, refractory grand
mal or petite mal, mixed seizures—*
Adults: 375 mg P.O., I.M., or I.V.
daily up to 250 mg q.i.d. Initial dose
when used with other anticonvulsants
usually 250 mg daily.

Children: 8 to 30 mg/Kg daily, divided t.i.d. or q.i.d. Maximum dose
1.5 g daily, or 300 to 900 mg/m²
daily.

SIDE EFFECTS
Blood: leukopenia, *aplastic anemia.*
CNS: paresthesias, drowsiness.
EENT: transient myopia.
GI: anorexia, nausea, vomiting.
GU: crystalluria, renal calculi.
Metabolic: *hyperchloremic acidosis.*
Skin: rash.
Local: *pain at injection site,* sterile
abscesses.

INTERACTIONS
Methenamine: antagonized methenamine effect. If used together, urine
must be kept at pH 5.5 or lower.

NURSING CONSIDERATIONS
• Contraindicated in sulfonamide
sensitivity, chronic pulmonary disease, renal or hepatic dysfunction,
Addison's disease (adrenocortical insufficiency), hyponatremia, hypokalemia, hyperchloremic acidosis,
chronic noncongestive narrow-angle
glaucoma. Use cautiously in hypercalciuria, diabetes mellitus, gout, and
respiratory acidosis.
• Obtain CBC and serum electrolytes
every 3 months; serum calcium every
6 months.
• Don't withdraw drug suddenly. Call
doctor if side effects develop.
• Warn patient to avoid activities that
require alertness and good psychomotor coordination until response to
drug has been determined.

- This drug is also a diuretic. Use diuretic precautions.
- Chronic use results in tolerance to drug.
- Reconstitute 500 mg vial with 5 ml sterile water for injection. Provides 100 mg/ml. Refrigerate reconstituted solution. Discard after 24 hours.
- Oral liquid: soften 1 tablet in 2 teaspoonfuls of very warm water and add to 2 teaspoonsful honey or syrup (chocolate, cherry). Don't use fruit juice.
- May cause hyperglycemia in prediabetics or diabetics on insulin or oral drugs. Monitor patients carefully.
- Observe and report signs of hypokalemia or metabolic acidosis.

bromides
Bromide, Lanabrom, Neurosine, Peacock's Bromides, Potassium Bromide, Sodium Bromide, Calcium Bromide

INDICATIONS & DOSAGE
Major motor and myoclonic seizures—
Adults: 1 to 2 g t.i.d.
Children: 50 to 100 mg/Kg daily, divided equally t.i.d. Or, 1.5 to 3g/m² daily in divided doses t.i.d.

SIDE EFFECTS
CNS: *drowsiness,* mental dullness, toxic psychosis.
Skin: *rashes* (acneform, morbilliform, granulomatous), Stevens-Johnson syndrome.

INTERACTIONS
None significant.

NURSING CONSIDERATIONS
- Contraindicated in cerebral arteriosclerosis, organic brain damage, impaired renal function, debilitated or dehydrated patients, alcoholics, severe depression, neurologic or psychologic disorders, tuberculosis or skin disorders (acne, dermatitis herpetiformis). Especially in adults, use may lead to chronic toxicity (mental, psychic, GI, and neurologic disturbances; skin eruptions). May be mistaken for acute alcohol intoxication, tabes dorsalis, cerebral tumor, uremia, or multiple sclerosis.
- Watch closely for toxicity In adults, serum levels above 5 mEq/liter may cause toxicity.
- Therapeutic serum level in children usually 20 to 25 mEq/liter (200 mg/100 ml), but range is 10 to 35 mEq/liter.
- Effect may not be seen for 2 to 3 weeks.
- Notify doctor if side effects develop.

carbamazepine
Tegretol♦

INDICATIONS & DOSAGE
Psychomotor, temporal lobe, grand mal, mixed seizure patterns—
Adults, and children over 12 years: 200 mg P.O. b.i.d. on day 1. May increase by 200 mg P.O. per day, in divided doses at 6- to 8-hour intervals. Adjust to minimum effective level when control achieved. Usual maintenance 800 to 1,200 mg daily. Don't exceed 1 g total daily dose in 12- to 15-year-olds and 1,200 mg P.O. daily in patients over 15 years.
Children under 12 years: 10 to 20 mg/Kg P.O daily in 2 to 4 divided doses.
Trigeminal neuralgia—
Adults: 100 mg P.O. b.i.d. with meals on day 1. Increase by 100 mg q 12 hours until pain relieved. Don't exceed 1.2 g daily. Maintenance dose 200 to 400 mg P.O. b.i.d.

SIDE EFFECTS
Blood: *aplastic anemia, agranulocytosis,* eosinophilia, leukocytosis, *thrombocytopenia.*

CNS: dizziness, *vertigo*, *drowsiness*, fatigue, *ataxia*.
CV: congestive heart failure, hypertension, hypotension, aggravation of coronary artery disease.
EENT: conjunctivitis, dry mouth and pharynx, blurred vision, diplopia, nystagmus.
GI: *nausea*, vomiting, abdominal pain, diarrhea, anorexia, *stomatitis*, glossitis, *dry mouth*.
GU: urinary frequency or retention, impotence, albuminuria, glycosuria, elevated blood urea nitrogen levels, microscopic deposits in urine.
Hepatic: abnormal liver function.
Metabolic: water intoxication.
Skin: rash, urticaria.
Other: diaphoresis, fever, chills.

INTERACTIONS
Troleandomycin, erythromycin: may increase carbamazepine blood levels. Use cautiously.
Propoxyphene: may raise carbamazepine levels. Use another analgesic.

NURSING CONSIDERATIONS
• Contraindicated in bone marrow depression, lactation, hypersensitivity to carbamazepine or tricyclic antidepressants. Use cautiously in cardiac, renal, or hepatic damage, or increased intraocular pressure.
• Warn patient to avoid activities that require alertness and good psychomotor coordination until response to drug has been determined.
• Never stop suddenly when treating seizures or status epilepticus. Notify doctor immediately if side effects occur.
• Obtain CBC, platelet and reticulocyte counts, and serum iron weekly for first 3 months, then monthly. If bone marrow depression develops, stop drug. Obtain urinalysis, BUN, and liver function tests every 3 months. Periodic eye examinations recommended.
• Tell patient to notify doctor imme-

diately if fever, sore throat, mouth ulcers, or easy bruising occurs.
• Therapeutic anticonvulsant serum level is 3 to 9 mcg/ml.
• When used for trigeminal neuralgia, an attempt should be made every 3 months to decrease dose or stop drug.

---

clonazepam
Controlled Substance Schedule IV
Clonopin, Rivotril♦

INDICATIONS & DOSAGE
Petit mal and petit mal variant (Lennox syndrome); akinetic and myoclonic seizures—
Adults: initial dose should not exceed 1.5 mg P.O. per day, divided into 3 doses. May be increased by 0.5 to 1 mg q 3 days until seizures controlled. Maximum recommended daily dose is 20 mg.
Children up to 10 years or 30 Kg: 0.01 to 0.03 mg/Kg P.O. daily (not to exceed 0.05 mg/Kg daily), divided q 8 hours. Increase dosage by 0.25 to 0.5 mg q third day to a maximum maintenance dose of 0.1 mg to 0.2 mg/Kg daily.

SIDE EFFECTS
Blood: leukopenia, thrombocytopenia, eosinophilia.
CNS: *drowsiness, ataxia, behavioral disturbances (especially in children)*, slurred speech, tremor, confusion.
EENT: *increased salivation*, diplopia, nystagmus, abnormal eye movements.
GI: constipation, gastritis, change in appetite, nausea, abnormal thirst, sore gums.
GU: dysuria, enuresis, nocturia, urinary retention.
Skin: rash.
Other: respiratory depression.

Italicized side effects are common or life-threatening.

INTERACTIONS
None significant.

NURSING CONSIDERATIONS
• Contraindicated in hepatic disease; chlordiazepoxide, diazepam, or other benzodiazepine sensitivity; acute narrow-angle glaucoma; or lactation. Use with caution in chronic respiratory disease, impaired renal function, open-angle glaucoma.
• Warn patient to avoid activities that require alertness and good psychomotor coordination until response to drug has been determined.
• Never withdraw suddenly. Call doctor at once if side effects develop.
• Obtain periodic CBC and liver function tests.
• Monitor patient for oversedation.
• Withdrawal symptoms similar to barbiturates.

diazepam
Controlled Substance Schedule IV
Valium♦

INDICATIONS & DOSAGE
Status epilepticus—
Adults: 5 to 10 mg slow I.V. push 5 mg/minute; may repeat q 10 minutes up to maximum total dose of 30 mg. Use 2 to 5 mg in elderly or debilitated patients. May repeat therapy in 2 to 4 hours with caution if seizures recur.
Children: 0.1 to 0.3 mg/Kg slow I.V. push (1 mg/minute over 3 minutes). May repeat q 15 minutes for 2 doses. Maximum single dose: children under 5 years—5 mg; children over 5 years—10 mg.
Adjunctive use in convulsive disorders—
Adults and children: 2 to 10 mg P.O. b.i.d., t.i.d., or q.i.d.

SIDE EFFECTS
Blood: neutropenia.

CNS: fatigue, *drowsiness, ataxia,* dizziness, headache, dysarthria, slurred speech, tremor.
CV: hypotension, bradycardia, *cardiovascular collapse.*
EENT: diplopia, blurred vision, nystagmus.
GI: nausea, constipation, change in salivation.
GU: incontinence, urinary retention.
Local: *pain, phlebitis at injection site.*
Skin: rash, urticaria.

INTERACTIONS
None significant.

NURSING CONSIDERATIONS
• Contraindicated in shock, psychosis, coma, acute alcohol intoxication with depression of vital signs, acute narrow-angle glaucoma. Use cautiously in elderly or debilitated patients, those with limited pulmonary reserve, and those in whom blood pressure drop might cause cardiovascular complications; also in history of anxiety states with suicidal tendencies, blood dyscrasias, hepatic or renal damage, open-angle glaucoma, or alcoholism.
• Monitor respirations every 5 to 15 minutes and before each I.V. repeated dose. Have emergency resuscitative equipment and oxygen at bedside.
• Do not mix with other drugs or I.V. fluids.
• Do not use small veins such as those on dorsum of hand or wrist.
• Avoid extravasation.
• Give slowly I.V. at rate not exceeding 5 mg/minute. Watch for phlebitis at injection site.
• Do not infuse through plastic tubing. Do not store in plastic syringe.
• Drug should not be withdrawn abruptly.
• Avoid heavy use of alcohol or other CNS depressants.

Unmarked trade names available in the United States only.
♦ Also available in Canada   ♦♦ Available in Canada only.

ethosuximide
Zarontin♦

INDICATIONS & DOSAGE
Petit mal—
Adults, and children over 6 years: initially, 250 mg P.O. b.i.d. May increase by 250 mg q 4 to 7 days up to 1.5 g daily.
Children 3 to 6 years: 250 mg P.O. daily or 125 mg P.O. b.i.d. May increase by 250 mg q 4 to 7 days up to 1.5 g daily.

SIDE EFFECTS
Blood: leukopenia, eosinophilia, *agranulocytosis,* pancytopenia, *aplastic anemia.*
CNS: *drowsiness,* headache, *fatigue, dizziness,* ataxia, irritability, hiccups, *euphoria, lethargy.*
EENT: myopia.
GI: *nausea, vomiting,* diarrhea, gum hypertrophy, weight loss, cramps, tongue swelling, *anorexia, epigastric and abdominal pain.*
GU: vaginal bleeding.
Skin: urticaria, pruritic and erythematous rashes, hirsutism.

INTERACTIONS
None significant.

NURSING CONSIDERATIONS
• Contraindicated in hypersensitivity to succinimide derivatives. Use cautiously in hepatic or renal disease.
• Never withdraw drug suddenly. Abrupt withdrawal may precipitate petit mal seizures. Call doctor immediately if side effects develop.
• Warn patient to avoid activities that require alertness and good psychomotor coordination until response to drug has been determined.
• Obtain CBC every 3 months.
• Therapeutic serum levels 40 to 80 mcg/ml.
• May increase frequency of grand mal seizures when used alone in mixed epilepsy.
• May cause positive direct Coombs' test.

ethotoin
Peganone

INDICATIONS & DOSAGE
Grand mal or psychomotor seizures—
Adults: initially, 250 mg P.O. q.i.d. after meals. May increase slowly over several days to 3 g daily divided q.i.d.
Children: initially, 250 mg P.O. b.i.d. May increase up to 250 mg P.O. q.i.d.

SIDE EFFECTS
Blood: thrombocytopenia, leukopenia, *agranulocytosis,* pancytopenia, megaloblastic anemia.
CNS: fatigue, insomnia, dizziness, headache, numbness.
CV: chest pain.
EENT: diplopia, nystagmus.
GI: nausea, vomiting, diarrhea, gingival hyperplasia (rare).
Skin: rash.
Other: fever, lymphadenopathy.

INTERACTIONS
Alcohol, folic acid, Loxitane: monitor for decreased ethotoin activity.
Oral anticoagulants, antihistamines, chloramphenicol, diazepam, diazoxide, disulfiram, isoniazid, phenylbutazone, phenyramidol, salicylates, sulfamethizole, valproate: monitor for increased ethotoin activity and toxicity.

NURSING CONSIDERATIONS
• Contraindicated in hydantoin hypersensitivity and in hepatic or hematologic disorders. Use cautiously in patients receiving other hydantoin derivatives.
• Never withdraw suddenly. Call doctor at once if side effects develop.

Italicized side effects are common or life-threatening.

- Warn patient to avoid activities that require alertness and good psycho-motor coordination until response to drug has been determined.
- Obtain CBC and urinalysis when therapy starts and monthly thereafter.
- Give after meals. Schedule doses as evenly as possible over 24 hours.
- Stop at once if lymphadenopathy or lupus-like syndrome develops.
- Heavy use of alcohol may diminish benefits of drug.
- Hydantoin derivative of choice in young adults who are prone to gingival hyperplasia caused by phenytoin.

magnesium sulfate

INDICATIONS & DOSAGE
Hypomagnesemic seizures—
Adults: 1 to 2 g (as 10% solution) I.V. over 15 minutes, then 1 g I.M. q 4 to 6 hours, based on patient's response and serum magnesium levels.
Children: seizures secondary to hypomagnesemia in acute nephritis—0.2 ml/Kg of 50% solution I.M. q 4 to 6 hours, p.r.n. or 100 mg/Kg of 10% solution I.V. very slowly. Titrate dosage according to serum magnesium levels and seizure response.
Prevention or control of seizures in pre-eclampsia or eclampsia—
Women: initially, 4 g I.V. in 250 ml 5% dextrose in water and 4 g deep I.M. each buttock; then 4 g deep I.M. into alternate buttock q 4 hours, p.r.n. Subsequent doses based on serum magnesium levels and urinary magnesium excretion. Do not exceed 40 g daily.

SIDE EFFECTS
CNS: sweating, drowsiness, depressed reflexes, flaccid paralysis, hypothermia.
CV: hypotension, flushing, *circulatory collapse*, depressed cardiac function, heart block.

Other: *respiratory paralysis*, hypocalcemia.

INTERACTIONS
Neuromuscular blocking agents: may cause increased neuromuscular blockade. Use cautiously.

NURSING CONSIDERATIONS
- Use cautiously in impaired renal function, myocardial damage, heart block, women in labor.
- Keep I.V. calcium gluconate available to reverse magnesium intoxication; however, don't use in digitalized patient due to danger of arrhythmias.
- Monitor vital signs every 15 minutes when giving drug I.V.
- Watch for respiratory depression and signs of heart block. Respirations should be approximately 16 per minute before each dose given.
- Monitor intake and output. Urinary output should be 100 ml or more in 4-hour period before each dose.
- Check serum magnesium levels after repeated doses. Disappearance of knee jerk and patellar reflexes is a sign of pending magnesium toxicity.
- Maximum infusion rate is 150 mg per minute. Rapid drip will induce uncomfortable feeling of heat.
- Call doctor if side effects develop.
- Especially when given I.V. to toxemic mothers within 24 hours before delivery, observe newborn for signs of magnesium toxicity, including neuromuscular or respiratory depression.
- Signs of hypermagnesemia begin to appear at blood levels of 4 mEq/liter.
- I.V. infusion should not be faster than 150 mg/minute.

mephenytoin
Mesantoin♦

INDICATIONS & DOSAGE
Refractory grand mal, focal, or psychomotor seizures—

Adults: 50 to 100 mg P.O. daily. May increase by 50 to 100 mg at weekly intervals up to 200 mg P.O. t.i.d.
Children: initial dose 50 to 100 mg P.O. daily or 100 to 450 mg/m² P.O. daily in 3 divided doses. May increase slowly by 50 to 100 mg at weekly intervals up to 200 mg P.O. t.i.d., divided q 8 hours. Dosage must be adjusted individually.

SIDE EFFECTS
Blood: *leukopenia*, neutropenia, *agranulocytosis*, thrombocytopenia, pancytopenia, eosinophilia.
CNS: ataxia, *drowsiness*, fatigue, irritability, choreiform movements, depression, tremor, sleeplessness, dizziness (usually transient).
EENT: photophobia, conjunctivitis, diplopia, nystagmus.
GI: gingival hyperplasia, nausea and vomiting (with prolonged use).
Skin: *rashes, exfoliative dermatitis.*
Other: hypertrichosis, edema, dysarthria, lymphadenopathy, polyarthropathy, pulmonary fibrosis.

INTERACTIONS
Alcohol, folic acid, Loxitane: monitor for decreased mephenytoin activity.
Oral anticoagulants, antihistamines, chloramphenicol, diazepam, diazoxide, disulfiram, isoniazid, phenylbutazone, phenyramidol, salicylates, sulfamethizole, valproate: monitor for increased mephenytoin activity and toxicity.

NURSING CONSIDERATIONS
• Contraindicated in hydantoin hypersensitivity. Use cautiously in patients receiving other hydantoin derivatives.
• Tell patient to notify doctor if fever, sore throat, bleeding, or rash occurs.
• Check CBC and platelet count initially and every 2 weeks thereafter, up to 2 weeks after full dose attained; then monthly for first year and every

3 months thereafter. Stop drug if neutrophils less than 1,600/mm³.
• Never withdraw drug suddenly. Call doctor if side effects develop.
• Warn patient to avoid activities that require alertness and good psychomotor coordination until response to drug has been determined.
• Therapeutic serum level is 5 to 20 mcg/ml.
• Heavy use of alcohol may diminish benefit of drug.

mephobarbital
Controlled Substance Schedule IV
Mebaral♦, Mentabal, Mephoral

INDICATIONS & DOSAGE
Grand or petit mal—
Adults: 400 to 600 mg P.O. daily or in divided doses.
Children: 6 to 12 mg/Kg P.O. daily, divided q 6 to 8 hours (smaller doses are given initially and increased over 4 to 5 days as needed).

SIDE EFFECTS
Blood: megaloblastic anemia, agranulocytosis, thrombocytopenia.
CNS: dizziness, headache, hangover, confusion, paradoxical excitation, exacerbation of existing pain, drowsiness.
CV: hypotension.
GI: nausea, vomiting, epigastric pain.
Skin: urticaria, morbilliform rash, blisters, purpura, erythema multiforme.
Other: allergic reactions (facial edema).

INTERACTIONS
Alcohol and other CNS depressants, including narcotic analgesics: excessive CNS depression. Use cautiously.
MAO inhibitors: potentiated barbiturate effect. Monitor patient for increased CNS and respiratory

---

Italicized side effects are common or life-threatening.

depression.
Rifampin: may decrease barbiturate levels. Monitor for decreased effect.

NURSING CONSIDERATIONS
• Contraindicated in barbiturate hypersensitivity, porphyria, and respiratory disease with dyspnea or obstruction. Use cautiously in hepatic, renal, cardiac, or respiratory function impairment, and in myasthenia gravis and myxedema.
• Never withdraw suddenly. Call doctor at once if side effects develop.
• Warn patient to avoid activities that require alertness and good psychomotor coordination until response to drug has been determined.
• Store in light-resistant container.
• In adults, give total or largest dose at night if seizures occur then.
• Three quarters of drug metabolized to phenobarbital; therapeutic serum levels as phenobarbital are 15 to 40 mcg/ml.
• Monitor prothrombin times carefully when patient on mephobarbital starts or ends anticoagulant therapy. Anticoagulant dose may need to be adjusted.

---

metharbital
Controlled Substance Schedule III
Gemonil

INDICATIONS & DOSAGE
Grand or petit mal; myoclonic or mixed seizures—
Adults: initially, 100 mg P.O. daily to t.i.d. May increase to 800 mg daily in divided doses.
Children: 5 to 15 mg/Kg P.O. daily, divided t.i.d. May increase to 50 to 100 mg P.O. daily, b.i.d., or t.i.d.

SIDE EFFECTS
Blood: megaloblastic anemia, *agranulocytosis,* thrombocytopenia.

CNS: dizziness, irritability, drowsiness, headache, confusion, excitation.
CV: hypotension.
GI: nausea, vomiting, discomfort.
Skin: rash, urticaria, purpura, erythema multiforme.

INTERACTIONS
Alcohol and other CNS depressants, including narcotic analgesics: excessive CNS depression. Use cautiously.
MAO inhibitors: potentiated barbiturate effect. Monitor patient for increased CNS and respiratory depression.
Rifampin: may decrease barbiturate levels. Monitor for decreased effect.

NURSING CONSIDERATIONS
• Contraindicated in barbiturate hypersensitivity, in manifest or latent porphyria, and in respiratory disease with dyspnea or obstruction. Use cautiously in hepatic, cardiac, or renal impairment.
• Don't stop drug abruptly.
• Warn patient to avoid activities that require alertness and good psychomotor coordination until response to drug is determined.
• Monitor prothrombin times carefully when patient on metharbital starts or ends anticoagulant therapy. Anticoagulant dose may need to be adjusted.

---

methsuximide
Celontin♦

INDICATIONS & DOSAGE
Refractory petit mal—
Adults and children: initially, 300 mg P.O. daily. May increase by 300 mg weekly. Maximum daily dosage of 1.2 g in divided doses.

SIDE EFFECTS
Blood: eosinophilia, leukopenia, monocytosis, pancytopenia.

CNS: *drowsiness, ataxia, dizziness,* irritability, nervousness, headache, insomnia, confusion, depression, aggressiveness.
EENT: blurred vision, photophobia, periorbital edema.
GI: *nausea, vomiting, anorexia,* diarrhea, weight loss, abdominal or epigastric pain.
Skin: urticaria, pruritic and erythematous rashes.

INTERACTIONS
None significant.

NURSING CONSIDERATIONS
• Contraindicated in hypersensitivity to succinimide derivatives. Use cautiously in hepatic or renal dysfunction.
• Never change or withdraw drug suddenly. Abrupt withdrawal may precipitate petit mal seizures. Call doctor immediately if side effects develop.
• Warn patient to avoid activities that require alertness and good psychomotor coordination until response to drug has been determined.
• Obtain CBC every 3 months; urinalysis and liver function tests every 6 months.
• May color urine pink or brown.
• Therapeutic serum levels 40 to 100 mcg/ml.

paraldehyde
Controlled Substance Schedule IV
Paral

INDICATIONS & DOSAGE
Refractory grand mal seizures, status epilepticus—
Adults: 5 to 10 ml I.M. (divide 10 ml dose into 2 injections); 0.2 to 0.4 ml/Kg in 0.9% saline injection I.V.
Children: 0.15 ml/Kg dose deep I.M. q 4 to 6 hours, p.r.n.; or 0.3 ml/Kg rectally in olive oil q 4 to 6 hours;

or 1 ml per year of age not to exceed 5 ml, repeated in 1 hour, p.r.n.; or dilute 5 ml in 95 ml 0.9% saline injection for I.V. infusion and titrate dose beginning at 5 ml/hour.

SIDE EFFECTS
CV: *I.V. administration may cause pulmonary edema or hemorrhage,* dilatation of right side of heart, *circulatory collapse.*
GI: irritation, *foul breath odor.*
GU: nephrosis with prolonged use.
Skin: *erythematous rash.*
Local: *pain,* sterile abscesses, sloughing of skin, fat necrosis, muscular irritation, nerve damage (if injection is near nerve trunk) at I.M. injection site.
Other: respiratory depression.

INTERACTIONS
Alcohol: increased CNS depression. Use with caution.
Disulfiram: increased paraldehyde and acetaldehyde blood levels; possible toxic disulfiram reaction. Use together cautiously.

NURSING CONSIDERATIONS
• Contraindicated in gastroenteritis with ulceration. Use cautiously in impaired hepatic function or in asthma or other pulmonary disease.
• Use fresh supply. Don't expose to air. Don't use if liquid is brown, has a vinegary odor, or if container has been opened longer than 24 hours.
• Watch closely for respiratory depression, especially in repeated doses.
• Drug reacts with plastic. Use glass syringe and bottle for parenteral dose. Prepare fresh I.V. solution every 4 hours. I.V. administration very hazardous.
• Give I.M. dose deeply, away from nerve trunks; massage injection site.
• Dilute paraldehyde in olive oil or cottonseed oil 1:2 for rectal administration. Give as retention enema. May

---

Italicized side effects are common or life-threatening.

also use 200 ml normal saline to prepare enema.
- Keep patient's room well ventilated to remove exhaled paraldehyde.
- Long-term high dosage may cause drug dependence and severe withdrawal symptoms.
- Oral or rectal administration of decomposed paraldehyde may cause severe corrosion of stomach or rectum.

---

paramethadione
Paradione♦

INDICATIONS & DOSAGE
Refractory petit mal—
Adults: initially, 300 mg P.O. t.i.d. May increase by 300 mg weekly, up to 600 mg q.i.d., if needed.
Children over 6 years: 0.9 g P.O. daily in divided doses t.i.d. or q.i.d.
Children 2 to 6 years: 0.6 g P.O. daily in divided doses t.i.d. or q.i.d.
Children under 2 years: 0.3 g P.O. daily in divided doses b.i.d.

SIDE EFFECTS
Blood: neutropenia, leukopenia, eosinophilia, thrombocytopenia, pancytopenia, *agranulocytosis, hypoplastic and aplastic anemia.*
CNS: *drowsiness,* fatigue, vertigo, headache, paresthesias, irritability.
CV: hypertension, hypotension.
EENT: hemeralopia, photophobia, diplopia, epistaxis, retinal hemorrhage.
GI: nausea, vomiting, abdominal pain, weight loss, bleeding gums.
GU: albuminuria, vaginal bleeding.
Hepatic: abnormal liver function.
Skin: acneiform or morbilliform rash, *exfoliative dermatitis,* erythema multiforme, petechiae, alopecia.
Other: lymphadenopathy, lupus erythematosus.

INTERACTIONS
None significant.

NURSING CONSIDERATIONS
- Contraindicated in renal and hepatic dysfunction, severe blood dyscrasias. Use cautiously in retinal or optic nerve diseases.
- Never withdraw suddenly. Call doctor at once if side effects develop.
- Therapeutic serum levels 6 to 71 mcg/ml.
- Stop drug if scotomata or signs of hepatitis, SLE, lymphadenopathy, skin rash, nephrosis, hair loss, or grand mal seizures appear.
- Tell patient to report sore throat, fever, malaise, bruises, petechiae, or epistaxis to doctor immediately. Advise patient to wear dark glasses if photophobia occurs. Warn him not to drive car or operate machinery.
- Obtain liver function studies and urinalysis before therapy; then monthly.
- Dilute oral solution with water before giving.
- Monitor CBC. Discontinue if neutrophil count falls below 2,500/mm³.
- 300 mg capsule contains tartrazine. May cause allergy in susceptible individuals.

---

phenacemide
Phenurone

INDICATIONS & DOSAGE
Refractory, mixed psychomotor, grand mal, petit mal, and petit mal variant seizures—
Adults: 500 mg P.O. t.i.d. May increase by 500 mg weekly up to 5 g daily, p.r.n.
Children 5 to 10 years: 250 mg P.O. t.i.d. May increase by 250 mg weekly, up to 1.5 g daily, p.r.n.

SIDE EFFECTS
Blood: *aplastic anemia, agranulocytosis,* leukopenia.
CNS: drowsiness, dizziness, insomnia, headaches, parethesias, *depres-*

sion, suicidal tendencies, aggressiveness.
GI: anorexia, weight loss.
GU: nephritis with marked albuminuria.
Hepatic: hepatitis, jaundice.
Skin: rashes.

INTERACTIONS
None significant.

NURSING CONSIDERATIONS
• Contraindicated in preexisting personality disturbances. Use with caution in hepatic dysfunction, history of allergy, and when a hydantoin is used concomitantly.
• Obtain liver function tests, CBC, and urinalysis before and at monthly intervals during therapy.
• Tell patient to report sore throat or fever to doctor immediately.
• Warn patient to avoid activities that require alertness or good psychomotor coordination until response to drug determined.
• Never withdraw suddenly. Call doctor at once if side effects develop.
• Tell patient's family to watch for personality or psychologic changes and report them to doctor at once.
• Extremely toxic. Use only when other anticonvulsants are ineffective.
• Notify doctor if patient develops jaundice or other signs of hepatitis, abnormal urinary findings, or WBC below 4,000/mm^3.

phenobarbital
Bar, Barbipil, Barbita, Eskabarb♦, Floramine, Gardenal♦♦, Henomint, Luminal♦, Nova-Pheno♦♦, Orprine, PB, PBR, Pheno-Squar, Solfoton, Solu-Barb, Stental
phenobarbital sodium
Controlled Substance Schedule IV
Luminal Sodium♦

INDICATIONS & DOSAGE
All forms of epilepsy, febrile seizures in children—
Adults: 100 to 200 mg P.O. daily, divided t.i.d. or given as single dose at bedtime.
Children: 4 to 6 mg/Kg P.O. daily, divided q 12 hours.
Status epilepticus—
Adults: 90 to 120 mg I.V., followed by 30 to 60 mg q 10 to 15 minutes, as needed, up to 500 mg total.
Children: 5 to 10 mg/Kg I.V. May repeat q 10 to 15 minutes up to total of 20 mg/Kg. I.V. injection rate should not exceed 60 mg/min.

SIDE EFFECTS
CNS: *drowsiness, lethargy, hangover,* paradoxical excitement in elderly patients.
GI: nausea, vomiting.
Skin: rash, urticaria.
Other: Stevens-Johnson syndrome, angioedema.

INTERACTIONS
Alcohol and other CNS depressants, including narcotic analgesics: excessive CNS depression. Use cautiously.
MAO inhibitors: potentiated barbiturate effect. Monitor for increased CNS and respiratory depression.
Rifampin: may decrease barbiturate levels. Monitor for decreased effect.
Primidone: monitor for excessive phenobarbital blood levels.
Valproic acid: increased phenobarbital levels. Monitor for toxicity.

NURSING CONSIDERATIONS

• Contraindicated in barbiturate hypersensitivity, porphyria, hepatic dysfunction, respiratory disease with dyspnea or obstruction, lactation, nephritis. Use cautiously in hyperthyroidism, diabetes mellitus, anemia, and in elderly or debilitated patients.

• I.V. injection should be reserved for emergency treatment and should be given slowly under close supervision. Monitor respirations closely.

• Watch for barbiturate toxicity signs, such as coma, asthmatic breathing, cyanosis, clammy skin, hypotension. Overdose can be fatal.

• Warn patient to avoid activities that require alertness and good psychomotor coordination until response to drug is determined.

• Don't stop drug abruptly. Call doctor immediately if side effects develop.

• Full therapeutic effects not seen for 2 to 3 weeks, except when loading dose is used.

• Do not use injection solution if it contains a precipitate.

• Therapeutic serum levels are 15 to 40 mg/ml.

• Monitor prothrombin times carefully when patient on phenobarbital starts or ends anticoagulant therapy. Anticoagulant dose may need to be adjusted.

• Do not mix parenteral form with acidic solutions: precipitation may result.

phensuximide
Milontin♦

INDICATIONS & DOSAGE

Petit mal—
Adults and children: 500 mg to 1 g P.O. b.i.d. to t.i.d.

SIDE EFFECTS

Blood: transient leukopenia, pancytopenia, *agranulocytosis.*
CNS: muscular weakness, *drowsiness,* dizziness, ataxia, headache.
GI: nausea, vomiting, anorexia.
GU: urinary frequency, renal damage, hematuria.
Skin: pruritus, eruptions, erythema.

INTERACTIONS
None significant.

NURSING CONSIDERATIONS

• Contraindicated in hypersensitivity to succinimide derivatives. Use cautiously in hepatic or renal disease.

• Never withdraw suddenly. Abrupt withdrawal may precipitate petit mal seizures. Call doctor immediately if side effects develop.

• Obtain CBC every 3 months; urinalysis and liver function tests every 6 months.

• May color urine pink or red to reddish brown.

• Therapeutic serum level 40 to 80 mcg/ml.

• May increase incidence of grand mal seizures if used alone to treat mixed epilepsy.

phenytoin sodium (extended)
Dilantin♦
phenytoin sodium (prompt)
Di-Phen, Diphenylan, Ditan

INDICATIONS & DOSAGE

Grand mal and psychomotor seizures, nonepileptic seizures (post head trauma, Reye's syndrome)—
Adults: loading dose 900 mg to 1.5 g I.V. at 50 mg/min or P.O. divided t.i.d., then start maintenance dose of 300 mg P.O. daily (extended only) or divided t.i.d. (extended or prompt).
Children: loading dose 15 mg/Kg I.V. at 50 mg/min or P.O. divided q 8 to 12 hours, then start maintenance

dose of 5 to 7 mg/Kg P.O. or I.V.
daily, divided q 12 hours.
*A loading dose is given if patient has
not taken phenytoin in the past or has
no detectible status epilepticus. If patient has not received phenytoin previously or has no detectible serum level,
use loading dose—*
Adults: 900 mg to 1.5 g I.V. divided
into t.i.d. at 50 mg/min. Do not exceed 500 mg each dose.
Children: 15 mg/Kg I.V. at
50 mg/min.
*If patient has been receiving phenytoin
but has missed one or more doses and
has subtherapeutic levels—*
Adults: 100 to 300 mg I.V. at
50 mg/min.
Children: 5 to 7 mg/Kg I.V. at
50 mg/min. May repeat lower dose in
30 minutes if needed.
*Neuritic pain (migraine, trigeminal
neuralgia, Bell's palsy)—*
Adults: 200 to 400 mg P.O. daily.

SIDE EFFECTS
Blood: thrombocytopenia, leukopenia, *agranulocytosis,* pancytopenia,
macrocytosis, megaloblastic anemia.
CNS: *ataxia,* slurred speech, confusion, dizziness, insomnia, nervousness, twitching, headache.
CV: hypotension, *ventricular
fibrillation.*
EENT: *nystagmus, diplopia,* blurred
vision.
GI: *nausea, vomiting, gingival hyperplasia (especially children).*
Hepatic: *toxic hepatitis.*
Skin: scarlatiniform or morbilliform
rash; bullous, *exfoliative* or purpuric
dermatitis; Stevens-Johnson syndrome; lupus erythematosus; hirsutism, toxic epidermal necrolysis.
Local: pain, necrosis, and inflammation at injection site.
Other: periarteritis nodosa, lymphadenopathy, hyperglycemia, osteoma-
lacia, hypertrichosis.

INTERACTIONS
Alcohol, folic acid, loxapine: monitor
for decreased phenytoin activity.
*Oral anticoagulants, antihistamines,
chloramphenicol, diazepam, diazoxide, disulfiram, isoniazid, phenylbutazone, phenyramidol, salicylates,
sulfamethizole, valproate:* monitor for
increased phenytoin activity and
toxicity.

NURSING CONSIDERATIONS
• Contraindicated in phenacemide or
hydantoin hypersensitivity, bradycardia, S-A and A-V block, Stokes-Adams syndrome. Use cautiously in hepatic or renal dysfunction, elderly or
debilitated patients, hypotension,
myocardial insufficiency, respiratory
depression, patients receiving other
hydantoin derivatives.
• Don't withdraw suddenly. Call doctor at once if side effects develop.
• Warn patient to avoid activities that
require alertness and good psychomotor coordination until response to
drug is determined.
• Don't mix drug with 5% dextrose in
water because it will precipitate.
Clear I.V. tubing first with normal saline solution. Never use cloudy solution. May mix with normal saline at a
concentration of 100 mg/50 ml if necessary.
• Do not give I.M. unless dosage adjustments are made. Drug may precipitate at injection site, cause pain, and
give erratic blood levels.
• Obtain CBC and serum calcium every 6 months. Doctor may order folic
acid and vitamin B_{12} if megaloblastic
anemia is evident.
• Drug may color urine pink or red to
reddish brown.
• Tell patient to carry identification
stating that he's taking phenytoin.
• Stress importance of good oral hygiene and regular dental exams.
• Drug should be stopped if rash appears. If rash is scarlet or measleslike, drug may be resumed after rash

Italicized side effects are common or life-threatening.

clears. If rash reappears, therapy should be stopped. If rash is exfoliative, purpuric, or bullous, don't resume drug.
• Use only clear solution for injection. Slight yellow color acceptable. Don't refrigerate.
• Divided doses given with or after meals may decrease GI side effects.
• Available as suspension. Shake well before each dose. Use solid form (chewable tablets or capsules) if possible.
• Therapeutic serum level is 10 to 20 mcg/ml.
• Heavy use of alcohol may diminish benefits of drug.
• Phenytoin levels may be decreased in mononucleosis. Monitor for increased seizure activity.
• Dilantin brand is the only oral form that can be given on a once-daily basis. Toxic levels may result if any other brand is given once daily.
• Advise patient not to change brands once stabilized on therapy.
• The drug was formerly known as diphenylhydantoin.

primidone
Mysoline♦, Sertan♦♦

INDICATIONS & DOSAGE
Grand mal, psychomotor, and focal seizures—
Adults, and children over 8 years: 250 mg P.O. daily. Increase by 250 mg weekly, up to maximum 2 g daily, divided q.i.d.
Children under 8 years: 125 mg P.O. daily. Increase by 125 mg weekly, up to maximum 1 g daily, divided q.i.d.

SIDE EFFECTS
Blood: leukopenia, eosinophilia.
CNS: *drowsiness, ataxia,* emotional disturbances, vertigo, hyperirritability, fatigue.

EENT: *diplopia,* nystagmus, edema of the eyelids.
GI: anorexia, *nausea, vomiting.*
GU: impotence, polyuria.
Skin: morbilliform rash, alopecia.
Other: edema, thirst.

INTERACTIONS
Phenytoin: stimulated conversion of primidone to phenobarbital. Observe for increased phenobarbital effect.

NURSING CONSIDERATIONS
• Contraindicated in phenobarbital hypersensitivity, porphyria.
• Don't withdraw suddenly. Call doctor at once if side effects develop.
• Warn patient to avoid activities that require alertness and good psychomotor coordination until response to drug determined.
• Therapeutic serum levels of primidone 7 to 15 mcg/ml. Therapeutic serum levels of phenobarbital 15 to 40 mcg/ml.
• CBC and routine blood chemistry should be done every 6 months.
• Partially converted to phenobarbital; use cautiously with phenobarbital.
• Shake liquid suspension well.

trimethadione
Tridione, Trimedone♦♦

INDICATIONS & DOSAGE
Refractory petit mal—
Adults: initially, 300 mg P.O. t.i.d. May increase by 300 mg weekly up to 600 mg P.O. q.i.d.
Children: 20 to 50 mg/Kg P.O. daily, divided q 6 to 8 hours. May increase by 150 to 300 mg. Usual maintenance 40 mg/Kg or 1 g/m² P.O. daily in divided doses t.i.d. or q.i.d.

SIDE EFFECTS
Blood: neutropenia, leukopenia, eosinophilia, thrombocytopenia, pancy-

topenia, *agranulocytosis, hypoplastic and aplastic anemia.*
CNS: *drowsiness,* fatigue, *malaise,* insomnia, dizziness, headache, paresthesias, irritability.
CV: hypertension, hypotension.
EENT: *hemeralopia,* diplopia, photophobia, epistaxis, retinal hemorrhage.
GI: nausea, vomiting, anorexia, abdominal pain, bleeding gums.
GU: nephrosis, albuminuria, vaginal bleeding.
Hepatic: abnormal liver function.
Skin: acneiform and morbilliform rash, *exfoliative dermatitis,* erythema multiforme, petechiae, alopecia.
Other: lymphadenopathy.

INTERACTIONS
None significant.

NURSING CONSIDERATIONS
• Contraindicated in paramethadione and trimethadione hypersensitivity, severe blood dyscrasias, severe hepatic dysfunction. Use with extreme caution in retinal and optic nerve diseases.
• Don't withdraw drug suddenly. Abrupt withdrawal may precipitate petit mal seizures. Call doctor immediately if side effects develop.
• Check CBC, hepatic function, and urinalysis before starting therapy and monthly thereafter. Drug should be stopped if neutrophil count falls below 2,500/mm³.
• Watch for impending toxicity; may precipitate grand mal seizure.
• Warn patient to report skin rash, alopecia, sore throat, fever, bruises, or epistaxis to doctor immediately.
• Warn patient to avoid activities requiring alertness and good psychomotor coordination.
• Suggest sunglasses if vision blurs in bright light. Notify doctor.
• If scotomata or rash occurs, drug should be stopped.

• Therapeutic serum levels 20 to 40 mcg/ml.
• May increase incidence of grand mal seizures if used alone to treat mixed epilepsy.

---

valproic acid
Depakene
valproate sodium
Depakene Syrup

INDICATIONS & DOSAGE
Simple and complex absence seizures (including petit mal), mixed seizure types (including absence seizures), investigationally in major motor (grand mal, tonic clonic) seizures—
Adults and children: initially, 15 mg/Kg P.O. daily divided b.i.d. or t.i.d.; then may increase by 5 to 10 mg/Kg daily at weekly intervals up to maximum of 30 mg/Kg daily, divided b.i.d. or t.i.d.

SIDE EFFECTS
Because drug usually used in combination with other anticonvulsants, side effects reported may not be caused by valproic acid alone.
Blood: inhibited platelet aggregation, thrombocytopenia, increased bleeding time.
CNS: *sedation,* emotional upset, depression, psychosis, aggression, hyperactivity, behavioral deterioration, muscle weakness, tremors.
GI: *nausea, vomiting,* indigestion, diarrhea, abdominal cramps, constipation, increased appetite and weight gain, *anorexia,* pancreatitis.
Hepatic: *enzyme elevations, toxic hepatitis.*
Other: alopecia.

INTERACTIONS
None significant.

NURSING CONSIDERATIONS

• Use cautiously in hepatic dysfunction.

• Don't withdraw suddenly. Call doctor at once if side effects develop.

• Obtain liver function studies, platelet counts, and prothrombin time before starting drug and every 2 months thereafter.

• Warn patient to avoid activities that require alertness and good psychomotor coordination until response to drug is determined.

• May give drug with food or milk to reduce GI side effects. Advise against chewing capsules; causes irritation of mouth and throat.

• Tremors may indicate the need for dosage reduction.

• Available as tasty red syrup. Keep out of reach of children.

• Syrup is more rapidly absorbed. Peak effect within 15 minutes.

• Advise patients to take with meals; will produce more uniform blood levels.

• May produce false positive test for ketones in urine.

• Syrup shouldn't be mixed with carbonated beverages; may be irritating to mouth and throat.

25

Antidepressants

amitriptyline hydrochloride
desipramine hydrochloride
doxepin hydrochloride
imipramine hydrochloride
isocarboxazid
nortriptyline hydrochloride
phenelzine sulfate
protriptyline hydrochloride
tranylcypromine sulfate
trimipramine maleate

---

amitriptyline hydrochloride
Amavil, Amiline♦♦, Amitid, Amitril, Deprex♦♦, Elavil♦, Endep, Levate♦♦, Meravil♦♦, Novotriptyn♦♦, Rolavil

INDICATIONS & DOSAGE
Endogenous and other depression—
Adults: 50 to 100 mg P.O., h.s. increasing to 200 mg daily; maximum 300 mg daily if needed; or 20 to 30 mg I.M. q.i.d. Alternatively, the entire dosage can be given at bedtime.
Elderly and adolescents: 30 mg P.O. daily in divided doses. May be increased to 150 mg.

SIDE EFFECTS
Blood: *agranulocytosis.*
CNS: *drowsiness,* excitation, seizures, tremors, weakness, confusion, headache.
CV: *orthostatic hypotension, tachycardia, EKG changes,* hypertension.
EENT: *blurred vision,* tinnitus, mydriasis.
GI: *dry mouth, constipation,* nausea, vomiting, anorexia, paralytic ileus.

GU: *urinary retention.*
Skin: rash, urticaria.
Other: *sweating, weight gain and craving for sweets,* allergy.
Abrupt cessation after long-term therapy: nausea, headache, malaise. (Does not indicate addiction.)

INTERACTIONS
MAO inhibitors: may cause severe excitation, hyperpyrexia, convulsions, usually with high dose. Use together cautiously.
Epinephrine, levarterenol: increased hypertensive effect. Use with caution.
Barbiturates: decreased TCA blood levels. Monitor for decreased antidepressant effect.
Methylphenidate: increased TCA blood levels. Monitor for enhanced antidepressant effect.

NURSING CONSIDERATIONS
• Contraindicated in acute recovery phase of myocardial infarction, and in prostatic hypertrophy. Use with caution in history of seizures, urinary retention, narrow-angle glaucoma, increased intraocular pressure, cardiovascular disease, impaired hepatic function, hyperthyroidism, patients receiving thyroid medications, suicide risk, electroshock therapy, before elective surgery.
• Reduce dose in elderly or debilitated persons and adolescents.
• Do not withdraw abruptly.
• If psychotic signs increase, reduce dose. Chart mood changes. Watch for suicidal tendencies. Allow minimum supply of tablets to lessen suicide risk.

• Check for urinary retention and constipation. Increase fluids to lessen constipation. Suggest stool softener, if needed.

• Warn patient to avoid activities that require alertness and good psycho-motor coordination until response to drug is determined. Drowsiness and dizziness usually subside after first few weeks.

• Has strong anticholinergic effects; one of the most sedating tricyclic antidepressants. Avoid combining with alcohol or other depressants.

• Expect time lag of up to 10 to 14 days before noticeable effect. Full effect usually appears in 30 days.

• Dry mouth may be relieved with sugarless hard candy or gum.

---

desipramine hydrochloride
Norpramin♦, Pertofrane♦

INDICATIONS & DOSAGE

Endogenous and other depression—
Adults: 75 to 150 mg P.O. daily in divided doses, increasing to maximum 200 mg daily. Alternatively, the entire dosage can be given at bedtime.
Elderly and adolescents: 25 to 50 mg P.O. daily, increasing gradually to maximum 100 mg daily.

SIDE EFFECTS

Blood: *agranulocytosis.*
CNS: *drowsiness,* excitation, seizures, tremors, weakness, confusion, headache.
CV: *orthostatic hypotension, tachycardia, EKG changes,* hypertension.
EENT: *blurred vision,* tinnitus, mydriasis.
GI: *dry mouth, constipation,* nausea, vomiting, anorexia, paralytic ileus.
GU: *urinary retention.*
Skin: rash, urticaria.
Other: *sweating, weight gain and craving for sweets,* allergy.
Abrupt cessation after long-term

therapy: nausea, headache, malaise. (Does not indicate addiction.)

INTERACTIONS

MAO inhibitors: may cause severe excitation, hyperpyrexia, convulsions, usually with high dose. Use together cautiously.
Epinephrine, levarterenol: increased hypertensive effect. Use with caution.
Barbiturates: decreased TCA blood levels. Monitor for decreased antidepressant effect.
Methylphenidate: increased TCA blood levels. Monitor for enhanced antidepressant effect.

NURSING CONSIDERATIONS

• Contraindicated in acute recovery phase of myocardial infarction, in prostatic hypertrophy. Use with caution in cardiovascular disease, urinary retention, narrow-angle glaucoma, thyroid disease or medication, seizure disorders, electroshock therapy, blood dyscrasias, suicide risk, before elective surgery, impaired hepatic function.

• Reduce dose in elderly or debilitated persons, and adolescents.

• Do not withdraw abruptly.

• Orthostatic hypotension not as severe with this drug compared to that with other tricyclics.

• If psychotic signs increase, reduce dose. Chart mood changes. Watch for suicidal tendencies. To lessen suicide risk, allow minimum supply of tablets.

• Check for urinary retention and constipation. Increase fluids to lessen constipation. Suggest stool softener, if needed.

• Warn patient to avoid activities that require alertness and good psycho-motor coordination until response to drug is determined. Drowsiness and dizziness usually subside after a few weeks.

• Dry mouth may be relieved with sugarless hard candy or gum.

• Drug has anticholinergic effect, is a metabolite of imipramine, and produces less sedation than amitriptyline or doxepin. Alcohol may antagonize effects of desipramine.
• Because it produces less tachycardia and other anticholinergic effects compared with other tricyclics, desipramine is often prescribed in heart patients.
• Expect time lag of 10 to 14 days before noticeable effects. Full effect usually appears in 30 days.

---

doxepin hydrochloride
Adapin, Sinequan♦

INDICATIONS & DOSAGE
Endogenous and other depression—
Adults: initially, 50 to 75 mg P.O. daily in divided doses, to maximum 300 mg daily. Alternatively, entire dosage may be given at bedtime.

SIDE EFFECTS
Blood: *agranulocytosis.*
CNS: *drowsiness,* excitation, seizures, tremors, weakness, confusion, headache.
CV: *orthostatic hypotension, tachycardia, EKG changes,* hypertension.
EENT: *blurred vision,* tinnitus, mydriasis.
GI: *dry mouth, constipation,* nausea, vomiting, anorexia, paralytic ileus.
GU: *urinary retention.*
Skin: rash, urticaria.
Other: *sweating, weight gain and craving for sweets,* allergy.
Abrupt cessation after long-term therapy: nausea, headache, malaise. (Does not indicate addiction.)

INTERACTIONS
MAO inhibitors: may cause severe excitation, hyperpyrexia, convulsions, usually with high dose. Use together cautiously.
Barbiturates: decreased TCA blood levels. Monitor for decreased antidepressant effect.
Methylphenidate: increased TCA blood levels. Monitor for enhanced antidepressant effect.

NURSING CONSIDERATIONS
• Contraindicated in urinary retention, narrow-angle glaucoma, and prostatic hypertrophy. Use with caution in suicide risk.
• Reduce dose in elderly or debilitated persons, adolescents, and those receiving other medications (especially anticholinergics).
• Dilute oral concentrate with 120 ml water, milk, or juice (orange, grapefruit, tomato, prune, or pineapple). Avoid carbonated beverages.
• Have patient take most of daily dose at bedtime.
• If psychotic symptoms increase, reduce dose. Chart mood changes. Watch for suicidal tendencies.
• Check for urinary retention and constipation. Increase fluids to lessen constipation. Suggest stool softener, if needed.
• Warn patient to avoid activities that require alertness and good psychomotor coordination until response to drug is determined. Drowsiness and dizziness usually subside after a few weeks.
• Expect time lag of 10 to 14 days before noticeable effect. Full effect usually appears within 30 days.
• Dry mouth may be relieved with sugarless hard candy or gum.
• Has strong anticholinergic effects; one of the most sedating tricyclic antidepressants. Avoid combining with alcohol or other depressants.

Italicized side effects are common or life-threatening.

imipramine hydrochloride

Antipress, Imavate, Impril♦♦, Janimine, Novopramine♦♦, Praminil♦♦ Presamine, Ropramine, SK-Pramine, Tofranil♦, W.D.D.

INDICATIONS & DOSAGE

Endogenous and other depression—
Adults: 75 to 100 mg P.O. or I.M. daily in divided doses, with 25 to 50 mg increments up to 200 mg. Maximum 300 mg daily. Alternatively, the entire dosage may be given at bedtime. (I.M. route rarely used.)
Childhood enuresis—
25 to 75 mg P.O. daily.

SIDE EFFECTS

Blood: *agranulocytosis.*
CNS: *drowsiness,* excitation, seizures, tremors, weakness, confusion, headache.
CV: *orthostatic hypotension, tachycardia, EKG changes,* hypertension.
EENT: *blurred vision,* tinnitus, mydriasis.
GI: *dry mouth, constipation,* nausea, vomiting, anorexia, paralytic ileus.
GU: *urinary retention.*
Skin: rash, urticaria.
Other: *sweating, weight gain and craving for sweets,* allergy.
Abrupt cessation after long-term therapy: nausea, headache, malaise. (Does not indicate addiction.)

INTERACTIONS

MAO inhibitors: may cause severe excitation, hyperpyrexia, convulsions, usually with high dose. Use together cautiously.
Epinephrine, levarterenol: increased hypertensive effect. Use with caution.
Barbiturates: decreased TCA blood levels. Monitor for decreased antidepressant effect.
Methylphenidate: increased TCA blood levels. Monitor for enhanced antidepressant effect.

NURSING CONSIDERATIONS

• Contraindicated in acute recovery phase of myocardial infarction; in prostatic hypertrophy. Use with extreme caution in cardiovascular disease, urinary retention, narrow-angle glaucoma or increased intraocular pressure, thyroid disease or medication, seizure disorders, electroshock therapy, blood dyscrasias, suicide risk, before elective surgery, impaired hepatic function.
• Reduce dose in elderly or debilitated persons, adolescents, and patients with aggravated psychotic symptoms.
• Do not withdraw abruptly.
• If psychotic signs increase, reduce dose. Chart mood changes. Watch for suicidal tendencies. To lessen suicide risk, allow minimum tablet supply.
• Check for urinary retention and constipation. Increase fluids to lessen constipation. Suggest stool softener, if needed.
• Warn patient to avoid activities that require alertness and good psychomotor coordination until response to drug is determined. Drowsiness and dizziness usually subside after a few weeks.
• Expect time lag of 10 to 14 days before noticeable effect. Full effect usually appears in 30 days.
• Dry mouth may be relieved with sugarless hard candy or gum.
• Avoid combining with alcohol or other depressants.

isocarboxazid

Marplan♦

INDICATIONS & DOSAGE

Depression—
Adults: 30 mg P.O. daily in divided doses. Reduce to 10 to 20 mg daily when condition improves.
Not recommended for children under 16 years.

SIDE EFFECTS

CNS: dizziness, vertigo, weakness, headache, overactivity, hyperreflexia, tremors, muscle twitching, mania, *insomnia*, confusion, memory impairment, fatigue.
CV: *orthostatic hypotension*, arrhythmias, paradoxical hypertension.
EENT: blurred vision.
GI: dry mouth, *anorexia*, nausea, diarrhea, constipation.
GU: changed libido.
Skin: rash.
Other: peripheral edema, sweating, weight changes.

INTERACTIONS

Amphetamines, ephedrine, levodopa, meperidine, metaraminol, methotrimeprazine, methylphenidate, phenylephrine, phenylpropanolamine: pressor effects of these drugs are enhanced by isocarboxazid. Use together very cautiously.
Alcohol, barbiturates, and other sedatives; tranquilizers; narcotics; dextromethorphan; tricyclic antidepressants: unpredictable interaction. Use with caution and in reduced dosage.

NURSING CONSIDERATIONS

• Contraindicated in severe hepatic or renal impairment; congestive heart failure; pheochromocytoma; foods containing tryptophan or tyramine; excess caffeine; elderly or debilitated persons; hypertensive, cardiovascular, or cerebrovascular disease; severe or frequent headaches; therapy with other MAO inhibitor (including pargyline HCl, phenelzine sulfate, tranylcypromine sulfate) or within 10 days of such therapy; within 10 days of elective surgery requiring general anesthetic, cocaine, or local anesthetic containing sympathomimetic vasoconstrictors. Use cautiously with other psychotropic drugs or with spinal anesthetic; in hyperactive, agitated, or schizophrenic patients; in suicide risk, diabetes, epilepsy.
• Recommended only when TCA or electroshock therapy is ineffective or contraindicated.
• Hold dose and notify doctor if patient develops symptoms of overdosage: palpitations or frequent headaches, or severe orthostatic hypotension.
• Watch for suicidal tendencies.
• Dose is usually reduced to maintenance level as soon as possible.
• Do not withdraw drug abruptly.
• Weigh patient biweekly; check for edema and urinary retention.
• Warn patient to avoid foods high in tyramine or tryptophan; large amounts of caffeine; and self-medication with over-the-counter cold, hay fever, or reducing preparations.
• Incidence of orthostatic hypotension is high. Supervise walking. Tell patient to get out of bed slowly, sitting up first for 1 minute.
• Have phentolamine (Regitine) available to counteract severe hypertension.
• Continue precautions 10 days after stopping drug; long-lasting effects.
• Expect time lag of 1 to 4 weeks before noticeable effect.
• Drug is MAO inhibitor and is generally less effective than tricyclic antidepressant. Avoid combining with alcohol or other depressant.

nortriptyline hydrochloride
Aventyl♦, Pamelor

INDICATIONS & DOSAGE

Endogenous and other depression—
Adults: 25 mg P.O. t.i.d. or q.i.d., gradually increasing to maximum 100 mg daily. Alternatively, entire dose may be given at bedtime.

SIDE EFFECTS

Blood: *agranulocytosis*.
CNS: *drowsiness*, excitation, sei-

zures, tremors, weakness, confusion, headache.

CV: *orthostatic hypotension, tachycardia, EKG changes,* hypertension.

EENT: *blurred vision,* tinnitus, mydriasis.

GI: *dry mouth, constipation,* nausea, vomiting, anorexia, paralytic ileus.

GU: *urinary retention.*

Skin: rash, urticaria.

Other: *sweating, weight gain and craving for sweets,* allergy.

Abrupt cessation after long-term therapy: nausea, headache, malaise. (Does not indicate addiction.)

INTERACTIONS

MAO inhibitors: may cause severe excitation, hyperpyrexia, convulsions, usually with high dose. Use together cautiously.

Epinephrine, levarterenol: increased hypertensive effect. Use with caution.

Barbiturates: decreased TCA blood levels. Monitor for decreased antidepressant effect.

Methylphenidate: increased TCA blood levels. Monitor for enhanced antidepressant effect.

NURSING CONSIDERATIONS

- Contraindicated in acute recovery phase of myocardial infarction and in prostatic hypertrophy. Use with caution in cardiovascular disease, urinary retention, glaucoma, thyroid disease or medication, seizure disorders, electroshock therapy, blood dyscrasias, suicide risk, before elective surgery.
- Reduce dose in elderly or debilitated persons, or adolescents.
- Do not withdraw abruptly.
- If psychotic signs increase, reduce dose. Chart mood changes. Watch for suicidal tendencies. To lessen suicide risk, allow minimum tablet supply.
- Check for urinary retention and constipation. Increase fluids to lessen constipation. Suggest stool softener, if needed.
- Warn patient to avoid activities that require alertness and good psychomotor coordination until response to drug is determined. Drowsiness and dizziness usually subside after a few weeks.
- Expect time lag of 10 to 14 days before noticeable effects. Full effect usually appears in 30 days.
- Dry mouth may be relieved with sugarless hard candy or gum.
- Drug is tricyclic antidepressant, similar in anticholinergic effects to other tricyclics. Avoid combining with alcohol or other depressants.

---

phenelzine sulfate
Nardil ◆

INDICATIONS & DOSAGE

Endogenous and other depression—

Adults: 45 mg P.O. daily in divided doses, increasing rapidly to 60 mg daily. Maximum 90 mg daily.

Not recommended for children under 16 years.

SIDE EFFECTS

CNS: dizziness, vertigo, headache, overactivity, hyperreflexia, tremors, muscle twitching, mania, jitteriness, *insomnia,* confusion, memory impairment, drowsiness, weakness, fatigue.

CV: paradoxical hypertension, *orthostatic hypotension,* arrhythmias.

GI: dry mouth, *anorexia,* nausea, constipation.

Other: peripheral edema, sweating, weight changes.

INTERACTIONS

Amphetamines, ephedrine, levodopa, meperidine, metaraminol, methotrimeprazine, methylphenidate, phenylephrine, phenylpropanolamine: enhanced pressor effects. Use together cautiously.

Alcohol, barbiturates, and other sedatives; tranquilizers; narcotics; dextromethorphan; tricyclic antidepres-

sants: unpredictable interaction. Use with caution and in reduced dosage.

NURSING CONSIDERATIONS
• Contraindicated in hepatic impairment; congestive heart failure; pheochromocytoma; foods containing tryptophan (broad beans) or tyramine; excess caffeine or chocolate; elderly or debilitated persons; hypertension, cardiovascular, or cerebrovascular disease; severe or frequent headaches; therapy with other MAO inhibitor, including pargyline HCl, isocarboxazid, tranylcypromine sulfate, or within 10 days of such therapy; within 10 days of elective surgery requiring general anesthetic, cocaine, or local anesthetic containing sympathomimetic vasoconstrictors; hyperactive, agitated, or schizophrenic patients. Use cautiously with antihypertensive drugs containing thiazide diuretics or with spinal anesthetic; in suicide risk, diabetes, epilepsy.
• Use only when TCA or electroshock therapy is ineffective or contraindicated.
• Hold dose and notify doctor if patient develops symptoms of overdose: severe hypotension, palpitations, or frequent headaches.
• Watch for suicidal tendencies.
• Dose is usually reduced to maintenance level as soon as possible.
• Store drug in tight container, away from heat and light.
• Have phentolamine (Regitine) available to counteract severe hypertension.
• Warn patient to avoid foods high in tyramine or tryptophan; large amounts of caffeine; and self-medication with over-the-counter cold, hay fever, or reducing preparations.
• Incidence of orthostatic hypotension is high. Supervise walking. Tell patient to get out of bed slowly, sitting up first for 1 minute.
• Continue precautions 10 days after stopping drug; long-lasting effects.

• Expect time lag of 1 to 4 weeks before noticeable effect.
• Drug is MAO inhibitor and is generally less effective than tricyclic antidepressant. Avoid combining with alcohol or other depressants.

---

protriptyline hydrochloride
Triptil♦♦, Vivactil

INDICATIONS & DOSAGE
Endogenous and other depression—
Adults: 15 to 40 mg P.O. daily in divided doses, increasing gradually to maximum 60 mg daily.

SIDE EFFECTS
Blood: *agranulocytosis.*
CNS: excitation, seizures, tremors, weakness, confusion, headache.
CV: *orthostatic hypotension, tachycardia, EKG changes,* hypertension.
EENT: *blurred vision,* tinnitus, mydriasis.
GI: *dry mouth, constipation,* nausea, vomiting, anorexia, paralytic ileus.
GU: *urinary retention.*
Skin: rash, urticaria.
Other: *sweating, weight gain and craving for sweets,* allergy.
Abrupt cessation after long-term therapy: nausea, headache, malaise. (Does not indicate addiction.)

INTERACTIONS
MAO inhibitors: may cause severe excitation, hyperpyrexia, convulsions, and death, usually with high dose. Use together cautiously.
Epinephrine, levarterenol: increased hypertensive effect. Use with caution.
Barbiturates: decreased TCA blood levels. Monitor for decreased antidepressant effect.
Methylphenidate: increased TCA blood levels. Monitor for enhanced antidepressant effect.

Italicized side effects are common or life-threatening.

NURSING CONSIDERATIONS

• Contraindicated in acute recovery phase of myocardial infarction and in prostatic hypertrophy. Use with caution in cardiovascular disease, urinary retention, increased intraocular tension, elderly, thyroid disease or medication, seizure disorders, electroshock therapy, blood dyscrasias, suicide risk, before elective surgery.

• Reduce dose in elderly or debilitated persons, and adolescents.

• Do not withdraw abruptly.

• Watch for increased psychotic signs, anxiety, agitation, or cardiovascular reactions; reduce dose if they occur. Chart mood changes. Watch for suicidal tendencies. To lessen suicide risk, allow minimum supply of tablets.

• Check for urinary retention and constipation. Increase fluids to lessen constipation. Suggest stool softener, if needed.

• Warn patient to avoid activities that require alertness and good psychomotor coordination until response to drug is determined. Drowsiness and dizziness usually subside after a few weeks.

• Dry mouth may be relieved with sugarless hard candy or gum.

• Expect time lag of 7 to 14 days before noticeable effect.

• Drug is possibly the most rapid-acting but least sedating tricyclic antidepressant. May even have an amphetamine-like effect. Avoid combining with alcohol or other depressants.

• Do not give entire dose at bedtime as patient may develop insomnia.

---

tranylcypromine sulfate
Parnate♦

INDICATIONS & DOSAGE

Endogenous or other depression—
Adults: 10 mg P.O. b.i.d. Increase to maximum 30 mg daily, if necessary, after 2 weeks.
Not recommended for children under 16 years.

SIDE EFFECTS

CNS: dizziness, vertigo, headache, overactivity, hyperreflexia, tremors, muscle twitching, mania, jitteriness, confusion, memory impairment, fatigue.
CV: *orthostatic hypotension,* arrhythmias, paradoxical hypertension.
EENT: blurred vision.
GI: dry mouth, *anorexia,* nausea, diarrhea, constipation, abdominal pain.
GU: changed libido, impotence.
Skin: rash.
Other: peripheral edema, sweating, weight changes, chills.

INTERACTIONS

Amphetamines, ephedrine, levodopa, meperidine, metaraminol, methotrimeprazine, methylphenidate, phenylephrine, phenylpropanolamine: pressor effects of these drugs are enhanced by tranylcypromine. Use together cautiously.
Alcohol, barbiturates, and other sedatives; tranquilizers; narcotics; dextromethorphan; tricyclic antidepressants: use with caution and in reduced dosage.

NURSING CONSIDERATIONS

• Contraindicated in severe hepatic or renal impairment; congestive heart failure; pheochromocytoma; antihypertensive drugs; diuretics; patients for whom close supervision is not possible; with foods containing tryptophan or tyramine; with excess caffeine; elderly or debilitated persons; hypertension, cardiovascular, or cerebrovascular disease; severe or frequent headaches; therapy with other MAO inhibitor (including pargyline HCl, phenelzine sulfate, isocarboxazid) or within 7 days of such therapy;

---

within 7 days of elective surgery requiring general anesthetic, cocaine, or local anesthetic containing sympathomimetic vasoconstrictors; hyperactive, agitated, or schizophrenic patients. Use cautiously with anti-Parkinson drugs, spinal anesthetic, renal disease, suicide risk, diabetes, epilepsy, hyperthyroidism.
• Use only when TCA or electroshock therapy is ineffective or contraindicated.
• Hold dose and notify doctor if patient develops symptoms of overdose: palpitations, severe orthostatic hypotension.
• Watch for suicidal tendencies.
• Dose is usually reduced to maintenance level as soon as possible.
• Do not withdraw drug abruptly.
• Have phentolamine (Regitine) available to counteract severe hypertension.
• Warn patient to avoid foods high in tyramine or trytophan; large amounts of caffeine; and self-medication with over-the-counter cold, hay fever, or reducing preparations.
• Tell patient to get out of bed slowly, sitting up for 1 minute.
• Continue precautions for 7 days after stopping drug; effects last that long.
• Expect time lag of 1 to 3 weeks before noticeable effect.
• More rapid onset of action than isocarboxazid or phenelzine sulfate.
• MAO inhibitor most likely to cause hypertensive crisis in presence of high-tyramine ingestion. Generally less effective than a tricyclic antidepressant. Avoid combining with alcohol or other depressants.

---

trimipramine maleate
Surmontil

INDICATIONS & DOSAGE
Endogenous and other depression—
Adults: 75 mg daily in divided doses, increased to 200 mg per day. Dosages over 300 mg per day not recommended.
Enuresis—
Children over 6: initial dose 25 mg P.O. 1 hour before bedtime; if no response, increase dose to 50 mg in children under 12, and to 75 mg in children over 12.

SIDE EFFECTS
Blood: *agranulocytosis.*
CNS: *drowsiness,* excitation, seizures, tremors, weakness, confusion, headache.
CV: *orthostatic hypotension, tachycardia, EKG changes,* hypertension.
EENT: *blurred vision,* tinnitus, mydriasis.
GI: *dry mouth, constipation,* nausea, vomiting, anorexia, paralytic ileus.
GU: *urinary retention.*
Skin: rash, urticaria.
Other: *sweating, weight gain and craving for sweets,* allergy.
Abrupt cessation after long-term therapy: nausea, headache, malaise. (Does not indicate addiction.)

INTERACTIONS
MAO inhibitors: may cause severe excitation, hyperpyrexia, convulsions, usually with high dose. Use together cautiously.
Epinephrine, levarterenol: increased hypertensive effect. Use with caution.
Barbiturates: decreased TCA blood levels. Monitor for decreased antidepressant effect.
Methylphenidate: increased TCA blood levels. Monitor for enhanced antidepressant effects.

NURSING CONSIDERATIONS
• Contraindicated in acute recovery phase of myocardial infarction; in prostatic hypertrophy. Use with extreme caution in cardiovascular disease, urinary retention, narrow-angle glaucoma or increased intraocular

pressure, thyroid disease or medication, seizure disorders, electroshock therapy, blood dyscrasias, suicide risk, before elective surgery, impaired hepatic function.
• Reduce dose in elderly or debilitated persons, and adolescents.
• Do not withdraw abruptly.
• Watch for increased psychotic signs; reduce dose if they occur. Chart mood changes. Watch for suicidal tendencies. Allow only minimum supply of tablets to lessen suicide risk.
• Check for urinary retention and constipation. Increase fluids to lessen constipation. Suggest stool softener, if necessary.

• Warn patient to avoid activities that require alertness and good psychomotor coordination until response to drug has been determined. Drowsiness and dizziness usually subside after a few weeks.
• Don't combine with alcohol or other depressants.
• Expect time lag of 10 to 14 days before noticeable effect. Full effect usually appears in 30 days.
• Dry mouth may be relieved with sugarless hard candy or gum.
• Most common tricyclic used for enuresis, but effectiveness may decrease over time. Similar in anticholinergic effects to other tricyclics.

26

Tranquilizers

chlordiazepoxide hydrochloride
chlormezanone
clorazepate dipotassium
clorazepate monopotassium
diazepam
hydroxyzine hydrochloride
hydroxyzine pamoate
lorazepam
meprobamate
oxazepam
prazepam
tybamate

---

chlordiazepoxide hydrochloride
Controlled Substance Schedule IV
A-poxide, Chlordiazachel, Corax♦♦,
C-Tran♦♦, J-Liberty, Libritabs,
Librium♦, Medilium♦♦, Nack♦♦,
Novopoxide♦♦, Protensin♦♦,
Relaxil♦♦, Sereen, SK-Lygen, So-
lium♦♦, Tenax, Trilium♦♦, Zetran

INDICATIONS & DOSAGE
*Mild to moderate anxiety and
tension—*
Adults: 5 to 10 mg t.i.d. or q.i.d.
Children over 6 years: 5 mg P.O.
b.i.d. to q.i.d. Maximum 10 mg P.O.
b.i.d. to t.i.d.
Severe anxiety and tension—
Adults: 20 to 25 mg t.i.d. or q.i.d.
*Withdrawal symptoms of acute
alcoholism—*
Adults: 50 to 100 mg P.O., I.M., or
I.V. Maximum 300 mg daily.
Preop apprehension and anxiety—
Adults: 5 to 10 mg P.O. t.i.d. or
q.i.d. on days preceding surgery; or

50 to 100 mg I.M. 1 hour before surgery.
Note: parenteral form not recommended in children under 12.

SIDE EFFECTS
CNS: *drowsiness, lethargy, hangover,*
fainting.
CV: transient hypotension.
GI: nausea, vomiting, discomfort.
Local: *pain at injection site.*

INTERACTIONS
Cimetidine: increased sedation. Monitor carefully.

NURSING CONSIDERATIONS
• Use with caution in mental depres-
sion, blood dyscrasias, hepatic or
renal disease, or anticoagulant ther-
apy.
• Dosage should be reduced in elderly or debilitated patients.
• Do not withdraw drug abruptly.
• Possibility of abuse, addiction.
Withdrawal symptoms may occur.
• Warn patient to avoid activities that
require alertness and good psychomotor coordination until response to
drug is determined.
• Warn patient not to combine drug
with alcohol or other depressants.
• Although package recommends
I.M. use only, drug may be given I.V.
• Injectable form (as hydrochloride)
comes as two ampuls—diluent and
powdered drug. For I.M., add 2 ml of
diluent to powder and agitate gently
until clear. Use immediately. I.M.
form may be erratically absorbed. Do
not give packaged diluent I.V.

• For I.V., use 5 ml of saline injection or sterile water for injection as diluent; give slowly over 1 minute. Do not give such solution I.M.
• Keep powder away from light; mix just before use; discard remainder.
• Do not mix injectable form with any other parenteral drug.
• Caution patient against giving medication to others.
• Drug should not be prescribed regularly for everyday stress.

---

chlormezanone
Fenarol, Trancopal ◆

INDICATIONS & DOSAGE
Mild anxiety and tension, muscle relaxation—
Adults: 100 to 200 mg P.O. t.i.d. or q.i.d.
Children 5 to 12 years: 50 to 100 mg P.O. t.i.d. or q.i.d.

SIDE EFFECTS
CNS: *drowsiness,* mental depression, headache, dizziness, ataxia, lethargy, muscular weakness.
CV: edema.
GI: nausea, anorexia, dry mouth.
GU: urinary retention.
Skin: rash.

INTERACTIONS
None significant.

NURSING CONSIDERATIONS
• Use with caution in hepatic or renal disease.
• Dosage should be reduced in elderly or debilitated patients.
• Do not withdraw drug abruptly.
• Possibility of abuse, addiction exists.
• Warn patient to avoid activities that require alertness and good psychomotor coordination until response to drug is determined.

• Warn patient not to combine drug with alcohol or other depressants.
• Rapid onset of action (15 to 30 minutes), with effects lasting 4 to 6 hours.
• Chemically unrelated to other antianxiety agents.
• Suggest sugarless chewing gum or hard candy to relieve dry mouth.

---

clorazepate dipotassium
Controlled Substance Schedule IV
Tranxene ◆
clorazepate monopotassium
Controlled Substance Schedule IV
Azene

INDICATIONS & DOSAGE
Acute alcohol withdrawal (dipotassium)—
Adults: Day 1—30 mg P.O. initially, followed by 30 to 60 mg P.O. in divided doses; Day 2—45 to 90 mg P.O. in divided doses; Day 3—22.5 to 45 mg P.O. in divided doses; Day 4—15 to 30 mg P.O. in divided doses; gradually reduce daily dose to 7.5 to 15 mg.
Anxiety (dipotassium)—
Adults: 15 to 60 mg P.O. daily.
Acute alcohol withdrawal (monopotassium)—
Elderly or debilitated patients: 6.5 to 13 mg P.O. in divided doses.
Adults: Day 1—26 mg P.O. initially, followed by 26 to 52 mg P.O. in divided doses; Day 2—39 to 78 mg P.O. in divided doses; Day 3—19.5 to 39 mg P.O. in divided doses; Day 4—13 to 26 mg P.O. in divided doses; gradually reduce to 6.5 to 13 mg P.O., and stop when patient stable.
Anxiety (monopotassium)—
Adults: 13 to 52 mg P.O. in divided doses. Maximum—78 mg daily.

SIDE EFFECTS
CNS: *drowsiness, lethargy, hangover,* fainting.
CV: transient hypotension.

Unmarked trade names available in the United States only.
◆ Also available in Canada   ◆ ◆ Available in Canada only.

GI: nausea, vomiting, discomfort.

INTERACTIONS
Cimetidine: increased sedation. Monitor carefully.

NURSING CONSIDERATIONS
• Contraindicated in acute narrow-angle glaucoma, lactation, depressive neuroses, psychotic reactions, children under 18. Use with caution in hepatic or renal damage.
• Dosage should be reduced in elderly or debilitated patients.
• Do not withdraw drug abruptly.
• Possibility of abuse, addiction exists. Withdrawal symptoms may occur.
• Warn patient to avoid activities requiring alertness and good psychomotor coordination.
• Warn patient not to combine drug with alcohol or other depressants.
• Suggest sugarless chewing gum or hard candy to relieve dry mouth.
• Caution patient against giving medication to others.
• Drug should not be prescribed regularly for everyday stress.

---

diazepam
Controlled Substance Schedule IV
D-Tran♦♦, E-Pam♦♦, Erital♦♦, Meval♦♦, NeoCalme♦♦, Novodipam♦♦, Paxel♦♦, Serenack♦♦, Stress-Pam♦♦, Valium♦, Vivol♦♦

INDICATIONS & DOSAGE
Tension, anxiety, adjunct in convulsive disorders or skeletal muscle spasm—
Adults: 2 to 10 mg P.O. t.i.d. or q.i.d.
Children over 6 months: 1 to 2.5 mg P.O. t.i.d. or q.i.d.
Tension, anxiety, muscle spasm, endoscopic procedures, convulsive seizures—
Adults: 5 to 10 mg I.V. initially, up to

30 mg in 1 hour or possibly more for cardioversion or status epilepticus, depending on response.
Children 5 years and over: 1 mg I.V. or I.M. slowly q 2 to 5 minutes to maximum 10 mg. Repeat q 2 to 4 hours.
Children 30 days to 5 years: 0.2 to 0.5 mg I.V. or I.M. slowly q 2 to 5 minutes to maximum 5 mg. Repeat q 2 to 4 hours.
Tetanic muscle spasms—
Children over 5 years: 5 to 10 mg I.M. or I.V. q 3 to 4 hours, p.r.n.
Infants over 30 days: 1 to 2 mg I.M. or I.V. q 3 to 4 hours, p.r.n.

SIDE EFFECTS
CNS: *drowsiness, lethargy, hangover,* fainting.
CV: transient hypotension.
GI: nausea, vomiting, discomfort.
Local: desquamation, pain, phlebitis at injection site.

INTERACTIONS
Cimetidine: increased sedation. Monitor carefully.

NURSING CONSIDERATIONS
• Contraindicated in shock, coma, acute alcohol intoxication, acute narrow-angle glaucoma, psychosis; in oral form for children under 6 months. Use with caution in blood dyscrasias, hepatic or renal damage, depression, open-angle glaucoma, elderly and debilitated patients, those with limited pulmonary reserve.
• Dosage should be reduced in elderly or debilitated patients.
• Do not withdraw drug abruptly.
• Possibility of abuse, addiction exists. Withdrawal symptoms may occur.
• Warn patient to avoid activities that require alertness and good psychomotor coordination until response to drug is determined.
• Warn patient not to combine drug with alcohol or other depressants.

Italicized side effects are common or life-threatening.

- Do not dilute with solutions or mix with other drugs: incompatible.
- Avoid extravasation. Do not inject into small veins.
- Watch for phlebitis at injection site.
- Give I.V. slowly, at rate not exceeding 5 mg per minute.
- I.V. route more reliable; I.M. absorption variable, to be discouraged.
- Drug of choice (I.V. form) for status epilepticus.
- Do not store diazepam in plastic syringes.
- Caution patient against giving medication to others.
- Drug should not be prescribed regularly for everyday stress.

hydroxyzine hydrochloride
Atarax♦, Hyzine-50, Quiess, Vistaril (parenteral)
hydroxyzine pamoate
Vistaril (oral)

INDICATIONS & DOSAGE
Anxiety and tension—
Adults: 25 to 100 mg P.O. t.i.d. or q.i.d.
Anxiety, tension, hyperkinesis—
Children over 6 years: 50 to 100 mg P.O. daily in divided doses.
Children under 6 years: 50 mg P.O. daily in divided doses.
Preop and postop adjunctive therapy—
Adults: 25 to 100 mg I.M. q 4 to 6 hours.
Children: 1.1 mg/Kg I.M. q 4 to 6 hours.

SIDE EFFECTS
CNS: *drowsiness*, involuntary motor activity.
GI: *dry mouth.*
Local: marked discomfort at site of I.M. injection.

INTERACTIONS
None significant.

NURSING CONSIDERATIONS
- Dosage should be reduced in elderly or debilitated patients.
- Do not withdraw drug abruptly.
- Possibility of abuse, addiction exists.
- Warn patient to avoid activities that require alertness and good psychomotor coordination until response to drug is determined.
- Warn patient not to combine drug with alcohol or other depressants.
- Observe for excessive sedation due to potentiation with other CNS drugs.
- Used as an antiemetic and anti-anxiety drug.
- Used in psychogenically induced allergic conditions, such as chronic urticaria and pruritus.
- Parenteral form (hydroxyzine HCl) for I.M. use only, never I.V.
- Aspirate injection carefully to prevent inadvertent intravascular injection.

lorazepam
Controlled Substance Schedule IV
Ativan♦

INDICATIONS & DOSAGE
Anxiety, tension, agitation, irritability, especially in anxiety neuroses or organic (especially GI or CV) disorders—
Adults: 2 to 6 mg P.O. daily in divided doses. Maximum 10 mg daily.
Insomnia—
Adults: 2 to 4 mg h.s.

SIDE EFFECTS
CNS: *drowsiness, lethargy, hangover,* fainting.
CV: transient hypotension.
GI: distress.

INTERACTIONS
Cimetidine: increased sedation. Monitor carefully.

NURSING CONSIDERATIONS

• Contraindicated in myasthenia gravis, acute narrow-angle glaucoma, psychosis, mental depression. Use with caution in organic brain syndrome, renal or hepatic impairment.
• Dosage should be reduced in elderly or debilitated patients.
• Do not withdraw drug abruptly.
• Possibility of abuse, addiction exists. Withdrawal symptoms may occur.
• Warn patient to avoid activities that require alertness or good psychomotor coordination until response to drug is determined.
• Warn patient not to combine drug with alcohol or other depressants.
• Caution patient against giving medication to others.
• Drug should not be prescribed regularly for everyday stress.

---

meprobamate

Controlled Substance Schedule IV
Arcoban, Bamate, Bamo-400, Equanil, Kalmm, Lan-Dol♦♦, Maso-Bamate, Meditran, Mep-E, Mepriam, Meprocon, Meprotabs, Meribam, Miltown♦, Neo-Tran♦♦, Novomepro♦♦, Pax-400, Quietal♦♦, Saronil, Sedabamate, SK-Bamate, Tranmep

INDICATIONS & DOSAGE

Anxiety and tension—
Adults: 1.2 to 1.6 g P.O. in 3 or 4 equally divided doses. Maximum 2.4 g daily.
Children 6 to 12 years: 100 to 200 mg P.O. b.i.d. or t.i.d.
Not recommended for children under 6 years.

SIDE EFFECTS

Blood: *thrombocytopenia, leukopenia,* eosinophilia.
CNS: *drowsiness,* ataxia, dizziness, slurred speech, headache, vertigo.
CV: palpitation, tachycardia.
GI: anorexia, nausea, vomiting, diarrhea, stomatitis.
Skin: pruritus, urticaria, erythematous maculopapular rash.

INTERACTIONS

None significant.

NURSING CONSIDERATIONS

• Contraindicated in hypersensitivity to meprobamate, carisoprodol, mebutamate, tybamate, carbromal; renal insufficiency; porphyria. Use with caution in impaired hepatic or renal function, in lactation, and in patients with suicidal tendencies.
• Dosage should be reduced in elderly or debilitated patients.
• Withdraw drug gradually (over 2 weeks).
• Possibility of abuse, addiction exists.
• Warn patient to avoid activities that require alertness or good psychomotor coordination until response to drug is determined.
• Warn patient not to combine drug with alcohol or other depressants.
• Give I.M. deeply.
• Give P.O. with meals to reduce gastric distress.
• Therapeutic blood levels 0.5 to 2 mg/100 ml; levels above 20 mg/100 ml may cause coma and death.

---

oxazepam

Controlled Substance Schedule IV
Serax♦

INDICATIONS & DOSAGE

Alcohol withdrawal—
Adults: 15 to 30 mg P.O. t.i.d. or q.i.d.
Severe anxiety—
Adults: 15 to 30 mg P.O. t.i.d. or q.i.d.
Tension, mild to moderate anxiety—

Italicized side effects are common or life-threatening.

Adults: 10 to 15 mg P.O. t.i.d. or q.i.d.

SIDE EFFECTS
CNS: *drowsiness, lethargy, hangover,* fainting.
CV: transient hypotension.
GI: nausea, vomiting, discomfort.

INTERACTIONS
Cimetidine: increased sedation. Monitor carefully.

NURSING CONSIDERATIONS
• Contraindicated in psychoses. Use cautiously in history of convulsive disorders, drug allergies, blood dyscrasias, hepatic or renal disease, depression.
• Dose should be reduced in elderly or debilitated patients.
• Do not withdraw drug abruptly.
• Possibility of abuse, addiction exists. Withdrawal symptoms may occur.
• Warn patient to avoid activities that require alertness or good psychomotor coordination until response to drug is determined.
• Warn patient not to combine drug with alcohol or other depressants.
• Fewer cumulative effects due to short half-life.
• Caution patient against giving medication to others.
• Drug should not be prescribed for everyday stress.

prazepam
Controlled Substance Schedule IV
Verstran, Centrax

INDICATIONS & DOSAGE
Anxiety—
Adults: 30 mg P.O. in divided doses. Range 20 to 60 mg daily. May be administered as single daily dose at bedtime. Start with 20 mg.

SIDE EFFECTS
CNS: *drowsiness, lethargy, hangover,* fainting.
CV: transient hypotension.
GI: nausea, vomiting, discomfort.

INTERACTIONS
Cimetidine: increased sedation. Monitor carefully.

NURSING CONSIDERATIONS
• Contraindicated in acute narrow-angle glaucoma, psychosis, and psychiatric disorders not showing anxiety. Use with caution in renal or hepatic impairment.
• Dosage should be reduced in elderly or debilitated patients.
• Do not withdraw drug abruptly.
• Possibility of abuse, addiction exists. Withdrawal symptoms may occur.
• Warn patient to avoid activities that require alertness and good psychomotor coordination until response to drug is determined.
• Warn patient not to combine drug with alcohol or other depressants.
• Caution patient against giving medication to others.
• Drug should not be prescribed for everyday stress.

tybamate
Controlled Substance Schedule IV
Tybatran

INDICATIONS & DOSAGE
Anxiety and tension—
Adults: 750 mg to 2 g P.O. daily in divided doses; maximum 3 g daily.
Children 6 to 12 years: 20 to 25 mg/Kg daily, divided into 3 or 4 doses.

SIDE EFFECTS
Blood: dyscrasias.
CNS: *drowsiness,* dizziness, fatigue, weakness, ataxia, depressive or panic reactions, paradoxical irritability, ex-

citement, confusion, euphoria, insomnia, headache, paresthesia.
CV: flushing, light-headedness, hypotension, palpitation, tachycardia, fainting.
GI: nausea, anorexia, dry mouth, glossitis.
Skin: urticaria, pruritus, pruritus ani, rash.

INTERACTIONS
None significant.

NURSING CONSIDERATIONS
• Contraindicated in history of hypersensitivity to tybamate or related compounds, such as meprobamate, carisoprodol, or mebutamate; convulsive disorders; drug allergies; blood dyscrasias; lactation; porphyria. Use with caution in hepatic or renal dysfunction.
• Dosage should be reduced in elderly or debilitated patients.
• Do not withdraw drug abruptly.
• Possibility of abuse, addiction exists.
• Warn patient to avoid activities that require alertness and good psychomotor coordination until response to drug is determined.
• Warn patient not to combine drug with alcohol or other depressants.
• Shorter acting than meprobamate.

Italicized side effects are common or life-threatening.

27

Antipsychotics

acetophanazine maleate
butaperazine maleate
carphenazine maleate
chlorpromazine hydrochloride
chlorprothixene
droperidol
fluphenazine decanoate
fluphenazine enanthate
fluphenazine hydrochloride
haloperidol
loxapine succinate
mesoridazine besylate
molindone hydrochloride
perphenazine
piperacetazine
prochlorperazine edisylate
prochlorperazine maleate
promazine hydrochloride
thioridazine hydrochloride
thiothixene
thiothixene hydrochloride
trifluoperazine hydrochloride
triflupromazine hydrochloride

---

acetophenazine maleate
Tindal

INDICATIONS & DOSAGE

Psychotic disorders—
Adults: initially, 20 mg P.O. t.i.d. or
q.i.d. Daily dosage ranges from 40 to
80 mg in outpatients, or 80 to 120 mg
in hospitalized patients, but in severe
psychotic states up to 600 mg daily
has been safely administered. Smallest effective dose should be used at all
times.

SIDE EFFECTS

Blood: *transient leukopenias, agranulocytosis.*
CNS: *extrapyramidal reactions (high
incidence),* sedation (low incidence),
pseudoparkinsonism, EEG changes,
dizziness.
CV: *orthostatic hypotension,* tachycardia, EKG changes.
EENT: *ocular changes, blurred
vision.*
GI: *dry mouth, constipation.*
GU: *urinary retention,* dark urine,
menstrual irregularities, gynecomastia, inhibited ejaculation.
Hepatic: *cholestatic jaundice.*
Metabolic: hyperprolactinemia.
Skin: *mild photosensitivity,* dermal
allergic reactions, *exfoliative dermatitis.*
Other: weight gain, increased
appetite.
After abrupt withdrawal: gastritis,
nausea, vomiting, dizziness, tremors,
feeling of warmth or cold, sweating,
tachycardia, headache, insomnia.

INTERACTIONS

Antacids: inhibited absorption of oral
phenothiazines. Separate antacid and
phenothiazine dosage by at least
2 hours.
Barbiturates: may decrease phenothiazine effect. Observe patient.

NURSING CONSIDERATIONS

• Contraindicated in history of coma;
CNS depression; bone marrow
depression; subcortical damage; use
of spinal or epidural anesthetic, or adrenergic blocking agents. Use cau-

tiously with other CNS depressants, anticholinergics; in hepatic disease, elderly or debilitated patients, arteriosclerosis or cardiovascular disease (may cause sudden drop in blood pressure), exposure to extreme heat or cold (including antipyretic therapy), respiratory disorders, hypocalcemia, convulsive disorders, severe reactions to insulin or electroshock therapy, suspected brain tumor or intestinal obstruction, glaucoma, or prostatic hypertrophy.

• Hold dose and notify doctor if patient develops symptoms of blood dyscrasias (fever, sore throat, infection, cellulitis, weakness), persistent (longer than a few hours) extrapyramidal reactions, or any such reaction during pregnancy.

• Dose of 20 mg is therapeutic equivalent of 100 mg chlorpromazine.

• Monitor therapy by weekly bilirubin tests during first month; periodic blood tests (CBC, hepatic function); and ophthalmic tests (long-term use).

• Check intake/output for urinary retention or constipation.

• Tell patient to use sunscreening agents and protective clothing to avoid photosensitivity reactions.

• Warn against activities requiring alertness or good psychomotor coordination until response to drug determined.

• Watch for orthostatic hypotension. Advise patient to get up slowly.

• Dry mouth may be relieved with sugarless gum, sour hard candy, or rinsing with mouthwash.

• Avoid combining with alcohol or other depressants.

• Do not withdraw abruptly unless required by severe side effects.

• Patient on maintenance may take medication at bedtime to facilitate sleep and decrease sedation during daytime.

---

butaperazine maleate
Repoise

INDICATIONS & DOSAGE
Psychotic disorders—
Adults: initially, 5 to 10 mg P.O. t.i.d. Increase gradually to maximum 100 mg daily. Use lowest effective dose.

SIDE EFFECTS
Blood: *transient leukopenia, agranulocytosis.*
CNS: *extrapyramidal reactions (high incidence),* sedation (low incidence), pseudoparkinsonism, EEG changes, dizziness.
CV: *orthostatic hypotension,* tachycardia, EKG changes.
EENT: *ocular changes, blurred vision.*
GI: *dry mouth, constipation.*
GU: *urinary retention,* dark urine, menstrual irregularities, gynecomastia, inhibited ejaculation.
Hepatic: *cholestatic jaundice.*
Metabolic: hyperprolactinemia.
Skin: *mild photosensitivity,* dermal allergic reactions, *exfoliative dermatitis.*
Other: weight gain, increased appetite.
After abrupt withdrawal: gastritis, nausea, vomiting, dizziness, tremors, feeling of warmth or cold, sweating, tachycardia, headache, insomnia.

INTERACTIONS
Antacids: inhibited absorption of oral phenothiazines. Separate antacid and phenothiazine dosage by at least 2 hours.
Barbiturates: may decrease phenothiazine effect. Observe patient.

NURSING CONSIDERATIONS
• Contraindicated in history of coma; CNS depression; bone marrow depression; subcortical damage; use

of spinal or epidural anesthetic, or adrenergic blocking agents. Use cautiously with other CNS depressants, anticholinergics; in hepatic disease, elderly or debilitated patients, arteriosclerosis or cardiovascular disease (may cause sudden drop in blood pressure), exposure to extreme heat or cold (including antipyretic therapy), respiratory disorders, hypocalcemia, acutely ill or dehydrated children, convulsive disorders, severe reactions to insulin or electroshock therapy, suspected brain tumor or intestinal obstruction, glaucoma, or prostatic hypertrophy.

• Hold dose and notify doctor if patient develops symptoms of jaundice, blood dyscrasias (fever, sore throat, infection, cellulitis, weakness), persistent (longer than a few hours) extrapyramidal reactions, or any such reaction in children.

• Patients on maintenance may take medication at bedtime to facilitate sleep and decrease sedation during the daytime.

• Monitor therapy by weekly bilirubin tests during first month; periodic blood tests (CBC, hepatic function); and ophthalmic tests (long-term use).

• Check intake/output for urinary retention or constipation.

• Watch patient for possible addiction.

• Tell patient to use sunscreening agents and protective clothing to avoid photosensitivity reactions.

• Warn against activities that require alertness or good psychomotor coordination until response to drug is determined. Drowsiness and dizziness usually subside after first few weeks.

• Watch for orthostatic hypotension. Advise patient to get up slowly.

• If dry mouth or nasal congestion occurs, symptoms may diminish in a week or two. Dry mouth may be relieved with sugarless gum, sour hard candy, or rinsing with mouthwash.

• Do not withdraw abruptly unless required by severe side effects.

• Avoid combining with alcohol or other depressants.

• Dose of 10 mg is therapeutic equivalent of 100 mg chlorpromazine.

---

carphenazine maleate
Proketazine

INDICATIONS & DOSAGE
Psychotic disorders—
Adults: initially, 12.5 to 50 mg P.O., b.i.d. or t.i.d. Increase gradually to maximum 100 mg daily.

SIDE EFFECTS
Blood: *transient leukopenias, agranulocytosis.*
CNS: *extrapyramidal reactions (high incidence),* sedation (low incidence), pseudoparkinsonism, EEG changes, dizziness.
CV: *orthostatic hypotension,* tachycardia, EKG changes.
EENT: *ocular changes, blurred vision.*
GI: *dry mouth, constipation.*
GU: *urinary retention,* dark urine, menstrual irregularities, gynecomastia, inhibited ejaculation.
Hepatic: *cholestatic jaundice.*
Metabolic: hyperprolactinemia.
Skin: *mild photosensitivity,* dermal allergic reactions, *exfoliative dermatitis.*
Other: weight gain, increased appetite.
After abrupt withdrawal: gastritis, nausea, vomiting, dizziness, tremors, feeling of warmth or cold, sweating, tachycardia, headache, insomnia.

INTERACTIONS
Antacids: inhibited absorption of oral phenothiazines. Separate antacid and phenothiazine dosage by at least 2 hours.

Barbiturates: may decrease phenothiazine effect. Observe patient.

NURSING CONSIDERATIONS

• Contraindicated in history of coma; CNS depression; bone marrow depression; subcortical damage; use of spinal or epidural anesthetic, or adrenergic blocking agents. Use cautiously with other CNS depressants, anticholinergics; in hepatic disease, elderly or debilitated patients, arteriosclerosis or cardiovascular disease (may cause sudden drop in blood pressure), exposure to extreme heat or cold (including antipyretic therapy), respiratory disorders, hypocalcemia, acutely ill or dehydrated children, convulsive disorders, severe reactions to insulin or electroshock therapy, suspected brain tumor or intestinal obstruction, glaucoma, or prostatic hypertrophy.

• Hold dose and notify doctor if patient develops symptoms of jaundice, blood dyscrasias (fever, sore throat, infection, cellulitis, weakness) or persistent (longer than a few hours) extrapyramidal reactions.

• Monitor therapy by weekly bilirubin tests during first month; periodic blood tests (CBC, hepatic function); and ophthalmic tests (long-term use).

• Check intake/output for urinary retention or constipation.

• Tell patient to use sunscreening agents and protective clothing to avoid photosensitivity reactions.

• Warn against activities that require alertness or good psychomotor coordination until response to drug is determined. Drowsiness and dizziness usually subside after a few weeks.

• Watch for orthostatic hypotension. Advise patient to get up slowly.

• Avoid combining with alcohol or other depressants.

• Do not withdraw abruptly unless required by severe side effects.

• Dry mouth may be relieved by sugarless gum, sour hard candy, or rinsing with mouthwash.

• Dose of 25 mg is therapeutic equivalent of 100 mg chlorpromazine.

chlorpromazine hydrochloride

Chlorprom♦♦, Chlor-Promanyl♦♦, Chlorzine, Klorazine, Klomazine, Largactil♦♦, Ormazine, Promachel, Promachlor, Promapar, Promaz, Sonazine, Terpium, Thoradex, Thorazine

INDICATIONS & DOSAGE

Intractable hiccups—
Adults: 25 to 50 mg P.O. or I.M. t.i.d. or q.i.d.
Mild alcohol withdrawal, acute intermittent porphyria, and tetanus—
Adults: 25 to 50 mg I.M. t.i.d. or q.i.d.
Nausea and vomiting—
Adults: 10 to 25 mg P.O. or I.M. q 4 to 6 hours, p.r.n.; or 50 to 100 mg rectally q 6 to 8 hours, p.r.n.
Children: 0.25 mg/Kg P.O. q 4 to 6 hours; or 0.25 mg/Kg I.M. q 6 to 8 hours; or 0.5 mg/Kg rectally q 6 to 8 hours.
Psychosis—
Adults: 500 mg P.O. daily in divided doses, increasing gradually to 2 g; or 25 to 50 mg I.M. q 1 to 4 hours, p.r.n.
Children: 0.25 mg/Kg P.O. q 4 to 6 hours; or 0.25 mg/Kg I.M. q 6 to 8 hours; or 0.5 mg/Kg rectally q 6 to 8 hours. Maximum dose is 40 mg in children under 5 years, and 75 mg in children 5 to 12 years.

SIDE EFFECTS

Blood: *transient leukopenias, agranulocytosis.*
CNS: *extrapyramidal reactions (moderate incidence), sedation (high incidence),* pseudoparkinsonism, EEG changes, dizziness.
CV: *orthostatic hypotension,* tachycardia, EKG changes.

Italicized side effects are common or life-threatening.

EENT: *ocular changes, blurred vision.*

GI: *dry mouth, constipation.*

GU: *urinary retention,* dark urine, menstrual irregularities, gynecomastia, inhibited ejaculation.

Hepatic: *cholestatic jaundice.*

Metabolic: hyperprolactinemia.

Skin: *mild photosensitivity,* dermal allergic reactions, *exfoliative dermatitis.*

Local: pain on I.M. injection, sterile abscess.

Other: weight gain, increased appetite.

After abrupt withdrawal: gastritis, nausea, vomiting, dizziness, tremors, feeling of warmth or cold, sweating, tachycardia, headache, insomnia.

INTERACTIONS

Antacids: inhibited absorption of oral phenothiazines. Separate antacid and phenothiazine dosage by at least 2 hours.

Anticholinergics (including antidepressant and antiparkinson agents): increased anticholinergic activity, aggravated parkinson-like symptoms. Use with caution.

Barbiturates: may decrease phenothiazine effect. Observe patient.

Lithium: possible decreased response to chlorpromazine. Observe patient.

NURSING CONSIDERATIONS

• Contraindicated in history of coma; CNS depression; bone marrow depression; subcortical damage; use of spinal or epidural anesthetic, or adrenergic blocking agents; Reye's syndrome. Use cautiously with other CNS depressants, anticholinergics; in hepatic disease, elderly or debilitated patients, arteriosclerosis or cardiovascular disease (may cause sudden drop in blood pressure), exposure to extreme heat or cold (including antipyretic therapy), respiratory disorders, hypocalcemia, acutely ill or dehydrated children, convulsive disorders,

severe reactions to insulin or electroshock therapy, suspected brain tumor or intestinal obstruction, glaucoma, or prostatic hypertrophy.

• Hold dose and notify doctor if patient develops jaundice, symptoms of blood dyscrasias (fever, sore throat, infection, cellulitis, weakness), persistent (longer than a few hours) extrapyramidal reactions, or any such reaction in pregnancy or in children.

• Monitor therapy by weekly bilirubin tests during first month; periodic blood tests (CBC, hepatic function); and ophthalmic tests (long-term use).

• Check intake/output for urinary retention or constipation.

• Tell patient to use sunscreening agents and protective clothing to avoid photosensitivity reactions.

• Warn against activities that require alertness or good psychomotor coordination until response to drug is determined. Drowsiness and dizziness usually subside after first few weeks.

• Watch for orthostatic hypotension, especially with parenteral administration. Monitor blood pressure before and after I.M. administration. Keep patient supine for 1 hour afterward. Advise patient to get up slowly.

• Avoid combining with alcohol or other depressants.

• Give I.M. only in upper outer quadrant of buttocks. Massage slowly afterward to prevent sterile abscess. Injection may sting.

• Prevent contact dermatitis by keeping drug off patient's skin and clothes.

• Protect liquid concentrate from light. Dilute with fruit juice, milk, or semisolid food just before administration.

• Slight yellowing of injection or concentrate is common; does not affect potency. Discard markedly discolored solutions.

• Do not withdraw abruptly unless required by severe side effects.

• Dry mouth may be relieved by sug-

arless gum, sour hard candy, or rinsing with mouthwash.
• An aliphatic; has greater tendency to cause anticholinergic side effects.

chlorprothixene
Taractan, Tarasan♦ ♦

INDICATIONS & DOSAGE
Psychotic disorders—
Adults: initially, 10 mg P.O. t.i.d. or q.i.d. Increase gradually to maximum 600 mg daily.
Children over 6 years: 10 to 25 mg P.O. t.i.d. or q.i.d.
Agitation of severe neurosis, depression, schizophrenia—
Adults: 25 to 50 mg P.O. or I.M. t.i.d. or q.i.d. Increase as needed up to maximum 600 mg.

SIDE EFFECTS
Blood: *transient leukopenias, agranulocytosis.*
CNS: *extrapyramidal reactions (high incidence)*, sedation (low incidence), pseudoparkinsonism, EEG changes, dizziness.
CV: *orthostatic hypotension*, tachycardia, EKG changes.
EENT: *ocular changes, blurred vision*.
GI: *dry mouth, constipation*.
GU: *urinary retention*, dark urine, menstrual irregularities, gynecomastia, inhibited ejaculation.
Hepatic: *cholestatic jaundice*.
Metabolic: hyperprolactinemia.
Skin: *mild photosensitivity*, dermal allergic reactions, *exfoliative dermatitis*.
Local: pain on I.M. injection, sterile abscess.
Other: weight gain, increased appetite.
After abrupt withdrawal: gastritis, nausea, vomiting, dizziness, tremors, feeling of warmth or cold, sweating, tachycardia, headache, insomnia.

INTERACTIONS
None significant.

NURSING CONSIDERATIONS
• Contraindicated in coma, CNS depression, bone marrow depression, circulatory collapse, congestive failure, cardiac decompensation, coronary artery or cerebral vascular disorders, subcortical damage, use of spinal or epidural anesthetic or adrenergic blocking agents. Use cautiously with other CNS depressants, anticholinergics; in hepatic or renal disease, elderly or debilitated patients, arteriosclerosis or cardiovascular disease (may cause sudden drop in blood pressure), exposure to extreme heat or cold (including antipyretic therapy), respiratory disorders, hypocalcemia, acutely ill or dehydrated children, convulsive disorders, severe reactions to insulin or electroshock therapy, suspected brain tumor or intestinal obstruction, glaucoma, or prostatic hypertrophy.
• Hold dose and notify doctor if patient develops symptoms of blood dyscrasias (fever, sore throat, infection, cellulitis, weakness), jaundice, persistent (longer than a few hours) extrapyramidal reactions, or any such reactions in children.
• Monitor therapy by weekly bilirubin tests during first month; periodic blood tests (CBC, hepatic function) before and during therapy; and ophthalmic tests (long-term therapy).
• Check intake/output for urinary retention or constipation.
• Tell patient to use sunscreening agents and protective clothing to avoid photosensitivity reactions.
• Warn against activities that require alertness or good psychomotor coordination until response to drug is determined. Drowsiness and dizziness usually subside after first few weeks.
• Watch for orthostatic hypotension, especially with parenteral administration, since adrenergic blockage is

---

Italicized side effects are common or life-threatening.

high. Keep patient supine for 1 hour
afterward. Advise patient to change
positions slowly.
• Avoid combining with alcohol or
other depressants.
• Give deep I.M. only in upper outer
quadrant of buttocks or midlateral
thigh. Massage slowly afterward to
prevent sterile abscess. Injection may
sting.
• Dilute liquid concentrate with fruit
juice, milk, or semisolid food just before administration.
• Protect medication from light.
Slight yellowing of injection or concentrate is common; does not affect
potency. Discard markedly discolored
solutions.
• Do not withdraw abruptly unless required by severe side effects.
• Prevent contact dermatitis by keeping drug off patient's skin and clothes.
• Dry mouth may be relieved by sugarless gum, sour hard candy, or rinsing with mouthwash.
• Dose of 100 mg is therapeutic
equivalent of 100 mg chlorpromazine.

droperidol
Inapsine♦

INDICATIONS & DOSAGE
Premedication—
Adults: 2.5 to 10 mg (1 to 4 ml) I.M.
30 to 60 minutes preop.
Children 2 to 12 years: 1 to 1.5 mg
(0.4 to 0.6 ml) I.M. per 20 to 25 lbs
of body weight.
As induction agent—
Adults: 2.5 mg (1 ml) per 20 to 25 lbs
I.V. with analgesic and/or general an-
esthetic.
Children 2 to 12 years: 1 to 1.5 mg
(0.4 to 0.6 ml) per 20 to 25 lbs I.V.
Dose should be titrated.
Elderly, debilitated: initial dose
should be decreased.
Maintenance dose in general anes-

*thesia—*1.25 to 2.5 mg (0.5 to 1 ml)
I.V.

SIDE EFFECTS
CNS: extrapyramidal reactions (dys-
tonia, akathisia), upward rotation of
eyes and oculogyric crises, extended
neck, flexed arms, fine tremor of
limbs, dizziness, chills or shivering,
facial sweating, restlessness.
CV: hypotension, tachycardia.

INTERACTIONS
None significant.

NURSING CONSIDERATIONS
• Use cautiously in elderly or debilitated patients; hypotension or other
cardiovascular disease; impaired hepatic or renal function; Parkinson's
disease.
• Watch for extrapyramidal reactions.
Call doctor at once if any occur.
• Approved by FDA *only* for use
preop and during induction and maintenance of anesthesia.
• A butyrophenone compound,
related to haloperidol; has greater
tendency to cause extrapyramidal reactions.
• Keep intravenous fluids and vasopressors handy for hypotension.
• If used with a narcotic analgesic
such as fentamyl (Sublimaze), be familiar with the special properties of
each drug, particularly the widely dif-
fering durations of action. Watch for
respiratory depression, apnea, and
muscular rigidity, which could lead to
respiratory arrest if untreated. Have
narcotic antagonist and CPR equipment on hand.
• Monitor vital signs frequently; notify doctor of any changes immediately.
• Give intravenous injections slowly.
• Do not place patient in head-down
position (i.e., shock); severe hypotension and deeper anesthesia may result,
causing respiratory arrest.

• Has been used to prevent cis-platinum-associated nausea and vomiting.

fluphenazine decanoate
Modecate, Decanoate♦♦, Prolixin Decanoate
fluphenazine enanthate
Moditen♦, Prolixin Enanthate
fluphenazine hydrochloride
Moditen Hydrochloride♦♦, Permitil Hydrochloride, Prolixin Hydrochloride

INDICATIONS & DOSAGE
Psychotic disorders—
Adults: initially, 0.5 to 10 mg fluphenazine HCl P.O. daily in divided doses q 6 to 8 hours; may increase cautiously to 20 mg. Higher doses (50 to 100 mg) have been given. Maintenance: 1 to 5 mg P.O. daily. I.M. doses are ⅓ to ½ oral doses. Lower doses for geriatric patients (1 to 2.5 mg daily).
Children: 0.25 to 3.5 mg fluphenazine HCl P.O. daily in divided doses q 4 to 6 hours; or ⅓ to ½ of oral dose I.M.; maximum 10 mg daily.
Adults, and children over 12 years: 12.5 to 25 mg of long-acting esters (fluphenazine decanoate and enanthate) I.M. or S.C. q 1 to 6 weeks. Maintenance: 25 to 100 mg, p.r.n.

SIDE EFFECTS
Blood: *transient leukopenias, agranulocytosis.*
CNS: *extrapyramidal reactions (high incidence),* sedation (low incidence), pseudoparkinsonism, EEG changes, dizziness.
CV: *orthostatic hypotension,* tachycardia, EKG changes.
EENT: *ocular changes, blurred vision.*
GI: *dry mouth, constipation.*
GU: *urinary retention,* dark urine,

menstrual irregularities, gynecomastia, inhibited ejaculation.
Hepatic: *cholestatic jaundice.*
Metabolic: hyperprolactinemia.
Skin: *mild photosensitivity,* dermal allergic reactions, *exfoliative dermatitis.*
Other: weight gain, increased appetite.
After abrupt withdrawal: gastritis, nausea, vomiting, dizziness, tremors, feeling of warmth or cold, sweating, tachycardia, headache, insomnia.

INTERACTIONS
Antacids: inhibited absorption of oral phenothiazines. Separate antacid and phenothiazine dosage by at least 2 hours.
Barbiturates: may decrease phenothiazine effect. Observe patient.

NURSING CONSIDERATIONS
• Contraindicated in coma, CNS depression, bone marrow depression or other blood dyscrasia, subcortical damage, use of spinal or epidural anesthetic or adrenergic blocking agents, hepatic damage, renal insufficiency. Use cautiously with other CNS depressants, anticholinergics; in hepatic disease, elderly or debilitated patients, pheochromocytoma, arteriosclerotic, cerebrovascular, or cardiovascular disease (may cause sudden drop in blood pressure), peptic ulcer, exposure to extreme heat or cold (including antipyretic therapy), respiratory disorders, hypocalcemia, acutely ill or dehydrated children, convulsive disorders, severe reactions to insulin or electroshock therapy, suspected brain tumor or intestinal obstruction, glaucoma, or prostatic hypertrophy.
• Hold dose and notify doctor if patient develops symptoms of blood dyscrasias (fever, sore throat, infection, cellulitis, weakness), persistent (longer than a few hours) extrapyramidal reactions, or any such reactions in pregnancy or in children.

Italicized side effects are common or life-threatening.

- Monitor therapy by weekly bilirubin tests during first month; periodic blood tests (CBC, hepatic function); periodic renal function and ophthalmic tests (long-term use).
- Check intake/output for urinary retention or constipation.
- Tell patient to use sunscreening agents and protective clothing to avoid photosensitivity reactions.
- Warn against activities that require alertness and good psychomotor coordination until response to drug is determined. Drowsiness and dizziness usually subside after first few weeks.
- Avoid combining with alcohol or other depressants.
- Watch for orthostatic hypotension, especially with parenteral administration. Monitor blood pressure before and after I.M. administration. Keep patient supine for 1 hour afterward. Advise him to change positions slowly.
- Decanoate and enanthate may be given subcutaneously.
- For long-acting forms (decanoate and enanthate), which are oil preparations, use a dry needle of at least 21 gauge. Allow 24 to 96 hours for onset of action.
- Prevent contact dermatitis by keeping drug off patient's skin and clothes.
- Dilute liquid concentrate with water, fruit juice, milk, or semisolid food just before administration.
- Protect medication from light. Slight yellowing of injection or concentrate is common; does not affect potency. Discard markedly discolored solutions.
- Dry mouth may be relieved by sugarless gum, sour hard candy, or rinsing with mouthwash.
- Do not withdraw abruptly unless required by severe side effects.
- Dose of 2 mg is therapeutic equivalent of 100 mg chlorpromazine.

haloperidol
Haldol♦

INDICATIONS & DOSAGE
Psychotic disorders—
Adults: dosage varies for each patient. Initial range is 0.5 to 5 mg P.O. b.i.d. or t.i.d.; or 2 to 5 mg I.M. q 4 to 8 hours, increasing rapidly if necessary for prompt control. Maximum 100 mg P.O. daily. Doses over 100 mg have been used for severely resistant patients.
Control of tics, vocal utterances in Gilles de la Tourette's syndrome—
Adults: 0.5 to 5 mg P.O. b.i.d. or t.i.d., increasing p.r.n.

SIDE EFFECTS
Blood: transient leukopenia and leukocytosis.
CNS: *high incidence of severe extrapyramidal reactions,* low incidence of sedation.
CV: low incidence of cardiovascular effects.
EENT: blurred vision, dry mouth.
GU: urinary retention.
Skin: rash.

INTERACTIONS
Lithium: lethargy and confusion with high doses. Observe patient.
Methyldopa: possible symptoms of dementia. Observe patient.

NURSING CONSIDERATIONS
- Contraindicated in seizures, parkinsonism, coma, or CNS depression. Use with caution in severe cardiovascular disorders; allergies; elderly and debilitated patients; conjunction with anticonvulsant, anticoagulant, antiparkinson, or lithium medications; glaucoma; urinary retention.
- Warn patient against activities that require alertness and good psychomotor coordination until response to drug is determined. Drowsiness and

dizziness usually subside after a few weeks.
- Avoid combining with alcohol or other depressants.
- Protect medication from light. Slight yellowing of injection or concentrate is common; does not affect potency. Discard markedly discolored solutions.
- Do not withdraw abruptly unless required by severe side effects.
- Dry mouth may be relieved by sugarless gum, sour hard candy, and rinsing with mouthwash.
- Dose of 2 mg is therapeutic equivalent of 100 mg chlorpromazine.
- Only butyrophenone compound used as an antipsychotic in the U.S.

loxapine succinate
Daxolin, Loxapac♦♦, Loxitane, Loxitane-C

INDICATIONS & DOSAGE
Psychotic disorders—
Adults: 10 mg P.O. or I.M. b.i.d. to q.i.d., rapidly increasing to 60 to 100 mg P.O. daily for most patients; dose varies from patient to patient.

SIDE EFFECTS
Blood: *transient leukopenias.*
CNS: *extrapyramidal reactions (moderate incidence), sedation (moderate incidence),* pseudoparkinsonism, EEG changes, dizziness.
CV: *orthostatic hypotension,* tachycardia, EKG changes.
EENT: *blurred vision.*
GI: *dry mouth, constipation.*
GU: *urinary retention,* dark urine, menstrual irregularities, gynecomastia, inhibited ejaculation.
Hepatic: *cholestatic jaundice.*
Metabolic: hyperprolactinemia.
Skin: *mild photosensitivity,* dermal allergic reactions, *exfoliative dermatitis.*
Other: weight gain, increased appetite.

INTERACTIONS
None significant.

NURSING CONSIDERATIONS
- Contraindicated in convulsive disorders, coma, severe CNS depression, drug-induced depressed states. Use with caution in epilepsy, cardiovascular disorders, glaucoma, urinary retention, suspected intestinal obstruction or brain tumor, renal damage.
- Warn against activities that require alertness and good psychomotor coordination until response to drug is determined. Drowsiness and dizziness usually subside after first few weeks.
- Avoid combining with alcohol or other depressants.
- Advise patient to get up slowly to avoid orthostatic hypotension.
- Dilute liquid concentrate with orange or grapefruit juice just before giving.
- Dry mouth may be relieved by sugarless gum, sour hard candy, or rinsing with mouthwash.
- Monitor blood pressure.
- Periodic ophthalmic tests recommended.
- Tricyclic dibenzoxazepine; the only dibenzoxazepine derivative.
- Dose of 10 mg is therapeutic equivalent of 100 mg chlorpromazine.

mesoridazine besylate
Serentil♦

INDICATIONS & DOSAGE
Alcoholism—
Adults, and children over 12 years: 25 mg P.O. b.i.d. up to maximum 200 mg daily.
Behavioral problems associated with chronic brain syndrome—
Adults, and children over 12 years: 25 mg P.O. t.i.d. up to maximum of 300 mg daily.

Italicized side effects are common or life-threatening.

Psychoneurotic manifestations (anxiety)—
Adults, and children over 12 years:
10 mg P.O. t.i.d. up to maximum
150 mg daily.
Schizophrenia—
Adults, and children over 12 years:
initially, 50 mg P.O. t.i.d. or 25 mg
I.M. repeated in 30 to 60 minutes,
p.r.n.

SIDE EFFECTS
Blood: *transient leukopenias, agranulocytosis.*
CNS: extrapyramidal reactions (low incidence), *sedation (high incidence),* EEG changes, dizziness.
CV: *orthostatic hypotension,* tachycardia, EKG changes.
EENT: *ocular changes, blurred vision,* pigmentary retinopathy.
GI: *dry mouth, constipation.*
GU: *urinary retention,* dark urine, menstrual irregularities, gynecomastia, inhibited ejaculation.
Hepatic: *cholestatic jaundice.*
Metabolic: hyperprolactinemia.
Skin: *mild photosensitivity,* dermal allergic reactions, *exfoliative dermatitis.*
Local: pain on I.M. injection, sterile abscess.
Other: weight gain, increased appetite.
After abrupt withdrawal: gastritis, nausea, vomiting, dizziness, tremors, feeling of warmth or cold, sweating, tachycardia, headache, insomnia.

INTERACTIONS
Antacids: inhibited absorption of oral phenothiazines. Separate antacid and phenothiazine dosage by at least 2 hours.
Barbiturates: may decrease phenothiazine effect. Observe patient.

NURSING CONSIDERATIONS
• Contraindicated in coma, CNS depression, bone marrow depression, subcortical damage, use of spinal or epidural anesthetic or adrenergic blocking agents. Use cautiously with other CNS depressants, anticholinergics; in hepatic disease, elderly or debilitated patients, arteriosclerosis or cardiovascular disease (may cause sudden drop in blood pressure), exposure to extreme heat or cold (including antipyretic therapy), respiratory disorders, hypocalcemia, acutely ill or dehydrated children, convulsive disorders, severe reactions to insulin or electroshock therapy, suspected brain tumor or intestinal obstruction, glaucoma, or prostatic hypertrophy.
• Hold dose and notify doctor if patient develops jaundice, symptoms of blood dyscrasias (fever, sore throat, infection, cellulitis, weakness), persistent (longer than a few hours) extrapyramidal reactions, or any such reactions in pregnancy or in children over 12 years.
• Monitor therapy by weekly bilirubin tests during first month; periodic blood tests (CBC, hepatic function); and ophthalmic tests (long-term use).
• Check intake/output for urinary retention or constipation.
• Tell patient to use sunscreening agents and protective clothing to avoid photosensitivity reactions.
• Warn against activities that require alertness and good psychomotor coordination until response to drug is determined. Drowsiness and dizziness usually subside after a few weeks.
• Avoid combining with alcohol or other depressants.
• Watch for orthostatic hypotension, especially with parenteral administration. Advise patient to change positions slowly.
• Give I.M. only in upper outer quadrant of buttocks. Massage slowly afterward to prevent sterile abscess. Injection may sting.
• Protect medication from light. Slight yellowing of injection or concentrate is common; does not affect

potency. Discard markedly discolored solutions.
• Prevent contact dermatitis by keeping drug off patient's skin and clothes.
• Dry mouth may be relieved with sugarless gum, sour hard candy, or rinsing with mouthwash.
• Do not withdraw abruptly unless required by severe side effects.
• Drug is a piperidine phenothiazine (a metabolite of thioridazine).
• Dose of 50 mg is therapeutic equivalent of 100 mg chlorpromazine.

molindone hydrochloride
Lidone, Moban

INDICATIONS & DOSAGE
Psychotic disorders—
Adults: 50 to 75 mg P.O. daily, increasing to maximum 225 mg daily. Doses up to 400 mg may be required.

SIDE EFFECTS
Blood: *transient leukopenias.*
CNS: *extrapyramidal reactions (moderate incidence), sedation (moderate incidence),* pseudoparkinsonism, EEG changes, dizziness.
CV: *orthostatic hypotension,* tachycardia, EKG changes.
EENT: *blurred vision.*
GI: *dry mouth, constipation.*
GU: *urinary retention,* dark urine, menstrual irregularities, gynecomastia, inhibited ejaculation.
Hepatic: *cholestatic jaundice.*
Metabolic: hyperprolactinemia.
Skin: *mild photosensitivity,* dermal allergic reactions, *exfoliative dermatitis.*
Other: weight gain, increased appetite.

INTERACTIONS
None significant.

NURSING CONSIDERATIONS
• Contraindicated in coma or severe

CNS depression. Use with caution when increased physical activity would be harmful, as this agent increases activity; in seizures, suicide risk, suspected brain tumor, or intestinal obstruction.
• Warn against activities that require alertness or good psychomotor coordination until response to drug is determined. Drowsiness and dizziness usually subside after first few weeks.
• Avoid combining with alcohol or other depressants.
• Dry mouth may be relieved with sugarless gum, sour hard candy, or rinsing with mouthwash.
• Drug is the only dihydroindolone derivative.
• Dose of 20 mg is therapeutic equivalent of 100 mg chlorpromazine.
• No injection available.
• Liquid oral concentrate is available.
• Lidone capsules contain tartrazine dye. May cause allergy in susceptible individuals.

perphenazine
Phenazine♦♦, Trilafon♦

INDICATIONS & DOSAGE
Hospitalized psychiatric patients—
Adults: initially, 8 to 16 mg P.O. b.i.d., t.i.d., or q.i.d., increasing to 64 mg daily.
Children over 12 years: 6 to 12 mg P.O. daily in divided doses.
Mental disturbances, acute alcoholism, nausea, vomiting, hiccups—
Adults, and children over 12 years: 5 to 10 mg I.M., p.r.n. Maximum 15 mg daily in ambulatory, 30 mg daily in hospitalized patients.

SIDE EFFECTS
Blood: *transient leukopenias, agranulocytosis.*
CNS: *extrapyramidal reactions (high incidence),* sedation (low incidence),

pseudoparkinsonism, EEG changes, dizziness.
CV: *orthostatic hypotension,* tachycardia, EKG changes.
EENT: *ocular changes, blurred vision.*
GI: *dry mouth, constipation.*
GU: *urinary retention,* dark urine, menstrual irregularities, gynecomastia, inhibited ejaculation.
Hepatic: *cholestatic jaundice.*
Metabolic: hyperprolactinemia.
Skin: *mild photosensitivity,* dermal allergic reactions, *exfoliative dermatitis.*
Local: pain on I.M. injection, sterile abscess.
Other: weight gain, increased appetite.
After abrupt withdrawal: gastritis, nausea, vomiting, dizziness, tremors, feeling of warmth or cold, sweating, tachycardia, headache, insomnia.

INTERACTIONS

Antacids: inhibited absorption of oral phenothiazines. Separate antacid and phenothiazine dosage by at least 2 hours.
Barbiturates: may decrease phenothiazine effect. Observe patient.

NURSING CONSIDERATIONS

• Contraindicated in coma, CNS depression, bone marrow depression, subcortical damage, use of spinal or epidural anesthetic or adrenergic blocking agents. Use cautiously with other CNS depressants, anticholinergics; in hepatic disease, elderly or debilitated patients, arteriosclerosis or cardiovascular disease (may cause sudden drop in blood pressure), exposure to extreme heat or cold (including antipyretic therapy), respiratory disorders, hypocalcemia, acutely ill or dehydrated children, convulsive disorders, severe reactions to insulin or electroshock therapy, suspected brain tumor or intestinal obstruction, glaucoma, prostatic hypertrophy.

• Hold dose and notify doctor if patient develops jaundice, symptoms of blood dyscrasias (fever, sore throat, infection, cellulitis, weakness), persistent (longer than a few hours) extrapyramidal reactions, or any such reactions in pregnancy or in children.
• Monitor therapy by weekly bilirubin tests during first month; periodic blood tests (CBC, hepatic function); and ophthalmic tests (long-term use).
• Check intake/output for urinary retention or constipation.
• Tell patient to use sunscreening agents and protective clothing to avoid photosensitivity reactions.
• Warn against activities that require alertness or good psychomotor coordination until response to drug is determined. Drowsiness and dizziness usually subside after a few weeks.
• Avoid combining with alcohol or other depressants.
• Watch for orthostatic hypotension, especially with parenteral administration. Keep patient supine for 1 hour afterward. Advise patient to change positions slowly.
• Give deep I.M. only in upper outer quadrant of buttocks. Massage slowly afterward to prevent sterile abscess. Injection may sting.
• Do not withdraw abruptly unless required by severe side effects.
• Protect from light. Slight yellowing of injection or concentrate is common; does not affect potency. Discard markedly discolored solutions.
• Prevent contact dermatitis by keeping drug off patient's skin and clothes.
• Dilute liquid concentrate with fruit juice, milk, carbonated beverage, or semisolid food just before giving. Exceptions: oral concentrate causes turbidity or precipitation in colas, black coffee, grape or apple juice, or tea. Do not mix with these liquids.
• Dry mouth may be relieved with sugarless gum, sour hard candy, or rinsing with mouthwash.

• Dose of 8 mg is therapeutic equivalent of 100 mg chlorpromazine.

---

piperacetazine
Quide♦

INDICATIONS & DOSAGE
Psychotic disorders—
Adults: initially, 10 mg P.O. b.i.d. to q.i.d. Dosage may be gradually increased to 160 mg daily if necessary.

SIDE EFFECTS
Blood: *transient leukopenias, agranulocytosis.*
CNS: extrapyramidal reactions (low incidence), *sedation (high incidence),* EEG changes, dizziness.
CV: *orthostatic hypotension,* tachycardia, EKG changes.
EENT: *ocular changes, blurred vision,* pigmentary retinopathy.
GI: *dry mouth, constipation.*
GU: *urinary retention,* dark urine, menstrual irregularities, gynecomastia, inhibited ejaculation.
Hepatic: *cholestatic jaundice.*
Metabolic: hyperprolactinemia.
Skin: *mild photosensitivity,* dermal allergic reactions, *exfoliative dermatitis.*
Other: weight gain, increased appetite.
After abrupt withdrawal: gastritis, nausea, vomiting, dizziness, tremors, feeling of warmth or cold, sweating, tachycardia, headache, insomnia.

INTERACTIONS
Antacids: inhibited absorption of oral phenothiazines. Separate antacid and phenothiazine dosage by at least 2 hours.
Barbiturates: may decrease phenothiazine effect. Observe patient.

NURSING CONSIDERATIONS
• Contraindicated in coma, CNS depression, bone marrow depression, thrombocytopenia and other blood dyscrasias, subcortical damage, use of spinal or epidural anesthetic or adrenergic blocking agents. Use cautiously with other CNS depressants, anticholinergics; in hepatic disease, elderly or debilitated patients, arteriosclerosis or cardiovascular disease (may cause sudden drop in blood pressure), exposure to extreme heat or cold (including antipyretic therapy), respiratory disorders, hypocalcemia, convulsive disorders, severe reactions to insulin or electroshock therapy, suspected brain tumor or intestinal obstruction, glaucoma, or prostatic hypertrophy.
• Hold dose and notify doctor if patient develops jaundice, symptoms of blood dyscrasias (fever, sore throat, infection, cellulitis, weakness), persistent (longer than a few hours) extrapyramidal reactions, or any such reactions during pregnancy.
• Monitor therapy by weekly bilirubin tests during first month; periodic blood tests (CBC, hepatic function); and ophthalmic tests (long-term use).
• Check intake/output for urinary retention or constipation.
• Tell patient to use sunscreening agents and protective clothing to avoid photosensitivity reactions.
• Monitor blood pressure.
• Warn against activities that require alertness or good psychomotor coordination until response to drug is determined. Drowsiness and dizziness usually subside after a few weeks.
• Avoid combining with alcohol or other depressants.
• Watch for orthostatic hypotension.
• Protect tablets from light.
• Do not withdraw abruptly unless required by severe side effects.
• Dry mouth may be relieved with sugarless gum, sour hard candy, or rinsing with mouthwash.
• Drug is a piperidine phenothiazine.
• Dose of 10 mg is therapeutic equivalent of 100 mg chlorpromazine.

Italicized side effects are common or life-threatening.

prochlorperazine edisylate

prochlorperazine maleate
Compazine, Stemetil◆ ◆

INDICATIONS & DOSAGE
*Mild to moderate emotional distur-
bances—*
Adults: 5 to 10 mg P.O. t.i.d. or
q.i.d.; extended-release 15 mg P.O.
in a.m. or 10 mg q 12 hours; 25 mg
rectally b.i.d.; 5 to 10 mg I.M. q 3 to
4 hours.
Children weighing 18 to 38.5 Kg:
5 mg P.O. or rectally b.i.d., to maximum of 15 mg daily.
Children weighing 13.5 to 17.5 Kg:
2.5 mg P.O. or rectally b.i.d. or
t.i.d., up to maximum 10 mg daily.
Children weighing 9 to 13 Kg: 2.5
mg P.O. or rectally daily or b.i.d. to
maximum 7.5 mg daily. I.M. dose
0.13 mg/Kg; repeat if necessary.
Not recommended in children under
9 Kg.
*Psychomotor agitation in schizophre-
nia; manic phase of manic-depressive
psychosis; involutional toxic and senile psychoses—*
Adults: initially, 10 mg P.O. t.i.d. to
q.i.d., increasing up to 50 to 150 mg
daily; or 10 to 20 mg I.M. q 1 to 4
hours, p.r.n., up to 100 mg daily, until
symptoms are controlled. Prolonged
I.M. dosage 10 to 20 mg q 4 to 6
hours.

SIDE EFFECTS
Blood: *transient leukopenias, agranulocytosis.*
CNS: *extrapyramidal reactions (high
incidence),* sedation (low incidence),
pseudoparkinsonism, EEG changes,
dizziness.
CV: *orthostatic hypotension,* tachycardia, EKG changes.
EENT: *ocular changes, blurred vision.*
GI: *dry mouth, constipation.*

GU: *urinary retention,* dark urine,
menstrual irregularities, gynecomastia, inhibited ejaculation.
Hepatic: *cholestatic jaundice.*
Metabolic: hyperprolactinemia.
Skin: *mild photosensitivity,* dermal
allergic reactions, *exfoliative dermatitis.*
Local: pain on I.M. injection, sterile
abscess.
Other: weight gain, increased appetite.
After abrupt withdrawal: gastritis,
nausea, vomiting, dizziness, tremors,
feeling of warmth or cold, sweating,
tachycardia, headache, insomnia.

INTERACTIONS
Antacids: inhibited absorption of oral
phenothiazines. Separate antacid and
phenothiazine dosage by at least
2 hours.
Barbiturates: may decrease phenothiazine effect. Observe patient.

NURSING CONSIDERATIONS
• Contraindicated in coma, depression, CNS depression, bone marrow
depression, subcortical damage, pediatric surgery, use of spinal or epidural
anesthetic or adrenergic blocking
agents, alcohol usage. Use cautiously
with other CNS depressants, anticholinergics; in hepatic disease, elderly
or debilitated patients, arterioscloro-
sis or cardiovascular disease (may
cause sudden drop in blood pressure),
exposure to extreme heat or cold
(including antipyretic therapy), respiratory disorders, hypocalcemia, vomiting in children, acutely ill or dehydrated children, convulsive disorders
or severe reactions to insulin or electroshock therapy, suspected brain tumor or intestinal obstruction, glaucoma, or prostatic hypertrophy.
• Hold dose and notify doctor if patient develops jaundice, symptoms of
blood dyscrasias (fever, sore throat,
infection, cellulitis, weakness), persistent (longer than a few hours) ex-

trapyramidal reactions, or any such reactions during pregnancy or in children.

• Monitor therapy by weekly bilirubin tests during first month; periodic blood tests (CBC, hepatic function); and ophthalmic tests (long-term use).

• Check intake/output for urinary retention or constipation.

• Monitor blood pressure and heart rate.

• Tell patient to use sunscreening agents and protective clothing to avoid photosensitivity reactions.

• Warn against activities that require alertness or good psychomotor coordination until response to drug is determined. Drowsiness and dizziness usually subside after a few weeks.

• Avoid combining with alcohol or other depressants.

• Watch for orthostatic hypotension, especially with parenteral administration. Advise patient to change positions slowly.

• Give deep I.M. only in upper outer quadrant of buttocks. Massage slowly afterward to prevent sterile abscess. Injection may sting.

• Do not mix in same syringe with another drug.

• Do not give S.C.

• Protect from light. Slight yellowing of injection or concentrate is common; does not affect potency. Discard markedly discolored solutions.

• Prevent contact dermatitis by keeping drug off patient's skin and clothes.

• Dilute liquid concentrate with fruit juice, milk, coffee, tea, carbonated beverages, or semisolid food just before giving.

• Do not withdraw abruptly unless required by severe side effects.

• Dry mouth may be relieved with sugarless gum, sour hard candy, or rinsing with mouthwash.

• Piperazine phenothiazine; most commonly used as an antiemetic.

• If more than 4 doses are needed in 24-hour period, notify doctor.

promazine hydrochloride
Promabec♦♦, Promanyl♦♦, Promazettes♦♦, Sparine♦

INDICATIONS & DOSAGE
Psychosis—
Adults: 25 to 200 mg P.O. or I.M. q 4 to 6 hours, up to 1 g daily. I.V. dose in concentrations no greater than 25 mg/ml for acutely agitated patients. Initial dose 50 to 150 mg; repeat within 5 to 10 minutes if necessary.
Children over 12: 10 to 25 mg P.O. or I.M. q 4 to 6 hours.

SIDE EFFECTS
Blood: *transient leukopenias, agranulocytosis.*
CNS: *extrapyramidal reactions (moderate incidence), sedation (high incidence),* pseudoparkinsonism, EEG changes, dizziness.
CV: *orthostatic hypotension,* tachycardia, EKG changes.
EENT: *ocular changes, blurred vision.*
GI: *dry mouth, constipation.*
GU: *urinary retention,* dark urine, menstrual irregularities, gynecomastia, inhibited ejaculation.
Hepatic: *cholestatic jaundice.*
Metabolic: hyperprolactinemia.
Skin: *mild photosensitivity,* dermal allergic reactions, *exfoliative dermatitis.*
Local: pain on I.M. injection, sterile abscess.
Other: weight gain, increased appetite.
After abrupt withdrawal: gastritis, nausea, vomiting, dizziness, tremors, feeling of warmth or cold, sweating, tachycardia, headache, insomnia.

INTERACTIONS
Antacids: inhibited absorption of oral phenothiazines. Separate antacid and phenothiazine dosage by at least 2 hours.

Italicized side effects are common or life-threatening.

Anticholinergics (including antidepressant and antiparkinson agents): increased anticholinergic activity, aggravated parkinson-like symptoms. Use with caution.

Barbiturates: may decrease phenothiazine effect. Observe patient.

NURSING CONSIDERATIONS

• Contraindicated in coma, CNS depression, bone marrow depression, subcortical damage, use of spinal or epidural anesthetic or adrenergic blocking agents. Use cautiously with other CNS depressants, anticholinergics; in hepatic disease, elderly or debilitated patients, arteriosclerosis or cardiovascular disease (may cause sudden drop in blood pressure), exposure to extreme heat or cold (including antipyretic therapy), respiratory disorders, hypocalcemia, acutely ill or dehydrated children, convulsive disorders, severe reactions to insulin or electroshock therapy, suspected brain tumor or intestinal obstruction, glaucoma, prostatic hypertrophy.
• Hold dose and notify doctor if patient develops jaundice, symptoms of blood dyscrasias (fever, sore throat, infection, cellulitis, weakness), persistent (longer than a few hours) extrapyramidal reactions, or such reactions during pregnancy or in children.
• Monitor therapy by weekly bilirubin tests during first month; periodic blood tests (CBC, hepatic function); and ophthalmic tests (long-term use).
• Check intake/output for urinary retention or constipation.
• Tell patient to use sunscreening agents and protective clothing to avoid photosensitivity reactions.
• Warn against activities that require alertness or good psychomotor coordination until response to drug is determined. Drowsiness and dizziness usually subside after a few weeks.
• Avoid combining with alcohol or other depressants.

• Monitor blood pressure lying and standing.
• Watch for orthostatic hypotension, especially with parenteral administration. Keep patient supine for 1 hour afterward. Advise patient to change positions slowly.
• Give I.M. only in upper outer quadrant of buttocks. Massage slowly afterward to prevent sterile abscess. Injection may sting.
• Protect from light. Slight yellowing of injection or concentrate is common; does not affect potency. Discard markedly discolored solutions.
• Prevent contact dermatitis by keeping drug off patient's skin and clothes.
• Dilute liquid concentrate with fruit juice, milk, semisolid food, or chocolate-flavored drinks just before giving. For best taste, use at least 10 ml diluent per 25 mg drug.
• Do not withdraw abruptly unless required by severe side effects.
• Dry mouth may be relieved with sugarless gum, sour hard candy, or rinsing with mouthwash.
• Drug is an aliphatic phenothiazine; rarely used for psychiatric treatment.

thioridazine hydrochloride
Mellaril♦, Novoridazine♦♦

INDICATIONS & DOSAGE
Psychosis—
Adults: initially, 50 to 100 mg P.O. t.i.d., with gradual increments up to 800 mg daily in divided doses, if needed. Dosage varies. Dose above 800 mg may be associated with ocular toxicity (pigmentary retinopathy).
Depressive neurosis, alcohol withdrawal, dementia in geriatrics, behavioral problems in children—
Adults: initially, 25 mg P.O. t.i.d. Maintenance dose is 20 to 200 mg daily.
Children over 2 years: 0.5 to 3 mg/ Kg daily in divided doses.

SIDE EFFECTS
Blood: *transient leukopenias, agranulocytosis.*
CNS: extrapyramidal reactions (low incidence), *sedation (high incidence),* EEG changes, dizziness.
CV: *orthostatic hypotension,* tachycardia, EKG changes.
EENT: *ocular changes, blurred vision,* pigmentary retinopathy.
GI: *dry mouth, constipation.*
GU: *urinary retention,* dark urine, menstrual irregularities, gynecomastia, inhibited ejaculation.
Hepatic: *cholestatic jaundice.*
Metabolic: hyperprolactinemia.
Skin: *mild photosensitivity,* dermal allergic reactions, *exfoliative dermatitis.*
Other: weight gain, increased appetite.
After abrupt withdrawal: gastritis, nausea, vomiting, dizziness, tremors, feeling of warmth or cold, sweating, tachycardia, headache, insomnia.

INTERACTIONS
Antacids: inhibited absorption of oral phenothiazines. Separate antacid and phenothiazine dosage by at least 2 hours.
Barbiturates: may decrease phenothiazine effect. Observe patient.

NURSING CONSIDERATIONS
• Contraindicated in coma, CNS depression, bone marrow depression, hypertensive or hypotensive cardiac disease, subcortical damage, use of spinal or epidural anesthetic or adrenergic blocking agents. Use cautiously with other CNS depressants, anticholinergics; in hepatic disease, elderly or debilitated patients, arteriosclerosis or cardiovascular disease (may cause sudden drop in blood pressure), exposure to extreme heat or cold (including antipyretic therapy), respiratory disorders, hypocalcemia, acutely ill or dehydrated children, convulsive disorders, severe reactions to insulin or electroshock therapy, suspected brain tumor or intestinal obstruction, glaucoma, or prostatic hypertrophy.
• Hold dose and notify doctor if patient develops jaundice, symptoms of blood dyscrasias (fever, sore throat, infection, cellulitis, weakness), persistent (longer than a few hours) extrapyramidal reactions, or such reactions during pregnancy or in children.
• Monitor therapy by weekly bilirubin tests during first month; periodic blood tests (CBC, hepatic function); and ophthalmic tests (long-term therapy).
• Check intake/output for urinary retention or constipation.
• Watch for blurred vision, dry mouth; high incidence of anticholinergic effects.
• Tell patient to use sunscreening agents and protective clothing to avoid photosensitivity reactions.
• Monitor blood pressure.
• Warn against activities that require alertness or good psychomotor coordination until response to drug is determined. Drowsiness and dizziness usually subside after a few weeks.
• Avoid combining with alcohol or other depressants.
• Watch for orthostatic hypotension, especially with parenteral administration. Advise patient to change positions slowly.
• Prevent contact dermatitis by keeping drug off patient's skin and clothes.
• Dilute liquid concentrate with water or fruit juice just before giving.
• Do not withdraw abruptly unless required by severe side effects.
• Dry mouth may be relieved with sugarless gum, sour hard candy, or rinsing with mouthwash.
• Piperidine phenothiazine; used to continue antipsychotic therapy when parkinsonian effects require withdrawal of other phenothiazines.
• Dose of 100 mg is therapeutic equivalent of 100 mg chlorpromazine.

Italicized side effects are common or life-threatening.

thiothixene

thiothixene hydrochloride
Navane♦

INDICATIONS & DOSAGE
Acute agitation—
Adults: 4 mg I.M. b.i.d. to q.i.d.
Maximum 30 mg daily I.M. Change
to P.O. as soon as possible.
Mild to moderate psychosis—
Adults: initially, 2 mg P.O. t.i.d. May
increase gradually to 15 mg daily.
Severe psychosis—
Adults: initially, 5 mg P.O. b.i.d.
May increase gradually to 15 to 30 mg
daily. Maximum recommended daily
dose 60 mg.
Not recommended in children under
12.

SIDE EFFECTS
Blood: *transient leukopenias, agranulocytosis.*
CNS: *extrapyramidal reactions (high
incidence),* sedation (low incidence),
pseudoparkinsonism, EEG changes,
dizziness.
CV: *orthostatic hypotension,* tachycardia, EKG changes.
EENT: *ocular changes, blurred
vision.*
GI: *dry mouth, constipation.*
GU: *urinary retention,* dark urine,
menstrual irregularities, gynecomastia, inhibited ejaculation.
Hepatic: *cholestatic jaundice.*
Metabolic: hyperprolactinemia.
Skin: *mild photosensitivity,* dermal
allergic reactions, *exfoliative dermatitis.*
Local: pain on I.M. injection, sterile
abscess.
Other: weight gain, increased appetite.
After abrupt withdrawal: gastritis,
nausea, vomiting, dizziness, tremors,
feeling of warmth or cold, sweating,
tachycardia, headache, insomnia.

INTERACTIONS
None significant.

NURSING CONSIDERATIONS
• Contraindicated in convulsive seizures, circulatory collapse, coma,
CNS depression, blood dyscrasias,
bone marrow depression, alcohol
withdrawal, akathisia or restlessness,
subcortical damage, use of spinal or
epidural anesthetic or adrenergic
blocking agents. Use cautiously with
other CNS depressants, anticholinergics; in hepatic disease, elderly or debilitated patients, arteriosclerosis or
cardiovascular disease (may cause
sudden drop in blood pressure), exposure to extreme heat or cold (including antipyretic therapy), or undue
sunlight, respiratory disorders, hypocalcemia, severe reactions to insulin
or electroshock therapy, suspected
brain tumor or intestinal obstruction,
glaucoma, or prostatic hypertrophy.
• Hold dose and notify doctor if patient develops jaundice, symptoms of
blood dyscrasias (fever, sore throat,
infection, cellulitis, weakness), persistent (longer than a few hours) extrapyramidal reactions, or any such
reactions during pregnancy.
• Monitor therapy by weekly bilirubin tests during first month; periodic
blood tests (CBC, hepatic function);
and ophthalmic tests (long-term
therapy).
• Check intake/output for urinary retention or constipation.
• Tell patient to use sunscreening
agents and protective clothing to
avoid photosensitivity reactions.
• Warn against activities that require
alertness or good psychomotor coordination until response to drug is determined. Drowsiness and dizziness
usually subside after a few weeks.
• Avoid combining with alcohol or
other depressants.
• Watch for orthostatic hypotension,
especially with parenteral administration. Keep patient supine for 1 hour

afterward. Advise patient to change positions slowly.
• Give I.M. only in upper outer quadrant of buttocks or midlateral thigh. Massage slowly afterward to prevent sterile abscess. Injection may sting.
• I.M. form must be stored in refrigerator.
• Slight yellowing of injection or concentrate is common; does not affect potency. Discard markedly discolored solutions.
• Prevent contact dermatitis by keeping drug off patient's skin and clothes.
• Dilute liquid concentrate with fruit juice, milk, or semisolid food just before giving.
• Do not withdraw abruptly unless required by severe side effects.
• Dry mouth may be relieved with sugarless gum, sour hard candy, or rinsing with mouthwash.
• Drug is a thioxanthene derivative but produces responses similar to phenothiazine, butyrophenones, and chlorprothixene.
• Dose of 4 mg is therapeutic equivalent of 100 mg chlorpromazine.

---

trifluoperazine hydrochloride
Clinazine♦♦, Novoflurazine♦♦, Pentazine♦♦, Solazine♦♦, Stelazine♦, Terfluzine♦♦, Triflurin♦♦, Tripazine♦♦

INDICATIONS & DOSAGE
Anxiety states—
Adults: 1 to 2 mg P.O. b.i.d.
Schizophrenia and other psychotic disorders—
Adults: outpatients—1 to 2 mg P.O. b.i.d., up to 4 mg daily;
hospitalized— 2 to 5 mg P.O. b.i.d.; may gradually increase to 40 mg daily. 1 to 2 mg I.M. q 4 to 6 hours, p.r.n. More than 6 mg daily is rarely needed.
Children 6 to 12 years (hospitalized or under close supervision): 1 mg P.O. daily or b.i.d.; may increase gradually to 15 mg daily.

SIDE EFFECTS
Blood: *transient leukopenias, agranulocytosis.*
CNS: *extrapyramidal reactions (high incidence),* sedation (low incidence), pseudoparkinsonism, EEG changes, dizziness.
CV: *orthostatic hypotension,* tachycardia, EKG changes.
EENT: *ocular changes, blurred vision.*
GI: *dry mouth, constipation.*
GU: *urinary retention,* dark urine, menstrual irregularities, gynecomastia, inhibited ejaculation.
Hepatic: *cholestatic jaundice.*
Metabolic: hyperprolactinemia.
Skin: *mild photosensitivity,* dermal allergic reactions, *exfoliative dermatitis.*
Local: pain on I.M. injection, sterile abscess.
Other: weight gain, increased appetite.
After abrupt withdrawal: gastritis, nausea, vomiting, dizziness, tremors, feeling of warmth or cold, sweating, tachycardia, headache, insomnia.

INTERACTIONS
Antacids: inhibited absorption of oral phenothiazines. Separate antacid and phenothiazine dosage by at least 2 hours.
Barbiturates: may decrease phenothiazine effect. Observe patient.

NURSING CONSIDERATIONS
• Contraindicated in coma, CNS depression, bone marrow depression, subcortical damage, use of spinal or epidural anesthetic or adrenergic blocking agents. Use cautiously with other CNS depressants, anticholinergics; in hepatic disease, elderly or debilitated patients, arteriosclerosis or cardiovascular disease (may cause drop in blood pressure), exposure to

---

Italicized side effects are common or life-threatening.

extreme heat or cold (including anti-pyretic therapy), respiratory disorders, hypocalcemia, acutely ill or dehydrated children, convulsive disorders, severe reactions to insulin or electroshock therapy, suspected brain tumor or intestinal obstruction, glaucoma, or prostatic hypertrophy.

• Hold dose and notify doctor if patient develops jaundice, symptoms of blood dyscrasias (fever, sore throat, infection, cellulitis, weakness), persistent (longer than a few hours) extrapyramidal reactions, or any such reactions during pregnancy or in children.

• Monitor therapy by weekly bilirubin tests during first month; periodic blood tests (CBC, hepatic function); and ophthalmic tests (long-term therapy).

• Check intake/output for urinary retention or constipation.

• Tell patient to use sunscreening agents and protective clothing to avoid photosensitivity reactions.

• Warn against activities that require alertness or good psychomotor coordination until response to drug is determined. Drowsiness and dizziness usually subside after a few weeks.

• Avoid combining with alcohol or other depressants.

• Watch for orthostatic hypotension, especially with parenteral administration. Keep patient supine for 1 hour afterward. Advise patient to change positions slowly.

• Give deep I.M. only in upper outer quadrant of buttocks. Massage slowly afterward to prevent sterile abscess. Injection may sting.

• Protect from light. Slight yellowing of injection or concentrate is common; does not affect potency. Discard markedly discolored solutions.

• Prevent contact dermatitis by keeping drug off patient's skin and clothes.

• Dilute liquid concentrate with 60 ml tomato or fruit juice, carbonated beverages, coffee, tea, milk, water, or semisolid food just before giving.

• Do not withdraw abruptly unless required by severe side effects.

• Dry mouth may be relieved with sugarless gum, sour hard candy, or rinsing with mouthwash.

• Drug is a prototype piperazine phenothiazine.

• Dose of 5 mg is therapeutic equivalent of 100 mg chlorpromazine.

---

triflupromazine hydrochloride
Vesprin

INDICATIONS & DOSAGE

Acute, severe agitation—
Adults: 60 to 150 mg I.M. in 2 or 3 divided doses.
Children over 2½ years: 0.2 to 0.25 mg/Kg in divided doses. Maximum dose 10 mg daily.
Nausea and vomiting—
Adults: 20 to 30 mg P.O. daily; or 1 to 3 mg I.V. daily; or 5 to 15 mg I.M. daily up to maximum 60 mg daily.
Children: 0.2 mg/Kg P.O. or I.M. up to maximum 10 mg daily.
Psychotic disorders (mild to moderate symptoms)—
Adults: 10 to 25 mg P.O. b.i.d.
Children over 2½ years: 10 mg P.O. t.i.d.
Elderly or debilitated: 10 mg b.i.d. or t.i.d.; increase gradually to desired effect.
Severe symptoms—
Adults: 50 mg P.O. b.i.d. or t.i.d.
Children over 2½ years: 2 mg/Kg P.O. in 3 divided doses; may increase gradually to 150 mg daily.

SIDE EFFECTS

Blood: *transient leukopenias, agranulocytosis.*
CNS: *extrapyramidal reactions (moderate incidence), sedation (high inci-*

dence), pseudoparkinsonism, EEG changes, dizziness.
CV: *orthostatic hypotension,* tachycardia, EKG changes.
EENT: *ocular changes, blurred vision.*
GI: *dry mouth, constipation.*
GU: *urinary retention,* dark urine, menstrual irregularities, gynecomastia, inhibited ejaculation.
Hepatic: *cholestatic jaundice.*
Metabolic: hyperprolactinemia.
Skin: *mild photosensitivity,* dermal allergic reactions, *exfoliative dermatitis.*
Local: pain on I.M. injection, sterile abscess.
Other: weight gain, increased appetite.
After abrupt withdrawal: gastritis, nausea, vomiting, dizziness, tremors, feeling of warmth or cold, sweating, tachycardia, headache, insomnia.

INTERACTIONS
Antacids: inhibited absorption of oral phenothiazines. Separate antacid and phenothiazine dosage by at least 2 hours.
Anticholinergics (including antidepressant and antiparkinson agents): increased anticholinergic activity, aggravated parkinson-like symptoms. Use with caution.
Barbiturates: may decrease phenothiazine effect. Observe patient.

NURSING CONSIDERATIONS
• Contraindicated in coma, CNS depression, blood dyscrasias, bone marrow depression, subcortical brain damage, use of spinal or epidural anesthestic or adrenergic blocking agents. Use cautiously with other CNS depressants, anticholinergics; in hepatic disease, elderly or debilitated patients, arteriosclerosis or cardiovascular disease (may cause sudden drop in blood pressure), exposure to extreme heat or cold (including antipyretic therapy), respiratory disorders, pheochromocytoma, hypocalcemia, acutely ill or dehydrated children, convulsive disorders, severe reactions to insulin or electroshock therapy, suspected brain tumor or intestinal obstruction, glaucoma, prostatic hypertrophy.
• Hold dose and notify doctor if patient develops jaundice, symptoms of blood dyscrasias (fever, sore throat, infection, cellulitis, weakness), persistent (longer than a few hours) extrapyramidal reactions, or any such reactions during pregnancy or in children.
• Monitor therapy by weekly bilirubin tests during first month; periodic blood tests (CBC, hepatic function); and ophthalmic tests in long-term therapy.
• Check intake/output for urinary retention or constipation.
• Watch for hypothermia reactions.
• Tell patient to use sunscreening agents and protective clothing to avoid photosensitivity reactions.
• Warn against activities that require alertness or good psychomotor coordination until response to drug is determined. Drowsiness and dizziness usually subside after a few weeks.
• Avoid combining with alcohol or other depressants.
• Watch for orthostatic hypotension, especially with parenteral administration. Keep patient supine for 1 hour afterward. Advise patient to change positions slowly.
• Give I.M. only in upper outer quadrant of buttocks. Massage slowly afterward to prevent sterile abscess. Injection may sting.
• Protect from light. Slight yellowing of injection or concentrate is common; does not affect potency. Discard markedly discolored solutions.
• Keep liquid suspension tightly closed.
• Prevent contact dermatitis by keeping drug off patient's skin and clothes.

Italicized side effects are common or life-threatening.

• Do not withdraw abruptly unless required by severe side effects.
• Dry mouth may be relieved with sugarless gum, sour hard candy, or rinsing with mouthwash.

• Drug is an aliphatic phenothiazine.
• Dose of 25 mg is therapeutic equivalent of 10 mg chlorpromazine.

28

Miscellaneous psychotherapeutics

lithium carbonate
lithium citrate

---

lithium carbonate
Carbolith♦♦, Eskalith, Lithane♦, Lithizine♦♦, Lithobid, Lithonate, Lithotabs
lithium citrate
Lithonate-S

INDICATIONS & DOSAGE
Prevention or control of mania—
Adults: 300 to 600 mg P.O. up to 4 times daily, increasing on the basis of serum levels to achieve optimal dosage. Recommended therapeutic serum lithium levels: 1 to 1.5 mEq/liter for acute mania; 0.6 to 1.2 mEq/liter for maintenance therapy; and 2 mEq/liter as maximum.
Adults: 5 ml lithium citrate (liquid) contains 8 mEq lithium equal to 300 mg lithium carbonate.

SIDE EFFECTS
Blood: *leukocytosis of 14,000 to 18,000 (reversible).*
CNS: tremors, drowsiness, headache, confusion, restlessness, dizziness, psychomotor and mental retardation, stupor, lethargy, coma, blackouts, epileptiform seizures, EEG changes, impaired speech, ataxia, muscle weakness, incoordination, hyperexcitability.
CV: *reversible EKG changes*, arrhythmia, hypotension, peripheral circulatory failure and collapse, allergic vasculitis, ankle and wrist edema.
EENT: tinnitus, impaired vision.
GI: nausea, vomiting, anorexia, diarrhea, fecal incontinence, dry mouth, thirst, metallic taste.
GU: *polyuria*, glycosuria, incontinence, renal toxicity.
Metabolic: transient hyperglycemia, goiter, hypothyroidism (lowered T_3, T_4, and PBI, but elevated ^{131}I uptake), hyponatremia.
Skin: pruritus, rash, diminished or lost sensation.

INTERACTIONS
Diuretics: increased reabsorption of lithium by kidneys, with possible toxic effect. Use with extreme caution, and monitor lithium and electrolyte levels (especially sodium).
Haloperidol: encephalopathic syndrome (lethargy, tremors, extrapyramidal symptoms). Watch for syndrome, and stop drug if it occurs.
Aminophylline, sodium bicarbonate and sodium chloride: ingestion of these salts increases lithium excretion. Avoid salt loads and monitor lithium levels.
Probenecid, methyldopa: increased effect of lithium. Monitor for lithium toxicity.

NURSING CONSIDERATIONS
• Contraindicated if therapy cannot be closely monitored. Use with caution with haloperidol; other antipsychotics; neuromuscular blocking agents; in elderly or debilitated persons; thyroid disease; epilepsy; in

renal or cardiovascular disease; brain damage; severe debilitation or dehydration; sodium depletion; with diuretic usage.

• Monitor baseline EKG, thyroid and renal studies, and electrolyte levels. Monitor serum lithium levels 8 to 12 hours after first dose, usually before a.m. dose, 2 to 3 times weekly first month, then weekly to monthly on maintenance.

• When serum levels of lithium are below 1.5 mEq/liter, side effects generally remain mild.

• Check fluid intake and output, especially when surgery is scheduled.

• Warn patient and family to watch for signs of toxicity (diarrhea, vomiting, drowsiness, muscular weakness, ataxia) and to expect transient nausea, polyuria, thirst, and discomfort during first few days. He should withhold 1 dose and call doctor if toxic symptoms appear, but not stop drug abruptly.

• Expect lag of 1 to 3 weeks before drug's beneficial effects are noticed.

• Adjust fluid and salt ingestion to compensate if excessive loss occurs through protracted sweating or diarrhea.

• Have outpatient follow-up of thyroid and renal functions every 6 to 12 months. Palpate thyroid to check for enlargement.

• Patient should carry identification/instruction card (available from pharmacy) with toxicity and emergency information.

• Warn ambulatory patient to avoid activities that require alertness and good psychomotor coordination until response to drug is determined.

• Check urine for specific gravity and report level below 1.015.

• Has been used to treat syndrome of inappropriate ADH.

• Tell patient not to switch brands of lithium without doctor's guidance.

• Investigationally used to increase white cells in patients undergoing cancer chemotherapy.

• Also used investigationally for treatment of cluster headaches, aggression, organic brain syndrome, and tardive dyskinesia.

29

Cerebral stimulants

amphetamine hydrochloride
amphetamine phosphate
amphetamine sulfate
benzphetamine hydrochloride
caffeine
caffeine, citrated
caffeine sodium benzoate
chlorphentermine hydrochloride
clortermine hydrochloride
deanol acetamidobenzoate
dextroamphetamine phosphate
dextroamphetamine sulfate
diethylpropion hydrochloride
fenfluramine hydrochloride
mazindol
methamphetamine hydrochloride
methylphenidate hydrochloride
pemoline
phendimetrazine tartrate
phenmetrazine hydrochloride
phentermine hydrochloride

---

amphetamine hydrochloride

amphetamine phosphate

amphetamine sulfate
Controlled Substance Schedule II
Benzedrine ♦

INDICATIONS & DOSAGE
Minimal brain dysfunction—
Children 6 years and older: 5 mg
P.O. daily, with 5 mg increments
weekly, p.r.n.
Children 3 to 5 years: 2.5 mg P.O.
daily, with 2.5 mg increments weekly,
p.r.n.
Narcolepsy—

Adults: 5 to 60 mg P.O. daily in divided doses.
Children over 12 years: 10 mg P.O.
daily, with 10 mg increments weekly,
p.r.n.
Children 6 to 12 years: 5 mg P.O.
daily, with 5 mg increments weekly,
p.r.n.
*Short-term adjunct in exogenous
obesity—*
Adults: single 10 or 15 mg long-acting capsule daily, or 2 if needed, up to
30 mg daily; or 5 to 30 mg daily in divided doses 30 to 60 minutes before
meals.
Not recommended for children under
12 years old.

SIDE EFFECTS
CNS: *restlessness,* tremor, *hyperactivity, talkativeness, insomnia,* irritability, dizziness, headache, chills, overstimulation, dysphoria.
CV: *tachycardia, palpitations,* hypertension, hypotension.
GI: nausea, vomiting, cramps, dry
mouth, diarrhea, constipation, metallic taste, anorexia, weight loss.
Other: urticaria, impotence, changes
in libido.

INTERACTIONS
MAO inhibitors: severe hypertension;
possible hypertensive crisis. Don't
use together.
Sodium bicarbonate, acetazolamide:
increased renal reabsorption. Monitor
for enhanced effect.
Ammonium chloride, ascorbic acid:
observe for decreased amphetamine
effect.

Phenothiazines, haloperidol: observe for decreased amphetamine effect.

NURSING CONSIDERATIONS
• Contraindicated in symptomatic cardiovascular diseases, hyperthyroidism, nephritis, diabetes mellitus, angina pectoris, moderate to severe hypertension, parkinsonism due to arteriosclerosis, certain types of glaucoma, advanced arteriosclerosis, agitated states, or history of drug abuse. Use with caution in elderly, debilitated, or hyperexcitable patients.
• Psychic dependence or habituation may occur, especially in patients with history of drug addiction. Avoid prolonged administration. When used long-term, lower dosage gradually to prevent acute rebound depression.
• When used for obesity, make sure patient is also on a weight reduction program. Give drug 30 to 60 minutes before meals.
• Fatigue may result as drug effects wear off. Patient will need more rest.
• Tell patient to avoid caffeine drinks, which increase the effects of amphetamines and related amines.
• Check vital signs regularly for signs of excessive stimulation.
• Urinary acidification enhances renal excretion; urinary alkalinization enhances renal reabsorption and recycling.
• When tolerance to anorexic effect develops, dosage should not be increased, but drug discontinued.
• Discourage use to combat fatigue.
• Warn patient to avoid activities that require alertness or good psychomotor coordination until response to drug is determined.
• May alter daily insulin needs. Monitor blood sugar and fractional urine.
• Use as analeptic is usually discouraged, since CNS stimulation superimposed on CNS depression can lead to neuronal instability and seizures.
• May reverse beneficial effect of

antihypertensives. Monitor blood pressure.

benzphetamine hydrochloride
Controlled Substance Schedule III
Didrex

INDICATIONS & DOSAGE
Short-term adjunct in exogenous obesity—
Adults: 25 to 50 mg P.O. daily, b.i.d., or t.i.d.

SIDE EFFECTS
CNS: *restlessness,* tremor, *hyperactivity, talkativeness, insomnia,* irritability, dizziness, headache, chills, overstimulation, dysphoria.
CV: *tachycardia, palpitations,* hypertension, hypotension.
GI: nausea, vomiting, cramps, dry mouth, diarrhea, constipation, metallic taste, anorexia, weight loss.
Other: urticaria, impotence, changes in libido.

INTERACTIONS
MAO inhibitors: severe hypertension; possible hypertensive crisis. Don't use together.
Sodium bicarbonate, acetazolamide: increased renal reabsorption. Monitor for enhanced effects.
Ammonium chloride, ascorbic acid: observe for decreased benzphetamine effects.
Phenothiazines, haloperidol: observe for decreased benzphetamine effects.

NURSING CONSIDERATIONS
• Contraindicated in symptomatic cardiovascular diseases, hyperthyroidism, nephritis, diabetes mellitus, angina pectoris, moderate to severe hypertension, parkinsonism due to arteriosclerosis, certain types of glaucoma, advanced arteriosclerosis, agitated states, or history of drug abuse.

Use with caution in elderly, debilitated, or hyperexcitable patients.
• Psychic dependence or habituation may occur, especially in patients with history of drug addiction. Avoid prolonged administration. When used long-term, lower dosage gradually to prevent acute rebound depression.
• Use in conjunction with weight reduction program. Give 30 to 60 minutes before meals.
• Fatigue may result as drug effects wear off. Patient will need more rest.
• Tell patient to avoid caffeine drinks, which increase the effects of amphetamines and related amines.
• Check vital signs regularly for signs of excessive stimulation.
• Urinary acidification enhances renal excretion; urinary alkalinization enhances renal reabsorption and recycling.
• When tolerance to anorexic effect develops, dosage should not be increased, but drug discontinued.
• Warn patient to avoid activities that require alertness or good psychomotor coordination until response to drug is determined.
• May alter daily insulin needs. Monitor blood sugar and fractional urine.

---

caffeine
Ban-Drowz, Kirkaffein, Nodoz, Stim 250, Stim-Tabs, Tirend, Vivarin
caffeine, citrated

caffeine sodium benzoate injection

INDICATIONS & DOSAGE
Respiratory and central nervous system stimulant—
Adults: 100 to 200 mg anhydrous caffeine P.O.; 500 mg to 1 g I.M. caffeine sodium benzoate or I.V. in emergency only.

SIDE EFFECTS
CNS: *stimulation, insomnia,* restlessness, nervousness, mild delirium, headache, excitement, agitation, muscle tremors, twitches.
CV: *tachycardia.*
GI: nausea, vomiting.
GU: *diuresis.*
Skin: hyperesthesia.

INTERACTIONS
None significant.

NURSING CONSIDERATIONS
• Contraindicated for patients with gastric or duodenal ulcer.
• Tolerance or psychological dependence may develop.
• Be alert for signs of overdose: GI pain, mild delirium, insomnia, diuresis, dehydration, and fever. Treat with short-acting barbiturates, gastric emesis, or lavage.
• Single dose should not exceed 1 g.
• Caffeine content in cola beverages, 17 to 55 mg/180 ml; tea, 40 to 100 mg/180 ml; instant coffee, 60 to 180 mg/180 ml; brewed coffee, 100 to 150 mg/180 ml.
• Caffeine does not reverse alcohol intoxication or depressant effects of alcohol. Overvigorous therapy with caffeine may aggravate depression in an already depressed patient.
• Use as analeptic is discouraged.

---

chlorphentermine hydrochloride
Controlled Substance Schedule III
Chlorophen, Pre-Sate♦

INDICATIONS & DOSAGE
Short-term adjunct in exogenous obesity—
Adults: 65 mg P.O. taken after breakfast.

SIDE EFFECTS
CNS: *insomnia,* overstimulation, ner-

---

vousness, dizziness, paradoxical sedation, headache.
CV: *tachycardia, palpitations,* increased blood pressure.
GI: nausea, dry mouth, constipation.
Skin: urticaria.

INTERACTIONS
MAO inhibitors: severe hypertension; possible hypertensive crisis. Don't use together.
Sodium bicarbonate, acetazolamide: increased renal reabsorption. Monitor for enhanced effects.
Ammonium chloride, ascorbic acid: observe for decreased chlorphentermine effects.

NURSING CONSIDERATIONS
• Contraindicated in hyperexcitability states, hyperthyroidism, hypertension, angina pectoris, severe cardiovascular disease, glaucoma, or history of drug abuse.
• Psychic dependence and habituation may occur. When tolerance to anorexic effect develops, dose should not be increased, but stop drug.
• May alter daily insulin needs. Monitor blood sugar and fractional urine.
• Teach patient a good dietary plan and exercise program.
• Withdraw drug gradually.
• Fatigue may result as drug effects wear off. Patient will need more rest.
• Tell patient to avoid caffeine drinks, which increase the effects of amphetamines and related amines.
• Check vital signs regularly. Observe for signs of excessive stimulation.
• Urinary acidification enhances renal excretion; urinary alkalinization enhances renal reabsorption and recycling.

clortermine hydrochloride
Controlled Substance Schedule III
Voranil

INDICATIONS & DOSAGE
Short-term adjunct in exogenous obesity—
Adults: 50 mg P.O. taken at midmorning.

SIDE EFFECTS
CNS: *restlessness,* dizziness, *insomnia,* euphoria, tremor, headache.
CV: *tachycardia, palpitations,* arrhythmias, increased blood pressure.
GI: dry mouth, diarrhea, constipation.
Skin: urticaria.
Other: impotence, libido changes.

INTERACTIONS
MAO inhibitors: severe hypertension; possible hypertensive crisis. Don't use together.
Sodium bicarbonate, acetazolamide: increased renal reabsorption. Monitor for enhanced effects.
Ammonium chloride, ascorbic acid: observe for decreased clortermine effects.

NURSING CONSIDERATIONS
• Contraindicated in hyperthyroidism, glaucoma, severe hypertension, cardiovascular diseases, agitated states, history of drug abuse. Use with caution in diabetes mellitus. Insulin requirements may be altered. Monitor blood sugar and fractional urine.
• Warn patient to avoid activities that require alertness or good psychomotor coordination until response to drug is determined.
• Be sure patient is following a sensible dietary regimen.
• Drug should be discontinued when tolerance develops.
• Fatigue may result as drug effects wear off. Patient will need more rest.

- Tell patient to avoid caffeine drinks, which increase the effects of amphetamines and related amines.
- Check vital signs regularly. Observe for signs of excessive stimulation.
- Urinary acidification enhances renal excretion; urinary alkalinization enhances renal reabsorption and recycling.

---

deanol acetamidobenzoate
Deaner, Deaner-100♦♦, Deaner-250

INDICATIONS & DOSAGE
Minimal brain dysfunction—
Children over 6 years: initially, 500 mg P.O. daily after breakfast; may reduce to maintenance 250 to 500 mg daily. Dose adjusted to patient's needs and response.
Dyskinesia, blepharospasm—
Adults: 600 mg to 1.6 g P.O. daily.

SIDE EFFECTS
CNS: insomnia, mild overstimulation, irritability, headache, muscle twitching, tenseness.
CV: postural hypotension.
EENT: increased nasal and oral secretions.
GI: constipation.
Skin: transient rash.
Other: dyspnea.

INTERACTIONS
None significant.

NURSING CONSIDERATIONS
- Contraindicated for patients with grand mal epilepsy.
- In long-term use, monitor child closely for signs of growth suppression.
- Beneficial effects may not appear until after several weeks of therapy.
- Used with some success in treatment of tardive dyskinesia.

---

dextroamphetamine phosphate

dextroamphetamine sulfate
Controlled Substance Schedule II
Dexampex, Dexedrine♦, Ferndex, Robese, Spancap #1 and #4, Tidex

---

INDICATIONS & DOSAGE
Narcolepsy—
Adults: 5 to 60 mg P.O. daily in divided doses.
Children over 12 years: 10 mg P.O. daily, with 10 mg increments weekly, p.r.n.
Children 6 to 12 years: 5 mg P.O. daily, with 5 mg increments weekly, p.r.n.
Short-term adjunct in exogenous obesity—
Adults: single 10 to 15 mg long-acting capsule, up to 30 mg daily; or in divided doses, 5 to 10 mg 1/2 hour before meals.
Minimal brain dysfunction—
Children 6 years and over: 5 mg once daily or b.i.d., with 5 mg increments weekly, p.r.n.
Children 3 to 5 years: 2.5 mg P.O. daily, with 2.5 mg increments weekly, p.r.n.

SIDE EFFECTS
CNS: *restlessness,* tremor, *hyperactivity, talkativeness, insomnia,* irritability, dizziness, headache, chills, overstimulation, dysphoria.
CV: *tachycardia, palpitations,* hypertension, hypotension.
GI: nausea, vomiting, cramps, dry mouth, diarrhea, constipation, metallic taste, anorexia, weight loss.
Other: urticaria, impotence, changes in libido.

INTERACTIONS
MAO inhibitors: severe hypertension; possible hypertensive crisis. Don't use together.
Sodium bicarbonate, acetazolamide:

---

increased renal reabsorption. Monitor for enhanced amphetamine effects.
Ammonium chloride, ascorbic acid: observe for decreased amphetamine effects.
Phenothiazines, haloperidol: observe for decreased amphetamine effects.

NURSING CONSIDERATIONS
• Contraindicated in hyperthyroidism, nephritis, diabetes mellitus, severe hypertension, angina pectoris or other severe cardiovascular disease, some types of glaucoma, or history of drug abuse. Use with caution in elderly, debilitated, or hyperexcitable patients.
• Psychic dependence or habituation may occur, especially in patients with history of drug addiction. Avoid prolonged administration. When used long-term, lower dosage gradually to prevent acute rebound depression.
• When used for obesity, be sure patient is also on a weight reduction program. Give 30 to 60 minutes before meals. Avoid giving within 6 hours of bedtime.
• Fatigue may result as drug effects wear off. Patient will need more rest.
• Tell patient to avoid caffeine drinks, which increase the effects of amphetamines and related amines.
• Check vital signs regularly. Observe for signs of excessive stimulation.
• Urinary acidification enhances renal excretion; urinary alkalinization enhances renal reabsorption and recycling.
• When tolerance to anorexic effect develops, dosage should not be increased, but drug discontinued.
• Discourage use to combat fatigue.
• Warn patient to avoid activities that require alertness or good psychomotor coordination until response to drug is determined.
• May alter daily insulin needs. Monitor blood sugar and fractional urine.
• Use as analeptic is usually discour-

aged, since CNS stimulation superimposed on CNS depression can lead to neuronal instability and seizures.

---

diethylpropion hydrochloride
Controlled Substance Schedule IV
Dietec♦♦, D.I.P.♦♦, Nobesine♦♦,
NuDispoz, o.b.c.t., Regibon♦♦, Ro-Diet, Tenuate♦, Tepanil

INDICATIONS & DOSAGE
Short-term adjunct in exogenous obesity—
Adults: 25 mg P.O. before meals, t.i.d.; or 75 mg controlled-release tablet P.O. in midmorning.

SIDE EFFECTS
CNS: headache, *nervousness, dizziness.*
CV: *tachycardia, palpitations,* rise in blood pressure.
EENT: blurred vision.
GI: nausea, abdominal cramps, dry mouth, diarrhea, constipation.
Skin: urticaria.
Other: impotence, libido changes, menstrual upset.

INTERACTIONS
MAO inhibitors: hypertension; possible hypertensive crisis. Don't use together.

NURSING CONSIDERATIONS
• Contraindicated in hyperthyroidism, hypertension, angina pectoris, severe cardiovascular disease, glaucoma, or history of drug abuse. Use with caution in epilepsy, diabetes mellitus, or hyperexcitability states. May alter insulin requirements. Monitor blood sugar and fractional urine.
• When tolerance to anorexic effect develops, dosage should not be increased, but drug discontinued.
• Habituation or psychic dependence may occur.

Unmarked trade names available in the United States only.
♦ Also available in Canada ♦♦ Available in Canada only.

- Be sure patient is also on a weight reduction program.
- Can be used to stop nighttime eating. Rarely causes insomnia.
- Fatigue may result as drug effects wear off. Patient will need more rest.
- Tell patient to avoid caffeine drinks, which increase the effects of amphetamines and related amines.
- Check vital signs regularly. Observe for signs of excessive stimulation.
- Urinary acidification enhances renal excretion; urinary alkalinization enhances renal reabsorption and recycling.
- Use as analeptic is usually discouraged, since CNS stimulation superimposed on CNS depression can lead to neuronal instability and seizures.

fenfluramine hydrochloride
Controlled Substance Schedule IV
Pondimin♦

INDICATIONS & DOSAGE
Short-term adjunct in exogenous obesity—
Adults: initially, 20 mg P.O. t.i.d. before meals. Maximum 40 mg t.i.d. Adjust dosage according to patient's response.

SIDE EFFECTS
CNS: dizziness, incoordination, headache, euphoria or depression, anxiety, *insomnia,* weakness or fatigue, agitation.
CV: *palpitations,* hypotension, hypertension, chest pain.
EENT: eye irritation, blurred vision.
GI: diarrhea, dry mouth, nausea, vomiting, abdominal pain, constipation.
GU: dysuria, increased urinary frequency, impotence, increased libido.
Skin: rashes, urticaria, burning sensation.
Other: sweating, chills, fever.

INTERACTIONS
MAO inhibitors: severe hypertension; possible hypertensive crisis. Don't use together.

NURSING CONSIDERATIONS
- Contraindicated in glaucoma, hypersensitivity to sympathomimetic amines, symptomatic cardiovascular disease, history of drug abuse, or alcoholism. Use with caution in hypertension, history of mental depression, diabetes mellitus.
- Because of possible hypoglycemia, diabetics may have altered insulin or sulfonylureas requirements. Monitor blood sugar and fractional urine.
- Check vital signs regularly. Observe patient for signs of excessive sedation, depression, or excessive stimulation. Closely monitor blood pressure.
- Be sure patient is on a weight reduction program.
- Tolerance or dependence may occur. Avoid prolonged administration.
- Fatigue may result as drug effects wear off. Patient will need more rest.
- Tell patient to avoid caffeine drinks, which increase the effects of amphetamines and related amines.

mazindol
Controlled Substance Schedule IV
Sanorex♦

INDICATIONS & DOSAGE
Short-term adjunct in exogenous obesity—
Adults: 1 mg t.i.d. 1 hour before meals, or 2 mg daily 1 hour before lunch. Use lowest effective dose.

SIDE EFFECTS
CNS: *nervousness,* restlessness, dizziness, *insomnia,* dysphoria, headache, depression, drowsiness, weakness, tremors.
CV: *palpitations, tachycardia.*

GI: dry mouth, nausea, constipation, diarrhea, unpleasant taste.
GU: difficulty initiating micturition, impotence, libido changes.
Skin: rash, clamminess, pallor.
Other: shivering, excessive sweating.

INTERACTIONS
MAO inhibitors: severe hypertension; possible hypertensive crisis. Don't use together.

NURSING CONSIDERATIONS
• Contraindicated in glaucoma, cardiovascular disease including arrhythmias, agitated states, history of drug abuse. Use with caution in diabetes mellitus, hypertension, hyperexcitability states.
• Warn patient to avoid activities that require alertness or good psychomotor coordination until response has been determined.
• Fatigue may result as drug effects wear off. Patient will need more rest.
• Tell patient to avoid caffeine drinks, which increase the effects of amphetamines and related amines.
• Check vital signs regularly. Observe for signs of excessive stimulation.
• Tolerance or dependence may develop. Avoid prolonged use.
• Be sure patient is also on a weight reduction program.
• May alter insulin needs. Monitor blood sugar and fractional urine.

---

methamphetamine hydrochloride
Controlled Substance Schedule II
Desoxyn, Methampex, Obedrin-LA

INDICATIONS & DOSAGE
Minimal brain dysfunction—
Children 6 years and over: 2.5 to 5 mg P.O. once daily or b.i.d., with 5 mg increments weekly, p.r.n. Usual effective dosage is 20 to 25 mg daily.
Short-term adjunct in exogenous obesity—
Adults: 2.5 to 5 mg P.O. once to t.i.d. 30 minutes before meals; or 1 long-acting 5 to 15 mg tablet daily before breakfast.

SIDE EFFECTS
CNS: *nervousness, insomnia,* irritability, *talkativeness,* dizziness, headache, hyperexcitability, tremor.
CV: hypertension or hypotension, *tachycardia, palpitations,* cardiac arrhythmias.
EENT: blurred vision, mydriasis.
GI: nausea, vomiting, abdominal cramps, diarrhea or constipation, dry mouth, anorexia, metallic taste.
GU: impotence, libido changes.
Skin: urticaria.

INTERACTIONS
MAO inhibitors: severe hypertension; possible hypertensive crisis. Don't use together.
Sodium bicarbonate, acetazolamide: increased renal reabsorption. Monitor for enhanced effects.
Ammonium chloride, ascorbic acid: observe for decreased amphetamine effects.
Phenothiazines, haloperidol: observe for decreased amphetamine effects.

NURSING CONSIDERATIONS
• Contraindicated in hypertension, hyperthyroidism, nephritis, angina pectoris or other severe cardiovascular disease, diabetes, glaucoma, parkinsonism due to arteriosclerosis, agitated states, or history of drug abuse. Use with caution in patients who are elderly, debilitated, asthenic, psychopathic, or who have a history of suicidal or homicidal tendencies.
• Warn that potential for abuse is high. Discourage use to combat fatigue.
• May alter insulin needs. Monitor blood sugar and fractional urine.
• When used for obesity, be sure

Unmarked trade names available in the United States only.
♦ Also available in Canada   ♦♦ Available in Canada only.

patient is on a weight reduction program.
• Tell patient to avoid caffeine drinks, which increase the effects of amphetamines and related amines.
• Check vital signs regularly. Observe for signs of excessive stimulation.
• Urinary acidification enhances renal excretion; urinary alkalinization enhances renal reabsorption and recycling.
• When tolerance to anorexic effect develops, dosage should not be increased, but drug discontinued.
• Warn patient to avoid activities that require alertness or good psychomotor coordination until response to drug is determined.

---

methylphenidate hydrochloride
Controlled Substance Schedule II
Methidate♦♦, Ritalin♦

INDICATIONS & DOSAGE
Minimal brain dysfunction (hyperkinetic behavior disorders)—
Children 6 years and over: initial dose 5 to 10 mg P.O. daily before breakfast and lunch, with 5 to 10 mg increments weekly as needed, up to 60 mg daily.
Narcolepsy—
Adults: 10 mg P.O. b.i.d. or t.i.d. ½ hour before meals. Dosage varies with patient needs. Dosage range is 5 to 50 mg daily.

SIDE EFFECTS
CNS: *nervousness, insomnia,* dizziness, headache, akathisia, dyskinesia.
CV: *palpitations,* angina, *tachycardia,* changes in blood pressure and pulse rate.
EENT: difficulty with accommodation and blurring of vision.
GI: nausea, dry throat, abdominal pain, anorexia, weight loss.

Skin: rash, urticaria, *exfoliative dermatitis,* erythema multiforme.

INTERACTIONS
MAO inhibitors: severe hypertension; possible hypertensive crisis. Don't use together.

NURSING CONSIDERATIONS
• Contraindicated in symptomatic cardiac disease; hyperthyroidism; moderate to severe hypertension; angina pectoris; advanced arteriosclerosis; severe depression of either endogenous or exogenous forms; glaucoma; history of drug abuse or dependency; history of marked anxiety, tension, or agitation; parkinsonism. Use with caution in elderly, debilitated, or hyperexcitable patients and those with history of cardiovascular disease, diabetes, or seizures.
• Closely monitor blood pressure. Observe for signs of excessive stimulation.
• Discourage use to combat fatigue.
• Observe for interactions, as treatment of other disease states may be affected. May alter daily insulin needs. Monitor blood sugar and fractional urine. May decrease seizure threshold in seizure disorder patients.
• Drug of choice for minimal brain dysfunction. Usually stopped postpuberty.
• Used in treatment for nocturnal enuresis in children.
• Periodic CBC, differential, and platelet counts advised with long-term use.
• Tolerance, psychic dependence or habituation may develop, especially in patients with history of drug addiction. High abuse potential. Avoid prolonged administration. When used long-term, lower dosage gradually to prevent acute rebound depression.
• Fatigue may result as drug effects wear off. Patient will need more rest.
• Tell patient to avoid caffeine drinks,

Italicized side effects are common or life-threatening.

which increase the effects of amphetamines and related amines.
• Warn patient to avoid activities that require alertness or good psychomotor coordination until response to drug is determined.

pemoline
Controlled Substance Schedule IV
Cylert

INDICATIONS & DOSAGE
Minimal brain dysfunction—
Children 6 years and over: initially, 37.5 mg P.O. given in the morning. Daily dose can be raised by 18.75 mg weekly. Effective dosage range 56.25 to 75 mg daily; maximum is 112.5 mg daily.

SIDE EFFECTS
CNS: *insomnia*, malaise, irritability, fatigue, mild depression, dizziness, headache, drowsiness, hallucinations, nervousness (large doses), seizures.
CV: tachycardia (large doses).
GI: anorexia, abdominal pain, nausea, diarrhea.
Hepatic: liver enzyme elevations.
Skin: rash.

INTERACTIONS
None significant.

NURSING CONSIDERATIONS
• Use with caution in impaired renal function. Drug may accumulate.
• Safety and efficacy for more than 2 years of administration has not been established. Closely monitor patients on long-term therapy for possible hepatic function abnormalities and for growth suppression.
• Structurally dissimilar to amphetamines or methylphenidate.
• Therapeutic effects may not be evident for 2 to 3 weeks.

phendimetrazine tartrate
Controlled Substance Schedule IV
Adphen, Anorex, Bacarate, Banobese, Bontril PDM, Delcozine, Di-Ap-Trol, Ex-Obese, Limit, Melfiat, Metra, Minus, Obalan, Obepar, Obeval, Obezine, Phenazine◆, Phenzine, Plegine, Ropledge, Sprx 1,2,3, Sprx-105, Statobex, Trimstat, Trimtabs, Weightrol

INDICATIONS & DOSAGE
Short-term adjunct in exogenous obesity—
Adults: 35 mg P.O. 2 to 3 times daily 1 hour before meals. Maximum dosage is 70 mg t.i.d. Use lowest effective dosage. Adjust dose to individual response.

SIDE EFFECTS
CNS: *nervousness, dizziness, insomnia,* tremor, headache.
CV: *tachycardia, palpitations,* rise in blood pressure.
EENT: blurred vision.
GI: dry mouth, nausea, abdominal cramps, diarrhea or constipation.
GU: dysuria.

INTERACTIONS
MAO inhibitors: severe hypertension; possible hypertensive crisis. Don't use together.
Sodium bicarbonate, acetazolamide: increased renal reabsorption. Monitor for enhanced effects.
Ammonium chloride, ascorbic acid: observe for decreased phendimetrazine effects.
Phenothiazines, haloperidol: observe for decreased effect.

NURSING CONSIDERATIONS
• Contraindicated in hyperthyroidism, hypertension, angina pectoris or other severe cardiovascular disease, glaucoma. Use with caution in hyperexcitability states or history of addiction.

Unmarked trade names available in the United States only.
◆ Also available in Canada   ◆◆ Available in Canada only.

- Warn patient to avoid activities that require alertness or good psycho-motor coordination until response to drug has been determined.
- Be sure patient is following weight reduction program.
- Tolerance or dependence can develop. Not advised for prolonged use.
- Fatigue may result as drug effects wear off. Patient will need more rest.
- Tell patient to avoid caffeine drinks, which increase the effects of amphetamines and related amines.
- Check vital signs regularly. Observe for signs of excessive stimulation.
- Urinary acidification enhances renal excretion; urinary alkalinization enhances renal reabsorption and recycling.
- May alter daily insulin needs. Monitor blood sugar and fractional urine.

---

phenmetrazine hydrochloride
Controlled Substance Schedule II
Preludin

INDICATIONS & DOSAGE
Short-term adjunct in exogenous obesity—
Adults: 25 mg P.O. b.i.d. or t.i.d. 1 hour before meals, up to 75 mg daily; or single 50 to 75 mg extended-release tablet daily in midmorning.

SIDE EFFECTS
CNS: *nervousness,* dizziness, *insomnia,* headache.
CV: *tachycardia, palpitations,* increased blood pressure.
EENT: blurred vision.
GI: dry mouth, nausea, abdominal cramps, constipation.
GU: libido changes, impotence.
Skin: urticaria.

INTERACTIONS
MAO inhibitors: severe hypertension;

possible hypertensive crisis. Don't use together.
Sodium bicarbonate, acetazolamide: increased renal reabsorption. Monitor for enhanced effects.
Ammonium chloride, ascorbic acid: observe for decreased phenmetrazine effects.
Phenothiazines, haloperidol: observe for decreased effect.

NURSING CONSIDERATIONS
- Contraindicated in hyperthyroidism, hypertension, angina pectoris or other cardiovascular disease, glaucoma, or history of drug abuse. Use with caution in hyperexcitability states.
- Tolerance or dependence may develop. High abuse potential. Not advised for prolonged use.
- Be sure patient is also following weight reduction program.
- Administer 1 hour before meals.
- Fatigue may result as drug effects wear off. Patient will need more rest.
- Tell patient to avoid caffeine drinks, which increase the effects of amphetamines and related amines.
- Check vital signs regularly. Observe for signs of excessive stimulation.
- Urinary acidification enhances renal excretion; urinary alkalinization enhances renal reabsorption and recycling.

---

phentermine hydrochloride
Controlled Substance Schedule IV
Adipex, Anoxine, Fastin, Ionamin♦, Parmine, Phentrol, Rolaphent, Wilpowr

INDICATIONS & DOSAGE
Short-term adjunct in exogenous obesity—
Adults: 8 mg P.O. t.i.d. ½ hour before meals; or 15 to 30 mg daily before breakfast (resin complex).

SIDE EFFECTS

CNS: *nervousness*, dizziness, *insomnia*.
CV: *palpitations, tachycardia*, increased blood pressure.
GI: dry mouth, unpleasant taste, nausea, constipation, diarrhea.
GU: libido changes, impotence.
Skin: urticaria.

INTERACTIONS

MAO inhibitors: severe hypertension; possible hypertensive crisis. Don't use together.
Sodium bicarbonate, acetazolamide: increased renal reabsorption. Monitor for enhanced effects.
Ammonium chloride, ascorbic acid: observe for decreased phentermine effects.
Phenothiazines, haloperidol: observe for decreased effect.

NURSING CONSIDERATIONS

• Contraindicated in hyperthyroidism, hypertension, angina pectoris or other severe cardiovascular disease, glaucoma. Use with caution in hyperexcitability states or history of drug addiction.
• Tolerance or dependence may develop. Avoid prolonged administration.
• Use with weight reduction program. Give 30 minutes before meals.
• Fatigue may result as drug effects wear off. Patient will need more rest.
• Tell patient to avoid caffeine drinks, which increase the effects of amphetamines and related amines.
• Check vital signs regularly. Observe for signs of excessive stimulation.
• Urinary acidification enhances renal excretion; urinary alkalinization enhances renal reabsorption and recycling.

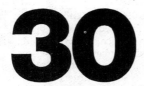

Respiratory stimulants

ammonia, aromatic spirits
doxapram hydrochloride
nikethamide
pentylenetetrazol

ammonia, aromatic spirits

INDICATIONS & DOSAGE
Fainting—
Adults and children: inhale as
needed.

SIDE EFFECTS
None reported.

INTERACTIONS
None significant.

NURSING CONSIDERATIONS
• Stimulates mucous membranes of
upper respiratory tract.

doxapram hydrochloride
Dopram♦

INDICATIONS & DOSAGE
*Postanesthesia respiratory stimulant,
drug-induced central nervous system
depression, and chronic pulmonary
disease associated with acute hypercapnia—*
Adults: 0.5 to 1 mg/Kg of body
weight (up to 2 mg/Kg in CNS
depression), I.V. injection or infusion.
Maximum 4 mg/Kg, up to 3 g in 1
day. Infusion rate 1 to 3 mg/min (initial: 5 mg/min for postanesthesia).

*Chronic obstructive pulmonary
disease—*
Adults: infusion, 1 to 2 mg/min.
Maximum 3 mg/min for a maximum
duration of 2 hours.

SIDE EFFECTS
CNS: headache, dizziness, apprehension, disorientation, pupillary dilation, bilateral Babinski signs, flushing, sweating, pruritus, paresthesias.
CV: chest pain and tightness, variations in heart rate.
GI: nausea, vomiting, diarrhea.
GU: urinary retention, or stimulation
of the urinary bladder with spontaneous voiding.
Other: sneezing, coughing, laryngospasm, bronchospasm, hiccups, rebound hypoventilation.

INTERACTIONS
MAO inhibitors: potentiated adverse
cardiovascular effects. Use together
cautiously.

NURSING CONSIDERATIONS
• Contraindicated in epilepsy, convulsive disorders, head injury, cardiovascular disorders, frank uncompensated heart failure, severe hypertension, cerebrovascular accidents, respiratory failure or incompetence secondary to neuromuscular disorders,
muscle paresis, flail chest, obstructed
airway, pulmonary embolism, pneu-
mothorax, restrictive respiratory disease, acute bronchial asthma, extreme
dyspnea, hypoxia not associated with
hypercapnia. Use with caution in
bronchial asthma, severe tachycardia

or cardiac arrhythmias, cerebral edema or increased cerebrospinal fluid pressure, hyperthyroidism, pheochromocytoma, or profound metabolic disorders.
• Establish adequate airway before administering drug. Prevent patient from aspirating vomitus.
• Monitor blood pressure, heart rate, deep tendon reflexes, and arterial blood gases before giving drug and every 30 minutes afterward.
• Be alert for signs of overdosage: hypertension, tachycardia, arrhythmias, skeletal muscle hyperactivity, dyspnea. Discontinue if patient shows signs of increased arterial carbon dioxide or oxygen tension, or if mechanical ventilation is started. May give I.V. injection of anticonvulsant for convulsions.
• Use only in surgical or emergency room situations.
• Do not combine with alkaline solutions.

nikethamide
Coramine♦, Kardonyl♦♦

INDICATIONS & DOSAGE
Adults:
Acute alcoholism—1.25 to 5 g I.V.; repeat as necessary.
Carbon monoxide poisoning—1.25 to 2.5 g I.V. initially, then 1.25 g q 5 minutes for first hour, depending on response.
Cardiac arrest—125 to 250 mg intracardially associated with anesthetic overdose.
Combat respiratory paralysis—3.75 g I.V.; repeat as required.
Overcome respiratory depression—1.25 to 2.5 g I.V.
Shock—2.5 to 3.75 g I.V. or I.M. initially; repeat as indicated.
Shorten narcosis—1 g I.V. or I.M.
Neonates:

Adjunct in neonatal asphyxia—375 mg injected into umbilical vein. Oral maintenance:
Adults and children: 3 to 5 ml oral solution q 4 to 6 hours.

SIDE EFFECTS
CNS: restlessness, muscle twitching or fasciculations.
CV: increase in heart rate, respiratory rate, and blood pressure.
EENT: unpleasant burning or itching at back of nose.
GI: nausea, vomiting.
Other: flushing, feeling of warmth, fear, sneezing, coughing, sweating.

INTERACTIONS
None significant.

NURSING CONSIDERATIONS
• Monitor patient's respiratory rate and volume.
• Mechanical support of breathing is often preferred over nikethamide.
• Don't inject intra-arterially; arterial spasm and thrombosis may result.
• Watch for signs of overdosage: muscle tremors or spasm, retching, tachycardia, arrhythmias, hyperpyrexia, hyperpnea, convulsions, psychotic reactions, postictal depression. May give I.V. injection of diazepam or barbiturate such as thiopental sodium for convulsions. Induced emesis and gastric lavage aren't effective.

pentylenetetrazol
Metrazol, Nelex-100, Nioric, Petrazole

INDICATIONS & DOSAGE
Overdose of CNS depressants—
Adults: 100 to 500 mg I.V. Repeat, if necessary, followed by 100 to 200 mg I.M., p.r.n.
In depression from barbiturates—5 ml of 10% solution I.V. within 3 to

5 seconds. If necessary, may be repeated until patient awakens.
To improve mental and physical activity in elderly patients—
Adults: 100 to 200 mg P.O. t.i.d.

SIDE EFFECTS

Few side effects with oral administration; narrow margin of safety with parenteral administration.
Signs of overdose:
CNS: fasciculations, clonic convulsions.
CV: slight increases in blood pressure, bradycardia.
GI: nausea, vomiting.
Other: hypersalivation, coughing, hyperthermia.

INTERACTIONS

None significant.

NURSING CONSIDERATIONS

• Use with caution in history of seizures or focal brain lesion. If dosage is high, use with caution in heart disease.
• Analeptic use is not recommended.
• False positive response to HCG pregnancy test.

31

Cholinergics (parasympathomimetics)

ambenonium chloride
bethanechol chloride
edrophonium chloride
neostigmine bromide
neostigmine methylsulfate
physostigmine salicylate
pyridostigmine bromide

---

ambenonium chloride
Mytelase♦

INDICATIONS & DOSAGE
Symptomatic treatment of myasthenia gravis in patients who cannot take neostigmine bromide and pyridostigmine bromide—
Adults: dose must be individualized for each patient, but usually ranges from 5 to 25 mg P.O. q 3 to 4 hours while awake. Starting dose usually 5 mg P.O. q 3 to 4 hours. Increase gradually and adjust at 1- to 2-day intervals to avoid drug accumulation and overdosage. May range from 5 to as much as 75 mg per dose.

SIDE EFFECTS
CNS: headache, dizziness, muscle weakness, convulsions, mental confusion, jitters, sweating, respiratory depression.
CV: bradycardia, hypotension.
EENT: miosis.
GI: *nausea, vomiting, diarrhea, abdominal cramps,* increased salivation.
GU: urinary frequency, incontinence.
Other: bronchospasm, *muscle cramps,* bronchoconstriction.

INTERACTIONS
Procainamide, quinidine: may reverse cholinergic effect on muscle. Observe for lack of drug effect.

NURSING CONSIDERATIONS
• Contraindicated in patients with mechanical obstruction of intestine or urinary tract, bradycardia, hypotension.
• Use with extreme caution in bronchial asthma.
• Use cautiously in patients with epilepsy, recent coronary occlusion, vagotonia, hyperthyroidism, cardiac arrhythmias, peptic ulcer.
• Avoid large dose in patients with decreased gastrointestinal motility or megacolon.
• Discontinue all other cholinergic drugs before administering this drug.
• Watch patient very closely for side effects, particularly if total dose is greater than 200 mg daily. Side effects may indicate drug toxicity. Notify doctor immediately if they develop.
• Monitor and document vital signs frequently, being especially careful to check respirations. Position patient to make breathing easier. Always have atropine injection readily available and be prepared to give atropine 0.5 mg S.C. or slow I.V. push, and provide respiratory support if needed.
• Administer each dose exactly as ordered, on time. Amount and frequency of dosage should vary with patient's activity level. The doctor will probably order larger doses to be given when patient is fatigued, for ex-

ample, in the afternoon and at meal-time.

• If muscle weakness is severe, doctor must determine if this is caused by drug toxicity or exacerbation of myasthenia gravis. A test dose of edrophonium I.V. will aggravate drug-induced weakness but will temporarily relieve weakness that results from the disease.

• Observe and record the patient's variations in muscle strength. Show him how to do it himself.

• When given for myasthenia gravis, explain to patient that this drug will relieve symptoms of lid drooping, double vision, difficulty in chewing and swallowing, trunk and limb weakness. Stress the importance of taking this drug exactly as ordered. Explain to patient and his family that he must take this drug for the rest of his life. Teach them about the disease and the drug's effect on symptoms.

• Monitor intake and output.

• Patient may develop resistance to drug.

• Seek approval when indicated for hospitalized patient to have bedside supply of tablets to take himself. Patients with long-standing disease often insist on this.

• Give with milk or food to produce fewer muscarinic side effects.

---

bethanechol chloride
Duvoid, Mictrol-10, Mictrol-25, Myotonachol, Urecholine♦, Urolax, Vesicholine

INDICATIONS & DOSAGE
Acute postop and postpartum nonobstructive (functional) urinary retention, neurogenic atony of urinary bladder with retention, abdominal distention, megacolon—
Adults: 10 to 30 mg P.O. t.i.d. to q.i.d. Never give I.M. or I.V. When used for urinary retention, some pa-

tients may require 50 to 100 mg P.O. per dose. Use such doses with extreme caution.
Test dose: 2.5 mg S.C. repeated at 15- to 30-minute intervals to total of 4 doses to determine the minimal effective dose; then use minimal effective dose q 6 to 8 hours. All doses must be adjusted individually.

SIDE EFFECTS
Dose-related:
CNS: headache, malaise.
CV: bradycardia, hypotension, *cardiac arrest,* tachycardia.
EENT: lacrimation, miosis.
GI: *abdominal cramps, diarrhea,* salivation, nausea, vomiting, belching, borborygmi.
GU: urinary urgency.
Skin: flushing.
Other: bronchoconstriction, sweating.

INTERACTIONS
Procainamide, quinidine: may reverse cholinergic effects on muscle. Observe for lack of drug effect.

NURSING CONSIDERATIONS
• Contraindicated in patients with uncertain strength or integrity of bladder wall; when increased muscular activity of GI or urinary tract is harmful; in mechanical obstructions of GI or urinary tract; in hyperthyroidism; peptic ulcer; latent or active bronchial asthma; cardiac or coronary artery disease; vagotonia; epilepsy; Parkinson's disease; bradycardia; chronic obstructive pulmonary disease; hypotension. Use cautiously in hypertension, vasomotor instability, peritonitis, or other acute inflammatory conditions of GI tract.
• NEVER give I.M. or I.V.; could cause circulatory collapse, hypotension, severe abdominal cramping, bloody diarrhea, shock, cardiac arrest.
• Should stop all other cholinergics before giving this drug.

Italicized side effects are common or life-threatening.

- Watch closely for side effects which may indicate drug toxicity, especially with S.C. administration.
- Monitor vital signs frequently, being especially careful to check respirations. Position patient to make breathing easier. Always have atropine injection readily available and be prepared to give atropine 0.5 mg S.C. or slow I.V. push, and provide respiratory support if needed.
- If used to treat urinary retention, make sure bedpan is handy. Monitor intake and output.
- When used to prevent abdominal distention and GI distress, the doctor may also order a rectal tube inserted to help passage of gas.
- Poor and variable oral absorption requires larger oral doses. Oral and S.C. doses are *NOT* interchangeable.
- Drug usually effective 5 to 15 minutes after injection and 30 to 90 minutes after oral use.
- Give on empty stomach; if taken after meals may cause nausea and vomiting.

---

edrophonium chloride
Tensilon◆

INDICATIONS & DOSAGE

As a curare antagonist (to reverse neuromuscular blocking action)—
Adults: 10 mg I.V. given over 30 to 45 seconds. Dose may be repeated as necessary to 40 mg maximum dose per patient. Larger doses may potentiate rather than antagonize effect of curare.
Diagnostic aid in myasthenia gravis (The "Tensilon Test")—
Adults: 1 to 2 mg I.V. within 15 to 30 seconds, then 8 mg if no response (increase in muscle strength).
Children over 34 Kg: 2 mg I.V. If no response within 45 seconds, give 1 mg q 45 seconds to maximum of 10 mg.

Children up to 34 Kg: 1 mg I.V. If no response within 45 seconds, give 1 mg q 45 seconds to maximum of 5 mg.
Infants: 0.5 mg I.V.
To differentiate myasthenic crisis from cholinergic crisis—
Adults: 1 mg I.V. If no response in 1 minute, repeat dose once. Increased muscular strength confirms myasthenic crisis; no increase or exaggerated weakness confirms cholinergic crisis.
Paroxysmal supraventricular tachycardia—
Adults: 10 mg I.V. given over 1 minute or less.

SIDE EFFECTS

CNS: weakness, respiratory paralysis.
CV: hypotension, bradycardia.
EENT: miosis.
GI: nausea, vomiting, *diarrhea, abdominal cramps,* excessive salivation.
Other: increased bronchial secretions, bronchospasm, muscle cramps, muscle fasciculation, sweating.

INTERACTIONS

Procainamide, quinidine: may reverse cholinergic effects on muscle. Observe for lack of drug effect.

NURSING CONSIDERATIONS

- Contraindicated in mechanical obstruction of intestine or urinary tract, bradycardia, hypotension. Use cautiously in hyperthyroidism, cardiac disease, peptic ulcer, bronchial asthma.
- Should stop all other cholinergics before giving this drug.
- Watch closely for side effects; may indicate toxicity.
- Monitor vital signs frequently, being especially careful to check respirations. Position patient to make breathing easier. Always have atropine injection readily available and be prepared to give atropine 0.5 mg S.C.

---

or slow I.V. push, and provide respiratory support if needed.
• When giving drug to differentiate myasthenic crisis from cholinergic crisis, observe patient's muscle strength closely.
• Edrophonium not effective against muscle relaxation induced by decamethonium bromide and succinylcholine chloride.
• This cholinergic has the most rapid onset but shortest duration; therefore not used for treatment of myasthenia gravis.
• For easier parenteral administration, use a tuberculin syringe with an I.V. needle and leave in situ.
• I.M. route may be used in children due to difficulty with I.V. route: for children under 34 Kg, inject 2 mg I.M.; children over 34 Kg, 5 mg I.M. Expect same reactions as with I.V. test, but these appear after 2- to 10-minute delay.
• When used as antidote for curariform drugs, record each dose given.

---

neostigmine bromide
Prostigmin Bromide♦
neostigmine methylsulfate
Prostigmin♦

INDICATIONS & DOSAGE

Antidote for tubocurarine—
Adults: 0.5 to 2 mg I.V. slowly. Repeat p.r.n. Give 0.6 to1.2 mg atropine sulfate I.V. before antidote dose.
*Functional amenorrhea—*1 mg I.M. or S.C. daily for 3 days.
Postop abdominal distention and bladder atony—
Adults: 0.5 to 1 mg I.M. or S.C. q 4 to 6 hours.
Postop ileus—
Adults: 0.25 to 1 mg I.M. or S.C. q 4 to 6 hours.
Treatment of myasthenia gravis—
Adults: 15 to 30 mg t.i.d. (range 15 to 375 mg per day); or 0.5 to 2 mg

I.M. or I.V. q 1 to 3 hours. Dose must be individualized, depending on response and tolerance of side effects. Therapy may be required day and night.
Children: 7.5 to 15 mg P.O. t.i.d. to q.i.d.
Note: 1:1,000 solution of injectable solution contains 1 mg/1 ml; 1:2,000 solution contains 0.5 mg/ml.

SIDE EFFECTS
CNS: dizziness, muscle weakness, mental confusion, jitters, sweating, respiratory depression.
CV: bradycardia, hypotension.
EENT: miosis.
GI: *nausea, vomiting, diarrhea, abdominal cramps,* excessive salivation.
Skin: rash (bromide).
Other: bronchospasm, *muscle cramps,* bronchoconstriction.

INTERACTIONS
Procainamide, quinidine: may reverse cholinergic effect on muscle. Observe for lack of drug effect.

NURSING CONSIDERATIONS
• Contraindicated in hypersensitivity to cholinergics or to bromide, mechanical obstruction of the intestine or urinary tract, bradycardia, hypotension. Use with extreme caution in bronchial asthma. Use cautiously in epilepsy, recent coronary occlusion, peritonitis, vagotonia, hyperthyroidism, cardiac arrhythmias, or peptic ulcer.
• Should stop all other cholinergics before giving this drug.
• Watch closely for side effects; may indicate toxicity.
• Monitor vital signs frequently, being especially careful to check respirations. Position patient to make breathing easier. Always have atropine injection readily available and be prepared to give atropine 0.5 mg S.C. or slow I.V. push, and provide respiratory support if needed.

Italicized side effects are common or life-threatening.

- Difficult to judge optimum dose. Help doctor by documenting patient's response after each dose. Show patient how to observe and record variations in muscle strength.
- When using for myasthenia gravis, explain that this drug will relieve lid drooping, double vision, difficulty in chewing and swallowing, trunk and limb weakness. Stress importance of taking drug exactly as ordered. Explain that drug may have to be taken for life. Explain drug's effect on myasthenic symptoms.
- If patient has dysphagia, schedule dose 30 minutes before each meal.
- When used to prevent abdominal distention and GI distress, the doctor may order a rectal tube inserted to help passage of gas.
- Patients sometimes develop a resistance to neostigmine.
- When used for functional amenorrhea, check for vaginal bleeding and instruct patient to report any vaginal bleeding. If no bleeding in 72 hours after third injection, patient has nonfunctional amenorrhea.
- If muscle weakness is severe, doctor determines if drug-induced toxicity or exacerbation of myasthenia gravis. Test dose of edrophonium I.V. will aggravate drug-induced weakness but will temporarily relieve weakness caused by disease.
- Hospitalized patients with long-standing myasthenia may request bedside supply of tablets. This will enable patient to take each dose precisely when ordered. Seek approval, if indicated, but continue to oversee medication regimen.

---

physostigmine salicylate
Antilirium♦

INDICATIONS & DOSAGE
Anticholinergic poisoning—

Adults: 0.5 to 4 mg I.M. or I.V. q 2 hours.
Tricyclic antidepressant poisoning—
Adults: 0.5 to 3 mg I.M. or I.V. (1 mg per minute I.V.) repeated as necessary if life-threatening signs recur (coma, convulsions, arrhythmias).

SIDE EFFECTS
CNS: hallucinations, muscular twitching, muscle weakness, ataxia, *restlessness, excitability, sweating.*
CV: irregular pulse, palpitations.
EENT: miosis.
GI: nausea, vomiting, epigastric pain, *diarrhea, excessive salivation.*
Other: bronchospasm, bronchial constriction, dyspnea.

INTERACTIONS
Procainamide, quinidine: may reverse cholinergic effects on muscle. Observe for lack of drug effect.

NURSING CONSIDERATIONS
- Use cautiously for preexisting conditions: mechanical obstruction of intestine or urogenital tract, bronchial asthma, gangrene, diabetes, cardiovascular disease, vagotonia, bradycardia, hypotension, epilepsy, Parkinson's disease, hyperthyroidism, peptic ulcer.
- Watch closely for side effects, particularly CNS disturbances. Use side rails if patient becomes restless or hallucinates. Side effects may indicate drug toxicity.
- Monitor vital signs frequently, being especially careful to check respirations. Position patient to make breathing easier. Always have atropine injection readily available and be prepared to give atropine 0.5 mg S.C. or slow I.V. push, and provide respiratory support if needed. Best administered in presence of doctor.
- Use only clear solution. Darkening may indicate loss of potency.
- Give I.V. at controlled rate; use

Unmarked trade names available in the United States only.
♦ Also available in Canada ♦♦ Available in Canada only.

slow, direct injection at no more than 1 mg/minute.
• Only cholinergic that crosses blood/brain barrier; therefore the only one useful for treating CNS effects of anticholinergic or tricyclic toxicity.
• Effectiveness often immediate and dramatic but may be transient and may require repeat dose.

pyridostigmine bromide
Mestinon♦, Regonol♦

INDICATIONS & DOSAGE
Curariform antagonist—
Adults: 10 to 30 mg I.V. preceded by atropine sulfate 0.6 to 1.2 mg I.V.
Myasthenia gravis—
Adults: 60 to 180 mg P.O. b.i.d. or q.i.d. Usual dose 600 mg daily but higher doses may be needed (up to 1,500 mg per day). Give 1/30 of oral dose I.M. or I.V. Dose must be adjusted for each patient, depending on response and tolerance of side effects.

SIDE EFFECTS
CNS: headache (with high doses), weakness, sweating, convulsions.
CV: bradycardia, hypotension.
EENT: miosis.
GI: abdominal cramps, nausea, vomiting, diarrhea, excessive salivation.
Skin: rash.
Local: thrombophlebitis.
Other: bronchospasm, bronchoconstriction, increased bronchial secretions, muscle cramps.

INTERACTIONS
Procainamide, quinidine: may reverse cholinergic effects on muscle. Observe for lack of drug effect.

NURSING CONSIDERATIONS
• Contraindicated in mechanical obstruction of intestine or urinary tract, bradycardia, hypotension. Use with extreme caution in bronchial asthma. Use cautiously in epilepsy, recent coronary occlusion, vagotonia, hyperthyroidism, cardiac arrhythmias, peptic ulcer. Avoid large doses in decreased gastrointestinal motility or megacolon.
• Difficult to judge optimum dosage. Help doctor by recording patient's response after each dose.
• Should stop all other cholinergics before giving this drug.
• Watch closely for side effects; may indicate toxicity.
• Monitor vital signs frequently, being especially careful to check respirations. Position patient to make breathing easier. Always have atropine injection readily available and be prepared to give atropine 0.5 mg S.C. or slow I.V. push, and provide respiratory support if needed.
• If muscle weakness is severe, doctor determines if drug-induced toxicity or exacerbation of myasthenia gravis. Test dose of edrophonium I.V. will aggravate drug-induced weakness but will temporarily relieve weakness caused by disease.
• When using for myasthenia gravis, stress importance of taking drug exactly as ordered, on time, in evenly spaced doses. If doctor has ordered extended-release tablets, explain how these work. Patient must take them at the same time each day, at least 6 hours apart. Explain that he may have to take this drug for life. Tell about drug's effect on myasthenic symptoms.
• Has longest duration of the cholinergics used for myasthenia gravis.
• Available in 60 mg tablets, sustained-release (180 mg) tablets, injection, and syrup.

Italicized side effects are common or life-threatening.

32

Cholinergic blockers (parasympatholytics)

atropine sulfate
benztropine mesylate
biperiden hydrochloride
chlorphenoxamine hydrochloride
cycrimine hydrochloride
glycopyrrolate
procyclidine hydrochloride
scopolamine hydrobromide
trihexyphenidyl hydrochloride

---

atropine sulfate

INDICATIONS & DOSAGE
Antidote for anticholinesterase insecticide poisoning—
Adults and children: 2 mg I.M. or I.V. repeated at hourly intervals until muscarinic symptoms disappear. Severe cases may require up to 6 mg I.M. or I.V. q 1 hour.
Preop for diminishing secretions and blocking cardiac vagal reflexes—
Adults: 0.4 to 0.6 mg I.M. 45 to 60 minutes before anesthesia.
Children: 0.01 mg/Kg I.M. up to a maximum dose of 0.4 mg 45 to 60 minutes before anesthesia.

SIDE EFFECTS
With usual doses of 0.4 to 0.6 mg, there are few side effects other than dry mouth. However, individual tolerance varies greatly.
CNS: disorientation, restlessness, irritability, incoherence, hallucinations, headache.
CV: palpitations, tachycardia, paradoxical bradycardia with doses less than 0.4 mg.

EENT: *dilated pupils, blurred vision,* photophobia, increased intraocular pressure, eye pain, dysphagia.
GI: *constipation, mouth dryness,* nausea, vomiting.
GU: *urinary hesitancy or retention.*
Skin: flushing, dryness.
Other: bronchial plugging, fever.
Side effects above may be due to pending atropine toxicity and are dose-related.

INTERACTIONS
None significant.

NURSING CONSIDERATIONS
• Contraindicated in narrow-angle glaucoma, obstructive uropathy, obstructive disease of GI tract, myasthenia gravis, paralytic ileus, intestinal atony, unstable cardiovascular status in acute hemorrhage, and toxic megacolon. Use with caution in autonomic neuropathy, hyperthyroidism, coronary heart disease, cardiac arrhythmias, congestive heart failure, hypertension, hiatal hernia associated with reflux esophagitis, hepatic or renal disease, ulcerative colitis, in patients over 40 because of the increased incidence of glaucoma, and in children under 6 years. Use with caution in hot or humid environments. Drug-induced heat stroke possible.
• Check all dosages carefully. Even slight overdose could lead to toxicity.
• Monitor vital signs carefully. Watch closely for side effects, especially in elderly or debilitated patients. Call doctor promptly.
• When given I.V., may cause para-

doxical initial bradycardia. Usually disappears within 2 minutes.
- Monitor intake/output. Drug causes urinary retention and hesitancy; have patient void before administering.
- Many of the side effects (such as dry mouth and constipation) are an extension of the drug's pharmacologic activity and may be expected.

benztropine mesylate
Cogentin♦

INDICATIONS & DOSAGE
Acute dystonic reaction—
Adults: 2 mg I.V. or I.M. followed by 1 to 2 mg P.O. b.i.d. to prevent recurrence.
Parkinsonism—
Adults: 0.5 to 6 mg P.O. daily. Initial dose 0.5 mg to 1 mg. Increase 0.5 mg every 5 to 6 days. Adjust dosage to meet individual requirements.

SIDE EFFECTS
CNS: disorientation, restlessness, irritability, incoherence, hallucinations, headache, sedation, depression, muscular weakness.
CV: palpitations, tachycardia, paradoxical bradycardia.
EENT: dilated pupils, blurred vision, photophobia, difficulty swallowing.
GI: *constipation, mouth dryness,* nausea, vomiting, epigastric distress.
GU: urinary hesitancy or retention. Some side effects may be due to pending atropine-like toxicity and are dose-related.

INTERACTIONS
Amantadine: anticholinergic side effects, such as confusion and hallucinations. Reduce dosage before administering amantadine.

NURSING CONSIDERATIONS
- Contraindicated in narrow-angle-glaucoma. Use cautiously in prostatic

hypertrophy, tendency to tachycardia, and in elderly or debilitated patients; produces atropine-like side effects.
- Monitor vital signs carefully. Watch closely for side effects, especially in elderly or debilitated patients. Call doctor promptly.
- Never discontinue this drug abruptly. Dosages must be reduced gradually.
- Warn patient to avoid activities that require alertness until response to drug determined. If patient is to receive single daily dose, give at bedtime.
- Explain that drug may take 2 to 3 days to exert full effect.
- Monitor intake/output.
- Watch for intermittent constipation, distention, abdominal pain; may be onset of paralytic ileus.
- Relieve dry mouth with cool drinks, ice chips, sugarless gum, or hard candy.
- To help prevent gastric irritation, administer after meals.

biperiden hydrochloride or lactate
Akineton♦

INDICATIONS & DOSAGE
Extrapyramidal disorders—
Adults: 2 to 6 mg P.O. daily, b.i.d., or t.i.d., depending on severity. Usual dose is 2 mg daily, or 2 mg I.M. or I.V. q ½ hour, not to exceed 4 doses or 8 mg total daily.
Parkinsonism—
Adults: 2 mg P.O. t.i.d. to q.i.d.

SIDE EFFECTS
CNS: disorientation, euphoria, restlessness, irritability, incoherence, dizziness, increased tremor.
CV: transient postural hypotension.
EENT: blurred vision.
GI: *constipation, mouth dryness,* nausea, vomiting, epigastric distress.

Italicized side effects are common or life-threatening.

GU: urinary hesitancy or retention. Side effects are dose-related and may resemble atropine toxicity.

INTERACTIONS
None significant.

NURSING CONSIDERATIONS
• Use with caution in prostatism, cardiac arrhythmias, narrow-angle glaucoma.
• Monitor vital signs carefully. Watch closely for side effects, especially in elderly or debilitated patients. Call doctor promptly.
• Give oral doses with or after meals to decrease GI side effects.
• When giving parenterally, keep patient supine. Parenteral administration may cause transient postural hypotension and coordination disturbances.
• Because of possible dizziness, assist patient when he gets out of bed.
• Tolerance may develop, requiring increased dosage.
• In severe parkinsonism, tremors may increase as spasticity is relieved.
• Relieve dry mouth with cool drinks, ice chips, sugarless gum, or hard candy.
• I.V. injections should be made very slowly.

---

chlorphenoxamine hydrochloride
Phenoxene♦

INDICATIONS & DOSAGE
Parkinsonism—
Adults: 50 mg P.O. t.i.d.; in severe cases, 300 to 400 mg daily, 100 mg t.i.d. to q.i.d.

SIDE EFFECTS
CNS: drowsiness, sedation, increased tremors.
EENT: blurred vision.

GI: *constipation, dry mouth,* nausea, vomiting, epigastric distress.

INTERACTIONS
None significant.

NURSING CONSIDERATIONS
• Use cautiously in narrow-angle glaucoma, tachycardia, or prostatic hypertrophy.
• Monitor vital signs carefully. Watch closely for side effects, especially in elderly or debilitated patients. Call doctor promptly.
• Warn patient to avoid activities that require alertness until reaction to drug is determined.
• Administer doses with milk after meals to decrease GI side effects.
• In severe parkinsonism, tremors may increase as spasticity is relieved.
• Tolerance may develop, requiring increased dosage.
• Relieve dry mouth with cool drinks, ice chips, sugarless gum, or hard candy.

---

cycrimine hydrochloride
Pagitane Hydrochloride

INDICATIONS & DOSAGE
Idiopathic and arteriosclerotic parkinsonism—
Adults: initially, 1.25 to 2.5 mg P.O. t.i.d.; gradually increase dosage to 5 mg q.i.d.
Postencephalitic parkinsonism—
Adults: 5 mg t.i.d. or up to 5 mg q 2 hours while awake.

SIDE EFFECTS
CNS: disorientation, incoherence, weakness, drowsiness, dizziness.
EENT: blurred vision.
GI: epigastric distress, sore mouth and tongue, *constipation, mouth dryness.* Also transient nausea and anorexia 30 minutes to 1 hour after administration.

Unmarked trade names available in the United States only.
♦ Also available in Canada   ♦♦ Available in Canada only.

Skin: flushing, dryness, rash.
Other: fever.

INTERACTIONS
None significant.

NURSING CONSIDERATIONS
• Use with caution in narrow-angle glaucoma; in the elderly with arteriosclerotic changes; in tachycardia or tendency toward urinary retention.
• Monitor vital signs carefully.
• Watch closely for side effects, especially vertigo, disorientation, and weakness. Call doctor promptly; he may want to stop or reduce dosage.
• Explain that mild side effects, such as dry mouth, blurred vision, epigastric distress, disappear with continued administration.
• Administer doses with milk or after meals to decrease GI side effects.
• Relieve dry mouth with cool drinks, ice chips, sugarless gum, or hard candy.

---

glycopyrrolate
Robinul

INDICATIONS & DOSAGE
To reverse neuromuscular blockade—
Adults: 0.2 mg I.V. for each 1 mg neostigmine or equivalent dose of pyridostigmine. May be given intravenously without dilution or may be added to dextrose injection and given by infusion.
Preop to diminish secretions and block cardiac vagal reflexes—
Adults: 0.002 mg/lb of body weight I.M. 30 to 60 minutes before anesthesia.

SIDE EFFECTS
CNS: disorientation, irritability, incoherence, weakness, nervousness, drowsiness, dizziness, headache.
CV: palpitations, tachycardia, paradoxical bradycardia.

EENT: *dilated pupils, blurred vision,* photophobia, increased intraocular pressure, difficulty swallowing.
GI: *constipation, mouth dryness,* nausea, vomiting, epigastric distress.
GU: urinary hesitancy or retention.
Skin: flushing, dryness, rash.
Local: burning at injection site.
Other: bronchial plugging, fever.

INTERACTIONS
None significant.

NURSING CONSIDERATIONS
• Contraindicated in narrow-angle glaucoma, obstructive uropathy, obstructive disease of the GI tract, myasthenia gravis, paralytic ileus, intestinal atony, unstable cardiovascular status in acute hemorrhage, toxic megacolon. Use with caution in autonomic neuropathy, hyperthyroidism, coronary heart disease, cardiac arrhythmias, congestive heart failure, hypertension, hiatal hernia associated with reflux esophagitis, hepatic or renal disease, ulcerative colitis, and patients over 40 because of increased incidence of glaucoma. Use with caution in hot or humid environments. Drug-induced heat stroke possible.
• Check all dosages carefully. Even slight overdose could lead to toxicity.
• Don't mix with I.V. solution containing sodium chloride or bicarbonate.
• Monitor vital signs carefully. Watch closely for side effects, especially in elderly or debilitated patients. Call doctor promptly.
• Monitor intake/output. Causes urinary retention or hesitancy.
• Side effects less likely than with other parasympatholytics, unless dosages are excessive.

---

procyclidine hydrochloride
Kemadrin♦, Procyclid♦♦

INDICATIONS & DOSAGE
Parkinsonism, muscle rigidity—
Adults: initially, 2 to 2.5 mg P.O. t.i.d., after meals. Increase as needed to maximum 60 mg daily.
Also used to relieve extrapyramidal dysfunction which accompanies treatment with phenothiazines and rauwolfia derivatives. Also controls sialorrhea from neuroleptic medications.

SIDE EFFECTS
CNS: light-headedness, giddiness.
EENT: blurred vision, mydriasis.
GI: *constipation, mouth dryness,* nausea, vomiting, epigastric distress.
Skin: rash.

INTERACTIONS
None significant.

NURSING CONSIDERATIONS
• Contraindicated in narrow-angle glaucoma. Use cautiously in tachycardia, hypotension, urinary retention, or prostatic hypertrophy.
• Watch closely for mental confusion, disorientation, agitation, hallucinations, and psychotic symptoms, especially in elderly. Call doctor promptly.
• In severe parkinsonism, tremors may increase as spasticity is relieved.
• Give after meals.
• Relieve dry mouth with cool drinks, ice chips, sugarless gum, or hard candy.

scopolamine hydrobromide

INDICATIONS & DOSAGE
Postencephalitic parkinsonism and other spastic states—
Adults: 0.5 to 1 mg P.O. t.i.d. to q.i.d.; 0.3 to 0.6 mg S.C., I.M., or I.V. (with suitable dilution) t.i.d. to q.i.d.
Children: 0.006 mg/Kg P.O. or S.C. t.i.d. to q.i.d.; or 0.2 mg/m².

SIDE EFFECTS
CNS: disorientation, restlessness, irritability, incoherence, headache.
CV: palpitations, tachycardia, paradoxical bradycardia.
EENT: dilated pupils, blurred vision, photophobia, increased intraocular pressure, difficulty swallowing.
GI: *constipation, mouth dryness,* nausea, vomiting, epigastric distress.
GU: urinary hesitancy or retention.
Skin: flushing, dryness.
Other: bronchial plugging, fever, depressed respirations.
Side effects may be due to pending atropine-like toxicity and are dose-related. Individual tolerance varies greatly.

INTERACTIONS
None significant.

NURSING CONSIDERATIONS
• Contraindicated in narrow-angle glaucoma, obstructive uropathy, obstructive disease of the GI tract, asthma, chronic lung disease, myasthenia gravis, paralytic ileus, intestinal atony, unstable cardiovascular status in acute hemorrhage, or toxic megacolon. Use with caution in autonomic neuropathy, hyperthyroidism, coronary heart disease, cardiac arrhythmias, congestive heart failure, hypertension, hiatal hernia associated with reflux esophagitis, hepatic or renal disease, ulcerative colitis, in patients over 40 because of the increased incidence of glaucoma, and in children under 6 years. Use with caution in hot or humid environments. Drug-induced heat stroke possible.
• Some patients become temporarily excited or disoriented. Symptoms disappear when sedative effect is complete. Use bed rails as precaution.

- Tolerance may develop when administered over a long period of time.
- Many of the side effects (such as dry mouth, constipation) are an extension of the drug's pharmacologic activity and may be expected.

---

trihexyphenidyl hydrochloride
Aparkane♦♦, Artane♦, Hexaphen, Novohexidyl♦♦, T.H.P., Tremin, Trihexane, Trihexidyl, Trihexy♦♦, Trixyl♦♦

INDICATIONS & DOSAGE
Drug-induced parkinsonism—
Adults: 1 mg P.O. 1st day, 2 mg 2nd day, then increase 2 mg every 3 to 5 days until total of 6 to 10 mg given daily. Usually given t.i.d. before meals and, if needed, q.i.d. (last dose should be before bedtime). Postencephalitic parkinsonism may require 12 to 15 mg total daily dose.

SIDE EFFECTS
CNS: nervousness, dizziness, headache, restlessness, agitation, hallucinations, euphoria, delusion, amnesia.
CV: tachycardia.
EENT: *dry mouth,* blurred vision, mydriasis, increased intraocular pressure.
GI: constipation.
GU: urinary hesitancy or retention.
Side effects are dose-related.

INTERACTIONS
Amantadine: anticholinergic side effects, such as confusion and hallucinations. Reduce dosage before administering amantadine.

NURSING CONSIDERATIONS
- Use cautiously in narrow-angle glaucoma; cardiac, hepatic, or renal disorders; hypertension; obstructive disease of the gastrointestinal and the genitourinary tracts; possible prostatic hypertrophy; patients over 60; and those with arteriosclerosis or history of drug hypersensitivities.
- Warn patient to avoid activities that require alertness until response to drug is determined.
- Causes nausea if given before meals.
- Relieve dry mouth with cool drinks, ice chips, sugarless gum, or hard candy.
- Patient may develop a tolerance to this drug.
- Gonioscopic evaluation and close monitoring of intraocular pressures advised, especially in patients over 40.

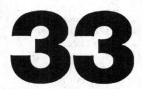

Adrenergics (sympathomimetics)

dobutamine hydrochloride
dopamine hydrochloride
ephedrine sulfate
epinephrine
epinephrine bitartrate
epinephrine hydrochloride
ethylnorepinephrine hydrochloride
isoetharine hydrochloride 1%
isoetharine mesylate
isoproterenol hydrochloride
isoproterenol sulfate
mephentermine sulfate
metaproterenol sulfate
metaraminol bitartrate
methoxamine hydrochloride
methoxyphenamine hydrochloride
norepinephrine injection
(formerly levarterenol bitartrate)
phenylephrine hydrochloride
pseudoephedrine hydrochloride
terbutaline sulfate

---

dobutamine hydrochloride
Dobutrex

INDICATIONS & DOSAGE
Refractory heart failure and as adjunct in cardiac surgery—
Adults: 2.5 to 10 mcg/Kg/min as an I.V. infusion. Rarely, infusion rates up to 40 mcg/Kg/min have been required. May be reconstituted with 5% dextrose in water, normal saline, or lactated Ringer's.

SIDE EFFECTS
CNS: headache.
CV: *increased heart rate, hypertension, premature ventricular beats,* angina.
GI: nausea, vomiting.
Other: nonspecific chest pain, shortness of breath.

INTERACTIONS
Propranolol, metoprolol: These beta-blockers may make dobutamine ineffective. Do not use together.

NURSING CONSIDERATIONS
• Contraindicated in idiopathic hypertrophic subaortic stenosis.
• A unique agent. Increases contractility of failing heart without inducing marked tachycardia, except at high doses.
• Dobutamine is chemical modification of isoproterenol.
• Often used with nitroprusside for additive effects.
• EKG, blood pressure, pulmonary wedge pressure, and cardiac output should be monitored continuously.
• Incompatible with alkaline solutions. Do not mix with sodium bicarbonate injection.
• Infusions of up to 72 hours produce no more adverse effects than shorter infusions.
• Oxidation of drug may slightly discolor admixtures containing dobutamine. This does not indicate a significant loss of potency.
• Intravenous solutions remain stable for 24 hours.

dopamine hydrochloride
Intropin◆

INDICATIONS & DOSAGE
To treat shock and correct hemody-
namic imbalances; to improve perfu-
sion to vital organs, increase cardiac
output; to correct hypotension—
Adults: 2 to 5 mcg/Kg/min I.V. infusion, up to 50 mcg/Kg/min.
Titrate the dosage to the desired he-
modynamic and/or renal response.

SIDE EFFECTS
CNS: headache.
CV: ectopic beats, tachycardia, an-
ginal pain, palpitations, *hypotension.*
Less frequently, bradycardia, widen-
ing of QRS intervals, conduction dis-
turbances, vasoconstriction.
GI: nausea, vomiting.
Local: necrosis and tissue sloughing
with extravasation.
Other: piloerection, dyspnea.

INTERACTIONS
Ergot alkaloids: extreme elevations in
blood pressure. Don't use together.
Phenytoin: may lower blood pressure
of dopamine-stabilized patients.
Monitor carefully.

NURSING CONSIDERATIONS
• Contraindicated in uncorrected
tachyarrhythmias, pheochromocytoma, ventricular fibrillation. Use
cautiously in occlusive vascular disease, cold injuries, diabetic endarteritis, arterial embolism; also, in pregnant patients and those taking MAO
inhibitors.
• Not a substitute for blood or fluid
volume deficit. If volume deficit exists, it should be replaced before vasopressors are administered.
• Don't mix with alkaline solutions.
Use 5% dextrose in water, normal saline, or combination of 5% dextrose in
water and saline. Mix just before use.

• Dopamine solutions deteriorate after 24 hours. Discard at that time or
earlier if solution is discolored.
• Use large vein, as in antecubital
fossa, to minimize risk of extravasation. Watch site carefully for signs of
extravasation. If it occurs, stop infusion immediately and call doctor. He
may want to counteract effect by infiltrating the area with 5 to 10 mg phentolamine and 10 to 15 ml normal
saline.
• Check blood pressure, pulse, urine
output, and extremity color and temperature often during infusion. Titrate
infusion rate according to findings,
using doctor's guidelines. Use a microdrip or infusion pump to regulate
flow rate.
• Observe patient closely for side
effects. If adverse effects develop,
dosage may need to be adjusted or
discontinued.
• If a disproportionate rise in the diastolic pressure (a marked decrease in
pulse pressure) is observed in patients
receiving dopamine, decrease infusion rate and observe carefully for
further evidence of predominant vasoconstrictor activity, unless such an effect is desired.
• Most patients satisfactorily maintained on less than 20 mcg/Kg/min.
• If doses exceed 50 mcg/Kg/min,
check urine output often. If urine flow
decreases without hypotension, consider reducing dose.
• If drug is stopped, watch closely for
sudden drop in blood pressure.
• Do not mix other drugs in bottle
containing dopamine.
• Do not give alkaline drugs (sodium
bicarbonate, phenytoin sodium)
through I.V. line containing dopamine.

Italicized side effects are common or life-threatening.

ephedrine sulfate
Ectasule Minus III

INDICATIONS & DOSAGE
To correct hypotensive states; to support ventricular rate in Adams-Stokes syndrome—
Adults: 25 to 50 mg I.M. or S.C., or 10 to 25 mg I.V. p.r.n. to maximum 150 mg/24 hours.
Children: 3 mg/Kg S.C. or I.V. daily, divided into 4 to 6 doses.
Bronchodilator or nasal decongestant—
Adults: 12.5 to 50 mg P.O. b.i.d., t.i.d., or q.i.d. Maximum 400 mg/day in 6 to 8 divided doses.
Children: 2 to 3 mg/Kg P.O. daily in 4 to 6 divided doses.

SIDE EFFECTS
CNS: *insomnia, nervousness,* dizziness, headache, muscle weakness, sweating, euphoria, confusion, delirium.
CV: *palpitations,* tachycardia, hypertension.
EENT: dryness of nose and throat.
GI: nausea, vomiting, anorexia.
GU: urinary retention, painful urination due to visceral sphincter spasm.

INTERACTIONS
MAO inhibitors and tricyclic antidepressants: when given with sympathomimetics, may cause severe hypertension (hypertensive crisis). Don't use together.
Methyldopa: may inhibit effect of ephedrine. Give together cautiously.

NURSING CONSIDERATIONS
• Contraindicated in porphyria, severe coronary artery disease, cardiac arrhythmias, patients on MAO inhibitor therapy, narrow-angle glaucoma, psychoneurosis. Use with caution in elderly patients, hypertension, hyperthyroidism, nervous or excitable states, cardiovascular disease, prostatic hypertrophy.
• Not a substitute for blood or fluid volume deficit. Volume deficit should be replaced before vasopressors are administered.
• Give I.V. injection slowly.
• Hypoxia, hypercapnia, and acidosis, which may reduce effectiveness or increase the incidence of adverse effects, must be identified and corrected before or during ephedrine administration.
• Effectiveness decreases after 2 to 3 weeks. Then increased dosage may be needed. Tolerance develops, but not known to cause addiction.
• To prevent insomnia, avoid giving within 2 hours before bedtime.
• Warn patient not to take over-the-counter drugs that contain ephedrine without informing doctor.

epinephrine
Inhalants:
Bronkaid Mist♦, Primatene Mist
epinephrine bitartrate
Inhalants:
AsthmaHaler, Medihaler-Epi♦
epinephrine hydrochloride
Adrenalin Chloride, Asmolin, Sus-Phrine♦

INDICATIONS & DOSAGE
Bronchospasm, hypersensitivity reactions, and anaphylaxis—
Adults: 0.1 to 0.5 ml of 1:1,000 S.C. or I.M. Repeat q 10 to 15 minutes, p.r.n. Or 0.1 to 0.25 ml 1:1,000 I.V.
Children: 0.01 ml (10 mcg) of 1:1,000/Kg S.C. Repeat q 20 minutes to 4 hours, p.r.n.; 0.005 ml/Kg of 1:200 (Sus-Phrine). Repeat q 8 to 12 hours, p.r.n.
Hemostatic—
Adults: 1:50,000 to 1:1,000, applied topically.
Acute asthmatic attacks (inhalation)—
Adults and children: 1 or

2 inhalations of 1:100 or 2.25% racemic, p.r.n.; 0.2 mg/dose usual content.
To prolong local anesthetic effect—
Adults and children: 0.2 to 0.4 ml of 1:1,000 intraspinal; 1:500,000 to 1:50,000 local mixed with local anesthetic.
To restore cardiac rhythm in cardiac arrest—
Adults: 0.5 to 1 mg I.V. or into endotracheal tube. May be given intracardiac if no I.V. route or intratracheal route available.
Children: 10 mcg/Kg I.V. or 5 to 10 mcg (0.05 to 0.1 ml of 1:10,000)/ Kg intracardiac.

Note: 1 mg = 1 ml of 1:1,000 or 10 ml of 1:10,000.

SIDE EFFECTS
CNS: *pallor, nervousness,* tremor, euphoria, anxiety, coldness of extremities, vertigo, *headache,* sweating, cerebral hemorrhage, disorientation, agitation. In patients with Parkinson's disease, the drug increases rigidity and tremor.
CV: *palpitations;* widened pulse pressure; hypertension; *tachycardia; ventricular fibrillation; CVA;* anginal pain; EKG changes, including a decrease in the T-wave amplitude.
Metabolic: *hyperglycemia,* glycosuria.
Other: pulmonary edema, dyspnea.

INTERACTIONS
Tricyclic antidepressants: when given with sympathomimetics, may cause severe hypertension (hypertensive crisis). Don't give together.
Propranolol: vasoconstriction and reflex bradycardia. Monitor patient carefully.

NURSING CONSIDERATIONS
• Contraindicated in narrow-angle glaucoma, shock (other than anaphylactic shock), during general anesthesia with halogenated hydrocarbons or cyclopropane, organic brain damage, labor (may delay second stage), cardiac dilatation and coronary insufficiency. Use with extreme caution in patients with long-standing bronchial asthma and emphysema who have developed degenerative heart disease. Use with caution in elderly patients, hyperthyroidism, angina, hypertension, psychoneurosis, diabetes, pregnancy.
• Don't mix with alkaline solutions. Use 5% dextrose in water, normal saline, or a combination of 5% dextrose in water and saline. Mix just before use.
• Epinephrine is rapidly destroyed by oxidizing agents, such as iodine, chromates, nitrates, nitrites, oxygen, and salts of easily reducible metals such as iron.
• Epinephrine solutions deteriorate after 24 hours. Discard after that time or before if solution is discolored or contains precipitate. Keep solution in light-resistant container, and don't remove before use.
• Massage site after injection to counteract possible vasoconstriction. Repeated local injection can cause necrosis at site due to vasoconstriction.
• Avoid intramuscular administration of oil injection into buttocks. Gas gangrene may occur because epinephrine reduces oxygen tension of the tissues, encouraging the growth of contaminating organisms.
• This drug may widen patient's pulse pressure.
• In the event of a sharp blood pressure rise, rapid-acting vasodilators, such as the nitrites or alpha-adrenergic blocking agents, can be given to counteract the marked pressor effect of large doses of epinephrine.
• Observe patient closely for side effects. If adverse effects develop, dosage may need to be adjusted or discontinued.
• If patient has acute hypersensitivity

reactions, it may be necessary to instruct him to self-inject epinephrine at home.
• Drug of choice in emergency treatment of acute anaphylactic reactions, including anaphylactic shock.

---

ethylnorepinephrine hydrochloride
Bronkephrine

INDICATIONS & DOSAGE
To relieve bronchospasm due to asthma—
Adults: 0.5 to 1 ml S.C. or I.M.
Children: 0.1 to 0.5 ml S.C. or I.M.

SIDE EFFECTS
CV: changes in blood pressure, *elevation in pulse rate,* palpitations.
Other: *headache, dizziness,* nausea.

INTERACTIONS
None significant.

NURSING CONSIDERATIONS
• Use with caution in cardiovascular disease or history of stroke.
• Safer than epinephrine for use in hypertensive or severely ill patients in whom significant pressor effects are undesirable.
• Valuable when used in children due to low incidence of adverse effects; may be useful in diabetic asthmatics due to low glycogenolytic activity.
• Choose anatomical injection site carefully to avoid inadvertent intraneural or intravascular injection.

---

isoetharine hydrochloride 1%
Bronkosol
isoetharine mesylate
Bronkometer

INDICATIONS & DOSAGE
Bronchial asthma and reversible bron-

chospasm that may occur with bronchitis and emphysema—
Adults: (hydrochloride): administered by hand nebulizer, oxygen aerosolization, or IPPB.

Method	Dose	Dilution
Hand	3 to 7 inhalations	undiluted
oxygen aerosolization	0.5 ml	1:3 with saline
IPPB	0.5 ml	1:3 with saline

Adults: (mesylate): 1 to 2 inhalations. Occasionally, more may be required.

SIDE EFFECTS
CNS: *tremor, headache,* dizziness, excitement.
CV: *palpitations,* increased heart rate.
GI: nausea, vomiting.

INTERACTIONS
None significant.

NURSING CONSIDERATIONS
• Use cautiously in patients with hyperthyroidism, hypertension, coronary disease, or those with sensitivity to sympathomimetics.
• Excessive use can lead to decreased effectiveness.
• Monitor for severe paradoxical bronchoconstriction after excessive use. Discontinue immediately if bronchoconstriction occurs.
• Although isoetharine has minimal effects on the heart, use cautiously in patients receiving general anesthetics that sensitize the myocardium to sympathomimetic drugs.
• Instruct patient in the use of aerosol and mouthpiece.

Unmarked trade names available in the United States only.
♦ Also available in Canada   ♦ ♦ Available in Canada only.

isoproterenol hydrochloride
Isuprel♦, Proternol (tabs)
Inhalants: Norisodrine, Vapo-Iso
isoproterenol sulfate
Iso-Autohaler, Luf-Iso Inhalation,
Medihaler-Iso♦, Norisodrine

INDICATIONS & DOSAGE
Bronchial asthma and reversible bronchospasm (hydrochloride)—
Adults: 10 to 20 mg S.L. q 6 to 8 hours.
Children: 5 to 10 mg S.L. q 6 to 8 hours. Not recommended for children under 6 years.
Bronchospasm (sulfate)—
Adults and children: acute dyspneic episodes: 1 inhalation initially. May repeat if needed after 2 to 5 minutes. Maintenance: 1 to 2 inhalations q.i.d. to 6 times daily. May repeat once more 10 minutes after second dose. Not more than 3 doses should be administered for each attack.
Heart block and ventricular arrhythmias (sulfate)—
Adults: initially, 0.02 to 0.06 mg I.V. Subsequent doses 0.01 to 0.2 mg I.V. or 5 mcg/min I.V.; or 0.2 mg I.M. initially, then 0.02 to 1 mg, p.r.n.
Children: may give ½ of initial adult dose.
Maintenance for Stokes-Adams disease or A-V block (sulfate)—
Adults: 30 to 180 mg timed-release tablets P.O. daily swallowed whole.
Shock (sulfate)—
Adults and children: 0.5 to 5 mcg/ min by continuous I.V. infusion. Usual concentration: 1 mg (5 ml) in 500 ml 5% dextrose in water. Adjust rate according to heart rate, central venous pressure, blood pressure, and urine flow.

SIDE EFFECTS
CNS: *headache,* mild tremor, dizziness, flushing of face, nervousness, insomnia.

CV: *palpitations,* tachycardia, anginal pain; blood pressure may be elevated and then fall.
GI: nausea, vomiting.
Metabolic: hyperglycemia.
Other: weakness, sweating, bronchial edema and inflammation.

INTERACTIONS
Propranolol and other beta-blockers: blocked effect of isoproterenol and vice versa. Monitor patient carefully if used together.

NURSING CONSIDERATIONS
• Contraindicated in tachycardia caused by digitalis intoxication and in patients with preexisting arrhythmias, especially tachycardia, because chronotropic effect on the heart may aggravate such disorders. Contraindicated in recent myocardial infarction. Use cautiously in coronary insufficiency, diabetes, hyperthyroidism.
• Not a substitute for blood or fluid volume deficit. If deficit exists, it should be replaced before vasopressors are administered.
• If heart rate exceeds 110 beats/minute, it may be advisable to decrease infusion rate or temporarily stop infusion. Doses sufficient to increase the heart rate to more than 130 beats/minute may induce ventricular arrhythmias.
• If precordial distress or anginal pain occurs, stop drug immediately.
• When administering I.V. isoproterenol for shock, closely monitor blood pressure, CVP, EKG, arterial blood gas measurements, and urinary output. Carefully adjust infusion rate according to these measurements.
• Oral and sublingual tablets are poorly and erratically absorbed.
• Teach patient how to take sublingual tablet properly. Tell him to hold tablet under tongue until it dissolves and is absorbed and not to swallow saliva until that time. Prolonged use of sublingual tablets can cause tooth de-

cay. Instruct patient to rinse mouth with water between doses. Will also help prevent dryness of oropharynx.
• If possible, don't give at bedtime because it interrupts sleep patterns.
• Oral tablets not for sublingual use; must be swallowed whole, not broken. Store in cool, dry place in airtight, light-resistant container. Keep bottle tightly capped after opening.
• This drug may cause slight rise in systolic blood pressure and slight to marked drop in diastolic blood pressure.
• Use a microdrip or infusion pump to regulate infusion flow rate.
• Observe patient closely for side effects. Dosage may need to be adjusted or discontinued.
• Teach patient to perform oral inhalation correctly. Give the following instructions for using a metered-dose nebulizer:
    —Clear nasal passages and throat.
    —Breathe out, expelling as much air from lungs as possible.
    —Place mouthpiece well into mouth as dose from nebulizer is released, and inhale deeply.
    —Hold breath for several seconds, remove mouthpiece, and exhale slowly.
• Instructions for metered powder nebulizer are the same, except that deep inhalation is not necessary.
• Patient may develop a tolerance to this drug. Warn against overuse.
• Warn patient using oral inhalant that drug may turn sputum and saliva pink.
• May aggravate ventilation perfusion abnormalities; even while ease of breathing is improved, arterial oxygen tension may fall paradoxically.
• Discard inhalation solution if it is discolored or contains precipitate.

mephentermine sulfate
Wyamine♦

INDICATIONS & DOSAGE
Hypotension following spinal anesthesia—
Adults: 30 to 45 mg I.V. in a single injection, then 30 mg I.V. repeated p.r.n. Maintenance of blood pressure: continuous I.V. infusion of 0.1% solution of mephentermine in 5% dextrose in water.
Hypotension following spinal anesthesia during obstetrical procedures—
Adults: initially, 15 mg I.V., p.r.n.
Prevention of hypotension during spinal anesthesia—
Adults: 30 to 40 mg I.M. 10 to 20 minutes prior to anesthesia.
Treatment of shock and hypotension—
Adults: 0.5 mg/Kg I.V.
Children: 0.4 mg/Kg I.V.

SIDE EFFECTS
CNS: euphoria, nervousness, anxiety, tremor, incoherence, drowsiness, convulsions.
CV: arrhythmias, marked elevation of blood pressure (with large doses).

INTERACTIONS
None significant.

NURSING CONSIDERATIONS
• Contraindicated in concealed hemorrhage or hypotension from hemorrhage, except in emergencies; also in patients receiving phenothiazines, or who have received MAO inhibitors within 2 weeks. Use cautiously with arteriosclerosis, cardiovascular disease, hyperthyroidism, hypertension, chronic illness.
• Not a substitute for blood or fluid volume deficit. If deficit exists, it should be replaced before vasopressors are administered.
• During infusion, check blood pres-

sure every 5 minutes until stabilized; then every 15 minutes.
• Observe patient closely for side effects. If adverse effects develop, dosage may need to be adjusted or discontinued.
• Monitor blood pressure even after stopping drug.
• I.M. route may be used since drug is not irritating to tissue.
• I.V. drug is not irritating to tissue, and extravasation is not dangerous. To prepare 0.1% I.V. solution: add 16.6 ml mephentermine (30 mg/ml) to 500 ml 5% dextrose in water.
• Can be given I.V. undiluted.
• May increase uterine contractions during 3rd trimester of pregnancy.
• Hypercapnia, hypoxia, and acidosis may reduce effectiveness or increase adverse effects. Identify and correct before and during administration.

metaproterenol sulfate
Alupent♦, Metaprel

INDICATIONS & DOSAGE
Acute episodes of bronchial asthma—
Adults and children: 2 to 3 inhalations. Should not repeat inhalations more often than q 3 to 4 hours. Should not exceed 12 inhalations daily.
Bronchial asthma and reversible bronchospasm—
Adults: 20 mg P.O. q 6 to 8 hours.
Children over 9 years or over 27 Kg: 20 mg P.O. q 6 to 8 hours. (0.4 mg to 0.9 mg/Kg/dose t.i.d.)
Children 6 to 9 years or less than 27 Kg: 10 mg P.O. q 6 to 8 hours. (0.4 mg to 0.9 mg/Kg/dose t.i.d.) Not recommended for children under 6 years.

SIDE EFFECTS
CNS: nervousness, weakness, drowsiness, tremor.

CV: tachycardia, hypertension, palpitations; *with excessive use, cardiac arrest.*
GI: vomiting, nausea, bad taste in mouth.
Other: paradoxical bronchiolar constriction with excessive use.

INTERACTIONS
None significant.

NURSING CONSIDERATIONS
• Contraindicated in tachycardia, and in arrhythmias associated with tachycardia. Use with caution in hypertension, coronary artery disease, hyperthyroidism, diabetes.
• Safe use of inhalant in children under 12 not established.
• Teach patient how to administer metered dose correctly. Instructions: shake container; exhale through nose; administer aerosol while inhaling deeply on mouthpiece of inhaler; hold breath for a few seconds, then exhale slowly. Allow 2 minutes between inhalations. Store drug in light-resistant container.
• Tell patient to notify doctor if no response to dosage. Warn against changing dose without calling doctor.

metaraminol bitartrate
Aramine♦

INDICATIONS & DOSAGE
Prevention of hypotension—
Adults: 2 to 10 mg I.M. or S.C.
Severe shock—
Adults: 0.5 to 5 mg direct I.V. followed by I.V. infusion.
Treatment of hypotension due to shock—
Adults: 15 to 100 mg in 500 ml normal saline or 5% dextrose in water I.V. infusion. Adjust rate to maintain blood pressure.
All indications—
Children: 0.01 mg/Kg as single I.V.

Italicized side effects are common or life-threatening.

injection; 1 mg/25 ml 5% dextrose in water as I.V. infusion. Adjust rate to maintain blood pressure in normal range. 0.1 mg/Kg I.M. as single dose, p.r.n. Allow at least 10 minutes to elapse before increasing dose because maximum effect is not immediately apparent.

SIDE EFFECTS
CNS: apprehension, restlessness, dizziness, headache, tremor, weakness; with excessive use, convulsions.
CV: hypertension; hypotension; precordial pain; palpitations; arrhythmias, including sinus or ventricular tachycardia; bradycardia; supraventricular premature beats; atrioventricular dissociation.
GI: nausea, vomiting.
GU: decreased urinary output.
Metabolic: hyperglycemia.
Skin: flushing, pallor, sweating.
Local: irritation upon extravasation.
Other: *metabolic acidosis in hypovolemia, increased body temperature, respiratory distress.*

INTERACTIONS
MAO inhibitors: may cause severe hypertension (hypertensive crisis). Don't use together.

NURSING CONSIDERATIONS
• Contraindicated in peripheral or mesenteric thrombosis; pulmonary edema; hypercarbia; and acidosis; during anesthesia with cyclopropane and halogenated hydrocarbon anesthetics. Use cautiously in hypertension, thyroid disease, diabetes, cirrhosis, or malaria, and those receiving digitalis.
• Not a substitute for blood or fluid volume deficit. Fluid deficit should be replaced before vasopressors are administered.
• Keep solution in light-resistant container, away from heat.
• Use large veins, as in antecubital fossa, to minimize risk of extravasa-

tion. Watch infusion site carefully for signs of extravasation. If it occurs, stop infusion immediately and call doctor.
• During infusion check blood pressure every 5 minutes until stabilized; then every 15 minutes. Check pulse rates, urinary output, and color and temperature of extremities. Titrate infusion rate according to findings, using doctor's guidelines.
• Use a microdrip or infusion pump to regulate infusion flow rate.
• Observe patient closely for side effects. If adverse effects develop, dosage may need to be adjusted or discontinued.
• For I.V. therapy, use 2-bottle setup so I.V. can run if this drug is stopped.
• Blood pressure should be raised to slightly less than the patient's normal level. Be careful to avoid excessive blood pressure response. Rapidly induced hypertensive response can cause acute pulmonary edema, arrhythmias, and cardiac arrest.
• Because of prolonged action, a cumulative effect is possible. With an excessive vasopressor response, elevated blood pressure may persist after stopping.
• Urinary output may decrease initially, then increase as blood pressure reaches normal level. Report persistent decreased urine output.
• When discontinuing therapy with this drug, slow infusion rate gradually. Continue monitoring vital signs, watching for possible severe drop in blood pressure. Keep equipment nearby to start drug again, if necessary. Pressor therapy should not be reinstated until the systolic blood pressure falls below 70 to 80 mm Hg.
• Keep emergency drugs on hand to reverse effects of metaraminol: atropine for reflex bradycardia; phentolamine to decrease vasopressor effects; propranolol for arrhythmias.
• Closely monitor diabetics. Adjustment in insulin dose may be needed.

- Metaraminol should not be mixed with other drugs.

---

methoxamine hydrochloride
Vasoxyl ♦

INDICATIONS & DOSAGE
Moderate fall in blood pressure—
Adults: 5 to 10 mg I.M.
Paroxysmal supraventricular tachycardia—
Adults: 5 to 15 mg I.V. injected slowly. 10 to 20 mg I.M. Allow 15 minutes before additional increased doses to evaluate effects of initial dose and prevent a cumulative effect.
Prevention of hypotension during spinal anesthesia—
Adults: 10 to 15 mg I.M. before or with spinal anesthesia.
Support and restoration of blood pressure during anesthesia (including cyclopropane); termination of paroxysmal supraventricular tachycardia; emergency situations; systolic falls below 60 mm Hg—
Adults: initially, 3 to 5 mg slow I.V. injection, followed by 10 to 15 mg I.M. to prolong effect.
Children: direct I.V. dose is 80 mcg/Kg of body weight or 2.5 mg/m^2 of body surface area, injected slowly.

SIDE EFFECTS
CNS: paresthesias, chills, severe headache, restlessness, tremors, dizziness, anxiety, nervousness.
CV: hypertension, bradycardia, cardiac depression, precordial pain, heart failure in diseased myocardium.
GI: projectile vomiting.
GU: urinary urgency, decreased urine output.
Skin: gooseflesh, pallor.
Other: respiratory distress, *metabolic acidosis.*

INTERACTIONS
None significant.

NURSING CONSIDERATIONS
- Contraindicated in severe heart disease or in those taking MAO inhibitors; in shock due to myocardial infarction, or peripheral or mesenteric vascular thrombosis; and in the elderly. Use cautiously in hyperthyroidism or hypertension; after use of ergot alkaloids; and in pregnancy.
- Should not be used with local anesthetics to prolong their effect.
- Not a substitute for blood volume or fluid volume deficit. If deficit exists, replace before vasopressors are given. Hypoxia and acidosis should also be corrected before or during therapy.
- Methoxamine solutions deteriorate after 24 hours. Discard after that time or before if discolored or contains precipitate.
- Has potent, prolonged pressor action. Does not increase cardiac rate or irritability of cyclopropane-sensitized heart.
- Does not stimulate CNS.
- Monitor response by checking blood pressure. Adjust dose accordingly. Blood pressure should be raised to slightly less than normal level. In previously normotensive patients, systolic blood pressure should be maintained at 80 to 100 mm Hg; in previously hypertensive patients, systolic blood pressure should be maintained at 30 to 40 mm Hg below usual level.
- Observe patient closely for side effects. Dosage may need to be adjusted or discontinued.
- Keep these emergency drugs on hand to reverse effects of methoxamine: atropine for reflex bradycardia and phentolamine for increased vasopressor effects.
- Monitor blood pressure and pulse rate even after stopping drug. Report sudden changes.

---

methoxyphenamine hydrochloride
Orthoxine Hydrochloride

INDICATIONS & DOSAGE
To treat allergies and bronchial asthma—
Adults: 100 mg P.O. q 4 to 6 hours. Maximum dose, 600 mg/day.
Children: 25 to 50 mg P.O. q 4 to 6 hours.

SIDE EFFECTS
CNS: insomnia, nervousness, dizziness, headache, sweating, anxiety, flushing.
CV: palpitations, tachycardia, hypertension.
GI: nausea, vomiting, dry mouth.

INTERACTIONS
None significant.

NURSING CONSIDERATIONS
• Contraindicated in those who have used MAO inhibitors within past 2 weeks. Use cautiously in hypertension, hyperthyroidism, acute coronary disease, cardiac decompensation, diabetes mellitus.
• Only "possibly effective" in treating bronchial asthma, acute urticaria, allergic rhinitis, gastrointestinal allergy, and allergic headaches.
• Effectiveness decreases after 2 to 3 weeks. Then increased dose may be needed.
• Avoid giving this drug within 2 hours of bedtime.
• Warn against using over-the-counter drugs containing sympathomimetics without informing doctor.

norepinephrine injection (formerly levarterenol bitartrate)
Levophed♦

INDICATIONS & DOSAGE
To restore blood pressure in acute hypotensive states—
Adults: initially, 8 to 12 mcg/min I.V. infusion, then adjust to maintain normal blood pressure. Average maintenance dose 2 to 4 mcg/min.

SIDE EFFECTS
CNS: *headache,* anxiety, weakness, dizziness, tremor, restlessness, insomnia.
CV: bradycardia, severe hypertension, marked increase in peripheral resistance, decreased cardiac output, arrhythmias, *ventricular tachycardia, fibrillation,* bigeminal rhythm, atrioventricular dissociation, precordial pain.
GU: *decreased urine output.*
Metabolic: *metabolic acidosis.*
Local: irritation upon extravasation.
Other: hyperglycemia, increased glycogenolysis, fever, respiratory difficulty.

INTERACTIONS
Tricyclic antidepressants: when given with sympathomimetics, may cause severe hypertension (hypertensive crisis). Don't give together.

NURSING CONSIDERATIONS
• Contraindicated in mesenteric or peripheral vascular thrombosis, pregnancy, profound hypoxia, hypercarbia, hypotension from blood volume deficits, or during cyclopropane and halothane anesthesia. Use cautiously in hypertension, hyperthyroidism, severe heart disease. Use with extreme caution in patients receiving MAO inhibitors or tricyclic antidepressants.
• Not a substitute for blood or fluid volume deficit. If deficit exists, it

should be replaced before vasopressors are administered.
• Norepinephrine solutions deteriorate after 24 hours. Discard after that time.
• Use large vein, as in antecubital fossa, to minimize risk of extravasation. Check site frequently for signs of extravasation. If it occurs, stop infusion immediately and call doctor. He may counteract effect by infiltrating area with 5 to 10 mg phentolamine and 10 to 15 ml normal saline. Also check for blanching along course of infused vein; may progress to superficial slough. During infusion, check blood pressure every 2 minutes until stabilized; then every 5 minutes. Also check pulse rates, urinary output, and color and temperature of extremities. Titrate infusion rate according to findings, using doctor's guidelines. In previously hypertensive patients, blood pressure should be raised no more than 40 mm Hg below preexisting systolic pressure.
• Never leave patient unattended.
• Use a microdrip or infusion pump to regulate infusion flow rate.
• For I.V. therapy, use bottle setup so I.V. can run if norepinephrine is stopped.
• Report decreased urinary output to doctor immediately.
• If prolonged I.V. therapy is necessary, change injection site frequently.
• When stopping drug, slow infusion rate gradually. Monitor vital signs, even after stopping. Watch for possible severe drop in blood pressure.
• Keep emergency drugs on hand to reverse effects of norepinephrine: atropine for reflex bradycardia; propranolol for arrhythmias; phentolamine for increased vasopressor effects.
• Administer in dextrose and saline; saline alone is not recommended.

phenylephrine hydrochloride
Neo-Synephrine♦

INDICATIONS & DOSAGE
Hypotensive emergencies during spinal anesthesia—
Adults: initially, 0.2 mg I.V., then subsequent doses of 0.1 to 0.2 mg.
Maintenance of blood pressure during spinal or inhalation anesthesia—
Adults: 2 to 3 mg S.C. or I.M. 3 or 4 minutes before anesthesia is administered.
Children: 0.04 mg to 0.088 mg/Kg S.C. or I.M.
Mild to moderate hypotension—
Adults: 2 to 5 mg S.C. or I.M; 0.1 to 0.5 mg I.V. Not to be repeated more often than 10 to 15 minutes.
Paroxysmal supraventricular tachycardia—
Adults: initially, 0.5 mg rapid I.V.; subsequent doses should not exceed the preceding dose by more than 0.1 to 0.2 mg and should not exceed 1 mg.
Prolongation of spinal anesthesia—
Adults: 2 to 5 mg added to anesthetic solution.
Severe hypotension and shock (including drug-induced)—
Adults: 10 mg in 500 ml 5% dextrose in water. Start 100 to 180 drops per minute I.V. infusion, then 40 to 60 drops per minute. Adjust to patient response.
Vasoconstrictor for regional anesthesia—
Adults: 1 mg phenylephrine added to 20 ml local anesthetic.

SIDE EFFECTS
CNS: trembling, sweating, pallor, sense of fullness in head, tingling in extremities, sleeplessness, dizziness, paresthesia in extremities from injection, light-headedness, weakness.
CV: palpitations, tachycardia, extrasystoles, short paroxysms of ventricu-

lar tachycardia, hypertension, anginal pain.
EENT: blurred vision.
Skin: gooseflesh, feeling of coolness.
Other: tachyphylaxis may occur with continued use.

INTERACTIONS

MAO inhibitors: may cause severe hypertension (hypertensive crisis). Don't use together.
Tricyclic antidepressants: increased pressor response. Observe patient carefully.

NURSING CONSIDERATIONS

• Contraindicated in narrow-angle glaucoma; with MAO inhibitors, tricyclic antidepressants; hypotension; ventricular tachycardia; severe coronary disease or cardiovascular disease (including myocardial infarction). Use with extreme caution in heart disease, hyperthyroidism, diabetes, severe atherosclerosis, bradycardia, partial heart block, myocardial disease, and the elderly.
• Longer acting than ephedrine and epinephrine.
• Causes little or no CNS stimulation.
• Monitor blood pressure frequently. Avoid excessive rise in blood pressure. Maintain blood pressure at slightly below the patient's normal level. In previously normotensive patients, maintain systolic blood pressure at 80 to 100 mm Hg; in previously hypertensive patients, maintain systolic blood pressure at 30 to 40 mm Hg below their usual level.
• May reverse severe increase in blood pressure with phentolamine.
• With I.V. infusions, avoid abrupt withdrawal. Monitor blood pressure throughout. Reverse therapy if blood pressure falls too rapidly.

pseudoephedrine hydrochloride
Besan, Cenafed, D-Feda, Eltor♦♦, First Sign, Gyrocaps, Novafed, Robidrine♦♦, Ro-Fedrin, Sudabid, Sudafed♦, Sudafed SA

INDICATIONS & DOSAGE

Nasal and eustachian tube decongestant—
Adults: 60 mg P.O. q 4 hours.
Children 6 to 12 years: 30 mg P.O. q 4 hours. Maximum 120 mg/day.
Children 2 to 6 years: 15 mg P.O. q 4 hours. Maximum 60 mg/day.
Extended-relief tablets:
Adults, and children over 12 years: 60 to 120 mg P.O. q 12 hours. This form contraindicated for children under 12.

SIDE EFFECTS

CNS: *anxiety,* transient stimulation, tremors, dizziness, headache, insomnia, *nervousness.*
CV: arrhythmias, *palpitations,* tachycardia.
GI: anorexia, nausea, vomiting, dry mouth.
GU: difficulty in urination.
Skin: pallor.

INTERACTIONS

MAO inhibitors: may cause severe hypertension (hypertensive crisis). Don't use together.

NURSING CONSIDERATIONS

• Contraindicated in severe hypertension or severe coronary artery disease; and in those receiving MAO inhibitors; nursing mothers. Use cautiously in hypertension, heart disease, glaucoma, hyperthyroidism, or prostatic hypertrophy.
• Tell patient to stop drug if he becomes unusually restless and to notify doctor promptly.
• Warn against using over-the-counter products containing ephed-

rine or other sympathomimetic
amines.
• Tell patient not to take drug within
2 hours of bedtime because it can
cause insomnia.
• Relieve dry mouth with sugarless
gum or sour hard candy.

---

terbutaline sulfate
Brethine, Bricanyl ♦

INDICATIONS & DOSAGE
Bronchodilator—
Adults: 2.5 to 5 mg P.O. q 8 hours;
or 0.25 mg S.C. If no improvement in
15 to 30 minutes, repeat dose. Do not
exceed 0.5 mg in 4 hours.
Children 12 to 15 years: 2.5 mg P.O.
t.i.d.
Not recommended for children under
12.

SIDE EFFECTS
CNS: *nervousness, tremors, headache,* drowsiness, sweating.

CV: palpitations, increased heart
rate.
GI: vomiting, nausea.

INTERACTIONS
MAO inhibitors: when given with
sympathomimetics may cause severe
hypertension (hypertensive crisis).
Don't use together.
Propranolol and other beta-blockers:
blocked effects of terbutaline. Monitor patient carefully if used together.

NURSING CONSIDERATIONS
• Use cautiously in patients with diabetes, hypertension, hyperthyroidism, severe heart disease, or cardiac
arrhythmias.
• Protect injection from light. Do not
use if discolored.
• Make sure patient's family understands why patient is taking drug, so
they can encourage continuation.
• Give subcutaneous injections in lateral deltoid area.
• Tolerance may develop with prolonged use.

Italicized side effects are common or life-threatening.

34

Adrenergic blockers (sympatholytics)

dihydroergotamine mesylate
ergotamine tartrate
methysergide maleate
phenoxybenzamine hydrochloride
phentolamine hydrochloride
phentolamine mesylate
propranolol

dihydroergotamine mesylate
D.H.E. 45

INDICATIONS & DOSAGE
Vascular or migraine headache—
Adults: 1 mg I.M. or I.V. May repeat
q 1 to 2 hours, p.r.n., up to total of
3 mg. Maximum weekly dose is
6 mg.

SIDE EFFECTS
CV: transient tachycardia or brady-
cardia, precordial distress and pain,
increased arterial pressure.
GI: nausea, vomiting.
Skin: itching.
Local: numbness and tingling in fin-
gers and toes, weakness in legs, mus-
cle pains in extremities.
Other: localized edema.

INTERACTIONS
Propranolol and other beta-blockers:
blocked natural pathway for vasodilation in patients receiving ergot alkaloids and thus could result in excessive vasoconstriction. Watch closely if
drugs are used together.

NURSING CONSIDERATIONS
• Contraindicated in peripheral and

occlusive vascular disease, coronary
artery disease, hypertension, hepatic
or renal dysfunction, sepsis.
• Avoid prolonged administration;
don't exceed recommended dosage.
• Tell patient to report any feeling of
coldness in extremities or tingling of
fingers and toes. These symptoms appear before onset of gangrene.
• Most effective when used to prevent
migraine or soon after onset. Provide
a quiet, low-light environment to help
patient relax.
• Help patient evaluate underlying
causes of stress.

ergotamine tartrate
Ergomar♦, Ergostat, Gynergen♦,
Medihaler-Ergotamine♦

INDICATIONS & DOSAGE
Vascular or migraine headache—
Adults: initially, 2 mg P.O. S.L., then
1 to 2 mg P.O. q hour or S.L. q
½ hour, to maximum 6 mg daily and
10 mg weekly; or initially, 0.25 mg
I.M. or S.C.; repeat in 40 minutes if
needed. Maximum dose 0.5 mg/24
hours and 1 mg/week; or 1 inhalation
initially, if not relieved in 5 minutes,
use another inhalation. May repeat inhalations at least 5 minutes apart up
to maximum of 6 per 24 hours.

SIDE EFFECTS
CV: transient tachycardia or bradycardia, precordial distress and pain,
increased arterial pressure, angina
pectoris.

GI: nausea, vomiting, diarrhea, abdominal cramps.
Skin: itching.
Local: numbness and tingling in fingers and toes, weakness in legs, muscle pains in extremities.
Other: localized edema.

INTERACTIONS

Propranolol and other beta-blockers: blocked natural pathway for vasodilation in patients receiving ergot alkaloids and thus could result in excessive vasoconstriction. Watch closely if drugs are used together.

NURSING CONSIDERATIONS

• Contraindicated in peripheral and occlusive vascular diseases, coronary artery disease, hypertension, hepatic or renal dysfunction, sepsis.
• Avoid prolonged administration; don't exceed recommended dosage.
• Most effective when used to prevent migraine or soon after onset.
• Provide a quiet, low-light environment to help patient relax.
• Help patient evaluate underlying causes of stress.
• Instruct patient on long-term therapy to check for and report feeling of coldness in extremities or tingling of fingers and toes. Symptoms appear before onset of gangrene.
• Store drug in light-resistant container.

---

methysergide maleate
Sansert♦

INDICATIONS & DOSAGE

Prevention of frequent, severe, uncontrollable, or disabling migraine or vascular headache—
Adults: 2 to 4 mg P.O. b.i.d. with meals.

SIDE EFFECTS

Blood: neutropenia, eosinophilia.

CNS: insomnia, drowsiness, *euphoria, vertigo,* ataxia, *light-headedness,* hyperesthesia, weakness, *hallucinations or feelings of disassociation.*
CV: *fibrotic thickening of cardiac valves and aorta, inferior vena cava, and common iliac branches;* vasoconstriction, causing chest pain, abdominal pain, vascular insufficiency of lower limbs; cold, numb, painful extremities with or without paresthesias and diminished or absent pulses; postural hypotension; tachycardia; peripheral edema; murmurs; bruits.
EENT: nasal stuffiness.
GI: nausea, vomiting, diarrhea, constipation, epigastric pain.
Skin: hair loss, dermatitis, sweating, flushing, rash.
Other: *retroperitoneal fibrosis,* causing general malaise, fatigue, weight gain, backache, low-grade fever, urinary obstruction; *pulmonary fibrosis,* causing dyspnea, tightness and pain in chest, pleural friction rubs and effusion, arthralgia, myalgia.

INTERACTIONS
None significant.

NURSING CONSIDERATIONS
• Contraindicated in severe hypertension, arteriosclerosis, peripheral vascular insufficiency, renal or hepatic disease, severe coronary artery diseases, thromboembolic disorders, phlebitis or cellulitis of lower limbs, fibrotic processes, valvular disease, debilitated patients. Use cautiously in peptic ulcers; in suspected coronary artery disease. EKG and cardiac status evaluation advisable before giving to patients over 40.
• Stop drug every 6 months; then restart after at least 3 or 4 weeks.
• Tell patient not to stop drug abruptly; may cause rebound headaches. Stop gradually over 2 to 3 weeks.
• Patient should keep daily weight record and report unusually rapid

---

Italicized side effects are common or life-threatening.

weight gain. Teach him to check for peripheral edema. Explain and suggest low-salt diet if necessary.
• Give drug for 3 weeks before evaluating effectiveness.
• Tell patient to report to doctor promptly if he experiences cold, numb, or painful hands and feet; leg cramps when walking; girdle, chest, or flank pain.
• Not for treatment of migraine or vascular headache in progress, or for treatment of tension (muscle contraction) headaches.
• Indicated only for patients who are unresponsive to other drugs and who can be kept under close medical supervision.

phenoxybenzamine hydrochloride
Dibenzyline

INDICATIONS & DOSAGE
To control or prevent hypertension and sweating associated with pheochromocytoma; Raynaud's syndrome; frostbite; acrocyanosis—
Adults: initially, 10 mg P.O., then increase by 10 mg q 4 days to a maximum of 60 mg daily.

SIDE EFFECTS
CNS: sedation, fatigue, lassitude.
CV: tachycardia, *postural hypotension with dizziness.*
EENT: miosis, nasal congestion.
GI: irritation.
GU: inhibition of ejaculation.

INTERACTIONS
None significant.

NURSING CONSIDERATIONS
• Contraindicated whenever a fall in blood pressure is undesirable. Use cautiously in cerebral or coronary arteriosclerosis, renal damage, or respiratory disease.

• May aggravate symptoms of respiratory infections.
• Safe use in pregnancy has not been established, but drug has been used during the third trimester to treat hypertension caused by pheochromocytoma without apparent harm to mother or fetus.
• Reduce gastric irritation by giving with milk or in divided doses.
• Place overdosed patient in Trendelenburg position; have I.V. solution ready. Treat hypotension with norepinephrine.
• Full therapeutic effect may not be seen for several weeks.

phentolamine hydrochloride
Regitine, Rogitine ♦ ♦
phentolamine mesylate

INDICATIONS & DOSAGE
To control or prevent hypertension before or during pheochromocytomectomy—
Adults: 50 to 100 mg P.O. 4 to 6 times daily; or 5 mg I.M. or I.V. 1 to 2 hours preop. May repeat if needed. During surgery, 5 mg I.V. may be given as needed.
Children: 25 mg P.O. daily, divided q 4 to 6 hours; or 1 mg I.M. or I.V. 1 to 2 hours preop. May repeat if needed. During surgery, 1 mg I.V. may be given as needed.
To treat extravasation— infiltrate area with 5 to 10 mg phentolamine in 10 ml 0.9% normal saline solution. Must be done within 12 hours.

SIDE EFFECTS
CV: acute and prolonged hypotension, tachycardia, cardiac arrhythmia, angina, orthostatic hypotension, flushing.
EENT: nasal congestion.
GI: nausea, vomiting, diarrhea, exacerbation of peptic ulcer.

INTERACTIONS
None significant.

NURSING CONSIDERATIONS
• Contraindicated in angina, coronary artery disease, or in history of myocardial infarction. Use with caution in gastritis or peptic ulcer.
• If cardiac arrhythmias occur, don't give digitalis glycosides until cardiac rhythm returns to normal.
• Place overdosed patient in Trendelenburg position; have I.V. solution ready. Treat hypotension with norepinephrine.
• Monitor blood pressure closely, especially after parenteral administration.
• To reconstitute injection, add 1 ml sterile water for injection to 5 mg vial of drug. Use immediately after reconstitution.

propranolol
Inderal♦

INDICATIONS & DOSAGE
Prevention of frequent, severe, uncontrollable, or disabling migraine or vascular headache—
Adults: initially, 80 mg daily in divided doses. Usual maintenance dose: 160 to 240 mg daily, divided t.i.d. or q.i.d.

SIDE EFFECTS
CNS: *fatigue, lethargy,* vivid dreams, hallucinations.
CV: *bradycardia, hypotension, congestive heart failure,* peripheral vascular disease.
GI: nausea, vomiting, diarrhea.
Metabolic: hypoglycemia without symptoms.
Skin: rash.
Other: *increased airway resistance,* fever.

INTERACTIONS
Insulin, hypoglycemic drugs (oral): can alter requirements for these drugs in previously stabilized diabetics. Monitor for hypoglycemia.
Cardiac glycosides: excessive bradycardia and increased depressant effect on myocardium. Monitor pulse.
Aminophylline: antagonized beta-blocking effects of propranolol. Use together cautiously.
Isoproterenol, glucagon: antagonized propranolol effect. May be used therapeutically and in emergencies.

NURSING CONSIDERATIONS
• Contraindicated in diabetes mellitus, asthma, or allergic rhinitis; during ethyl ether anesthesia; in sinus bradycardia and in heart block greater than first degree; in cardiogenic shock; in right ventricular failure secondary to pulmonary hypertension. Use with caution in congestive heart failure or respiratory disease.
• Withdraw drug slowly in patients with coronary artery disease. Abrupt withdrawal might precipitate myocardial infarction or aggravate angina or pheochromocytoma. Abrupt withdrawal in thyrotoxicosis may exacerbate hyperthyroidism or precipitate thyroid storm. In thyrotoxicosis, propranolol may mask clinical signs of hyperthyroidism.
• Don't stop before surgery for pheochromocytoma. Before any surgical procedure, notify anesthesiologist that patient is receiving propranolol.
• Monitor blood pressure frequently. If patient develops excessive hypotension, notify doctor. Tell patient that orthostatic hypotension can be minimized by rising slowly and avoiding sudden position changes.
• Relieve mouth dryness with sugarless gum, sour hard candy, or ice chips.
• Drug masks common signs of shock and hypoglycemia.

Italicized side effects are common or life-threatening.

35

Skeletal muscle relaxants

baclofen
carisoprodol
chlorphenesin carbamate
chlorzoxazone
cyclobenzaprine
dantrolene sodium
metaxalone
methocarbamol
orphenadrine citrate

---

baclofen
Lioresal

INDICATIONS & DOSAGE
Spasticity in multiple sclerosis, spinal cord injury—
Adults: initially, 5 mg t.i.d. for 3 days, 10 mg t.i.d. for 3 days, 15 mg t.i.d. for 3 days, 20 mg t.i.d. for 3 days. Increase according to response up to maximum 80 mg daily.

SIDE EFFECTS
CNS: *drowsiness, dizziness,* headache, *weakness, fatigue,* confusion, insomnia.
CV: hypotension.
EENT: nasal congestion.
GI: *nausea,* constipation.
GU: urinary frequency.
Hepatic: increased SGOT, alkaline phosphatase.
Metabolic: hyperglycemia.
Skin: rash, pruritus.
Other: ankle edema, excessive perspiration, weight gain.

INTERACTIONS
None significant.

NURSING CONSIDERATIONS
• Use cautiously in impaired renal function, stroke patients (minimal benefit, poor tolerance), epilepsy, spasticity used to sustain upright balance and locomotion or to obtain increased body function.
• Give with meals or milk to prevent gastric distress.
• Amount of relief determines if dosage (and drowsiness) can be reduced.
• Watch for increased seizures in epileptics.
• Watch for sensitivity reactions such as fever, skin eruptions, respiratory distress.
• Tell patient to avoid activities that require alertness until response to drug is determined. Drowsiness usually transient.
• Patient should follow doctor's orders regarding rest, physical therapy.
• Do not withdraw abruptly unless required by severe side effects; may precipitate hallucinations or rebound spasticity.
• Overdosage treatment supportive only; do not induce emesis or use respiratory stimulant in obtunded patients.
• Used investigationally for treatment of unstable bladder.

---

carisoprodol
Rela♦, Soma♦

INDICATIONS & DOSAGE
As an adjunct in acute, painful musculoskeletal conditions—

Adults, and children over 12:
350 mg P.O. t.i.d. and at bedtime.
Not recommended for children
under 12.

SIDE EFFECTS
CNS: *drowsiness, dizziness,* vertigo,
ataxia, tremor, agitation, irritability,
headache, depressive reactions,
insomnia.
CV: orthostatic hypotension, tachycardia, facial flushing.
GI: nausea, vomiting, increased
bowel activity, epigastric distress.
Skin: rash, *erythema multiforme,*
pruritus.
Other: hiccups, asthmatic episodes,
fever, angioneurotic edema, *anaphylaxis.*

INTERACTIONS
None significant.

NURSING CONSIDERATIONS
• Contraindicated in hypersensitivity
to related compounds (including meprobamate, tybamate); or intermittent
porphyria. Use with caution in impaired hepatic or renal function.
• Watch for idiosyncratic reactions
after first to fourth dose (weakness,
ataxia, visual and speech difficulties,
fever, skin eruptions, mental changes)
or severe reactions, including bronchospasm, hypotension, anaphylactic
shock. Hold dose and notify doctor
immediately of any unusual reactions.
• Record amount of relief to determine whether dosage can be reduced.
• Warn patient to avoid activities that
require alertness until response to
drug is determined. Drowsiness is
transient.
• Avoid combining with alcohol or
other depressants.
• Patient should follow doctor's orders regarding rest, physical therapy.

---

chlorphenesin carbamate
Maolate

INDICATIONS & DOSAGE
*As an adjunct in short-term, acute,
painful musculoskeletal conditions—*
Adults: initial dose 800 mg P.O.
t.i.d. Maintenance 400 mg P.O.
q.i.d. for maximum of 8 weeks.

SIDE EFFECTS
Blood: blood dyscrasia.
CNS: *drowsiness, dizziness,* confusion, headache, weakness. Dose-
related side effects include paradoxical stimulation, agitation, insomnia,
nervousness, headache.
GI: *nausea, epigastric distress.*
Other: *anaphylaxis.*

INTERACTIONS
None significant.

NURSING CONSIDERATIONS
• Use cautiously in hepatic disease or
impaired renal function.
• Safe use for periods over 8 weeks
not established.
• Take with meals or milk to prevent
gastric distress.
• Amount of relief determines if dosage (and drowsiness) can be reduced.
• Watch for sensitivity reactions such
as fever, skin eruptions, and respiratory distress. Hold dose and notify
doctor of unusual reactions.
• Monitor blood studies.
• Watch for unusual bleeding and infectious problems which may indicate
blood dyscrasia.

---

chlorzoxazone
Paraflex

INDICATIONS & DOSAGE
*As an adjunct in acute, painful muscu-
loskeletal conditions—*

Adults: 250 to 750 mg t.i.d. or q.i.d.
Children: 20 mg/Kg daily divided
t.i.d. or q.i.d.

SIDE EFFECTS
CNS: *drowsiness, dizziness, light-headedness,* malaise, headache, over-stimulation.
GI: anorexia, nausea, vomiting, heartburn, abdominal distress, constipation, diarrhea.
GU: urinary color change (orange or purple-red).
Hepatic: liver dysfunction.
Skin: urticaria, redness, itching, petechiae, bruising.

INTERACTIONS
None significant.

NURSING CONSIDERATIONS
• Contraindicated in impaired hepatic function. Use cautiously in drug allergies.
• Record amount of relief to determine whether dosage can be reduced.
• Watch for signs of hepatic damage. Hold dose and notify doctor.
• Warn patient to avoid activities that require alertness until response to drug is determined. Drowsiness is transient.
• Avoid combining with alcohol or other depressants.
• Expect urine color to change.
• Patient should follow doctor's orders regarding rest, physical therapy.
• Give with meals or milk to prevent gastric distress.

---

cyclobenzaprine
Flexeril♦

INDICATIONS & DOSAGE
Short-term treatment of muscle spasm—
Adults: 10 mg P.O. t.i.d. for 7 days.

Maximum: 60 mg/day for 2 to 3 weeks.

SIDE EFFECTS
CNS: *drowsiness,* euphoria, weakness, headache, insomnia, nightmares, paresthesias, dizziness.
CV: tachycardia.
EENT: blurred vision.
GI: abdominal pain, dyspepsia, peculiar taste, constipation, dry mouth.
GU: urinary retention.
Skin: rash, urticaria, pruritus.
Other: in high doses, watch for side effects like those of other tricyclic drugs (amitriptyline, imipramine).

INTERACTIONS
None significant.

NURSING CONSIDERATIONS
• Contraindicated in patients who have received MAO inhibitors within 14 days; during acute recovery phase of myocardial infarction; in heart block; arrhythmias; conduction disturbances; or congestive heart failure. Use cautiously in urinary retention, narrow-angle glaucoma, increased intraocular pressure, cardiovascular disease, impaired hepatic function, elderly or debilitated patients, or seizures.
• Withdrawal symptoms (nausea, headache, malaise) may occur if drug stopped abruptly after long-term use.
• Watch for symptoms of overdose, including possible cardiotoxicity. Notify doctor immediately and have physostigmine available.
• Check intake and output. Be alert for urinary retention. If constipation is a problem, increase fluid intake and get an order for a stool softener.
• Warn patient to avoid activities that require alertness until drug response is determined. Drowsiness and dizziness usually subside after 2 weeks.
• Avoid combining alcohol or other depressants with cyclobenzaprine.

• Patient may relieve dry mouth with sugarless candy or gum.

dantrolene sodium
Dantrium♦, Dantrium I.V.

INDICATIONS & DOSAGE
Spasticity and sequelae secondary to severe chronic disorders (multiple sclerosis, cerebral palsy, spinal cord injury, stroke)—
Adults: 25 mg P.O. daily. Increase gradually in increments of 25 mg, up to 100 mg b.i.d. to q.i.d. to maximum of 400 mg/day for 4 to 7 days.
Children: 1 mg/Kg/day P.O. b.i.d. to q.i.d. Increase gradually as needed by 1 mg/Kg/day to maximum of 100 mg q.i.d.
Management of malignant hyperthermia—
Adults and children: 1 mg/Kg I.V. initially; may repeat dose up to cumulative dose of 10 mg/Kg.

SIDE EFFECTS
Blood: eosinophilia.
CNS: *muscle weakness, drowsiness,* dizziness, light-headedness, malaise, headache, confusion, nervousness, insomnia.
CV: tachycardia, blood pressure changes.
EENT: excessive tearing, visual disturbances.
GI: anorexia, constipation, cramping, dysphagia.
GU: urinary frequency, incontinence, nocturia, dysuria, crystalluria, difficult erection.
Hepatic: *hepatocellular injury.*
Skin: eczematoid eruption, pruritus, urticaria.
Other: abnormal hair growth, drooling, sweating, pleural effusion, myalgia, chills, fever.

INTERACTIONS
None significant.

NURSING CONSIDERATIONS
The following are considerations for the P.O. form only.
• Contraindicated when spasticity is used to sustain upright balance and locomotion or to maintain increased body function; in spasms in rheumatic disorders; lactation. Use with caution in severely impaired cardiac or pulmonary function; preexisting hepatic disease; in females; and in patients over 35.
• Safety and efficacy in long-term use not established; value may be determined by therapeutic trial. Do not give more than 45 days if no benefits observed.
• Give with meals or milk to prevent gastric distress.
• Prepare oral suspension for single dose by dissolving capsule contents in juice or other suitable liquid. For multiple dose, use acid vehicle, such as citric acid in USP Syrup; refrigerate. Use in several days.
• Record amount of relief to determine whether dosage can be reduced.
• Watch for hepatitis (fever, jaundice), severe diarrhea or weakness, or sensitivity reactions (fever, skin eruptions). Hold dose and notify doctor.
• Warn patient to avoid driving and other hazardous activities until response to drug is determined. Side effects should subside after 4 days.
• Tell patient to avoid combining with alcohol or other depressants; to avoid photosensitivity reactions by using sunscreening agents and protective clothing; to report abdominal discomfort or GI problems immediately; and to follow doctor's orders regarding rest, physical therapy.
The following are considerations for the I.V. form only.
• Administer as soon as malignant hyperthermia reaction is recognized.
• Reconstitute each vial by adding 60 ml of sterile water for injection and shaking vial until clear.

Italicized side effects are common or life-threatening.

• Protect contents from light and use within 6 hours.

metaxalone
Skelaxin♦

INDICATIONS & DOSAGE
As an adjunct in acute, painful musculoskeletal conditions—
Adults, and children over 12 years:
800 mg P.O. t.i.d. or q.i.d.

SIDE EFFECTS
Blood: leukopenia, hemolytic anemia.
CNS: *drowsiness,* dizziness, headache, nervousness, irritability, exacerbation of grand mal epilepsy.
GI: *nausea, vomiting,* jaundice.
Skin: light rash with or without pruritus.

INTERACTIONS
None significant.

NURSING CONSIDERATIONS
• Contraindicated in impaired hepatic or renal function; history of drug-induced hemolytic or other anemias.
• Test hepatic function periodically. May cause abnormalities in liver function studies; repeat tests after drug is discontinued.
• Record amount of relief to determine if dosage can be reduced.
• Watch for sensitivity reactions such as rash with pruritus.
• Warn patient to avoid combining with alcohol or other depressants.
• Patient should follow doctor's orders regarding rest, physical therapy.
• Give with meals or milk to prevent gastric distress.
• False positive results in glucose tests if cupric sulfate is used. Use glucose oxidase instead.

methocarbamol
Delaxin, Forbaxin, Metho-500, Robamol, Robaxin♦, Romethocarb, Spenaxin

INDICATIONS & DOSAGE
As an adjunct in acute, painful musculoskeletal conditions—
Adults: 1.5 g P.O. for 2 to 3 days, then 1 g P.O. q.i.d., or not more than 500 mg (5 ml) I.M. into each gluteal region. May repeat q 8 hours. Or 1 to 3 g/day (10 to 30 ml) I.V. directly into vein at 3 ml/minute, or 10 ml may be added to no more than 250 ml of 5% dextrose in water or normal saline. Maximum dose 3 g/day.
Supportive therapy in tetanus management—
Adults: 1 to 2 g into tubing of running I.V. or 1 to 3 g in infusion bottle q 6 hours.
Children: 15 mg/Kg I.V. q 6 hours.

SIDE EFFECTS
Blood: hemolysis, increased hemoglobin (I.V. only).
CNS: drowsiness, dizziness, lightheadedness, headache, vertigo, mild muscular incoordination (I.M. or I.V. only), convulsions (I.V. only).
CV: hypotension, bradycardia (I.M. or I.V. only).
GI: *nausea, anorexia, GI upset.*
GU: red blood cells in urine (I.V. only).
Skin: urticaria, pruritus, rash.
Local: thrombophlebitis, extravasation (I.V. only).
Other: fever, metallic taste, flushing, *anaphylactic reactions (I.M. or I.V. only).*

INTERACTIONS
None significant.

NURSING CONSIDERATIONS
• Contraindicated in impaired renal function (injectable form), children

under 12 years (except in tetanus), myasthenia gravis, patients receiving anticholinesterase agents, epilepsy (injectable form).
• I.V. irritates veins, may cause phlebitis, aggravates seizures, may cause fainting if injected rapidly.
• In tetanus management, use methocarbamol with tetanus antitoxin, penicillin, tracheotomy, and aggressive supportive care. Long course of I.V. methocarbamol required.
• Watch for sensitivity reactions such as fever, skin eruptions.
• Warn patient to avoid activities that require alertness until response to drug is determined. Drowsiness subsides.
• Avoid combining with alcohol or other depressants.
• Patient should follow doctor's orders regarding rest, physical therapy.
• Tell patient urine may turn green, black, or brown.
• Give with meals or milk to prevent gastric distress.
• Watch for orthostatic hypotension, especially with parenteral administration. Keep patient supine for 15 minutes afterward, and supervise ambulation. Advise patient to get up slowly.
• Give I.V. slowly. Maximum rate 300 mg (3 ml)/minute. Give I.M. deeply, only in upper outer quadrant of buttocks, with maximum of 5 ml in each buttock, and inject slowly. Do not give S.C.
• Have epinephrine, antihistamines, corticosteroids available.
• Prepare liquid by crushing tablets into water or saline solution. Give through nasogastric tube.

orphenadrine citrate
Flexon, Myolin, Norflex♦, Ro-Orphena, Tega-Flex, X-Otag

INDICATIONS & DOSAGE
Adjunctive treatment in painful, acute musculoskeletal conditions—
Adults: 100 mg P.O. b.i.d., or 60 mg I.V. or I.M. q 12 hours, p.r.n.

SIDE EFFECTS
CNS: disorientation, restlessness, irritability, weakness, *drowsiness*, headache.
CV: palpitations, tachycardia.
EENT: dilated pupils, blurred vision, difficulty swallowing.
GI: constipation, *dry mouth*, nausea, vomiting, paralytic ileus, epigastric distress.
GU: urinary hesitancy or retention.

INTERACTIONS
None significant.

NURSING CONSIDERATIONS
• Contraindicated in narrow-angle glaucoma; prostatic hypertrophy; pyloric, duodenal, or bladder neck obstruction; myasthenia gravis; tachycardia; severe hepatic or renal disease; ulcerative colitis; lactation. Use cautiously in elderly or debilitated patients with cardiac disease; those exposed to high temperatures; arrhythmias.
• Check all dosages carefully. Even a slight overdose can lead to toxicity. Early signs are excessive dry mouth, dilated pupils, blurred vision, skin flushing, fever.
• Monitor vital signs carefully.
• When given I.V., may cause paradoxical initial bradycardia. Usually disappears in 2 minutes.

Italicized side effects are common or life-threatening.

• Monitor intake and output. Causes urinary retention and hesitancy; have patient void before administering.
• Relieve dry mouth with cool drinks, ice chips, sugarless gum, or hard candy.

• Monitor blood, urine, and hepatic function periodically, especially with long-term use.
• Patient may develop a tolerance to this drug.

36

Neuromuscular blockers

decamethonium bromide
gallamine triethiodide
hexafluorenium bromide
metocurine iodide
pancuronium bromide
succinylcholine chloride
tubocurarine chloride

decamethonium bromide
Syncurine♦

INDICATIONS & DOSAGE
Adjunct to anesthesia to induce skeletal muscle relaxation; facilitate intubation, lessen muscle contractions in pharmacologically or electrically induced convulsions; assist with mechanical ventilation—
Dose depends on anesthetic used, individual needs, and response. Doses are representative and must be adjusted.
Adults: initially, 0.5 to 3 mg I.V., at a rate of 0.5 mg to 1 mg per minute, then 0.5 to 1 mg q 10 to 30 minutes for sustained relaxation.
Children and infants: initially, 0.05 to 0.08 mg/Kg I.V., then 0.02 to 0.03 mg/Kg at intervals.

SIDE EFFECTS
CV: bradycardia, tachycardia, hypo- and hypertension.
Other: *dose-related prolonged apnea,* residual muscle weakness, increased oropharyngeal secretions, allergic or idiosyncratic hypersensitivity reactions, *postoperative muscle pain.*

INTERACTIONS
Aminoglycoside antibiotics (including amikacin, gentamicin, kanamycin, neomycin, streptomycin); polymyxin antibiotics (polymyxin B sulfate, colistin); clindamycin, quinidine: potentiated neuromuscular blockade, leading to increased skeletal muscle relaxation and possible respiratory paralysis. Use cautiously during surgical and postop periods.
Narcotic analgesics: potentiated neuromuscular blockade, leading to increased skeletal muscle relaxation and possible respiratory paralysis. Use with extreme caution.

NURSING CONSIDERATIONS
• Contraindicated in hypersensitivity to bromides, impaired renal function, shock, myasthenia gravis, surgical procedures lasting longer than 20 minutes. Use cautiously in patients undergoing surgery in Trendelenburg or lithotomy positions; patients recently digitalized; elderly or debilitated patients; in hepatic or pulmonary impairment; respiratory depression; myasthenic syndrome of lung cancer; dehydration; thyroid disorders; collagen disease; porphyria; electrolyte disturbances; fractures; muscular spasms; and (in large doses) cesarean section.
• Seldom used due to uncertain effects and lack of suitable antidote.
• Multiple doses not often recommended; may cause reduced response, prolonged apnea.
• Monitor baseline electrolyte determinations (electrolyte imbalance, es-

pecially K, Ca, and Mg, can potentiate neuromuscular effects), vital signs, especially respiration.
• Check intake/output (renal dysfunction prolongs duration of action, since drug is unchanged before excretion).
• Maintain clear airway. Have emergency respiratory support (endotracheal equipment, respirator, oxygen, atropine, neostigmine, or edrophonium) on hand.
• Reassure patient that postop stiffness is normal and will soon subside.
• Use only fresh solutions.
• Give I.V. slowly (not more than 1 mg/minute).
• Do not give without direct supervision of doctor or experienced clinician.

---

gallamine triethiodide
Flaxedil♦

INDICATIONS & DOSAGE
Adjunct to anesthesia to induce skeletal muscle relaxation; facilitate intubation; reduction of fractures and dislocations; lessen muscle contractions in pharmacologically or electrically induced convulsions; assist with mechanical ventilation—
Dose depends on anesthetic used, individual needs, and response. Doses are representative and must be adjusted.
Adults, and children over 1 month: initially, 1 mg/Kg I.V. to maximum of 100 mg, regardless of patient's weight; then 0.5 mg to 1 mg/Kg q 30 to 40 minutes.
Children under 1 month but over 5 Kg (11 lbs): initially, 0.25 to 0.75 mg/Kg I.V., then 0.01 to 0.05 mg/Kg q 30 to 40 minutes.

SIDE EFFECTS
CV: tachycardia.
Other: *respiratory paralysis, dose-re-*
lated prolonged apnea, residual muscle weakness, increased oropharyngeal secretions, allergic or idiosyncratic hypersensitivity reactions.

INTERACTIONS
Aminoglycoside antibiotics (amikacin, gentamicin, kanamycin, neomycin, streptomycin); polymyxin antibiotics (polymyxin B sulfate, colistin); clindamycin; quinidine: potentiated neuromuscular blockade, leading to increased skeletal muscle relaxation and possible respiratory paralysis. Use cautiously during surgical and postop periods.
Narcotic analgesics: potentiated neuromuscular blockade, leading to increased skeletal muscle relaxation and possible respiratory paralysis. Use with extreme caution, and reduce dose of gallamine.

NURSING CONSIDERATIONS
• Contraindicated in hypersensitivity to iodides; patients in whom tachycardia may be hazardous; impaired renal function; shock; myasthenia gravis. Use cautiously in cesarean section, hepatic or pulmonary impairment, respiratory depression, elderly or debilitated patients, myasthenic syndrome of lung cancer, dehydration, thyroid disorders, collagen diseases, porphyria, electrolyte disturbances, fractures, muscular spasm.
• Monitor baseline electrolyte determinations (electrolyte imbalance can potentiate neuromuscular effects).
• Watch respiration for early symptoms of paralysis, inability to keep eyelids open and eyes focused, difficulty in swallowing and speaking. Notify doctor immediately.
• Take vital signs every 15 minutes, especially for developing tachycardia. Notify doctor immediately of changes.
• Measure intake/output (renal dysfunction prolongs duration of action, since drug is unchanged before

---

excretion).
• Keep airway clear. Have emergency respiratory support (endotracheal equipment, respirator, oxygen, atropine, neostigmine) on hand.
• Reassure patient that postop stiffness is normal and will soon subside.
• Determine whether patient has iodide allergy.
• Protect drug from light or excessive heat; use only fresh solutions.
• Do not mix solution with meperidine HCl or barbiturate solutions.
• Give I.V. slowly (over 30 to 90 seconds).
• Do not give without direct supervision of doctor.

---

hexafluorenium bromide
Mylaxen

INDICATIONS & DOSAGE
Adjunct for use with succinylcholine to prolong neuromuscular blockade and reduce muscular fasciculations—
Dose depends on individual needs and response. Doses are representative and must be adjusted.
Adults and children: use in ratio of 2 mg/1 mg succinylcholine. Maximum hexafluorenium bromide 10 to 36 mg; should not be administered more frequently than q 15 to 30 minutes.

SIDE EFFECTS
CNS: *prolonged neuromuscular blockade.*
CV: hypotension, hypertension, tachycardia, bradycardia.
EENT: increased intraocular pressure.
Other: increased bronchial tone, *bronchospasm.*

INTERACTIONS
None reported for this drug alone; always used with succinylcholine. See succinylcholine.

NURSING CONSIDERATIONS
• Contraindicated in hypersensitivity to bromides, in bronchial asthma. Use cautiously in renal, hepatic, or pulmonary impairment, or respiratory depression; in elderly or debilitated patients; in myasthenia gravis; myasthenic syndrome of lung cancer; dehydration; thyroid disorders; collagen diseases; porphyria; electrolyte disturbances; (in large doses) cesarean section; glaucoma; or during ocular surgery.
• Not used extensively in clinical practice.
• Monitor baseline electrolyte determinations (electrolyte imbalance potentiates neuromuscular effects) and vital signs (watch respirations closely).
• Keep airway clear. Have emergency respiratory support (endotracheal equipment, respirator, oxygen, atropine, neostigmine) on hand.
• Reassure patient that postop stiffness is normal and will soon subside.
• Determine whether patient has bromide allergy.
• Use only fresh solutions; do not give without direct supervision of doctor.

---

metocurine iodide
Metubine

INDICATIONS & DOSAGE
Adjunct to anesthesia to induce skeletal muscle relaxation; facilitate intubation, reduction of fractures and dislocations—
Dose depends on anesthetic used, individual needs, and response. Doses are representative and must be adjusted. Administer as sustained injection over 30 to 60 seconds.
Adults: given cyclopropane: 2 to 4 mg I.V. (2.68 mg average).
Given ether: 1.5 to 3 mg I.V. (2.1 mg average).

Italicized side effects are common or life-threatening.

Given nitrous oxide: 4 to 7 mg I.V. (4.79 mg average). Supplemental injections of 0.5 to 1 mg in 25 to 90 minutes, repeated p.r.n.
Lessen muscle contractions in pharmacologically or electrically induced convulsions—
Adults: 1.75 to 5.5 mg I.V.

SIDE EFFECTS
CV: hypotension secondary to histamine release, ganglionic blockade in rapid dose or overdose.
Other: *dose-related prolonged apnea,* residual muscle weakness, increased oropharyngeal secretions, allergic or idiosyncratic hypersensitivity reactions, *bronchospasm.*

INTERACTIONS
Aminoglycoside antibiotics (including amikacin, gentamicin, kanamycin, neomycin, streptomycin); polymyxin and polypeptide antibiotics (polymyxin B sulfate, colistin); clindamycin; quinidine: potentiated neuromuscular blockade, leading to increased skeletal muscle relaxation and possible respiratory paralysis. Use cautiously during surgical and postop periods.
Narcotic analgesics: potentiated neuromuscular blockade, leading to increased skeletal muscle relaxation and possible respiratory paralysis. Use with extreme caution, and reduce dose of metocurine iodide.

NURSING CONSIDERATIONS
• Contraindicated in hypersensitivity to iodides; in patients in whom histamine release is a hazard (asthmatic or atopic patients). Use cautiously in myasthenia gravis; renal, hepatic, or pulmonary impairment; respiratory depression; elderly or debilitated patients; myasthenia gravis; myasthenic syndrome of lung cancer; dehydration; thyroid disorders; collagen diseases; porphyria; electrolyte disturbances; hyperthermia; (in large doses) cesarean section.
• Neostigmine, edrophonium, and epinephrine may be used to reverse effects of metocurine because of their anticurare effects.
• Doses of 1 mg therapeutic equivalent of 3 mg *d*-tubocurarine chloride.
• Monitor baseline electrolyte determinations (electrolyte imbalance, especially K, Ca, and Mg, can potentiate neuromuscular effects), vital signs, especially respiration.
• Measure intake and output (renal dysfunction prolongs duration of action, since drug is mainly unchanged before excretion).
• Keep airway clear. Have emergency respiratory support (endotracheal equipment, respirator, oxygen, atropine, edrophonium, epinephrine, and neostigmine) on hand.
• Reassure patient that postop stiffness is normal and will soon subside.
• Determine whether patient has iodide allergy.
• Store solution away from heat, sunlight; do not mix with barbiturates, methohexital, or thiopental (precipitate will form). Use fresh solutions only.
• Do not give without direct supervision of doctor.

---

pancuronium bromide
Pavulon♦

INDICATIONS & DOSAGE
Adjunct to anesthesia to induce skeletal muscle relaxation; facilitate intubation, lessen muscle contractions in pharmacologically or electrically induced convulsions; assist with mechanical ventilation—
Dose depends on anesthetic used, individual needs, and response. Doses are representative and must be adjusted.

Adults: initially, 0.04 to 0.1 mg/Kg I.V.; then 0.01 mg/Kg q 30 to 60 minutes.
Children over 10 years: initially, 0.04 to 0.1 mg/Kg I.V., then ¹/₅ initial dose q 30 to 60 minutes.

SIDE EFFECTS
CV: tachycardia, increased blood pressure.
Local: burning sensation.
Skin: transient rashes.
Other: excessive sweating and salivation, *prolonged dose-related apnea,* residual muscle weakness, allergic or idiosyncratic hypersensitivity reactions.

INTERACTIONS
Aminoglycoside antibiotics (including amikacin, gentamicin, kanamycin, neomycin, streptomycin); polymyxin and polypeptide antibiotics (polymyxin B sulfate, colistin); clindamycin; quinidine: potentiated neuromuscular blockade, leading to increased skeletal muscle relaxation and possible respiratory paralysis. Use cautiously during surgical and postop periods.
Lithium, narcotic analgesics: potentiated neuromuscular blockade, leading to increased skeletal muscle relaxation and possible respiratory paralysis. Use with extreme caution, and reduce dose of pancuronium.

NURSING CONSIDERATIONS
• Contraindicated in hypersensitivity to bromides; preexisting tachycardia; patients for whom even a minor increase in heart rate is undesirable. Use cautiously in renal, hepatic, or pulmonary impairment; respiratory depression; elderly or debilitated patients; myasthenic gravis; myasthenia syndrome of lung cancer; dehydration; thyroid disorders; collagen diseases; porphyria; electrolyte disturbances; hyperthermia; (in large

doses) cesarean section; or in toxemic states.
• Causes no histamine release or hypotension.
• Dose of 1 mg approximates therapeutic equivalent of 5 mg *d*-tubocurarine chloride.
• Monitor baseline electrolyte determinations (electrolyte imbalance can potentiate neuromuscular effects) and vital signs (watch respiration and heart rate closely).
• Measure intake and output (renal dysfunction may prolong duration of action, since 25% of the drug is unchanged before excretion).
• Have emergency respiratory support (endotracheal equipment, respirator, oxygen, atropine, neostigmine) on hand.
• Allow succinylcholine effects to subside before giving pancuronium.
• Store in refrigerator. Do not store in plastic containers or syringes, although plastic syringes may be used for administration.
• Do not mix with barbiturate solutions; use only fresh solutions.
• Do not give without direct supervision of doctor.

---

succinylcholine chloride
Anectine♦, Anectine Flo-Pack Powder, Sucostrin, Sux-Cert

INDICATIONS & DOSAGE
Adjunct to anesthesia to induce skeletal muscle relaxation; facilitate intubation and assist with mechanical ventilation or orthopedic manipulations (drug of choice); lessen muscle contractions in pharmacologically or electrically induced convulsions—
Dose depends on anesthetic used, individual needs, and response. Doses are representative and must be adjusted.
Adults: 25 to 75 mg I.V., then 2.5 mg/minute, p.r.n. or 2.5 mg/Kg

I.M. up to maximum 150 mg I.M. in deltoid muscle.

Children: 1 to 2 mg/Kg I.M. or I.V. Maximum I.M. dose 150 mg. (Children may be less sensitive to succinylcholine than adults.)

SIDE EFFECTS
CV: bradycardia, tachycardia, hypertension, hypotension, arrhythmias.
EENT: increased intraocular pressure.
Other: *prolonged respiratory depression, apnea, malignant hyperthermia,* muscle fasciculation, *postoperative muscle pain,* myoglobinemia, excessive salivation, allergic or idiosyncratic hypersensitivity reactions.

INTERACTIONS
Aminoglycoside antibiotics (including amikacin, gentamicin, kanamycin, neomycin, paromomycin, streptomycin); polymyxin and polypeptide antibiotics (polymyxin B sulfate, colistin); echothiophate: potentiated neuromuscular blockade, leading to increased skeletal muscle relaxation and possible respiratory paralysis. Use cautiously during surgical and postop periods.
Narcotic analgesics, lidocaine, procaine, methotrimeprazine: potentiated neuromuscular blockade, leading to increased skeletal muscle relaxation and possible respiratory paralysis. Use with extreme caution.
MAO inhibitors, lithium, echothiophate, cyclophosphamide: prolonged apnea. Use with caution.
Magnesium sulfate (parenterally): potentiated neuromuscular blockade, increased skeletal muscle relaxation, and possible respiratory paralysis. Use with caution, preferably with reduced doses.
Digitalis glycosides: possible cardiac arrhythmias. Use together cautiously.

NURSING CONSIDERATIONS
• Contraindicated in abnormally low plasma or pseudocholinesterase levels. Use with caution in severe burns or trauma; electrolyte imbalance; quinidine or digitalis therapy; hyperkalemia; paraplegia; spinal neuraxis injury; degenerative or dystrophic neuromuscular disease; patient with personal or family history of malignant hypertension or hyperthermia; hepatic, renal, or pulmonary impairment; respiratory depression; elderly or debilitated patients; myasthenia gravis; myasthenic syndrome of lung cancer; dehydration; thyroid disorders; collagen diseases; porphyria; fractures; muscular spasms; (in large doses) cesarean section; glaucoma; eye surgery or penetrating eye wounds; pheochromocytoma.
• Drug of choice for short procedures (less than 3 minutes) and for orthopedic manipulations; use caution in fractures or dislocations.
• Duration of action prolonged to 20 minutes by continuous I.V. infusion or single-dose administration, along with hexafluorenium bromide.
• Repeated or continuous infusions of succinylcholine alone not advised; may cause reduced response or prolonged apnea.
• Monitor baseline electrolyte determinations and vital signs (check respiration every 5 to 10 minutes during infusion).
• Keep airway clear. Have emergency respiratory support (endotracheal equipment, respirator, oxygen, atropine, neostigmine) on hand.
• Reassure patient that postop stiffness is normal and will soon subside.
• Store injectable form in refrigerator. Store powder form at room temperature, tightly closed. Use immediately after reconstitution. Do not mix with alkaline solutions (thiopental, sodium bicarbonate, barbiturates).
• Give test dose (10 mg I.M. or I.V.) after patient has been anesthetized.

Normal response (no respiratory depression or transient depression lasting less than 5 minutes) indicates drug may be given. Do not give if patient develops respiratory paralysis sufficient to permit endotracheal intubation. (Recovery within 30 to 60 minutes.)
• Do not give without direct supervision of doctor.

tubocurarine chloride
Tubarine♦ ♦

INDICATIONS & DOSAGE
Adjunct to anesthesia to induce skeletal muscle relaxation; facilitate intubation, orthopedic manipulations—
Dose depends on anesthetic used, individual needs, and response. Doses listed are representative and must be adjusted.
Adults: 1 unit/Kg or 0.15 mg/Kg I.V. slowly over 60 to 90 seconds. Average, initially, 40 to 60 units I.V. May give 20 to 30 units in 3 to 5 minutes. For longer procedures, give 20 units, p.r.n.
Children: 1 unit/Kg or 0.15 mg/Kg.
Assist with mechanical ventilation—
Adults and children: initially, 0.0165 mg/Kg I.V. (average 1 mg or 7 units), then adjust subsequent doses to patient's response.
Diagnose myasthenia gravis—
Adults and children: 0.0041 to 0.033 mg/Kg I.V. or $^1/_{15}$ to $^1/_5$ normal adult dose for electroshock. Positive result: profound exaggeration of myasthenic symptoms. Dose may also be given I.M. when necessary.
Lessen muscle contractions in pharmacologically or electrically induced convulsions—
Adults and children: 1 unit/Kg or 0.15 mg/Kg slowly over 60 to 90 seconds. Initial dose 20 units (3 mg) less than calculated dose.

SIDE EFFECTS
CV: hypotension, circulatory depression.
Other: profound and prolonged muscle relaxation, *respiratory depression to the point of apnea,* hypersensitivity, idiosyncrasy, residual muscle weakness, *bronchospasm.*

INTERACTIONS
Aminoglycoside antibiotics (including amikacin, gentamicin, kanamycin, neomycin, paromomycin, streptomycin); polymyxin and polypeptide antibiotics (polymyxin B sulfate, colistin): potentiated neuromuscular blockade, leading to increased skeletal muscle relaxation and possible respiratory paralysis. Use cautiously during surgical and postop periods.
Quinidine: prolonged neuromuscular blockade. Use together with caution. Monitor closely.
Thiazide diuretics, furosemide, ethacrynic acid, amphotericin B, propranolol, methotrimeprazine, narcotic analgesics: potentiated neuromuscular blockade, leading to increased respiratory paralysis. Use with extreme caution during surgical and postop periods.

NURSING CONSIDERATIONS
• Contraindicated in patients for whom histamine release is a hazard (asthmatics). Use cautiously in hepatic or pulmonary impairment; respiratory depression; elderly or debilitated patients; myasthenia gravis; myasthenic syndrome of lung cancer; dehydration; thyroid disorders; collagen diseases; porphyria; electrolyte disturbances; fractures; muscular spasms; and (in large doses) cesarean section.
• Small margin of safety between therapeutic dose and dose causing respiratory paralysis.
• Used to diagnose myasthenia gravis, but procedure is hazardous.

Italicized side effects are common or life-threatening.

- Allow succinylcholine effects to subside before giving tubocurarine.
- Monitor baseline electrolyte determinations (electrolyte imbalance can potentiate neuromuscular effects).
- Watch respiration closely for early symptoms of paralysis—inability to keep eyelids open and eyes focused or difficulty in swallowing and speaking; notify doctor immediately.
- Check vital signs every 15 minutes. Notify doctor at once of changes.
- Measure intake and output (renal dysfunction prolongs duration of action, since much of drug is unchanged before excretion).

- Keep airway clear. Have emergency respiratory support (endotracheal equipment, respirator, oxygen, atropine, edrophonium, epinephrine, and neostigmine) on hand.
- Reassure patient that postop stiffness is normal and will soon subside.
- Decrease dose if inhalation anesthetics are used.
- Do not mix with barbiturates. Use only fresh solutions and discard if discolored.
- Give I.V. slowly (60 to 90 seconds); give I.M. deeply in deltoid muscle.
- Do not give without direct supervision of doctor.

37

Antihistamines

azatadine maleate
brompheniramine maleate
carbinoxamine maleate
chlorpheniramine maleate
clemastine fumarate
cyproheptadine hydrochloride
dexchlorpheniramine maleate
dimethindene maleate
dimethothiazine mesylate
diphenhydramine hydrochloride
diphenylpyraline hydrochloride
doxylamine succinate
methdilazine hydrochloride
promethazine hydrochloride
trimeprazine tartrate
tripelennamine hydrochloride
triprolidine hydrochloride

---

azatadine maleate
Optimine♦

INDICATIONS & DOSAGE
Rhinitis, allergy symptoms, chronic urticaria—
Adults: 1 to 2 mg P.O. b.i.d. Maximum 4 mg daily.

SIDE EFFECTS
Blood: thrombocytopenia.
CNS (especially in the elderly): *drowsiness, dizziness,* vertigo, disturbed coordination, sedation.
CV: hypotension, palpitations.
GI: anorexia, *nausea,* vomiting, *dry mouth and throat.*
GU: urinary retention.
Skin: urticaria, rash.
Other: thickening of bronchial secretions.

INTERACTIONS
None significant.

NURSING CONSIDERATIONS
• Contraindicated in acute asthmatic attack. Use cautiously in increased intraocular pressure, hyperthyroidism, elderly patients, cardiovascular or renal disease, hypertension, bronchial asthma, narrow-angle glaucoma, urinary retention, prostatic hypertrophy, bladder neck obstruction.
• Warn patient against alcoholic beverages during therapy and against activities that require alertness until response to drug is determined.
• Reduce GI distress by giving with food or milk.
• Coffee or tea may reduce drowsiness. Sugarless gum, sour hard candy, or ice chips may relieve dry mouth.
• Titrate each patient's dose; response to drug varies.
• If tolerance develops, another antihistamine may be substituted.
• Warn patient to stop taking drug 4 days before allergy skin tests; otherwise, accuracy of tests may be affected.

---

brompheniramine maleate
Dimetane♦, Dimetane-Ten, Rolabromophen, Spentane, Veltane

INDICATIONS & DOSAGE
Rhinitis, allergy symptoms—
Adults: 4 to 8 mg P.O. t.i.d. or q.i.d.; or (timed-release) 8 to 12 mg P.O. b.i.d. or t.i.d.; or 5 to 20 mg q 6 to

12 hours I.M., I.V., or S.C. Maximum 40 mg daily.
Children over 6 years: 2 to 4 mg t.i.d. or q.i.d.; or (timed-release) 8 to 12 mg q 12 hours; or 0.5 mg/Kg daily I.M., I.V., or S.C. divided t.i.d. or q.i.d.
Children under 6 years: 0.5 mg/Kg daily P.O., I.M., I.V., or S.C. divided t.i.d. or q.i.d.

SIDE EFFECTS
Blood: thrombocytopenia, *agranulocytosis*.
CNS (especially in the elderly): dizziness, tremors, irritability, insomnia, *drowsiness*.
CV: hypotension, palpitations.
GI: anorexia, nausea, vomiting, *dry mouth and throat*.
GU: urinary retention.
Skin: urticaria, rash.
After parenteral administration: local reaction, sweating, syncope.

INTERACTIONS
None significant.

NURSING CONSIDERATIONS
• Contraindicated in acute asthmatic attack. Use cautiously in increased intraocular pressure, hyperthyroidism, elderly patients, cardiovascular or renal disease, hypertension, bronchial asthma, narrow-angle glaucoma, urinary retention, prostatic hypertrophy, bladder neck obstruction.
• Warn patient against alcoholic beverages during therapy and against activities that require alertness until response to drug is determined.
• Reduce GI distress by giving with food or milk.
• Coffee or tea may reduce drowsiness. Sugarless gum, sour hard candy, or ice chips may relieve dry mouth.
• Titrate each patient's dose; response to drug varies.
• If tolerance develops, another antihistamine may be substituted.
• Warn patient to stop taking drug

4 days before allergy skin tests; otherwise, accuracy of tests may be affected.
• Injectable form containing 10 mg per ml can be given diluted or undiluted very slowly I.V. The 100 mg/ml injection should not be given I.V.

---

carbinoxamine maleate
Clistin, Clistin RA

INDICATIONS & DOSAGE
Rhinitis, allergy symptoms—
Adults: 4 to 8 mg P.O. t.i.d. to q.i.d., or (timed-release) 8 to 12 mg q 8 to 12 hours.
Children over 6 years: 4 mg P.O. t.i.d. to q.i.d.
Children 3 to 6 years: 2 to 4 mg P.O. t.i.d. to q.i.d.
Children 1 to 3 years: 2 mg P.O. t.i.d. to q.i.d.

SIDE EFFECTS
CNS (especially in the elderly): *drowsiness, dizziness*.
GI: anorexia, nausea, vomiting, *dry mouth*.

INTERACTIONS
None significant.

NURSING CONSIDERATIONS
• Contraindicated in acute asthmatic attack. Use cautiously in increased intraocular pressure, hyperthyroidism, elderly patients, cardiovascular or renal disease, hypertension, bronchial asthma, narrow-angle glaucoma, urinary retention, prostatic hypertrophy, bladder neck obstruction.
• Warn patient against using alcoholic beverages during therapy and against driving or other activities that require alertness until response to drug is determined.
• Reduce GI distress by giving with food or milk.
• Coffee or tea may reduce drowsi-

---

ness. Sugarless gum, sour hard candy, or ice chips may relieve dry mouth.
• Titrate each patient's dose; response to drug varies.
• If tolerance develops, another antihistamine may be substituted.
• Warn patient to stop taking drug 4 days before allergy skin tests; otherwise, accuracy of tests may be affected.

chlorpheniramine maleate
Allerid-O.D., AL-R, Chloramate, Chlormene, Chlortab, Chlor-Trimeton, Chlor-Tripolon♦♦, Ciramine, Histalon♦♦, Histapan, Histex, Histrey, Novopheniram♦♦, Pyranistan, Teldrin

INDICATIONS & DOSAGE
Rhinitis, allergy symptoms—
Adults: 2 to 4 mg P.O. t.i.d. or q.i.d.; or (timed-release) 8 to 12 mg P.O. b.i.d. or t.i.d.; or 5 to 40 mg I.M., I.V., or S.C. Give I.V. injection over 1 minute.
Children 6 to 12 years: 2 mg P.O. t.i.d. or q.i.d.; or (timed-release) 8 mg P.O. daily or b.i.d.
Children 2 to 6 years: 1 mg P.O. t.i.d. or q.i.d.

SIDE EFFECTS
CNS (especially in the elderly): sedation, *drowsiness.*
CV: hypotension, palpitations.
GI: epigastric distress, *dry mouth.*
GU: urinary retention.
Other: thickening of bronchial secretions.
After parenteral administration: local stinging, burning sensation, pallor, weak pulse, transient hypotension.

INTERACTIONS
None significant.

NURSING CONSIDERATIONS
• Contraindicated in acute asthmatic attack. Use cautiously in increased intraocular pressure, hyperthyroidism, elderly patients, cardiovascular or renal disease, hypertension, bronchial asthma, narrow-angle glaucoma, urinary retention, prostatic hypertrophy, bladder neck obstruction.
• Warn patient against using alcoholic beverages and other CNS depressants during therapy and against driving or other activities that require alertness until response to drug is determined.
• Coffee or tea may reduce drowsiness.
• Titrate each patient's dose; response to drug varies.
• If tolerance develops, another antihistamine may be substituted.
• Warn patient to stop taking drug 4 days before allergy skin tests; otherwise, accuracy of tests may be affected.
• Only injectable forms *without* preservatives can be given I.V. Give *slowly.*
• If symptoms occur after parenteral dose, stop drug. Notify doctor.

clemastine fumarate
Tavist, Tavist-1

INDICATIONS & DOSAGE
Rhinitis, allergy symptoms—
Adults: 1.34 to 2.68 mg once daily. Maximum recommended daily dosage is 8.04 mg; or (timed-release) 1.34 mg (long-acting tablet) b.i.d., not to exceed 8.04 mg (6 long-acting tablets) per day.
Allergic skin manifestation of urticaria and angioedema—
Adults: 2.68 mg up to t.i.d. maximum.

Italicized side effects are common or life-threatening.

SIDE EFFECTS

Blood: hemolytic anemia, thrombo-cytopenia, *agranulocytosis.*
CNS (especially in the elderly): *sedation, drowsiness.*
CV: hypotension, palpitations, tachy-cardia.
GI: epigastric distress, anorexia, nausea, vomiting, constipation, *dry mouth.*
GU: urinary retention.
Skin: rash, urticaria.
Other: thickening of bronchial secretions.

INTERACTIONS

None significant.

NURSING CONSIDERATIONS

• Contraindicated in acute asthmatic attack. Use cautiously in increased intraocular pressure, hyperthyroidism, elderly patients, cardiovascular or renal disease, hypertension, bronchial asthma, narrow-angle glaucoma, urinary retention, prostatic hypertrophy, bladder neck obstruction.
• Warn patient against using alcoholic beverages during therapy and against driving or other activities that require alertness until response to drug is determined.
• Coffee or tea may reduce drowsiness. Sugarless gum, sour hard candy, or ice chips may relieve dry mouth.
• Titrate each patient's dose; response to drug varies.
• If tolerance develops, another anti-histamine may be substituted.
• Warn patient to stop taking drug 4 days before allergy skin tests; otherwise, accuracy of tests may be affected.
• Tablets are available as 1.34 and 2.68 mg. Long-acting tablets are 1.34 mg.

cyproheptadine hydrochloride
Periactin♦, Vimicon♦♦

INDICATIONS & DOSAGE

Allergy symptoms, pruritus—
Adults: 4 mg P.O. t.i.d. or q.i.d. Maximum 0.5 mg/Kg daily.
Children 7 to 14 years: 4 mg P.O. b.i.d. or t.i.d.
Children 2 to 6 years: 2 mg P.O. b.i.d. or t.i.d.

SIDE EFFECTS

CNS (especially in the elderly): sedation, *drowsiness,* dizziness, headache, fatigue.
GI: anorexia, nausea, vomiting, *dry mouth.*
Skin: rash.
Other: weight gain.

INTERACTIONS

None significant.

NURSING CONSIDERATIONS

• Contraindicated in acute asthmatic attack. Use cautiously in increased intraocular pressure, hyperthyroidism, cardiovascular or renal disease, hypertension, bronchial asthma, narrow-angle glaucoma, urinary retention, prostatic hypertrophy, bladder neck obstruction, and elderly patients.
• Warn patient against using alcoholic beverages during therapy and against driving or other activities that require alertness until response to drug is determined.
• Reduce GI distress by giving with food or milk.
• Coffee or tea may reduce drowsiness. Sugarless gum, sour hard candy, or ice chips may relieve dry mouth.
• Titrate each patient's dose; response to drug varies.
• If tolerance develops, another anti-histamine may be substituted.
• Warn patient to stop taking drug

4 days before allergy skin tests; otherwise, accuracy of tests may be affected.
• Used experimentally to stimulate appetite and increase weight gain in children.

• If tolerance develops, another antihistamine may be substituted.
• Warn patient to stop taking drug 4 days before allergy skin tests; otherwise, accuracy of tests may be affected.

---

dexchlorpheniramine maleate
Polaramine♦

INDICATIONS & DOSAGE
Rhinitis, allergy symptoms, contact dermatitis, pruritus—
Adults: 1 to 2 mg P.O. t.i.d. or q.i.d.; or (timed-release) 4 to 6 mg b.i.d. or t.i.d.
Children under 12: 0.15 mg/Kg P.O. daily divided into 4 doses.
Do not use timed-release tablets for children younger than 6 years.

SIDE EFFECTS
CNS (especially in the elderly): *drowsiness,* dizziness.
GI: nausea, *dry mouth.*
GU: polyuria, dysuria.

INTERACTIONS
None significant.

NURSING CONSIDERATIONS
• Contraindicated in acute asthmatic attack. Use cautiously in increased intraocular pressure, hyperthyroidism, elderly patients, cardiovascular or renal disease, hypertension, bronchial asthma, narrow-angle glaucoma, urinary retention, prostatic hypertrophy, bladder neck obstruction.
• Warn patient against using alcoholic beverages during therapy and against driving or other activities that require alertness until response to drug is determined.
• Coffee or tea may reduce drowsiness.
• Titrate each patient's dose; response to drug varies.

---

dimethindene maleate
Forhistal, Triten

INDICATIONS & DOSAGE
Allergy symptoms—
Adults, and children over 6 years: (timed-release) 2.5 mg P.O. daily b.i.d.

SIDE EFFECTS
CNS (especially in the elderly): *drowsiness,* dizziness, insomnia, irritability, headache.
GI: anorexia, nausea, vomiting, *dry mouth,* diarrhea.
GU: urinary frequency.

INTERACTIONS
None significant.

NURSING CONSIDERATIONS
• Contraindicated in acute asthmatic attack. Use cautiously in increased intraocular pressure, hyperthyroidism, elderly patients, cardiovascular or renal disease, hypertension, bronchial asthma, narrow-angle glaucoma, urinary retention, prostatic hypertrophy, bladder neck obstruction.
• Warn patient against using alcoholic beverages during therapy and against driving or other activities that require alertness until response to drug is determined.
• Reduce GI distress by giving with food or milk.
• Coffee or tea may reduce drowsiness. Sugarless gum, sour hard candy, or ice chips may relieve dry mouth.
• Titrate each patient's dose; response to drug varies.

- If tolerance develops, another antihistamine may be substituted.
- Warn patient to stop taking drug 4 days before allergy skin tests; otherwise, accuracy of tests may be affected.

dimethothiazine mesylate
Fonazine, Promaquid♦♦

INDICATIONS & DOSAGE
Allergy symptoms, pruritus—
Adults: 20 mg P.O. b.i.d. or t.i.d. Maximum 120 mg daily.
Children 12 to 15 years: 20 mg P.O. daily or b.i.d.

SIDE EFFECTS
CNS (especially in the elderly): *drowsiness,* dizziness, fatigue, headache, restlessness, insomnia.
CV: hypotension, palpitations, tachycardia, extrasystoles.
EENT: blurred vision.
GI: *dry mouth and throat.*
Skin: rash.

INTERACTIONS
Other phenothiazines: increased effects. Use together cautiously.

NURSING CONSIDERATIONS
- Contraindicated in narrow-angle glaucoma, peptic ulcer, intestinal obstruction, prostatic hypertrophy, bladder neck obstruction, epilepsy, bone marrow depression, coma, CNS depression, acutely ill or dehydrated children. Use cautiously in pulmonary, hepatic, or cardiovascular disease; asthma; hypertension; elderly or debilitated patients.
- Warn patient against driving or other activities that require alertness until response to drug is determined.
- Coffee or tea may reduce drowsiness.
- Titrate each patient's dose; response to drug varies.

- If tolerance develops, another antihistamine may be substituted.
- Warn patient to stop taking drug 4 days before allergy skin tests; otherwise, accuracy of tests may be affected.
- Blocks serotonin.

diphenhydramine hydrochloride
Allerdryl, Baramine, Bax, Benachlor, Benadryl♦, Benahist, Ben-Allergin, Bendylate, Bentrac, Bonyl, Eldadryl, Fenylhist, Hyrexin, Nordryl, Notose, Phen-Amin 50, Phenamine, Rodryl, Rohydra, SK-Diphenhydramine, Span-Lanin, Valdrene, Wehdryl

INDICATIONS & DOSAGE
Rhinitis, allergy symptoms, motion sickness, antiparkinsonism—
Adults: 25 to 50 mg P.O. t.i.d. to q.i.d.; or 10 to 50 mg deep I.M. or I.V. Maximum 400 mg daily.
Children under 12 years: 5 mg/Kg daily P.O., deep I.M., or I.V. divided q.i.d. Maximum 300 mg daily.
Sedation—
Adults: 25 to 50 mg P.O., deep I.M., p.r.n.

SIDE EFFECTS
CNS (especially in the elderly): *drowsiness,* confusion, insomnia, headache, vertigo.
CV: palpitations.
EENT: photosensitivity, diplopia, nasal stuffiness.
GI: *nausea,* vomiting, diarrhea, *dry mouth,* constipation.
GU: dysuria.
Skin: urticaria.

INTERACTIONS
None significant.

NURSING CONSIDERATIONS
- Contraindicated in acute asthmatic attack. Use cautiously in narrow-angle glaucoma, prostatic hypertrophy,

peptic ulcer, pyloroduodenal and bladder neck obstruction, newborns, and in asthmatic, hypertensive, or cardiac patients.
• Alternate injection sites to prevent irritation.
• Warn patient against alcoholic beverages during therapy and against driving or other hazardous activities until response to drug is determined.
• Reduce GI distress by giving with food or milk.
• Coffee or tea may reduce drowsiness. Sugarless gum, sour hard candy, or ice chips may relieve dry mouth.
• Titrate each patient's dose; response to drug varies.
• If tolerance develops, another antihistamine may be substituted.
• Warn patient to stop taking drug 4 days before allergy skin tests; otherwise, accuracy of tests may be affected.
• Used with epinephrine in anaphylaxis.
• One of most sedating antihistamines; often used as a nighttime sedative.

---

diphenylpyraline hydrochloride
Diafen, Hispril

INDICATIONS & DOSAGE
Rhinitis, allergy symptoms—
Adults: 2 mg P.O. q 4 hours, p.r.n.; or (timed-release) 5 mg P.O. q 12 hours.
Children over 6 years: 2 mg P.O. q 6 hours, p.r.n.; or (timed-release) 5 mg P.O. daily.
Children 2 to 6 years: 1 to 2 mg P.O. q 8 hours, p.r.n.

SIDE EFFECTS
CNS (especially in the elderly): *drowsiness*, dizziness, headache.
EENT: nasal congestion.
GI: *dry mouth and throat*, epigastric distress.

Skin: flushing.

INTERACTIONS
None significant.

NURSING CONSIDERATIONS
• Contraindicated in acute asthmatic attack. Use cautiously in increased intraocular pressure, hyperthyroidism, elderly patients, cardiovascular or renal disease, hypertension, diabetes mellitus, bronchial asthma, narrow-angle glaucoma, urinary retention, prostatic hypertrophy, bladder neck obstruction.
• Warn patient against using alcoholic beverages during therapy and against driving or other activities that require alertness until response to drug is determined.
• Reduce GI distress by giving with food or milk.
• Coffee or tea may reduce drowsiness. Sugarless gum, sour hard candy, or ice chips may relieve dry mouth.
• Titrate each patient's dose; response to drug varies.
• If tolerance develops, another antihistamine may be substituted.
• Warn patient to stop taking drug 4 days before allergy skin tests; otherwise, accuracy of tests may be affected.

---

doxylamine succinate
Bendectin, Decapryn, Unisom

INDICATIONS & DOSAGE
Rhinitis, allergy symptoms—
Adults: 12.5 to 25 mg P.O. q 4 to 6 hours, p.r.n.
Children 6 to 12 years: 6.25 to 12.5 mg P.O. q 4 to 6 hours, p.r.n.
Nausea and vomiting of pregnancy—
Adults: 2 Bendectin tablets at bedtime. Maximum 4 tablets daily.

SIDE EFFECTS
CNS (especially in the elderly):

Italicized side effects are common or life-threatening.

drowsiness, dizziness, insomnia, disorientation, confusion, tremor, irritability, vertigo.
CV: palpitations.
GI: *dry mouth and throat.*

INTERACTIONS
None significant.

NURSING CONSIDERATIONS
• Contraindicated in acute asthmatic attack. Use cautiously in increased intraocular pressure, hyperthyroidism, elderly patients, cardiovascular or renal disease, hypertension, bronchial asthma, narrow-angle glaucoma, urinary retention, prostatic hypertrophy, bladder neck obstruction.
• Warn patient against using alcoholic beverages during therapy and against driving or other activities that require alertness until response to drug is determined.
• Coffee or tea may reduce drowsiness. Sugarless gum, sour hard candy, or ice chips may relieve dry mouth.
• Titrate each patient's dose; response to drug varies.
• If tolerance develops, another antihistamine may be substituted.
• Warn patient to stop taking drug 4 days before allergy skin tests; otherwise, accuracy of tests may be affected.

---

methdilazine hydrochloride
Dilosyn♦♦, Tacaryl

INDICATIONS & DOSAGE
Pruritus—
Adults: 8 mg P.O. b.i.d. to q.i.d. or (chewable tablets) 7.2 mg P.O. b.i.d. to q.i.d.
Children over 3 years: 4 mg P.O. b.i.d. to q.i.d. or (chewable tablets) 3.6 mg P.O. b.i.d. to q.i.d.

SIDE EFFECTS
CNS (especially in the elderly):
drowsiness, dizziness, headache.
GI: nausea, *dry mouth and throat,* cholestatic jaundice.
Skin: rash.

INTERACTIONS
Phenothiazines: increased effects. Don't use together.

NURSING CONSIDERATIONS
• Contraindicated in acute asthmatic attack. Use cautiously in pulmonary, hepatic, or cardiovascular disease, asthma, hypertension, elderly or debilitated patients, narrow-angle glaucoma, peptic ulcer, prostatic hypertrophy, bladder neck obstruction, CNS depression, acutely ill or dehydrated children.
• Warn patient against using alcoholic beverages during therapy and against driving or other activities that require alertness until response to drug is determined.
• Reduce GI distress by giving with food or milk.
• Coffee or tea may reduce drowsiness. Sugarless gum, sour hard candy, or ice chips may relieve dry mouth.
• Titrate each patient's dose; response to drug varies.
• If tolerance develops, another antihistamine may be substituted.
• Available as chewable tablet for children. Instruct child to chew completely and swallow promptly; may cause local anesthetic effect in mouth.
• Warn patient to stop taking drug 4 days before allergy skin tests; otherwise, accuracy of tests may be affected.

promethazine hydrochloride
Ganphen, Histantil♦♦, K-Phen,
Methazine, Pentazine♦, Phencen-50,
Phenergan♦, Promethamead, Pro-
methazine, Prorex, Provigan,
Remsed, Rolamethazine, Sigazine

INDICATIONS & DOSAGE
Motion sickness—
Adults: 25 mg P.O. b.i.d.
Children: 12.5 to 25 mg P.O., I.M.,
or rectally b.i.d.
Nausea—
Adults: 12.5 to 25 mg P.O., I.M., or
rectally q 4 to 6 hours, p.r.n.
Children: 0.25 to 0.5 mg/Kg I.M. or
rectally q 4 to 6 hours, p.r.n.
Rhinitis, allergy symptoms—
Adults: 12.5 mg P.O. q.i.d.; or 25 mg
P.O. at bedtime.
Children: 6.25 to 12.5 mg P.O. t.i.d.
or 25 mg P.O. at bedtime.
Sedation—
Adults: 25 to 50 mg P.O., I.M. at
bedtime or p.r.n.
Children: 12.5 to 25 mg P.O., I.M.,
or rectally at bedtime.

SIDE EFFECTS
CNS (especially in the elderly):
sedation, confusion, restlessness,
tremors, *drowsiness.*
CV: hypotension.
EENT: transient myopia, nasal con-
gestion.
GI: anorexia, nausea, vomiting, con-
stipation, *dry mouth.*
Other: *photosensitization.*

INTERACTIONS
Phenothiazines: increased effects.
Don't give together.

NURSING CONSIDERATIONS
• Contraindicated in narrow-angle
glaucoma, peptic ulcer, intestinal obstruction, prostatic hypertrophy, bladder neck obstruction, epilepsy, bone
marrow depression, coma, CNS

depression, pregnancy (except during
labor), lactation, newborns, acutely
ill or dehydrated children. Use cautiously in pulmonary, hepatic, or cardiovascular disease, asthma, hypertension, elderly, or debilitated
patients.
• Warn patient against using alcoholic beverages during therapy and
against driving or other activities that
require alertness until response to
drug is determined.
• Reduce GI distress by giving with
food or milk.
• Coffee or tea may reduce drowsiness. Sugarless gum, sour hard candy,
or ice chips may relieve dry mouth.
• Titrate each patient's dose; response
to drug varies.
• If tolerance develops, another antihistamine may be substituted.
• Warn patient to stop taking drug
4 days before allergy skin tests; otherwise, accuracy of tests may be
affected.
• Pronounced sedative effect limits
use in many ambulatory patients.
• May cause false positive immuno-
logical urinary pregnancy test (Grav-
index). Also may interfere with blood
grouping in ABO system.
• When treating motion sickness, tell
patient to take first dose 30 to 60 minutes before travel. On succeeding
days of travel, he should take dose
upon arising and with evening meal.

trimeprazine tartrate
Panectyl♦♦, Temaril

INDICATIONS & DOSAGE
Pruritus—
Adults: 2.5 mg P.O. q.i.d.; or (timed-
release) 5 mg P.O. b.i.d.
Children 3 to 12 years: 2.5 mg P.O.
h.s. or t.i.d., p.r.n.
Children 6 months to 3 years:
1.25 mg P.O. h.s. or t.i.d., p.r.n.

SIDE EFFECTS

Blood: *agranulocytosis,* leukopenia.
CNS (especially in the elderly): *drowsiness,* dizziness, confusion, restlessness, tremors, irritability, insomnia.
CV: hypotension, headache, palpitations, tachycardia.
GI: anorexia, nausea, vomiting, *dry mouth and throat.*
GU: urinary frequency or retention.
Skin: urticaria, rash.

INTERACTIONS

Phenothiazines: increased effects. Don't use together.

NURSING CONSIDERATIONS

• Contraindicated in acute asthmatic attack. Use cautiously in pulmonary, hepatic, or cardiovascular disease, asthma, hypertension, elderly or debilitated patients, narrow-angle glaucoma, peptic ulcer, intestinal obstruction, prostatic hypertrophy, bladder neck obstruction, epilepsy, bone marrow depression, coma, CNS depression, acutely ill or dehydrated children.
• Warn patient against using alcoholic beverages during therapy and against driving or other activities that require alertness until response to drug is determined.
• Reduce GI distress by giving with food or milk.
• Coffee or tea may reduce drowsiness. Sugarless gum, sour hard candy, or ice chips may relieve dry mouth.
• Titrate each patient's dose; response to drug varies.
• If tolerance develops, another antihistamine may be substituted.
• Warn patient to stop taking drug 4 days before allergy skin tests; otherwise, accuracy of tests may be affected.

---

tripelennamine hydrochloride
PBZ-SR, Pyribenzamine♦, Ro-Hist

INDICATIONS & DOSAGE

Rhinitis, allergy symptoms—
Adults: 25 to 50 mg P.O. q 4 to 6 hours; or (timed-release) 100 mg b.i.d. to t.i.d. Maximum 600 mg daily.
Children over 5 years: 50 mg P.O. q 8 to 12 hours (timed-release).
Children under 5 years: 5 mg/Kg daily P.O. in 4 to 6 divided doses. Maximum 300 mg daily.

SIDE EFFECTS

CNS (especially in the elderly): *drowsiness,* dizziness, confusion, restlessness, tremors, irritability, insomnia.
CV: palpitations.
GI: anorexia, diarrhea or constipation, *nausea, vomiting, dry mouth.*
GU: urinary frequency or retention.
Skin: urticaria, rash.
Other: thickening of bronchial secretions.

INTERACTIONS

None significant.

NURSING CONSIDERATIONS

• Contraindicated in acute asthmatic attack. Use cautiously in increased intraocular pressure, hyperthyroidism, elderly patients, cardiovascular or renal disease, hypertension, or bronchial asthma, narrow-angle glaucoma, urinary retention, prostatic hypertrophy, bladder neck obstruction.
• Warn patient against using alcoholic beverages during therapy and against driving or other activities that require alertness until response to drug is determined.
• Reduce GI distress by giving with food or milk.
• Coffee or tea may reduce drowsi-

---

ness. Sugarless gum, sour hard candy, or ice chips may relieve dry mouth.
• Titrate each patient's dose; response to drug varies.
• If tolerance develops, another antihistamine may be substituted.
• Warn patient to stop taking drug 4 days before allergy skin tests; otherwise, accuracy of tests may be affected.

---

triprolidine hydrochloride
Actidil♦

INDICATIONS & DOSAGE
Colds and allergy symptoms—
Adults: 2.5 mg P.O. t.i.d. or q.i.d.
Children over 6 years: 1.25 mg t.i.d. or q.i.d.
Children under 6 years: 0.3 to 0.6 mg t.i.d. or q.i.d.

SIDE EFFECTS
CNS (especially in the elderly): *drowsiness,* dizziness, confusion, restlessness, insomnia.
GI: anorexia, diarrhea or constipation, nausea, vomiting, *dry mouth.*
GU: urinary frequency or retention.
Skin: urticaria, rash.

INTERACTIONS
None significant.

NURSING CONSIDERATIONS
• Contraindicated in acute asthma. Use cautiously in increased intraocular pressure, hyperthyroidism, elderly patients, cardiovascular or renal disease, hypertension, diabetes mellitus, or bronchial asthma, narrow-angle glaucoma, urinary retention, prostatic hypertrophy, bladder neck obstruction.
• Warn patient against using alcoholic beverages during therapy and against driving or other activities that require alertness until response to drug is determined.
• Reduce GI distress by giving with food or milk.
• Coffee or tea may reduce drowsiness. Sugarless gum, sour hard candy, or ice chips may relieve dry mouth.
• Titrate each patient's dose; response to drug varies.
• Warn patient to stop taking drug 4 days before allergy skin tests; otherwise, accuracy of tests may be affected.

Italicized side effects are common or life-threatening.

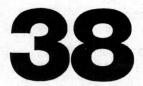

Expectorants and antitussives

acetylcysteine
ammonium chloride
benzonatate
chlophedianol hydrochloride
codeine
codeine phosphate
codeine sulfate
dextromethorphan hydrobromide
diphenhydramine hydrochloride
guaifenesin
hydriodic acid
hydrocodone bitartrate
hydromorphone hydrochloride
iodinated glycerol
levopropoxyphene napsylate
noscapine hydrochloride
potassium iodide (SSKI)
terpin hydrate
tyloxapol

acetylcysteine
Airbron♦♦, Mucomyst♦, NAC♦♦

INDICATIONS & DOSAGE
*Pneumonia, bronchitis, tuberculosis,
cystic fibrosis, emphysema, atelectasis
(adjunct), complications of thoracic
surgery and CV surgery—*
Adults and children: 1 to 2 ml 10%
to 20% solution by direct instillation
into trachea as often as every hour; or
3 to 5 ml 20% solution, or 6 to 10 ml
10% solution, by mouthpiece t.i.d. or
q.i.d.
Acetaminophen toxicity—
140 mg/Kg initially P.O., followed by
70 mg/Kg q 4 hours for 17 doses (a
total of 1,330 mg/Kg).

SIDE EFFECTS
EENT: *rhinorrhea, hemoptysis.*
GI: *stomatitis, nausea.*
Other: *bronchospasm (especially in
asthmatics).*

INTERACTIONS
None significant.

NURSING CONSIDERATIONS
• Use cautiously in asthma or severe
respiratory insufficiency, in elderly or
debilitated patients.
• A mucolytic.
• Use plastic, glass, stainless steel, or
another nonreactive metal when administering by nebulization. Hand-
bulb nebulizers not recommended be-
cause output too small and particle
size too large.
• After opening, store in refrigerator;
use within 96 hours.
• Incompatible with oxytetracycline,
tetracycline, and erythromycin lactobionate.
• Monitor cough type and frequency.
• Available in combination with isoproterenol in a 4-ml vial.
• Large doses are used P.O. to treat
acetaminophen overdose.

ammonium chloride

INDICATIONS & DOSAGE
As expectorant—
Adults: 250 to 500 mg P.O. q 2 to
4 hours.

SIDE EFFECTS
CNS: headache, drowsiness, confusion, excitation alternating with coma, twitching, hyperreflexia, EEG abnormalities.
CV: bradycardia.
GI: *anorexia, nausea, vomiting*.
GU: renal impairment, glycosuria.
Metabolic: decreased potassium, hypocalcemic tetany, hyperglycemia.
Skin: rash.
Other: thirst.

INTERACTIONS
Spironolactone: systemic acidosis. Use cautiously.

NURSING CONSIDERATIONS
• Contraindicated in hepatic or renal impairment. Use cautiously in pulmonary insufficiency, congestive heart failure.
• Give with full glass of water.
• Monitor cough type and frequency.
• Encourage deep-breathing exercises.
• Watch for potentiated diuresis when used with diuretics.
• Also used to acidify urine.

benzonatate
Tessalon♦

INDICATIONS & DOSAGE
Nonproductive cough—
Adults, and children over 10 years: 100 mg P.O. t.i.d.; up to 600 mg daily.
Children under 10 years: 8 mg/Kg P.O. in 3 to 6 divided doses.

SIDE EFFECTS
CNS: dizziness, drowsiness.
EENT: nasal congestion, sensation of burning in eyes.
GI: nausea, constipation.
Skin: rash.

INTERACTIONS
None significant.

NURSING CONSIDERATIONS
• Patient should not chew tablets or leave in mouth to dissolve; local anesthesia will result.
• A cough suppressant; don't use when cough is valuable as diagnostic sign or is beneficial (as after thoracic surgery).
• Use with percussion and chest vibration.
• Maintain fluid intake to help liquify sputum.
• Monitor cough type and frequency.

chlophedianol hydrochloride
Ulo, Ulone♦ ♦

INDICATIONS & DOSAGE
Nonproductive cough—
Adults, and children over 12 years: 25 mg P.O. t.i.d. or q.i.d.
Children 6 to 12 years: 12.5 to 25 mg P.O. t.i.d. or q.i.d.
Children 2 to 6 years: 12.5 mg P.O. t.i.d. or q.i.d.

SIDE EFFECTS
CNS: *drowsiness*, dizziness, excitation, irritability, nightmares, hallucinations.
GI: *nausea*, vomiting.

INTERACTIONS
None significant.

NURSING CONSIDERATIONS
• An antitussive; don't use when cough is valuable diagnostic sign or beneficial (as after thoracic surgery).
• Use with percussion and chest vibration.
• CNS side effects disappear when drug is stopped.
• Monitor cough type and frequency.

codeine

codeine phosphate

codeine sulfate
Controlled Substance Schedule II

INDICATIONS & DOSAGE
Nonproductive cough—
Adults: 8 to 20 mg P.O. q 4 to
6 hours. Maximum 120 mg/24 hours.
Children: 1 to 1.5 mg/Kg P.O. daily
in 4 divided doses. Maximum
60 mg/24 hours.

SIDE EFFECTS
CNS: *dizziness, sedation.*
CV: palpitations.
GI: *nausea,* vomiting; in repeated
doses, *constipation.*
Skin: pruritus.
Other: tolerance and physical
dependence.

INTERACTIONS
None significant.

NURSING CONSIDERATIONS
• Contraindicated in increased intracranial or CSF pressure. Use cautiously in asthma, emphysema, head
injury, after thoracotomies or laparot-
omies, in debilitated patients, in dehydrated postop patients; history of
drug abuse, hepatic or renal disease,
hypothyroidism, Addison's disease,
acute alcoholism, seizures, severe
CNS depression, COPD, psychosis,
and when other CNS depressants are
given. Monitor patient carefully.
• Use with percussion and chest
vibration.
• Warn patient against driving or
other activities that require alertness
until response to drug is determined.
• An antitussive; don't use when
cough is a valuable diagnostic sign or
beneficial (as after thoracic surgery).
• Monitor cough type and frequency.

dextromethorphan hydrobromide
Balminil DM♦♦, Broncho-Grippol-
DM♦♦, Contratuss♦♦, Pertussin 8-
hour, Romilar Chewable Tablets for
Children, St. Joseph's Cough Syrup
for Children, Sedatuss♦♦, Silence Is
Golden. More commonly available in
combination products such as Beny-
lin-DM, Coryban-D Cough Syrup,
Dimacol, Naldetuss, Novahistine
DMX, Ornacol, Phenergan Expectorant with Dextromethorphan, Robi-
tussin DM, Romilar CF, Rondec-DM,
Triaminicol, Trind-DM, Tussi-Organ-
idin-DM, 2G-DM

INDICATIONS & DOSAGE
Nonproductive cough—
Adults: 10 to 20 mg q 4 hours, or
30 mg q 6 to 8 hours. Maximum
120 mg/day.
Children 6 to 12 years: 5 to 10 mg q
4 hours, or 15 mg q 6 to 8 hours.
Maximum 60 mg/day.
Children 2 to 6 years: 2.5 mg q
4 hours, or 7.5 mg q 6 to 8 hours.
Maximum 30 mg/day.

SIDE EFFECTS
CNS: drowsiness.
GI: nausea.

INTERACTIONS
MAO inhibitors: hypotension, coma,
hyperpyrexia, and death have occurred. Do not use together.

NURSING CONSIDERATIONS
• Contraindicated in patients currently taking or within 2 weeks of
stopping MAO inhibitors.
• Produces no analgesia or addiction
and little or no CNS depression.
• An antitussive; don't use when
cough is valuable diagnostic sign or
beneficial (as after thoracic surgery).
• Instruct patient not to take fluids
immediately after taking drug.

Unmarked trade names available in the United States only.
♦ Also available in Canada   ♦♦ Available in Canada only.

- Use with percussion and chest vibration.
- Do not mix dextromethorphan syrups together with penicillins, tetracyclines, salicylates, phenobarbital, hydriodic acid, or high concentrations of sodium or potassium iodide.
- Monitor cough type and frequency.
- Available in most over-the-counter cough medicines.

diphenhydramine hydrochloride
Allerdryl, Baramine, Bax, Benachlor, Benadryl♦, Benahist, Ben-Allergin, Bendylate, Bentrac, Benylin Cough Syrup♦♦, Eldadryl, Fenylhist, Hyrexin, Nordryl, Notose, Phen-Amin 50, Phenamine, Rodryl, Rohydra, Valdrene, Wehdryl

INDICATIONS & DOSAGE
Nonproductive cough—
Adults: 25 mg P.O. q 4 hours (not to exceed 100 mg/day).
Children 6 to 12 years: 12.5 mg P.O. q 4 hours (not to exceed 50 mg/day).
Children 2 to 6 years: 6.25 mg P.O. q 4 hours (not to exceed 25 mg/day).

SIDE EFFECTS
CNS: *sedation,* confusion, restlessness, insomnia, headache.
CV: palpitations.
EENT: diplopia, blurred vision, nasal congestion.
GI: *dry mouth and throat,* nausea, vomiting, diarrhea, constipation.
GU: dysuria.
Skin: urticaria.

INTERACTIONS
None significant.

NURSING CONSIDERATIONS
- Contraindicated in acute asthma, narrow-angle glaucoma, prostatic hypertrophy, peptic ulcer, pyloroduodenal and bladder neck obstruction.

Use cautiously in asthmatic, hypertensive, or cardiac patients.
- Warn patient against using alcoholic beverages during therapy and against driving or other activities that require alertness until response to drug is determined.
- Liquid preparations are recommended for antitussive effect.
- Instruct patient not to take fluids immediately after taking drug.
- Coffee and tea may reduce drowsiness. Sugarless gum, sour hard candy, or ice chips may relieve dry mouth.
- If tolerance develops, another antihistamine may be substituted.
- Warn patient to stop taking drug 4 days before allergy skin tests; otherwise, accuracy of tests may be affected.

guaifenesin
(formerly glyceryl guaiacolate)
Anti-Tuss, Balminil♦♦, Bowtussin, Colrex, Cosin-GG, Demo-Cineol♦♦, Dilyn, 2/G, G-100, G-200, GG-CEN, Glycotuss, Gly-O-Tussin, Glytuss, G-Tussin, Guaiatussin, Hytuss, Malotuss, Motussin♦♦, Nortussin, Proco, Recsei-Tuss, Resyl♦♦, Robitussin♦, Sedatuss♦♦, Tursen, Tussanca♦♦, Wal-Tussin DM

INDICATIONS & DOSAGE
Productive and nonproductive cough—
Adults: 100 to 200 mg P.O. q 2 to 4 hours. Maximum 800 mg/day.
Children: 12 mg/Kg P.O. daily in 6 divided doses.

SIDE EFFECTS
CNS: drowsiness.
GI: vomiting and nausea occur with large doses.

INTERACTIONS
None significant.

Italicized side effects are common or life-threatening.

NURSING CONSIDERATIONS

• May interfere with certain laboratory tests for 5-hydroxyindoleacetic acid and vanillylmandelic acid.
• Watch for bleeding gums, hematuria, and bruising if given to patients on heparin. Should such symptoms appear, guaifenesin should be discontinued.
• Liquifies thick, tenacious sputum; maintain fluid intake. Advise patient to take with a glass of water whenever possible.
• Monitor cough type and frequency.
• An expectorant.
• Encourage deep-breathing exercises.
• Although very popular expectorant, many medical authorities doubt its efficacy.

---

hydriodic acid

INDICATIONS & DOSAGE
Chronic bronchitis, bronchial asthma—
Adults: 1.25 to 5 ml syrup well diluted in water P.O. b.i.d. or t.i.d.

SIDE EFFECTS
EENT: tooth damage.

INTERACTIONS
None significant.

NURSING CONSIDERATIONS
• Dilute well. Use straw to avoid injuring teeth; syrup is very acidic.
• Liquifies thick, tenacious sputum; maintain fluid intake. Advise patient to take with a glass of water whenever possible.
• Don't use if syrup is deep brown color.
• Monitor cough type and frequency.
• Encourage deep-breathing exercises.
• An expectorant.

---

hydrocodone bitartrate
Controlled Substance Schedule II
Coditrate, Codone, Corutol DH♦♦,
Dicodethal, Dicodid, Hycodan♦,
Robidone♦♦

INDICATIONS & DOSAGE
Nonproductive cough—
Adults: 5 to 10 mg P.O. t.i.d. or q.i.d,. p.r.n. Maximum single dose 15 mg.
Children: 0.6 mg/Kg P.O. daily in 3 or 4 divided doses.

SIDE EFFECTS
CNS: *drowsiness, dizziness.*
EENT: dryness of throat.
GI: *nausea, constipation.*
Other: tolerance and physical dependence after long-term use.

INTERACTIONS
CNS depressants: increased sedation. Use together cautiously.

NURSING CONSIDERATIONS
• Contraindicated in glaucoma. Use cautiously in asthma, emphysema, drug dependence, after thoracotomy or laparotomy, in debilitated or dehydrated patients.
• Warn patient against driving or other activities that require alertness until response to drug is determined.
• Evaluate patient's need for drug, which is addictive.
• An antitussive; don't use when cough is valuable diagnostic sign or beneficial (as after thoracic surgery).
• Use with percussion and chest vibration.
• Monitor cough type and frequency.

---

hydromorphone hydrochloride
Controlled Substance Schedule II
Dilaudid Cough Syrup♦

INDICATIONS & DOSAGE
Cough—
Adults: 1 mg P.O. q 3 to 4 hours,
p.r.n.
Children 6 to 12 years: 0.5 mg P.O.
q 3 to 4 hours, p.r.n.

SIDE EFFECTS
CNS: *dizziness, somnolence,* respiratory depression.
CV: hypotension.
GI: *nausea,* vomiting, anorexia,
constipation.

INTERACTIONS
CNS depressants: increased sedation.
Use together cautiously.

NURSING CONSIDERATIONS
• Contraindicated in increased intracranial pressure, status asthmaticus.
Use cautiously in hepatic or renal disease, hypothyroidism, Addison's disease, acute alcoholism, seizures, head injury, severe CNS depression, brain tumor, bronchial asthma, chronic obstructive pulmonary disease, or psychosis.
• Warn patient against driving and other activities that require alertness until response to drug is determined.
• Monitor respiration, pupil size, bowel function.
• An antitussive; don't use when cough is valuable diagnostic sign or beneficial (as after thoracic surgery).
• Use with percussion or chest vibration.
• Monitor cough type and frequency.
• Addictive.

iodinated glycerol
Organidin♦

INDICATIONS & DOSAGE
Bronchial asthma, bronchitis, emphysema (adjunct)—
Adults: 60 mg P.O. q.i.d.(tablets), or
20 drops (solution) P.O. q.i.d. with fluids, or 1 teaspoonful (elixir) P.O.
q.i.d.
Children: up to ½ adult dose based on child's weight.

SIDE EFFECTS
After long-term use:
GI: *nausea,* gastrointestinal distress.
Skin: *eruptions.*
Other: acute parotitis, thyroid enlargement.

INTERACTIONS
None significant.

NURSING CONSIDERATIONS
• Contraindicated in hypothyroidism,
iodine sensitivity.
• Skin rash or other hypersensitivity may require stopping drug.
• May liquify thick, tenacious sputum; maintain fluid intake.
• Monitor cough type and frequency.
• Encourage deep-breathing exercises.
• An expectorant.

levopropoxyphene napsylate
Novrad

INDICATIONS & DOSAGE
Nonproductive cough—
Adults: 50 to 100 mg q 4 hours.
Children 23 to 45 Kg: 50 mg q
4 hours.
Children up to 23 Kg: 25 mg q
4 hours.

Italicized side effects are common or life-threatening.

SIDE EFFECTS
CNS: *drowsiness,* jitters, *dizziness,* headache.
EENT: visual disturbances.
GI: dry mouth, *nausea,* vomiting, diarrhea, *epigastric burning.*
GU: urinary frequency or urgency.
Skin: rash, urticaria.

INTERACTIONS
None significant.

NURSING CONSIDERATIONS
• Contraindicated in first trimester of pregnancy.
• An antitussive; don't use when cough is valuable diagnostic sign or beneficial (as after thoracic surgery).
• Tell patient not to take fluids just after liquid preparation.
• Use with percussion or chest vibration.
• Monitor cough type and frequency.
• Warn patient against driving or other activities that require mental alertness until effect of drug is determined.

---

noscapine hydrochloride
Noscatuss♦♦, Tusscapine

INDICATIONS & DOSAGE
Nonproductive cough—
Adults: 15 to 30 mg P.O. q 4 to 6 hours as chewable tablet.
Children 6 to 12 years: 7.5 to 15 mg P.O. t.i.d. or q.i.d. as syrup.
Children 2 to 6 years: 5 to 10 mg P.O. t.i.d. or q.i.d. as syrup.

SIDE EFFECTS
CNS: slight drowsiness.
EENT: acute vasomotor rhinitis, conjunctivitis.
GI: nausea.

INTERACTIONS
None significant.

NURSING CONSIDERATIONS
• An antitussive; don't use when cough is valuable diagnostic sign or is beneficial (as after thoracic surgery). Use cautiously in sedated or debilitated patients.
• Tell patient not to take fluids just after liquid preparation.
• Use with percussion and chest vibration.
• Monitor cough type and frequency.

---

potassium iodide (SSKI)

INDICATIONS & DOSAGE
Chronic bronchitis, bronchial asthma—
Adults: 300 to 600 mg P.O. q 2 hours until desired response obtained.
Children: 0.25 to 1 ml of saturated solution (1 g/ml) b.i.d., t.i.d., or q.i.d.
Nuclear radiation protection—
Adults and children: 0.13 ml P.O. of SSKI immediately before or after initial exposure will block 90% of radioactive iodine. Same dose given 3 to 4 hours after exposure will provide 50% block. Should be administered for up to 10 days under medical supervision.
Infants under 1 year: ½ adult dose.

SIDE EFFECTS
GI: nonspecific small bowel lesions, *nausea,* vomiting, *epigastric pain,* metallic taste.
Metabolic: goiter, hyperthyroid adenoma, hypothyroidism (with excessive use), collagen disease-like syndrome.
Skin: rash.
Prolonged use: chronic iodine poisoning, soreness of mouth, coryza, sneezing, swelling of eyelids.

INTERACTIONS
Lithium carbonate: may cause hypothyroidism. Don't use together.

Unmarked trade names available in the United States only.
♦ Also available in Canada   ♦♦ Available in Canada only.

NURSING CONSIDERATIONS
• Contraindicated in iodine hypersensitivity, tuberculosis, hyperkalemia, acute bronchitis, hyperthyroidism.
• Maintain fluid intake to help liquify sputum.
• Has strong, salty, metallic taste. Dilute with milk or fruit juice to reduce GI distress.
• If given over long period, sudden withdrawal may precipitate thyroid storm.
• Monitor cough type and frequency.
• Encourage deep-breathing exercises.
• If skin rash appears, discontinue use. Contact doctor.
• An expectorant.

---

terpin hydrate
Creoterp, Terp

INDICATIONS & DOSAGE
Excessive bronchial secretions—
Adults: 5 to 10 ml P.O. of elixir.

SIDE EFFECTS
None.

INTERACTIONS
None significant.

NURSING CONSIDERATIONS
• Contraindicated on empty stomach, in peptic ulcer, or severe diabetes mellitus. Use cautiously in history of alcohol or drug abuse.
• Don't give in large doses; high alcoholic content of elixir (84 proof).

• Monitor cough type and frequency.
• Elixir contains 43% alcohol. Monitor for abuse.

---

tyloxapol
Alevaire

INDICATIONS & DOSAGE
Bronchitis, emphysema, pulmonary abscess, bronchiectasis, atelectasis (by inhalation only)—
Adults: up to 500 ml 0.125% solution q 12 to 24 hours by continuous aerosol inhalation, adjusting rate of flow, p.r.n.; or 10 to 20 ml 0.125% solution by intermittent inhalation for 30 to 90 minutes t.i.d. or q.i.d.

SIDE EFFECTS
GI: *nausea.*
Local: irritation.

INTERACTIONS
None significant.

NURSING CONSIDERATIONS
• Aerosols may induce bronchial spasm in some asthmatic patients.
• A surfactant with detergent properties.
• Lowers surface tension and reduces viscosity of thick, tenacious sputum to facilitate expectoration; maintain fluid intake. Most benefit results from humidification of inspired air.
• Monitor cough type and frequency.
• Encourage deep-breathing exercises.
• If used as a vehicle, add phenylephrine or isoproterenol just before use.

Italicized side effects are common or life-threatening.

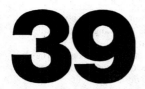

Antacids, adsorbents, and antiflatulents

activated charcoal
aluminum carbonate
aluminum hydroxide
aluminum phosphate
calcium carbonate
dihydroxyaluminum aminoacetate
dihydroxyaluminum sodium
  carbonate
magaldrate
magnesia magma (MOM)
magnesium carbonate
magnesium oxide
magnesium trisilicate
oxethazaine
simethicone
sodium bicarbonate

phenol, phenothiazines, potassium permanganate, propoxyphene, quinine, strychnine, sulfonamides, tricyclic antidepressants.

SIDE EFFECTS
GI: black stools.

INTERACTIONS
None significant.

NURSING CONSIDERATIONS
• Because activated charcoal absorbs and inactivates syrup of ipecac, give after emesis.
• Don't give in ice cream. Ice cream decreases absorptive capacity.
• Powder form most effective. Mix with tap water to form consistency of thick syrup. May add small amount of fruit juice or flavoring to make more palatable.
• Space doses at least 1 hour apart from other drugs if activated charcoal is being used for any indication other than poisoning.

---

activated charcoal
Charcocaps, Charcodote, Charcotabs, Digestalin

INDICATIONS & DOSAGE
Flatulence or dyspepsia—
Adults: 600 mg to 5 g P.O.
Poisoning—
Adults and children: 5 to 10 times estimated weight of drug or chemical ingested. Minimum dose 30 g in 250 ml water to make a slurry.
Give orally, preferably within 30 minutes of poisoning. Larger doses are necessary if food is in the stomach.
For treatment of overdosage with acetaminophen, amphetamines, aspirin, antimony, atropine, arsenic, barbiturates, camphor, cocaine, digitalis glycosides, glutethimide, ipecac, malathion, morphine, poisonous mushrooms, opium, oxalic acid, parathion,

---

aluminum carbonate
Basaljel ◆

INDICATIONS & DOSAGE
As antacid—
Adults: suspension: 5 to 10 ml, p.r.n.
Extra-strength suspension: 2.5 to 5 ml, p.r.n. Tablets: 1 to 2, p.r.n.
Capsules: 1 to 2, p.r.n.
To prevent formation of urinary phosphate stones (with low phosphate diet)—

Adults: suspension: 15 to 30 ml suspension in water or juice 1 hour after meals and h.s.; 5 to 15 ml extra strength in water or juice 1 hour after meals and h.s.; 2 to 6 tablets or capsules 1 hour after meals and h.s.

SIDE EFFECTS
Blood: hypophosphatemia.
GI: anorexia, *constipation*, intestinal obstruction.

INTERACTIONS
None significant.

NURSING CONSIDERATIONS
• Use cautiously in elderly patients, especially those with decreased bowel motility (those receiving antidiarrheals, antispasmodics, or anticholinergics), dehydration, fluid restriction, chronic renal disease, and suspected intestinal obstruction.
• Record amount and consistency of stools. Manage constipation with laxatives or stool softeners; alternate with magnesium-containing antacids (if not renal disease patient).
• Monitor serum phosphate levels.
• Shake suspension well; give with small amount of water or fruit juice to assure passage to stomach. When administering through nasogastric tube, be sure tube is placed correctly and is patent; follow antacid with water to ease passage.
• Watch long-term, high-dose use in patient on restricted sodium intake.
• Warn patient not to take aluminum carbonate indiscriminately and not to switch antacids without doctor's advice.
• Because it contains aluminum, it is used in renal failure patients to help control hyperphosphatemia. Binds phosphate in GI tract.
• Watch for symptoms of hypophosphatemia with prolonged use (anorexia, malaise, muscle weakness); can also lead to resorption of calcium and bone demineralization.

• If patient is able, he should be responsible for taking antacid while hospitalized.
• May cause enteric-coated drugs to be released prematurely in stomach. Separate doses by 1 hour.

---

aluminum hydroxide
ALternaGel, Alu-Cap, Al-U-Creme, Aluminett, Amphojel♦, Basaljel♦♦, Dialume, Hydroxal, No-Co-Gel, Nutrajel

INDICATIONS & DOSAGE
Antacid—
Adults: 600 mg P.O. (5 to 10 ml of most products) 1 hour after meals and h.s.; 300 or 600 mg tablet, chewed before swallowing, taken with milk or water 5 to 6 times daily after meals and h.s.
Hyperphosphatemia in renal failure—
Adults: 500 mg to 2 g b.i.d. to q.i.d.

SIDE EFFECTS
Blood: hypophosphatemia.
GI: anorexia, *constipation*, intestinal obstruction.

INTERACTIONS
None significant.

NURSING CONSIDERATIONS
• Use cautiously in elderly patients, especially those with decreased bowel motility (those receiving antidiarrheals, antispasmodics, or anticholinergics), dehydration, fluid restriction, chronic renal disease, and suspected intestinal obstruction.
• Record amount and consistency of stools. Manage constipation with laxatives or stool softeners; alternate with magnesium-containing antacids (if not renal disease patient).
• Monitor serum phosphate levels.
• Shake suspension well; give with small amount of milk or water to assure passage to stomach. When ad-

ministering through nasogastric tube, be sure tube is placed correctly and is patent. After instilling antacid, flush tube with water.
• Watch long-term, high-dose use in patient on restricted sodium intake.
• Warn patient not to take aluminum hydroxide indiscriminately and not to switch antacids without doctor's advice.
• Because it contains aluminum, it is used in renal failure patients to help control hyperphosphatemia. Binds phosphate in the GI tract.
• Watch for symptoms of hypophosphatemia with prolonged use (anorexia, malaise, muscle weakness); can also lead to resorption of calcium and bone demineralization.
• If patient is able, he should be responsible for taking antacid while hospitalized.
• May cause enteric-coated drugs to be released prematurely in stomach. Separate doses by 1 hour.

aluminum phosphate
Phosphaljel

INDICATIONS & DOSAGE
Antacid—
Adults: 15 to 30 ml undiluted q 2 hours between meals and h.s.

SIDE EFFECTS
GI: *constipation,* intestinal obstruction.

INTERACTIONS
None significant.

NURSING CONSIDERATIONS
• Use cautiously in elderly patients, especially those with decreased bowel motility (those receiving antidiarrheals, antispasmodics, or anticholinergics), dehydration, fluid restriction, chronic renal disease, and suspected intestinal obstruction.

• Record amount and consistency of stools. Manage constipation with laxatives or stool softeners; alternate with magnesium-containing antacids (if patient does not have renal disease).
• Shake well; give alone or with small amount of milk or water. When administering through nasogastric tube, be sure tube is placed correctly and is patent; after instilling, flush tube with water to facilitate passage to stomach.
• Watch long-term, high-dose use in patient on restricted sodium intake.
• Warn patient not to take aluminum phosphate indiscriminately and not to switch antacids without doctor's advice.
• This drug is a very weak antacid.
• Can reverse hypophosphatemia induced by aluminum hydroxide.
• If patient is able, he should be responsible for taking antacid while hospitalized.
• May cause enteric-coated drugs to be released prematurely in stomach. Separate doses by 1 hour.

calcium carbonate
Alka-2, Amitone, Calcilac, Calglycine, Dicarbosil, El-Da-Mint, Equilet, Gustalac, Mallamint, P.H. Tablets, Spentacid, Titracid, Titralac, Trialea, Tums

INDICATIONS & DOSAGE
Antacid—
Adults: 1 g tablet, 4 to 6 times daily, chewed well and taken with water; or 1 g of suspension (5 ml of most products) 1 hour after meals and h.s.

SIDE EFFECTS
Blood: *hypercalcemia;* if taken with milk—milk-alkali syndrome.
GI: *constipation,* gastric distention, flatulence, acid-rebound, *nausea.*

INTERACTIONS
None significant.

NURSING CONSIDERATIONS
• Contraindicated in severe renal disease. Use cautiously in elderly patients, especially those with decreased bowel motility (those receiving antidiarrheals, antispasmodics, anticholinergics), dehydration, fluid restriction, chronic renal disease, and suspected intestinal obstruction.
• Do not administer with milk. Can cause milk-alkali syndrome.
• Record amount and consistency of stools. Manage constipation with laxatives or stool softeners.
• Watch for symptoms of hypercalcemia (nausea, vomiting, headache, mental confusion, anorexia).
• Monitor serum calcium levels, especially in mild renal impairment.
• Warn patient not to take calcium carbonate indiscriminately and not to switch antacids without doctor's advice.
• If patient is able, he should be responsible for taking antacid while hospitalized.
• Has been known to cause rebound hyperacidity.
• Emphasize that it is *not* candy.
• May cause enteric-coated tablets to be released prematurely in stomach. Separate doses by 1 hour.

---

dihydroxyaluminum aminoacetate
Alkam, Hyperacid, Robalate♦

INDICATIONS & DOSAGE
Antacid—
Adults: 0.5 to 1 g (1 to 2 tablets) after meals and h.s., chewed before swallowing and taken with milk or water.

SIDE EFFECTS
Blood: hypophosphatemia.

GI: anorexia, *constipation*, intestinal obstruction.

INTERACTIONS
None significant.

NURSING CONSIDERATIONS
• Use cautiously in elderly patients, especially those with decreased bowel motility (those receiving antidiarrheals, antispasmodics, or anticholinergics), dehydration, fluid restriction, chronic renal disease, and suspected intestinal obstruction.
• Record amount and consistency of stools. Less constipating than aluminum hydroxide. Manage constipation with laxatives or stool softeners; alternate with magnesium-containing antacids (if not renal disease patient).
• Watch for symptoms of hypophosphatemia with prolonged use (anorexia, malaise, muscle weakness); can also lead to resorption of calcium and bone demineralization.
• Monitor serum phosphate levels.
• Watch long-term, high-dose use in patient on restricted sodium intake.
• Warn patient not to take dihydroxyaluminum aminoacetate indiscriminately and not to switch antacids without doctor's advice.
• If patient is able, he should be responsible for taking antacid while hospitalized.
• May cause enteric-coated drugs to be released prematurely in stomach. Separate doses by 1 hour.

---

dihydroxyaluminum sodium carbonate
Rolaids

INDICATIONS & DOSAGE
Antacid—
Adults: chew 1 to 2 tablets (334 mg to 668 mg), p.r.n.

SIDE EFFECTS
GI: anorexia, *constipation*, intestinal obstruction.

INTERACTIONS
None significant.

NURSING CONSIDERATIONS
• Use cautiously in elderly patients, especially those with decreased bowel motility (those receiving antidiarrheals, antispasmodics, or anticholinergics), dehydration, fluid restriction, chronic renal disease, and suspected intestinal obstruction.
• Has high sodium content and may increase sodium and water retention.
• Record amount and consistency of stools. Manage constipation with laxatives or stool softeners; alternate with magnesium-containing antacids (if patient does not have renal disease).
• Watch long-term, high-dose use in patient on restricted sodium intake.
• Warn patient not to take dihydroxyaluminum sodium carbonate indiscriminately.
• If patient is able, he should be responsible for taking antacid while hospitalized.
• Emphasize that it is *not* candy.
• May cause enteric-coated drugs to be released prematurely in stomach. Separate doses by 1 hour.

---

magaldrate (aluminum-magnesium complex)
Riopan♦

INDICATIONS & DOSAGE
Antacid—
Adults: suspension: 400 to 800 mg (5 to 10 ml) between meals and h.s. with water. Tablet: 400 to 800 mg (1 to 2 tablets) P.O. with water between meals and h.s.
Chewable tablet: 400 to 800 mg (1 to 2 tablets) chewed before swallowing, between meals and h.s.

SIDE EFFECTS
GI: mild constipation or diarrhea.

INTERACTIONS
None significant.

NURSING CONSIDERATIONS
• Contraindicated in severe renal disease. Use cautiously in elderly patients, especially those with decreased bowel motility (those receiving antidiarrheals, antispasmodics, or anticholinergics), dehydration, fluid restriction, and mild renal impairment.
• Record amount and consistency of stools.
• Shake suspension well; give with small amount of water to assure passage to stomach. When administering through nasogastric tube, be sure tube is placed properly and is patent. After instilling, flush tube with water.
• Monitor serum magnesium in mild renal impairment. Symptomatic hypermagnesemia usually occurs only in severe renal failure.
• Not usually used in renal failure patients (although it contains aluminum) to help control hypophosphatemia, since it contains magnesium, which may accumulate in renal failure.
• Good for patient on restricted sodium intake; very low sodium content.
• Warn patient not to take magaldrate indiscriminately and not to switch antacids without doctor's advice.
• If patient is able, he should be responsible for taking antacid while hospitalized.
• May cause enteric-coated drugs to be released prematurely in stomach. Separate doses by 1 hour.

---

magnesia magma (MOM)
(magnesium hydroxide)
Milk of Magnesia, Mint-O-Mag

INDICATIONS & DOSAGE
Antacid—
Adults: 5 to 10 ml or 1 to 2 tablets chewed before swallowing q.i.d., usually after meals and h.s.
Laxative—
Adults: 30 to 60 ml, usually h.s.
Children: 7.5 to 30 ml h.s.
Oral replacement therapy in mild hypomagnesemia—
Adults: 5 to 10 ml q.i.d., usually after meals and h.s. Monitor serum magnesium response.

SIDE EFFECTS
Blood: hypermagnesemia.
GI: *diarrhea,* abdominal pain, nausea.

INTERACTIONS
None significant.

NURSING CONSIDERATIONS
• Contraindicated in severe renal disease. Use cautiously in elderly patients and in mild renal impairment.
• Usually not used as antacid, even though it is very effective and potent, due to increased frequency of stools. Usually used as laxative.
• Record amount and consistency of stools.
• Shake suspension well; give with small amount of water when used as antacid, large amount of water when used as laxative. When administering through nasogastric tube, be sure tube is placed properly and is patent. After instilling, flush tube with water.
• Watch for symptoms of hypermagnesemia with prolonged use and some degree of renal impairment (hypotension, nausea, vomiting, depressed reflexes, respiratory depression, coma).

• Monitor serum magnesium in mild renal impairment.
• When used as laxative, don't give oral drugs 1 to 2 hours before or after.
• If diarrhea occurs with antacid doses, suggest alternative preparation.
• Subcathartic doses also used as oral magnesium replacement therapy in hypomagnesemia.
• Warn patient not to take magnesia magma indiscriminately and not to switch antacids without doctor's advice.
• If patient is able, he should be responsible for taking antacid while hospitalized.
• May cause enteric-coated drugs to be released prematurely in stomach. Separate doses by 1 hour.

magnesium carbonate

INDICATIONS & DOSAGE
Antacid—
Adults: 0.5 to 2 g of powder product or chewable tablets between meals with ½ glass of water.
Laxative—
Adults: 8 g of powder product or chewable tablets with water h.s.

SIDE EFFECTS
Blood: hypermagnesemia.
GI: *diarrhea,* gastric distention, flatulence, abdominal pain, nausea.

INTERACTIONS
None significant.

NURSING CONSIDERATIONS
• Contraindicated in severe renal disease. Use cautiously in elderly patients, mild renal impairment.
• Watch for symptoms of hypermagnesemia with prolonged use and some degree of renal impairment (hypotension, nausea, vomiting, depressed reflexes, respiratory depression, coma).

Italicized side effects are common or life-threatening.

- Monitor serum magnesium in mild renal impairment.
- When used as laxative, do not give other oral drugs 1 to 2 hours before or after.
- Record amount and consistency of stools.
- Warn patient not to take magnesium carbonate indiscriminately and not to switch antacids without doctor's advice.
- If patient is able, he should be responsible for taking antacid while hospitalized.
- May cause enteric-coated drugs to be released prematurely in stomach. Separate doses by 1 hour.

magnesium oxide
Mag-Ox, Maox, Niko-Mag, Oxabid, Par-Mag, Uro-Mag

INDICATIONS & DOSAGE
Antacid—
Adults: 250 mg to 1 g with water or milk after meals and h.s.
Laxative—
Adults: 4 g with water or milk, usually h.s.
Oral replacement therapy in mild hypomagnesemia—
Adults: 650 mg to 1.3 g tablet or capsule daily. Monitor serum magnesium response.

SIDE EFFECTS
Blood: hypermagnesemia.
GI: *diarrhea,* nausea, abdominal pain.

INTERACTIONS
None significant.

NURSING CONSIDERATIONS
- Contraindicated in severe renal disease. Use cautiously in elderly patients, mild renal impairment.
- Watch for symptoms of hypermagnesemia with prolonged use and some

degree of renal impairment (hypotension, nausea, vomiting, depressed reflexes, respiratory depression, coma).
- Monitor serum magnesium in mild renal impairment.
- When used as laxative, do not give other oral drugs 1 to 2 hours before or after.
- If diarrhea occurs on antacid doses, suggest alternate preparation.
- Warn patient not to take magnesium oxide indiscriminately and not to switch antacids without doctor's advice.
- If patient is able, he should be responsible for taking antacid while hospitalized.
- May cause enteric-coated drugs to be released prematurely in stomach. Separate doses by 1 hour.

magnesium trisilicate
Trisomin

INDICATIONS & DOSAGE
Antacid—
Adults: 1 to 4 g tablet t.i.d. chewed well and taken with ½ glass of water.

SIDE EFFECTS
Blood: hypermagnesemia.
GI: *diarrhea,* gastric distention, flatulence, nausea, abdominal pain.
GU: possible formation of silica renal calculi with prolonged use.

INTERACTIONS
None significant.

NURSING CONSIDERATIONS
- Contraindicated in severe renal disease. Use cautiously in elderly patients, mild renal impairment.
- Watch for symptoms of hypermagnesemia with prolonged use and some degree of renal impairment (hypotension, nausea, vomiting, depressed reflexes, respiratory depression, coma).

• Monitor serum magnesium in mild renal impairment.
• If diarrhea occurs on antacid doses, suggest alternate preparation.
• Warn patient not to take magnesium trisilicate indiscriminately and not to switch antacids without doctor's advice.
• If patient is able, he should be responsible for taking antacid while hospitalized.
• May cause enteric-coated drugs to be released prematurely in stomach. Separate doses by 1 hour.

---

oxethazaine
Oxaine (oxethazaine in aluminum hydroxide gel)

INDICATIONS & DOSAGE
Adjunct therapy for hyperacidity—
Adults: 10 to 20 mg suspended in 5 to 10 ml aluminum hydroxide gel (equivalent to 5 to 10 ml of commercial product) q.i.d. 15 minutes before meals and h.s.

SIDE EFFECTS
CNS: with high doses (120 mg oxethazaine daily): dizziness, faintness, drowsiness.
GI: anorexia, *constipation,* intestinal obstruction.

INTERACTIONS
None significant.

NURSING CONSIDERATIONS
• Use cautiously in elderly patients, especially those with decreased bowel motility (those receiving antidiarrheals, antispasmodics, or anticholinergics), dehydration, fluid restriction, chronic renal disease, suspected intestinal obstruction.
• Record amount and consistency of stools. Manage constipation with laxatives or stool softeners.
• Shake suspension well; give with

small amount of water to assure passage to stomach. When administering antacids through nasogastric tube, be sure tube is placed correctly and is patent; after instilling, flush tube with water.
• Caution: Local anesthetic can affect gastric mucosa for up to 6 hours. Prolonged use may mask extension of ulcerative disease and may lead to perforation. Also may mask symptoms of gastric neoplasm.
• Warn patient not to take oxethazaine indiscriminately and not to switch antacids without doctor's advice.
• If patient is able, he should be responsible for taking antacid while hospitalized.
• May cause enteric-coated drugs to be released prematurely in stomach. Separate doses by 1 hour.

---

simethicone
Mylicon, Silain

INDICATIONS & DOSAGE
Flatulence, functional gastric bloating—
Adults, and children over 12: 40 to 100 mg after each meal and h.s.

SIDE EFFECTS
GI: expulsion of excessive liberated gas as belching, rectal flatus.

INTERACTIONS
None significant.

NURSING CONSIDERATIONS
• Observe patient for effectiveness.
• Warn patient not to take simethicone indiscriminately.
• Tablets should be chewed, not swallowed whole.

Italicized side effects are common or life-threatening.

sodium bicarbonate
Bell-ans, Soda Mint

INDICATIONS & DOSAGE
Antacid—
Adults: 300 mg to 2 g tablets chewed well and taken with full glass of water, p.r.n.

SIDE EFFECTS
GI: *gastric distention, belching, flatulence.*
GU: renal calculi or crystals.
Metabolic: systemic alkalosis (prolonged use), sodium and water retention.

INTERACTIONS
None significant.

NURSING CONSIDERATIONS
• Contraindicated in congestive heart failure, hypertension, advanced renal disease, sodium restrictions, tendency toward edema, patients losing chloride from continuous GI suction, and patients receiving diuretics that cause hypochloremic alkalosis. Also contraindicated for long-term use. Use cautiously in elderly patients and in mild renal impairment.
• Discourage use as antacid. Offer nonabsorbable alternative antacid if it is to be used repeatedly.
• If patient is able, he should be responsible for taking antacid while hospitalized.
• Do not administer with milk; can cause milk-alkali syndrome.
• May be used cautiously to treat chronic metabolic acidosis.

40

Digestants

bile salts
dehydrocholic acid
glutamic acid hydrochloride
hydrochloric acid, diluted
ketocholanic acids
pancreatin
pancrelipase

bile salts
Biso, Chobile, Ox-Bile Extract
Enseals

INDICATIONS & DOSAGE
Uncomplicated constipation—
Adults and children: 300 to 500 mg
(enteric-coated tablets) b.i.d. or t.i.d.
after meals; or 150 to 450 mg capsules with or after meals.

SIDE EFFECTS
GI: loose stools and mild cramping
(in large doses).

INTERACTIONS
None significant.

NURSING CONSIDERATIONS
• Contraindicated in marked hepatic
dysfunction, except in malnutrition
with steatorrhea and vitamin K deficiency with hypoprothrombinemia.
• Use Ox-Bile Extract cautiously in
obstructive jaundice.
• Don't use Ox-Bile Extract if other
preparations are available, since it
doesn't provide an adequate amount
of conjugated bile salts.

dehydrocholic acid
Bio-Cholin♦♦, Cholan-DH, Choly-
phyl♦♦, Decholin♦, Dycholium♦♦,
Hepahydrin, Idrocrine♦♦, Neocholan

INDICATIONS & DOSAGE
*Constipation, biliary tract
conditions—*
Adults: 250 to 500 mg P.O. b.i.d. to
t.i.d. after meals for 4 to 6 weeks.

SIDE EFFECTS
None reported.

INTERACTIONS
None significant.

NURSING CONSIDERATIONS
• Contraindicated in complete mechanical biliary obstruction. Use cautiously in prostatic hypertrophy, acute
hepatitis, asthmatic bronchitis, elderly patients, partial GI or GU tract
obstruction.
• Do not use when patient is nauseated or vomiting, or has abdominal
pain.
• Simultaneous administration of bile
salts may be needed in biliary fistula.
• Used to prevent bacterial accumulation after biliary tract surgery.
• Probably much less effective than
natural bile salts in lowering surface
tension and promoting absorption.
• Don't use dehydrocholic acid to accelerate rate of healing in jaundice.
• Frequent use may result in dependence on laxatives.

glutamic acid hydrochloride
Acidulin♦

INDICATIONS & DOSAGE
Hypoacidity—
Adults: 1 to 3 capsules P.O. t.i.d. before meals.

SIDE EFFECTS
Metabolic: systemic acidosis in massive overdose.

INTERACTIONS
None significant.

NURSING CONSIDERATIONS
• Contraindicated in gastric hyperacidity or peptic ulcer.
• Use instead of hydrochloric acid so tooth enamel won't be damaged; however, glutamic acid HCl is not as effective in increasing gastric pH.
• Gastric acidifier.

hydrochloric acid, diluted

INDICATIONS & DOSAGE
Hypoacidity—
Adults: 2 to 8 ml P.O. well diluted in 25 to 50 ml water.

SIDE EFFECTS
Metabolic: systemic acidosis in massive overdose.
Other: *tooth enamel damage.*

INTERACTIONS
None significant.

NURSING CONSIDERATIONS
• Contraindicated in gastric hyperacidity or peptic ulcer.
• Sip, during meal, through glass straw to protect tooth enamel.
• Alleviates primary functional hypoacidity or hypoacidity caused by organic disease such as pernicious ane-

mia, certain allergies, chronic gastritis, other chronic debilitating diseases, or after gastric resection.
• Gastric acidifier; usual dose not sufficient to release free acid in stomach; no evidence that even larger doses are beneficial for this.

ketocholanic acids
Ketochol

INDICATIONS & DOSAGE
Constipation, biliary tract conditions—
Adults: 250 mg to 500 mg P.O. t.i.d. with meals.

SIDE EFFECTS
None reported.

INTERACTIONS
None significant.

NURSING CONSIDERATIONS
• Use cautiously in prostatic hypertrophy, acute hepatitis, asthmatic bronchitis, elderly patients, partial GI or GU tract obstruction.
• Bile salt; derived from beef bile.
• Approximately equivalent to 250 mg dehydrocholic acid.
• Do not use when patient is nauseated, vomiting, or has abdominal pain.
• Frequent use may result in dependence on laxatives.

pancreatin
Beef Viokase, Elzyme, Panteric Double Strength, Viokase

INDICATIONS & DOSAGE
Exocrine pancreatic secretion insufficiency, digestive aid in cystic fibrosis—
Adults and children: 325 mg to 1 g P.O. with meals.

SIDE EFFECTS
GI: nausea, diarrhea in high doses.

INTERACTIONS
None significant.

NURSING CONSIDERATIONS
• Use cautiously in sensitivity to pork.
• Balance fat, protein, and starch intake properly to avoid indigestion. Dosage varies according to degree of maldigestion and malabsorption, amount of fat in diet, and enzyme activity of individual preparations.
• Pancreatin therapy shouldn't delay or replace treatment of primary disorder.
• Adequate replacement decreases number of bowel movements and improves stool consistency.
• Use only after confirmed diagnosis of exocrine pancreatic insufficiency. Not effective in GI disorders unrelated to pancreatic enzyme deficiency.
• Bovine preparations available for use in pork sensitivity; less effective.
• For infants, mix powder with applesauce and give with meals. Older children may swallow capsules with food.
• Enteric coating on some products may reduce availability of enzyme in upper portion of jejunum where it is primarily required.

---

pancrelipase
Cotazym♦, Ilozyme, Ku-Zyme HP, Pancrease

INDICATIONS & DOSAGE
Dose must be titrated to patient's re-sponse. Exocrine pancreatic secretion insufficiency, cystic fibrosis in adults and children, steatorrhea and other disorders of fat metabolism secondary to insufficient pancreatic enzymes—
Adults and children: dosage range 1 to 3 capsules or tablets P.O. before or with meals and 1 capsule or tablet with snack; or 1 to 2 powder packets before meals or snacks.

SIDE EFFECTS
GI: *nausea,* diarrhea in high doses.

INTERACTIONS
None significant.

NURSING CONSIDERATIONS
• Contraindicated in severe pork sensitivity. Otherwise, use with caution.
• Pancrelipase therapy shouldn't delay or replace treatment of primary disorder.
• Use only after confirmed diagnosis of exocrine pancreatic insufficiency. Not effective in GI disorders unrelated to enzyme deficiency.
• Lipase activity greater than with other pancreatic enzymes.
• For infants, mix powder with applesauce and give at mealtime. Older children may swallow capsules with food.
• Dosage varies with degree of maldigestion and malabsorption, amount of fat in diet, and enzyme activity of individual preparations.
• Adequate replacement decreases number of bowel movements and improves stool consistency.
• Enteric coating on some products may reduce availability of enzyme in upper portion of jejunum where it is primarily required.

41

Antidiarrheals

bismuth subcarbonate
bismuth subgallate
bismuth subsalicylate
diphenoxylate hydrochloride
(with atropine sulfate)
kaolin and pectin mixtures
lactobacillus
loperamide
opium tincture
opium tincture, camphorated

INTERACTIONS
None significant.

NURSING CONSIDERATIONS
• GI adsorbent.
• Don't use in place of specific therapy for underlying cause.
• May reduce absorption of other P.O. drugs, requiring dosage adjustment.

---

bismuth subcarbonate

bismuth subgallate
Devrom

INDICATIONS & DOSAGE
Deodorize fecal odors in colostomy and ileostomy (subcarbonate)—
Adults: 600 mg P.O. t.i.d. after each meal.
Mild, nonspecific diarrhea (subgallate)—
Adults: 1 to 2 tablets chewed or swallowed whole t.i.d.

SIDE EFFECTS
CNS: personality changes. Prolonged use (especially in colostomy and ileostomy patients) may lead to reversible deterioration of mental ability, confusion, tremors, and impaired coordination.
GI: *transient darkened tongue and stool* (both with subgallate); fecal impaction or ulceration (in infants, elderly, or debilitated patients) after chronic use; *constipation.*

---

bismuth subsalicylate
Pepto-Bismol

INDICATIONS & DOSAGE
Mild, nonspecific diarrhea—
Adults: 30 ml or 2 tablets q ½ to 1 hour up to a maximum of 8 doses and for no longer than 2 days.
Children 10 to 14 years: 20 ml.
Children 6 to 10 years: 10 ml.
Children 3 to 6 years: 5 ml.

SIDE EFFECTS
GI: temporary darkening of tongue and stools.
Other: salicylism (high doses).

INTERACTIONS
None significant.

NURSING CONSIDERATIONS
• Has been used successfully to treat "turista" (traveler's diarrhea).
• Warn patient that this drug contains a large amount of salicylate. Should be used cautiously in patients already taking aspirin products.

diphenoxylate hydrochloride (with atropine sulfate)
Controlled Substance Schedule V
Colonaid, Diaction, Lofene, Loflo,
Lomo-Plus, Lomotil♦, Lonox,
Lotrol, Ro-Diphen-Atro,
SK-Diphenoxylate

INDICATIONS & DOSAGE
Acute, nonspecific diarrhea—
Adults: initially, 5 mg P.O. q.i.d.,
then adjust dose to individual response.
Children 2 to 12 years: 0.3 to
0.4 mg/Kg P.O. daily in divided
doses, using liquid form only.
Don't use in children under 2 years.

SIDE EFFECTS
CNS: *sedation, dizziness,* headache,
drowsiness, lethargy, restlessness,
depression, euphoria.
CV: tachycardia.
EENT: mydriasis.
GI: *dry mouth,* nausea, vomiting, abdominal discomfort or distention,
paralytic ileus, anorexia, fluid retention in bowel (may mask depletion of
extracellular fluid and electrolytes,
especially in young children treated
for acute gastroenteritis).
GU: urinary retention.
Skin: pruritus, giant urticaria, rash.
Other: possibly physical dependence
in long-term use, angioedema, respiratory depression.

INTERACTIONS
None significant.

NURSING CONSIDERATIONS
• Contraindicated in acute diarrhea
resulting from poison until toxic material is eliminated from GI tract; in
acute diarrhea caused by organisms
that penetrate intestinal mucosa; in
diarrhea resulting from antibiotic-induced pseudomembranous enterocolitis; in jaundiced patients. Use cau-

tiously in children, hepatic disease,
narcotic dependence, pregnancy. Use
cautiously in acute ulcerative colitis.
Stop therapy immediately if abdominal distention or other signs of toxic
megacolon develop.
• Risk of physical dependence increases with long-term use. Discourage long-term or unsupervised use.
Atropine sulfate is included to discourage abuse.
• Warn patient not to exceed recommended dosage.
• Dehydration, especially in young
children, may increase risk of delayed
toxicity. Correct fluid and electrolyte
disturbances before starting drug.
• Dose of 2.5 mg as effective as 5 ml
camphorated tincture of opium.
• Not indicated in treatment of antibiotic-induced diarrhea.

kaolin and pectin mixtures
Baropectin, Kaoparin, Kaopectate♦,
Kapectin, Keotin, Pargel, Pecto-
Kalin, Pectokay

INDICATIONS & DOSAGE
Mild, nonspecific diarrhea—
Adults: 60 to 120 ml after each bowel
movement.
Children over 12 years: 60 ml after
each bowel movement.
Children 6 to 12 years: 30 to 60 ml
after each bowel movement.
Children 3 to 6 years: 15 to 30 ml af-
ter each bowel movement.

SIDE EFFECTS
GI: drug absorbs nutrients and enzymes; fecal impaction or ulceration
in infants, elderly, debilitated patients
after chronic use; constipation.

INTERACTIONS
None significant.

Italicized side effects are common or life-threatening.

NURSING CONSIDERATIONS
• Contraindicated in suspected obstructive bowel lesions.
• Don't use for more than 2 days.
• Don't use in place of specific therapy for underlying cause.
• May reduce absorption of other P.O. drugs, requiring dosage adjustments.
• GI absorbent.

lactobacillus
Bacid♦, DoFUS, Lactinex♦

INDICATIONS & DOSAGE
Diarrhea, especially that caused by antibiotics—
Adults: 2 capsules (Bacid) P.O. b.i.d., t.i.d., or q.i.d., preferably with milk; or 4 tablets or 1 packet (Lactinex) P.O. t.i.d. or q.i.d., preferably with food, milk, or juice; or 1 tablet (DoFUS) P.O. daily before meals.

SIDE EFFECTS
GI: (with Bacid and DoFUS) increased intestinal flatus at beginning of therapy; subsides with continued therapy.

INTERACTIONS
None significant.

NURSING CONSIDERATIONS
• Bacid and DoFUS contraindicated in fever.
• Don't use Bacid for more than 2 days.
• Store in refrigerator.
• Diet containing large amounts of carbohydrate (up to 400 g), such as lactose, lactulose, and dextrin, may be more effective than lactobacillus in reestablishing normal flora after antibiotic therapy.
• Controversial form of diarrhea treatment.

• May be used prophylactically in history of antibiotic-induced diarrhea.

loperamide
Controlled Substance Schedule V
Imodium♦

INDICATIONS & DOSAGE
Acute, nonspecific diarrhea—
Adults: initially, 4 mg P.O., then 2 mg after each unformed stool. Maximum 16 mg daily.
Chronic diarrhea—
Adults: initially, 4 mg P.O., then 2 mg after each unformed stool until diarrhea subsides. Adjust dose to individual response.

SIDE EFFECTS
CNS: drowsiness, fatigue, dizziness.
GI: dry mouth; abdominal pain, distention, or discomfort; *constipation;* nausea; vomiting.
Skin: rash.

INTERACTIONS
None significant.

NURSING CONSIDERATIONS
• Contraindicated in acute diarrhea resulting from poison until toxic material is removed from GI tract, when constipation must be avoided, and in acute diarrhea caused by organisms that penetrate intestinal mucosa. Use cautiously in severe prostatic hypertrophy, hepatic disease, and history of narcotic dependence.
• Stop drug immediately if abdominal distention or other symptoms develop in patients with acute ulcerative colitis.
• In acute diarrhea, stop drug if no improvement within 48 hours; in chronic diarrhea, stop drug if no improvement after giving 16 mg daily for at least 10 days.

- Appears to have low potential for abuse.
- Warn patient not to exceed recommended dosage.
- Produces antidiarrheal action similar to diphenoxylate HCl but without as many CNS side effects; 3 times more potent than diphenoxylate HCl.

opium tincture

opium tincture, camphorated
Controlled Substance Schedule III
Paregoric♦

INDICATIONS & DOSAGE
Acute, nonspecific diarrhea—
Adults: 0.6 ml opium tincture (range 0.3 to 1 ml) P.O. q.i.d. Maximum dose 6 ml daily; or 5 to 10 ml camphorated opium tincture daily b.i.d., t.i.d., or q.i.d. until diarrhea subsides.
Children: 0.25 to 0.5 ml/Kg camphorated opium tincture daily, b.i.d., t.i.d., or q.i.d. until diarrhea subsides.

SIDE EFFECTS
GI: nausea, vomiting.
Other: physical dependence after long-term use.

INTERACTIONS
None significant.

NURSING CONSIDERATIONS
- Contraindicated in acute diarrhea resulting from poisons until toxic material is removed from GI tract, and in acute diarrhea caused by organisms that penetrate intestinal mucosa. Use cautiously in asthma, severe prostatic hypertrophy, hepatic disease, narcotic dependence.
- Risk of physical dependence increases with long-term use. Discourage long-term or unsupervised use.
- An effective and prompt-acting antidiarrheal.
- Opium content of opium tincture 25 times greater than camphorated tincture of opium. Camphorated opium tincture is more dilute, and teaspoonful doses easier to measure than dropper quantities of opium tincture.
- Not used as widely today as in past, but unique because dose can be adjusted precisely to patient's needs.
- Milky fluid forms when camphorated opium tincture is added to water.
- Camphorated opium tincture 0.06 to 0.5 ml daily has been used to treat infants with mild narcotic physical dependence.

42

Laxatives

barley-malt extract
bisacodyl
cascara sagrada
castor oil
danthron
docusate calcium (formerly dioctyl
   calcium sulfosuccinate)
docusate potassium (formerly
   dioctyl potassium sulfosuccinate)
docusate sodium (formerly dioctyl
   sodium sulfosuccinate)
glycerin
magnesium salts
methylcellulose
mineral oil
phenolphthalein
psyllium
senna
sodium biphosphate
sodium phosphate

---

barley-malt extract
Maltsupex

INDICATIONS & DOSAGE
Constipation—
Adults: 4 tablets P.O. with meals and
at bedtime for 4 days, then 2 to 4 tablets at bedtime; or 2 tablespoonfuls
powder or liquid b.i.d. for 3 to 4 days,
until stools become soft, then 1 to
2 tablespoonfuls at bedtime.
Children over 2 months: ½ to 2 tablespoonfuls in milk or on cereal daily
or b.i.d.
Infants 1 or 2 months:
½ tablespoonful daily with milk or
cereal. To prevent constipation, may

add 1 to 2 teaspoonfuls to each day's
feeding.

SIDE EFFECTS
GI: loose stools.
Other: laxative dependence in fre-
quent or long-term use.

INTERACTIONS
None significant.

NURSING CONSIDERATIONS
• Contraindicated in abdominal pain,
nausea, vomiting, or other symptoms
of appendicitis or acute surgical abdomen, and in intestinal obstruction or
ulceration, disabling adhesion, or difficulty swallowing.
• In diabetics, allow for carbohydrate
content of approximately 14 g/table-
spoon of liquid, 13 g/tablespoon of
powder, and 0.6 g/tablet.
• Tell patient to take with at least
8 ounces liquid.
• Rectal bleeding or failure to respond may indicate need for surgery.
• For short-term use. Before giving,
determine if patient has adequate
fluid intake, lacks exercise, or follows
proper diet. Tell him that dietary
sources of bulk include bran and other
cereals, fresh fruit, and vegetables.
• Infants usually need diet change to
increase bulk in addition to laxative.
• Laxative effect usually takes 12 to
24 hours; may be delayed 3 days.
• Bulk laxative; increases bulk and
water content of stool.
• Not absorbed systemically; nontoxic.
• Reduces fecal pH. Especially useful

in constipated postpartum mothers, debilitated patients, infants, chronic laxative abuse, irritable bowel syndrome, diverticular disease, and to empty colon before barium enema examination.

bisacodyl
Biscolax♦, Codylax, Dulcolax♦, Dulcolax Micro-enema♦♦, Fleet Bisacodyl, Rolax, Theralax

INDICATIONS & DOSAGE
Chronic constipation; preparation for delivery, surgery, or rectal or bowel examination—
Adults: 10 to 15 mg P.O. in evening or before breakfast. Up to 30 mg may be used for thorough evacuation needed for examinations or surgery.
Children: 5 to 10 mg P.O.
Rectal: **Adults, and children over 2 years:** 10 mg.
Under 2 years: 5 mg.
Enema: **Adults:** 1.25 oz.
Children under 6 years: approximately ½ contents of micro enema.

SIDE EFFECTS
CNS: muscle weakness in excessive use.
GI: *abdominal cramps,* diarrhea in high doses, *burning sensation in rectum with suppositories, nausea.*
Metabolic: alkalosis, hypokalemia, tetany, protein-losing enteropathy in excessive use.
Other: laxative dependence in long-term or excessive use.

INTERACTIONS
None significant.

NURSING CONSIDERATIONS
• Contraindicated in abdominal pain, nausea, vomiting, or other symptoms of appendicitis or acute surgical abdomen, or in rectal fissures or ulcerated hemorrhoids.

• Rectal bleeding or failure to respond may indicate need for surgery.
• Tell patient to swallow enteric-coated tablet whole to avoid GI irritation. Don't give with milk or antacids. Begins to act 6 to 12 hours after oral administration.
• Soft, formed stool usually produced 15 to 60 minutes after rectal administration.
• Tablets and suppositories may be used together to cleanse colon before and after surgery and before barium enema.
• Use for short-term treatment. Stimulant laxative, class of laxative most abused. Discourage excessive use.
• Before giving for constipation, determine if patient has adequate fluid intake, lacks exercise, or follows a proper diet. Tell him that dietary sources of bulk include bran and other cereals, fresh fruit, and vegetables.
• Store tablets and suppositories at temperature below 86°F. (30°C.).

cascara sagrada
Cas-Evac
cascara sagrada aromatic fluidextract

cascara sagrada fluidextract

INDICATIONS & DOSAGE
Acute constipation; preparation for bowel or rectal exam—
Adults: 325 mg cascara sagrada tablets P.O. h.s.; or 1 ml fluidextract daily; or 5 ml aromatic fluidextract daily; or 1.25 to 2.5 ml Cas-Evac liquid b.i.d.; or 2.5 to 5 ml Cas-Evac liquid h.s.
Children 2 to 12 years: ½ adult dose.
Children under 2 years: ¼ adult dose.

SIDE EFFECTS
GI: *nausea;* vomiting; diarrhea; loss

of normal bowel function in excessive use; *abdominal cramps,* especially in severe constipation; malabsorption of nutrients; "cathartic colon" (syndrome resembling ulcerative colitis radiologically and pathologically) after chronic misuse; discoloration of rectal mucosa after long-term use.
Metabolic: hypokalemia, protein enteropathy, electrolyte imbalance in excessive use.
Other: laxative dependence in long-term or excessive use.

INTERACTIONS
None significant.

NURSING CONSIDERATIONS
• Contraindicated in abdominal pain, nausea, vomiting, or other symptoms of appendicitis or acute surgical abdomen; in acute surgical delirium, fecal impaction, intestinal obstruction or perforation. Use cautiously in rectal bleeding.
• Failure to respond may indicate acute condition requiring surgery.
• Aromatic cascara fluidextract is less active and less bitter than nonaromatic fluidextract.
• Liquid preparations more reliable than solid dosage forms.
• Drug of choice among stimulant laxatives. Use for short-term treatment.
• Before giving for constipation, determine if patient has adequate fluid intake, lacks exercise, or follows a proper diet. Tell him that dietary sources of bulk include bran and other cereals, fresh fruit, and vegetables.
• May turn urine reddish-pink.

---

castor oil
Alphamul, Neoloid♦

INDICATIONS & DOSAGE
Preparation for rectal or bowel exam,
or surgery; acute constipation (rarely)—
Adults: 15 to 60 ml P.O. as liquid or 1.25 to 3.7 mg P.O. as tablet.
Children over 2 years: 5 to 15 ml P.O.
Children under 2 years: 1.25 to 7.5 ml P.O.
Infants: up to 4 ml P.O. Increased dose produces no greater effect.

SIDE EFFECTS
GI: *nausea;* vomiting; diarrhea; loss of normal bowel function in excessive use; *abdominal cramps,* especially in severe constipation; malabsorption of nutrients; "cathartic colon" (syndrome resembling ulcerative colitis radiologically and pathologically) in chronic misuse. May cause constipation after catharsis.
GU: pelvic congestion in menstruating women.
Metabolic: hypokalemia, protein enteropathy, other electrolyte imbalance in excessive use.
Other: laxative dependence in long-term or excessive use.

INTERACTIONS
None significant.

NURSING CONSIDERATIONS
• Contraindicated in ulcerative bowel lesions; during menstruation; in abdominal pain, nausea, vomiting, or other symptoms of appendicitis or acute surgical abdomen; in anal or rectal fissures; fecal impaction; intestinal obstruction or perforation. Use cautiously in rectal bleeding.
• Failure to respond may indicate acute condition requiring surgery.
• Give with juice or carbonated beverage to mask oily taste. Ice held in mouth before taking drug will help prevent tasting it.
• Shake emulsion well. Store below 4.4° C. (40° F.). Don't freeze.
• Give on empty stomach for best results.

• Produces complete evacuation after 3 hours. Tell patient that after castor oil has emptied bowel, he will not have bowel movement for 1 to 2 days.
• Generally used for diagnostic purposes or therapy requiring thorough evacuation of GI tract.
• Use for short-term treatment. Not recommended for routine use; useful for acute constipation not responsive to milder laxatives.
• Before giving for constipation, determine if patient has adequate fluid intake, lacks exercise, or follows a proper diet. Tell him that dietary sources of bulk include bran and other cereals, fresh fruit, and vegetables.
• Stimulant laxative.
• Increased intestinal motility lessens absorption of concomitantly administered P.O. drugs. Reschedule dosage.

danthron
Dorbane♦, Duolax, Modane♦, Modane Mild♦, Weslax

INDICATIONS & DOSAGE
Acute constipation, preparation for rectal or bowel exam, postsurgical and postpartum constipation—
Adults and children: 37.5 to 150 mg P.O. after or with evening meal.

SIDE EFFECTS
GI: *nausea;* vomiting; diarrhea; loss of normal bowel function in excessive use; *abdominal cramps,* especially in severe constipation; malabsorption of nutrients; "cathartic colon" (syndrome resembling ulcerative colitis radiologically and pathologically) in chronic misuse; discoloration of rectal mucosa in long-term use.
Metabolic: hypokalemia, protein enteropathy, electrolyte imbalance in excessive use.
Other: laxative dependence in long-term or excessive use.

INTERACTIONS
None significant.

NURSING CONSIDERATIONS
• Contraindicated in abdominal pain, nausea, vomiting, or other symptoms of appendicitis or acute surgical abdomen; in intestinal obstruction or perforation; and in hepatic dysfunction. Use cautiously in rectal bleeding or fecal impaction.
• Failure to respond may indicate acute condition requiring surgery.
• Give with fruit juice or carbonated beverage to mask oily taste.
• Give on empty stomach for best results.
• Produces complete evacuation of bowel in 6 to 24 hours. Tell patient that he will not have another bowel movement for 1 to 2 days.
• Generally used for diagnostic purposes or therapy requiring thorough evacuation of GI tract.
• Agent of choice for cardiac patients; reduces strain of evacuation.
• Use for short-term treatment. Not recommended for routine use; useful for acute constipation not responsive to milder laxatives.
• Before giving for constipation, determine if patient has adequate fluid intake, lacks exercise, or follows a proper diet. Tell him that dietary sources of bulk include bran and other cereals, fresh fruit, and vegetables.
• May discolor urine reddish-pink.
• Stimulant laxative.

docusate calcium (formerly dioctyl calcium sulfosuccinate)
Surfak♦
docusate potassium (formerly dioctyl potassium sulfosuccinate)
Kasof, Rectalad Enema
docusate sodium (formerly dioctyl sodium sulfosuccinate)
Bu-Lax, Colace, Comfolax, Disonate, Doctate, Doxinate, D.S.S., Dynoctol, Laxinate, Regutol, Roctate

INDICATIONS & DOSAGE
Stool softener—
Adults and older children: 50 to 300 mg (docusate sodium) P.O. daily or 240 mg (docusate calcium and docusate potassium) P.O. daily until bowel movements are normal; or 5 ml (250 mg) (docusate potassium) enema.
Children over 12: 2 ml (100 mg) (docusate potassium) enema.
Children 6 to 12 years: 40 to 120 mg (docusate sodium) P.O. daily.
Children 3 to 6 years: 20 to 60 mg (docusate sodium) P.O. daily.
Children under 3 years: 10 to 40 mg (docusate sodium) P.O. daily.
Higher doses are for initial therapy. Adjust dose to individual response. Usual dose in children and adults with minimal needs: 50 to 150 mg (docusate calcium) P.O. daily.

SIDE EFFECTS
EENT: throat irritation.
GI: bitter taste, mild abdominal cramping, diarrhea.
Other: laxative dependence in long-term or excessive use.

INTERACTIONS
None significant.

NURSING CONSIDERATIONS
• Sodium salts: use cautiously in so-dium-restricted diets, edema, congestive heart failure, renal dysfunction.
• Potassium salts: contraindicated in renal dysfunction.
• Give liquid in milk, fruit juice, or infant formula to mask bitter taste.
• Not for use in treating existing constipation, but prevents constipation from developing.
• Laxative of choice in patients who should not strain during defecation, such as those recovering from myocardial infarction or rectal surgery; in disease of rectum and anus that makes passage of firm stool difficult; or postpartum constipation.
• Acts within 24 to 48 hours to produce firm, semisolid stool.
• Instruct patient that dietary sources of bulk include bran and other cereals, fresh fruit, and vegetables.
• Emollient laxative or stool softener; doesn't stimulate intestinal peristaltic movements.
• Store at 15° to 30° C. (59° to 86° F.). Protect liquid from light.

glycerin

INDICATIONS & DOSAGE
Constipation—
Adults, and children over 6 years: 3 g as a suppository; or 5 to 15 ml as an enema.
Children under 6 years: 1 to 1.5 g as a suppository; or 2 to 5 ml as an enema.

SIDE EFFECTS
GI: *cramping pain,* rectal discomfort, hyperemia of rectal mucosa.

INTERACTIONS
None significant.

NURSING CONSIDERATIONS
• A hyperosmotic laxative used mainly to reestablish proper toilet habits in laxative-dependent patients.

magnesium salts
Concentrated Milk of Magnesia,
Magnesium Citrate, Magnesium
Sulfate, Milk of Magnesia

INDICATIONS & DOSAGE
*Constipation, to evacuate bowel before
surgery—*
Adults, and children over 6 years:
15 g magnesium sulfate P.O. in glass
of water; 10 to 20 ml concentrated
milk of magnesia P.O.; or 15 to 30 ml
milk of magnesia P.O.; or 5 to 10 oz
magnesium citrate at bedtime.

SIDE EFFECTS
GI: *abdominal cramping, nausea.*
Metabolic: fluid and electrolyte dis-
turbances if used daily.
Other: laxative dependence in long-
term or excessive use.

INTERACTIONS
None significant.

NURSING CONSIDERATIONS
• Contraindicated in abdominal pain,
nausea, vomiting, or other symptoms
of appendicitis or acute surgical abdomen; in myocardial damage, heart
block, imminent delivery, fecal impaction, rectal fissures, intestinal obstruction or perforation, renal disease.
Use cautiously in rectal bleeding.
• Failure to respond may indicate
acute condition requiring surgery.
• For short-term therapy; don't use
longer than 1 week.
• Saline laxative; produces watery
stool in 3 to 6 hours.
• Magnesium sulfate is more potent
than other saline laxatives.
• Before giving for constipation, determine if patient has adequate fluid
intake, lacks exercise, or follows a
proper diet. Tell him that dietary
sources of bulk include bran and other
cereals, fresh fruit, and vegetables.

• Magnesium may accumulate in
renal insufficiency.
• Chilling before use may make magnesium citrate more palatable.

methylcellulose
Cellothyl, Cologel, Hydrolose,
Syncelose

INDICATIONS & DOSAGE
Chronic constipation—
Adults: 5 to 20 ml liquid P.O. t.i.d.
with a glass of water; or 15 ml syrup
P.O. morning and evening.
Children: 5 to 10 ml P.O. daily or
b.i.d.

SIDE EFFECTS
GI: *nausea,* vomiting, diarrhea (all
after excessive use); esophageal, gastric, small intestinal, or colonic strictures when drug is chewed or taken in
dry form; *abdominal cramps,* especially in severe constipation.
Other: laxative dependence in long-
term or excessive use.

INTERACTIONS
None significant.

NURSING CONSIDERATIONS
• Contraindicated in abdominal pain,
nausea, vomiting, or other symptoms
of appendicitis or acute surgical abdomen; and in intestinal obstruction or
ulceration, disabling adhesion, or difficulty swallowing.
• Laxative effect usually takes 12 to
24 hours, but may be delayed 3 days.
• Tell patient to take drug with at
least 8 ounces of pleasant-tasting liquid to mask grittiness.
• Especially useful in postpartum
constipation, debilitated patients,
chronic laxative abuse, irritable bowel
syndrome, diverticular disease, colos-
tomies, and to empty colon before
barium enema examinations.

Italicized side effects are common or life-threatening.

• Rectal bleeding or failure to respond may indicate need for surgery.
• Use for short-term treatment.
• Before giving for constipation, determine if patient has adequate fluid intake, lacks exercise, or follows a proper diet. Tell him that dietary sources of bulk include bran and other cereals, fresh fruit, and vegetables.
• Not absorbed systemically; nontoxic.
• Bulk laxative; increases bulk and water content of stool.
• Instruct patient to notify doctor in 1 week about response to therapy.

mineral oil
Agoral Plain, Fleet Mineral Oil Enema, Kondremul Plain♦, Neo-Cultol, Petrogalar Plain, Saf-Tip Oil Retention Enema

INDICATIONS & DOSAGE
Constipation; preparation for bowel studies or surgery—
Adults: 15 to 30 ml P.O., usually h.s.; or 4 oz enema.
Children: 5 to 15 ml P.O. h.s.; or 1 to 2 oz enema.

SIDE EFFECTS
GI: *nausea;* vomiting; diarrhea in excessive use; *abdominal cramps,* especially in severe constipation; decreased absorption of nutrients and fat-soluble vitamins, resulting in deficiency; slowed healing after hemorrhoidectomy; and increased risk of rectal infections due to seepage from rectum.
Other: laxative dependence in long-term or excessive use.

INTERACTIONS
None significant.

NURSING CONSIDERATIONS
• Contraindicated in abdominal pain, nausea, vomiting, or other symptoms of appendicitis or acute surgical abdomen; in fecal impaction, intestinal obstruction or perforation. Use cautiously in young children; in elderly or debilitated patients due to susceptibility to lipid pneumonitis through aspiration, absorption, and transport from intestinal mucosa; in rectal bleeding. Enema contraindicated in children under 2 years.
• Failure to respond may indicate acute condition requiring surgery.
• Don't give drug with meals or immediately after, as it delays passage of food from stomach. More active on an empty stomach.
• A lubricant laxative.
• Give with fruit juices or carbonated drinks to disguise taste.
• Use when patient needs to ease the strain of evacuation.
• Before giving for constipation, determine if patient has adequate fluid intake, lacks exercise, or follows a proper diet. Tell him that dietary sources of bulk include bran and other cereals, fresh fruit, and vegetables.

phenolphthalein
Alophen, Espotabs, Evac-U-Lac, Ex-Lax, Feen-A-Mint, Phenolax, Evac-U-Gen

INDICATIONS & DOSAGE
Constipation—
Adults: 60 to 200 mg P.O., preferably h.s.

SIDE EFFECTS
GI: diarrhea; *colic in large doses;* factitious nausea; vomiting; loss of normal bowel function in excessive use; *abdominal cramps,* especially in severe constipation; malabsorption of nutrients; "cathartic colon" (syndrome resembling ulcerative colitis radiologically and pathologically) in chronic misuse; reddish discoloration in alkaline feces.

Skin: dermatitis, pruritus.
Other: laxative dependence in long-term or excessive use.

INTERACTIONS
None significant.

NURSING CONSIDERATIONS
• Contraindicated in abdominal pain, nausea, vomiting, or other symptoms of appendicitis or acute surgical abdomen; in fecal impaction, intestinal obstruction or perforation. Use cautiously in rectal bleeding.
• Failure to respond may indicate acute condition requiring surgery.
• Laxative effect may last up to 3 to 4 days.
• Produces semisolid stool within 6 to 8 hours, with little or no griping.
• Warn patient with rash to avoid sun and discontinue use.
• Before giving for constipation, determine if patient has adequate fluid intake, lacks exercise, or follows a proper diet. Tell him that dietary sources of bulk include bran and other cereals, fresh fruit, and vegetables.
• May discolor urine reddish-pink.
• Drug is available in many dosage forms. Most popular over-the-counter laxative; a frequent constituent of chewing gum and chocolate laxatives. Stimulant laxative, class of laxative most abused.

---

psyllium
Effersyllium Instant Mix, Konsyl, L.A. Formula, Metamucil♦, Metamucil Instant Mix♦, Modane Bulk, Mucillium, Mucilose, Plain Hydrocil, Siblin♦, Syllact

INDICATIONS & DOSAGE
Constipation; bowel management—
Adults: 1 to 2 rounded tsp. P.O. in full glass of liquid daily, b.i.d., or t.i.d., followed by second glass of liq-

uid; or 1 packet P.O. dissolved in water daily, b.i.d., or t.i.d.
Children over 6 years: 1 level tsp P.O. in ½ glass of liquid h.s.

SIDE EFFECTS
Blood: eosinophilia.
GI: nausea, vomiting, diarrhea, all after excessive use; esophageal, gastric, small intestinal, or colonic strictures when drug taken in dry form; abdominal cramps, especially in severe constipation.

INTERACTIONS
None significant.

NURSING CONSIDERATIONS
• Contraindicated in abdominal pain, nausea, vomiting, or other symptoms of appendicitis; and in intestinal obstruction or ulceration, disabling adhesion, or difficulty swallowing.
• Metamucil Instant Mix (effervescent form) contains a significant amount of sodium and should not be used for patients on sodium-restricted diets.
• Mix with at least 8 ounces of cold, pleasant-tasting liquid to mask grittiness, and stir only a few seconds. Patient should drink it immediately or mixture will solidify. Follow with additional glass of liquid.
• Rectal bleeding or failure to respond may indicate need for surgery.
• Use for short-term treatment. Don't use for maintenance.
• Frequent use of laxatives can cause drug dependence for evacuation.
• Before giving for constipation, determine if patient has adequate fluid intake, lacks exercise, or follows a proper diet. Tell him that dietary sources of bulk include bran and other cereals, fresh fruit, and vegetables.
• Laxative effect usually seen in 12 to 24 hours, but may be delayed 3 days.
• Popular bulk laxative; increases bulk and water content of stool.
• Highly refined, purified vegetable

mucilloid; from seeds of platango plant.
• Not absorbed systemically; nontoxic. Especially useful in postpartum constipation, debilitated patients, chronic laxative abuse, irritable bowel syndrome, diverticular disease, and in combination with other laxatives to empty colon before barium enema examinations.

senna
Black Draught, Glysennid, Senokot, X-Prep

INDICATIONS & DOSAGE
Acute constipation, preparation for bowel or rectal exam—
Adults: Dosage range for Senokot: 1 to 8 tablets P.O.; ½ to 4 teaspoonfuls of granules added to liquid; 1 to 2 suppositories h.s.; 1 to 4 teaspoonfuls syrup h.s. Black Draught: 7.5 to 15 ml.
Children over 27 Kg: ½ adult dose of tablets, granules, or syrup (except Black Draught tablets and granules not recommended for children).
Children 1 month to 1 year: 1.25 to 2.5 ml Senokot syrup P.O. h.s.
X-Prep used solely as single dose for preradiographic bowel evacuation. Give ¾ oz powder dissolved in juice or 2.5 oz liquid between 2 to 4 p.m. on day before X-ray procedure. May be given in divided doses for elderly or debilitated patients.

SIDE EFFECTS
GI: *nausea;* vomiting; diarrhea; loss of normal bowel function in excessive use; *abdominal cramps,* especially in severe constipation; malabsorption of nutrients; "cathartic colon" (syndrome resembling ulcerative colitis radiologically in chronic misuse; may cause constipation after catharsis); yellow, yellow-greenish cast feces, diarrhea in nursing infants of mothers on senna; darkened pigmentation of rectal mucosa in long-term use, which is usually reversible within 4 to 12 months after stopping drug.
GU: reddish-pink discoloration in alkaline urine; yellowish-brown color to acid urine.
Metabolic: hypokalemia, protein enteropathy, electrolyte imbalance with excessive use.
Other: laxative dependence in long-term or excessive use.

INTERACTIONS
None significant.

NURSING CONSIDERATIONS
• Contraindicated in ulcerative bowel lesions; in nausea, vomiting, abdominal pain, or other symptoms of appendicitis or acute surgical abdomen; in fecal impaction, intestinal obstruction, or perforation.
• Use for short-term treatment.
• Failure to respond may indicate acute condition requiring surgery.
• More potent than cascara sagrada; produces more griping. Acts in 6 to 10 hours. X-Prep gives thorough, strong bowel action beginning in 6 hours.
• Most recommended stimulant laxative.
• Before giving for constipation, determine if patient has adequate fluid intake, lacks exercise, or follows a proper diet. Tell him that dietary sources of bulk include bran and other cereals, fresh fruit, and vegetables.
• After X-Prep liquid is taken, diet should be confined to clear liquids.

sodium biphosphate
Enemeez, Fleet Enema♦, Phospho-
Soda, Saf-Tip Phosphate Enema,
Travad Enema♦
sodium phosphate
Sal-Hepatica

INDICATIONS & DOSAGE
Constipation—
Adults: 5 to 20 ml liquid P.O. with
water; or 4 g powder P.O. dissolved in
warm water; or 20 to 46 ml solution
mixed with 4 oz cold water; or 2 to
4.5 oz enema.

SIDE EFFECTS
GI: *abdominal cramping.*
Metabolic: fluid and electrolyte disturbances (hypernatremia, hyperphosphatemia) if used daily.
Other: laxative dependence in long-
term or excessive use.

INTERACTIONS
None significant.

NURSING CONSIDERATIONS
• Contraindicated in abdominal pain,
nausea, vomiting, or other symptoms
of appendicitis or acute surgical abdomen; in intestinal obstruction or perforation; edema; congestive heart failure; megacolon; impaired renal function; and in patients on salt-restricted
diets.
• Failure to respond may indicate
acute condition requiring surgery.
• Available in oral and rectal forms.
• Before giving for constipation, determine if patient has adequate fluid
intake, lacks exercise, or follows a
proper diet. Tell him that dietary
sources of bulk include bran and other
cereals, fresh fruit, and vegetables.
• Saline laxative; up to 10% of sodium content may be absorbed.
• Enema form elicits response in 5 to
10 minutes.
• Used in preparation for barium
enema and for fecal impaction.

43

Emetics and antiemetics

apomorphine hydrochloride
benzquinamide hydrochloride
buclizine hydrochloride
cyclizine hydrochloride
cyclizine lactate
dimenhydrinate
diphenidol
ipecac syrup
meclizine hydrochloride
prochlorperazine edisylate
prochlorperazine maleate
thiethylperazine maleate
trimethobenzamide hydrochloride

---

apomorphine hydrochloride
Controlled Substance Schedule II

INDICATIONS & DOSAGE

To induce vomiting in poisoning—
Adults: 2 to 10 mg S.C. preceded by
200 to 300 ml water. Don't repeat.
Children over 1 year: 0.07 mg/Kg
S.C. preceded by up to 2 glasses of
water.
Children under 1 year: 0.07 mg/Kg
S.C. preceded by ½ to 1 glass of
water.

SIDE EFFECTS

CNS: *depression, euphoria,* restlessness, tremors.
CV: *acute circulatory failure in elderly or debilitated patients,* tachycardia.
Other: *depressed respiratory center in
large or repeated doses.*

INTERACTIONS

None significant.

NURSING CONSIDERATIONS

• Contraindicated in hypersensitivity
to narcotics; impending shock; corrosive poisoning; narcosis resulting
from opiates, barbiturates, alcohol, or
other CNS depressants; and in patients too inebriated to stand unaided.
Use cautiously in children and in patients who are debilitated, have cardiac decompensation, or are predisposed to nausea and vomiting.
• Don't give after ingestion of petroleum distillates (e.g., kerosene, gasoline) or volatile oils; retching and
vomiting may cause aspiration and
lead to bronchospasm, pulmonary
edema, or aspiration pneumonitis.
Vegetable oil will delay absorption of
these substances.
• Don't give after ingestion of caustic
substances, such as lye; additional injury to the esophagus and mediastinum can occur.
• Keep narcotic antagonists, such as
naloxone, available to help stop vomiting and to alleviate drowsiness.
• When absorbable poison is ingested
or if delay in giving emetic is expected, give activated charcoal P.O.
immediately after apomorphine HCl.
• Vomiting occurs in 5 to 10 minutes
in adults. If vomiting doesn't occur
within 15 minutes, gastric lavage
should begin. Apomorphine HCl is
emetic of choice when rapid removal
of poisons is necessary, and when
identification of enteric-coated tablets
or other ingested toxic material in
vomitus is important. Stomach contents are usually expelled completely;

vomitus may also contain material from upper portion of intestinal tract.
• Don't administer if solution for injection is discolored or if precipitate is present.

benzquinamide hydrochloride
Emete-Con

INDICATIONS & DOSAGE
Nausea and vomiting associated with anesthesia and surgery—
Adults: 50 mg I.M. (0.5 mg/Kg to 1 mg/Kg). May repeat in 1 hour, and thereafter q 3 to 4 hours, p.r.n.; or 25 mg (0.2 mg/Kg to 0.4 mg/Kg) I.V. as single dose, administered slowly.

SIDE EFFECTS
CNS: *drowsiness,* fatigue, insomnia, restlessness, headache, excitation, tremors, twitching, dizziness.
CV: sudden rise in blood pressure and transient arrhythmias (premature atrial and ventricular contractions, atrial fibrillation) after I.V. administration; hypertension; hypotension.
EENT: dry mouth, salivation, blurred vision.
GI: anorexia, nausea.
Skin: urticaria, rash.
Other: muscle weakness, flushing, hiccups, sweating, chills, fever. May mask signs of overdose of toxic agents or underlying conditions (intestinal obstruction, brain tumor).

INTERACTIONS
None significant.

NURSING CONSIDERATIONS
• I.V. use contraindicated in cardiovascular disease. Don't give I.V. within 15 minutes of preanesthetic or concomitant cardiovascular drugs.
• Give I.M. injections in large muscle mass. Use deltoid area only if well developed. Don't inject into lower and midthird of upper arm. Aspirate syringe for I.M. injection to avoid inadvertent intravascular injection.
• Reconstituted solution stable for 14 days at room temperature. Store dry powder and reconstituted solution in light-resistant container.
• Monitor blood pressure frequently.
• Excellent antiemetic if prochlorperazine (Compazine) is contraindicated.

buclizine hydrochloride
Bucladin-S, Softran

INDICATIONS & DOSAGE
Motion sickness (prevention)—
Adults: 50 mg P.O. at least ½ hour before beginning travel. If needed, may repeat another 50 mg P.O. after 4 to 6 hours.
Nausea (treatment)—
Adults: 50 mg P.O., up to 150 mg P.O. daily in severe cases. Maintenance dose is 50 mg b.i.d.

SIDE EFFECTS
CNS: *drowsiness,* headache, dizziness, jitters.
EENT: blurred vision, dry mouth.
GU: urinary retention.
Other: may mask symptoms of ototoxicity, intestinal obstruction, or brain tumor.

INTERACTIONS
None significant.

NURSING CONSIDERATIONS
• Warn patient against driving and other activities that require alertness until response to drug is established.
• Tablets may be placed in mouth and allowed to dissolve without water. May also be chewed or swallowed whole.

Italicized side effects are common or life-threatening.

cyclizine hydrochloride

cyclizine lactate
Marezine, Marzine♦♦

INDICATIONS & DOSAGE
Motion sickness (prevention and treatment)—
Adults: 50 mg P.O. (hydrochloride) ½ hour before travel, then q 4 to 6 hours, p.r.n., to maximum of 200 mg daily; or 50 mg I.M. (lactate) q 4 to 6 hours, p.r.n.
Postop vomiting (prevention)—
50 mg I.M. (lactate) preop or 20 to 30 minutes before expected termination of surgery; then postop 50 mg I.M. (lactate) q 4 to 6 hours, p.r.n.; or 100 mg rectally (hydrochloride) q 4 to 6 hours.
Motion sickness and postop vomiting—
Children 6 to 12 years: 3 mg/Kg (lactate) I.M. divided t.i.d., or 25 mg (hydrochloride) P.O. q 4 to 6 hours p.r.n. to a maximum of 75 mg daily.

SIDE EFFECTS
CNS: *drowsiness,* dizziness, auditory and visual hallucinations.
CV: hypotension.
EENT: blurred vision, dry mouth.
GI: constipation.
GU: urinary retention.
Other: may mask symptoms of ototoxicity, brain tumor, or intestinal obstruction.

INTERACTIONS
None significant.

NURSING CONSIDERATIONS
• Use cautiously in glaucoma, GU or GI obstruction, in elderly males with possible prostatic hypertrophy.
• Warn patient against driving and other activities that require alertness until response to drug is determined.
• Antihistamine.
• Store in cool place. When stored at room temperature, injection may turn slightly yellow, but this color change does not indicate loss of potency.

dimenhydrinate
Dimate, Dimen, Dimentabs, Dipendrate, Dramaject, Dramamine♦, Dramamine Junior, Dramocen, Dymenate, Eldodram, Gravol♦♦, Hydrate, Hypo-emesis, Marmine, Nauseal♦♦, Nauseatol♦♦, Novodimenate♦♦, Ram, Reidamine, Signate, Travamine♦♦, Trav-Arex, Traveltabs, Vertiban, Wehamine

INDICATIONS & DOSAGE
Nausea, vomiting, dizziness of motion sickness (treatment and prevention)—
Adults: 50 mg P.O. q 4 hours, or 100 mg q 4 hours if drowsiness is not objectionable; or 100 mg rectally daily or b.i.d. if oral route is not practical; or 50 mg I.M., p.r.n.; or 50 mg I.V. diluted in 10 ml NaCl solution, injected over 2 minutes.
Children: 5 mg/Kg P.O. or I.M. or rectally, divided q.i.d. Maximum 300 mg daily.

SIDE EFFECTS
CNS: *drowsiness,* headache, incoordination, dizziness.
CV: palpitations, hypotension.
EENT: blurred vision, tinnitus, dry mouth and respiratory passages.
Other: may mask symptoms of ototoxicity, brain tumor, or intestinal obstruction.

INTERACTIONS
None significant.

NURSING CONSIDERATIONS
• Use cautiously in seizures, narrow-angle glaucoma, enlargement of prostate gland.
• Undiluted solution is irritating to veins; may sclerose.
• Antihistamine.

Unmarked trade names available in the United States only.
♦ Also available in Canada   ♦♦ Available in Canada only.

• Warn patient against driving and other activities that require alertness until response to drug is determined.
• May mask ototoxicity of aminoglycoside antibiotics.

diphenidol
Vontrol ♦

INDICATIONS & DOSAGE
Peripheral (labyrinthine) dizziness; nausea and vomiting—
Adults: 25 to 50 mg P.O. q 4 hours, p.r.n., or 20 to 40 mg deep I.M. injection (for rapid control of acute symptoms), then another 20 mg I.M. after 1 hour if symptoms persist. Thereafter 20 to 40 mg I.M. q 4 hours, p.r.n., or 20 mg I.V. injected directly through venoclysis already in operation (for rapid control of acute symptoms). May inject another 20 mg I.V. after 1 hour if symptoms persist, then switch to P.O. or I.M. route. Total daily dosage should not exceed 300 mg.
Nausea and vomiting—
Children: 0.9 mg/Kg P.O. or rectally, or 0.4 mg/Kg I.M. Give children's doses no more frequently than q 4 hours unless symptoms persist after 1 dose. An oral or I.M. dose may be repeated after 1 hour. Thereafter, doses may be given p.r.n. Maximum children's dose 5.5 mg/Kg P.O. daily; or 3.3 mg/Kg I.M. daily.

SIDE EFFECTS
CNS: drowsiness, dizziness, *confusion.*
CV: transient hypotension.
EENT: *auditory and visual hallucinations, disorientation occur within 3 days of starting drug; subside within 3 days after stopping drug.*
GI: dry mouth, nausea, indigestion, heartburn.
Skin: urticaria.
Other: antiemetic effect may mask

signs of overdose of drugs, or may obscure diagnosis of intestinal obstruction, brain tumor, or other conditions.

INTERACTIONS
None significant.

NURSING CONSIDERATIONS
• Contraindicated in anuria. Use cautiously in glaucoma, pyloric stenosis, pylorospasm, obstructive lesions of GI or GU tract, prostatic hypertrophy, or organic cardiospasm.
• I.V. use contraindicated in children and in sinus tachycardia.
• Don't give S.C.
• Drug should be stopped if auditory or visual hallucinations, or disorientation or confusion occurs.
• Closely supervise patient. Patients are usually hospitalized when receiving this drug.
• Treatment of toxicity is symptomatic and supportive.
• Used in Meniere's disease, following middle and inner ear surgery, labyrinthine disturbances, and to control nausea and vomiting associated with infectious disease, malignancies, radiation sickness, general anesthetics, and antineoplastic agents.

ipecac syrup

INDICATIONS & DOSAGE
To induce vomiting in poisoning—
Adults: 15 ml P.O., followed by 200 to 300 ml of water.
Children 1 year or older: 15 ml P.O., preceded by about 200 ml of water or milk.
Children under 1 year: 5 to 10 ml P.O., preceded by about 200 ml of water or milk.
May repeat dose once after 20 minutes, if necessary.

SIDE EFFECTS
CV: *cardiac disturbances, atrial fi-*

---

brillation, or fatal myocarditis if drug is absorbed (e.g., if patient doesn't vomit within 30 minutes) after ingestion of excessive dose.

INTERACTIONS
Activated charcoal: neutralized emetic effect. Don't give together but may give activated charcoal after vomiting has occurred.

NURSING CONSIDERATIONS
• Contraindicated in semicomatose or unconscious patients, severe inebriation, convulsions, shock, loss of gag reflex.
• Don't give after ingestion of petroleum distillates (e.g., kerosene, gasoline) or volatile oils; retching and vomiting may cause aspiration and lead to bronchospasm, pulmonary edema, or aspiration pneumonitis. Vegetable oil will delay absorption of these substances.
• Don't give after ingestion of caustic substances, such as lye; additional injury to the esophagus and mediastinum can occur.
• Clearly indicate ipecac *syrup*, not single word "ipecac," to avoid confusion with fluidextract. Fluidextract is 14 times more concentrated and if advertently used instead of syrup may cause death.
• Induces vomiting within 30 minutes in more than 90% of patients; average time usually less than 20 minutes.
• Stomach is usually emptied completely; vomitus may contain some intestinal material as well.
• In antiemetic toxicity, ipecac syrup is usually effective if less than 1 hour has passed since ingestion of antiemetic.
• Recommend that 1 ounce of syrup be readily available in the home when child becomes 1 year old for immediate use in case of emergency.
• No systemic toxicity with doses of 30 ml or less.

• If 2 doses do not induce vomiting, gastric lavage is necessary.

---

meclizine hydrochloride
Antivert♦, Bonamine♦♦, Bonine, Lamine, Roclizine, Vertrol, Whevert

INDICATIONS & DOSAGE
Dizziness—
Adults: 25 to 100 mg P.O. daily in divided doses. Dose varies with patient response.
Motion sickness—
Adults: 25 to 50 mg P.O. 1 hour before travel, repeated daily for duration of journey.

SIDE EFFECTS
CNS: *drowsiness,* fatigue.
EENT: dry mouth, blurred vision.
Other: may mask symptoms of ototoxicity, brain tumor, or intestinal obstruction.

INTERACTIONS
None significant.

NURSING CONSIDERATIONS
• Warn patient against driving and other activities that require alertness until response to drug is determined.
• Antihistamine with a slower onset and longer duration of action than other antihistamine antiemetics.

---

prochlorperazine edisylate

prochlorperazine maleate
Compazine, Stemetil♦♦

INDICATIONS & DOSAGE
*Preop nausea control—*5 to 10 mg I.M. 1 to 2 hours before induction of anesthetic, repeat once in 30 minutes, if necessary; or 5 to 10 mg I.V. 15 to 30 minutes before induction of anesthetic (repeat once if necessary); or

20 mg/liter isotonic solution by I.V. infusion, added to infusion 15 to 30 minutes before induction. Maximum parenteral dose 40 mg daily.
Severe nausea, vomiting—
Adults: 5 to 10 mg P.O. t.i.d. or q.i.d.; or 15 mg sustained-release form P.O. on arising; or 10 mg sustained-release form P.O. q 12 hours; or 25 mg rectally b.i.d. or 5 to 10 mg I.M. injected deeply into upper outer quadrant of gluteal region. Repeat q 3 to 4 hours, p.r.n.
Children 18 to 39 Kg: 2.5 mg P.O. or rectally t.i.d.; or 5 mg P.O. or rectally b.i.d. Maximum 15 mg daily; or 0.132 mg/Kg deep I.M. injection. (Control usually obtained with 1 dose.)
Children 14 to 17 Kg: 2.5 mg P.O. or rectally b.i.d. or t.i.d. Maximum 10 mg daily; or 0.132 mg/Kg deep I.M. injection. (Control usually obtained with 1 dose.)
Children 9 to 13 Kg: 2.5 mg P.O. or rectally daily or b.i.d. Maximum 7.5 mg daily; or 0.132 mg/Kg deep I.M. injection. (Control usually obtained with 1 dose.)

SIDE EFFECTS
Blood: *transient leukopenia, agranulocytosis.*
CNS: *extrapyramidal reactions (high incidence),* sedation (low incidence), pseudoparkinsonism, EEG changes, dizziness.
CV: *orthostatic hypotension,* tachycardia, EKG changes.
EENT: *ocular changes, blurred vision.*
GI: *dry mouth, constipation.*
GU: *urinary retention,* dark urine, menstrual irregularities, gynecomastia, inhibited ejaculation.
Hepatic: *cholestatic jaundice.*
Metabolic: hyperprolactinemia.
Skin: *mild photosensitivity,* dermal allergic reactions, *exfoliative dermatitis.*

Other: weight gain, increased appetite.

INTERACTIONS
Anticholinergics, including antidepressant and antiparkinson agents: increased anticholinergic activity, aggravated parkinson-like symptoms. Use together cautiously.
Antacids: inhibited absorption of oral phenothiazines. Separate antacid and phenothiazine dosage by at least 2 hours.
Barbiturates: may decrease phenothiazine effect. Monitor patient for decreased antiemetic effect.

NURSING CONSIDERATIONS
• Contraindicated in phenothiazine hypersensitivity, coma, depression, CNS depression, bone marrow depression, subcortical damage, pediatric surgery, use of spinal or epidural anesthetic or adrenergic blocking agents, alcohol usage. Use with caution in combination with other CNS depressants, hepatic disease, elderly or debilitated patients, arteriosclerosis or cardiovascular disease (may cause sudden drop in blood pressure), exposure to extreme heat or cold (including antipyretic therapy), respiratory disorders, hypocalcemia, vomiting in children, acutely ill or dehydrated children, convulsive disorders or severe reactions to insulin or electroshock therapy, suspected brain tumor or intestinal obstruction, glaucoma or prostatic hypertrophy.
• Store in light-resistant container. Slight yellowing does not affect potency; discard very discolored solutions.
• Since drug has a very long duration of action, timed-release capsules have no significant advantage over ordinary oral dosage forms.
• Use only when vomiting can't be controlled by other measures, or when only a few doses are required. If more

---

Italicized side effects are common or life-threatening.

than 4 doses needed in 24-hour period, notify doctor.
• Not effective in motion sickness.
• To prevent contact dermatitis, avoid getting concentrate or injection solution on hands or clothing.
• Dilute concentrate with tomato or fruit juice, milk, coffee, carbonated beverage, tea, water, soup, or pudding.
• Monitor CBC and liver function studies.
• Watch for orthostatic hypotension.
• Do not give S.C. or mix in syringe with another drug.

thiethylperazine maleate
Torecan♦

INDICATIONS & DOSAGE
Nausea, vomiting—
Adults: 10 mg P.O., I.M., or rectally daily, b.i.d. or t.i.d.

SIDE EFFECTS
Blood: *transient leukopenia, agranulocytosis.*
CNS: *extrapyramidal reactions (high incidence),* sedation (low incidence), pseudoparkinsonism, EEG changes, dizziness.
CV: *orthostatic hypotension,* tachycardia, EKG changes.
EENT: *ocular changes, blurred vision.*
GI: *dry mouth, constipation.*
GU: *urinary retention,* dark urine, menstrual irregularities, gynecomastia, inhibited ejaculation.
Hepatic: *cholestatic jaundice.*
Metabolic: hyperprolactinemia.
Skin: *mild photosensitivity,* dermal allergic reactions, *exfoliative dermatitis.*
Other: weight gain, increased appetite.

INTERACTIONS
Anticholinergics, including antide-pressants and antiparkinson agents: increased anticholinergic activity, aggravated parkinson-like symptoms. Use together cautiously.
Antacids: inhibited absorption of oral phenothiazines. Separate antacid and phenothiazine dosage by at least 2 hours.
Barbiturates: may decrease phenothiazine effect. Monitor for decreased antiemetic effect.

NURSING CONSIDERATIONS
• Contraindicated in severe CNS depression, hepatic disease, coma, phenothiazine hypersensitivity.
• Don't give I.V.
• For nausea and vomiting associated with anesthesia and surgery, give deep I.M. injection on or shortly before terminating anesthesia.
• Possibly effective in dizziness; not effective in motion sickness.
• Use only when vomiting can't be controlled by other measures, or when only a few doses are required.
• If drug gets on skin, wash off at once to prevent contact dermatitis.

trimethobenzamide hydrochloride
Tigan

INDICATIONS & DOSAGE
Nausea and vomiting (treatment)—
Adults: 250 mg P.O. t.i.d. or q.i.d.; or 200 mg I.M. or rectally t.i.d. or q.i.d.
Postop nausea and vomiting (prevention)—
Adults: 200 mg I.M. or rectally (single dose) before or during surgery; may repeat 3 hours after termination of anesthesia, p.r.n.
Children 13 to 40 Kg: 100 to 200 mg P.O. or rectally t.i.d. or q.i.d.
Children under 13 Kg: 100 mg rectally t.i.d. or q.i.d. Limited to prolonged vomiting of known etiology.

SIDE EFFECTS
CNS: drowsiness, dizziness (in large doses).
CV: hypotension.
GI: diarrhea, exaggeration of preexisting nausea (in large doses).
Hepatic: *liver toxicity.*
Local: pain, stinging, burning, redness, swelling at I.M. injection site.
Skin: skin hypersensitivity reactions.
Other: antiemetic effect may mask signs of overdosage of toxic agents, or intestinal obstruction, brain tumor, or other conditions.

INTERACTIONS
None significant.

NURSING CONSIDERATIONS
• Contraindicated in children with viral illness (a possible cause of vomiting in children); may contribute to the development of Reye's syndrome, a potentially fatal acute childhood encephalopathy, characterized by fatty degeneration of the liver.
• Suppositories contraindicated in hypersensitivity to benzocaine hydrochloride or similar local anesthetic.
• Stop drug if allergic skin reaction occurs.
• Give I.M. dose by deep injection into upper outer quadrant of gluteal region to reduce pain and local irritation.
• Store suppositories in refrigerator.
• Has little or no value in preventing motion sickness; limited value as antiemetic.

44

Gastrointestinal anticholinergics

anisotropine methylbromide
atropine sulfate
belladonna alkaloids
belladonna leaf
clidinium bromide
dicyclomine hydrochloride
diphemanil methylsulfate
glycopyrrolate
hexocyclium methylsulfate
homatropine methylbromide
isopropamide iodide
levorotatory alkaloids of belladonna
l-hyoscyamine sulfate
mepenzolate bromide
methantheline bromide
methixene hydrochloride
methscopolamine bromide
oxyphencyclimine hydrochloride
oxyphenonium bromide
propantheline bromide
thiphenamil hydrochloride
tridihexethyl chloride

anisotropine methylbromide
Valpin 50

INDICATIONS & DOSAGE

Adjunctive treatment of peptic ulcer—
Adults: 50 mg P.O. t.i.d. To be effective should be titrated to individual patient needs.

SIDE EFFECTS

CNS: headache, insomnia, drowsiness, dizziness, *confusion or excitement in elderly patients,* nervousness, weakness.
CV: *palpitations,* tachycardia.
EENT: *blurred vision,* mydriasis, in-

creased ocular tension, cycloplegia, photophobia.
GI: *dry mouth,* dysphagia, heartburn, loss of taste, nausea, vomiting, *paralytic ileus, constipation.*
GU: *urinary hesitancy and retention,* impotence.
Skin: urticaria, decreased sweating and possible anhidrosis, other dermal manifestations.
Other: fever, allergic reactions. Overdosage may cause curare-like symptoms.

INTERACTIONS
None significant.

NURSING CONSIDERATIONS
• Contraindicated in narrow-angle glaucoma, obstructive uropathy, obstructive disease of the GI tract, severe ulcerative colitis, myasthenia gravis, hypersensitivity to anticholinergics, paralytic ileus, intestinal atony, unstable cardiovascular status in acute hemorrhage, and toxic megacolon. Use cautiously in autonomic neuropathy, hyperthyroidism, coronary artery disease, cardiac arrhythmias, congestive heart failure, hypertension, hiatal hernia associated with reflux esophagitis, hepatic or renal disease, ulcerative colitis, or patients over 40 because of increased incidence of glaucoma.
• Use with caution in hot or humid environments. Drug-induced heat stroke can develop.
• Give 30 minutes to 1 hour before meals.
• Administer smaller doses to the

elderly.
• Monitor patient's vital signs and urinary output carefully.
• Instruct patient to avoid driving and other hazardous activities if he is drowsy, dizzy, or has blurred vision; to drink plenty of fluids to help prevent constipation; to report any skin rash or local eruption. Gum or sugarless hard candy may relieve mouth dryness.

---

atropine sulfate

INDICATIONS & DOSAGE
Adjunctive therapy in peptic ulcers, irritable bowel syndrome, neurogenic bowel disturbances, and functional gastrointestinal disorders—
Adults: 0.4 to 0.6 mg P.O. q 4 to 6 hours.
Children: the following dosages P.O. q 4 to 6 hours:
3 to 7 Kg—0.1 mg (1/600 gr)
8 to 11 Kg—0.15 mg (1/400 gr)
11 to 18 Kg—0.2 mg (1/300 gr)
18 to 30 Kg—0.3 mg (1/200 gr)
30 to 41 Kg—0.4 mg (1/150 gr)
over 41 Kg—0.4 to 0.6 mg (1/150 to 1/100 gr)

SIDE EFFECTS
CNS: headache, insomnia, drowsiness, dizziness, *confusion or excitement in elderly patients,* nervousness, weakness.
CV: *palpitations,* tachycardia.
EENT: *blurred vision,* mydriasis, increased ocular tension, cycloplegia, photophobia.
GI: *dry mouth,* dysphagia, heartburn, loss of taste, nausea, vomiting, paralytic ileus.
GU: *urinary hesitancy and retention,* impotence.
Skin: urticaria, decreased sweating or anhidrosis, other dermal manifestations.
Other: fever, allergic reactions.

Overdosage may cause curare-like symptoms.

INTERACTIONS
None significant

NURSING CONSIDERATIONS
• Contraindicated in narrow-angle glaucoma, obstructive uropathy, obstructive disease of GI tract, severe ulcerative colitis, myasthenia gravis, hypersensitivity to anticholinergics, paralytic ileus, intestinal atony, unstable cardiovascular status in acute hemorrhage, toxic megacolon. Use cautiously in autonomic neuropathy, hyperthyroidism, coronary artery disease, cardiac arrhythmias, congestive heart failure, hypertension, hiatal hernia associated with reflux esophagitis, hepatic or renal disease, ulcerative colitis, or patients over 40 because of increased incidence of glaucoma.
• Use with caution in hot or humid environments. Drug-induced heat stroke can develop.
• Give 30 minutes to 1 hour before meals and at bedtime. Bedtime dose can be larger and should be given at least 2 hours after last meal of day.
• Administer smaller doses to the elderly.
• Monitor patient's vital signs and urinary output carefully.
• Instruct patient to avoid driving and other hazardous activities if he is drowsy, dizzy, or has blurred vision; to drink plenty of fluids to help prevent constipation; to report any skin rash. Gum, sugarless hard candy, or pilocarpine syrup may relieve mouth dryness.
• Other anticholinergic drugs may increase vagal blockage.

Italicized side effects are common or life-threatening.

belladonna alkaloids

INDICATIONS & DOSAGE
Adjunctive therapy in gastric, peptic, duodenal, or intestinal ulcers to control excess motor activity, hyperirritability or spasm of the gastrointestinal tract—
Adults: 0.4 to 0.8 mg (timed-release capsules) P.O. q 12 hours.

SIDE EFFECTS
CNS: headache, insomnia, drowsiness, dizziness, *confusion or excitement in elderly patients,* nervousness, weakness.
CV: *palpitations,* tachycardia.
EENT: *blurred vision,* mydriasis, increased ocular tension, cycloplegia, photophobia.
GI: *dry mouth,* dysphagia, heartburn, loss of taste.
GU: *urinary hesitancy and retention,* impotence.
Skin: urticaria, decreased sweating or anhidrosis, other dermal manifestations.
Other: fever, allergic reactions.
Overdosage may cause curare-like symptoms.

INTERACTIONS
None significant.

NURSING CONSIDERATIONS
• Contraindicated in narrow-angle glaucoma, obstructive uropathy, obstructive disease of GI tract, severe ulcerative colitis, myasthenia gravis, hypersensitivity to anticholinergics, paralytic ileus, intestinal atony, unstable cardiovascular status in acute hemorrhage, toxic megacolon. Use cautiously in autonomic neuropathy, hyperthyroidism, coronary artery disease, cardiac arrhythmias, congestive heart failure, hypertension, hiatal hernia with reflux esophagitis, hepatic or renal disease, ulcerative coli-

tis, or patients over 40 because of increased incidence of glaucoma.
• Use with caution in hot or humid environments. Drug-induced heat stroke can develop.
• Administer smaller doses to the elderly.
• Monitor patient's vital signs and urinary output carefully.
• Instruct patient to avoid driving and other hazardous activities if he is drowsy, dizzy, or has blurred vision; to drink plenty of fluids to help prevent constipation; and to report any skin rash.

belladonna leaf
(used to prepare extract, fluidextract, and tincture)
Belladonna Tincture USP, Belladonna Fluidextract

INDICATIONS & DOSAGE
Adjunctive therapy for peptic ulcer, irritable bowel syndrome, functional gastrointestinal disorders, and neurogenic bowel disturbances—
Adults: 10.8 to 21.6 mg P.O. t.i.d. or q.i.d. of the extract; 0.06 ml P.O. t.i.d. or q.i.d. of the Fluidextract; 0.6 to 1 ml t.i.d. or q.i.d. of tincture.

SIDE EFFECTS
CNS: headache, insomnia, drowsiness, dizziness, *confusion or excitement in elderly patients,* nervousness, weakness.
CV: *palpitations,* tachycardia.
EENT: *blurred vision,* mydriasis, increased ocular tension, cycloplegia, photophobia.
GI: *dry mouth,* dysphagia, heartburn, loss of taste, *constipation,* nausea, vomiting.
GU: *urinary hesitancy and retention,* impotence.
Skin: urticaria, decreased sweating or anhidrosis, other dermal manifestations.

Other: fever, allergic reactions. Overdosage may cause curare-like symptoms.

INTERACTIONS
None significant.

NURSING CONSIDERATIONS
• Contraindicated in narrow-angle glaucoma, obstructive uropathy, obstructive disease of GI tract, severe ulcerative colitis, myasthenia gravis, hypersensitivity to anticholinergics, paralytic ileus, intestinal atony, unstable cardiovascular status in acute hemorrhage, and toxic megacolon. Use cautiously in autonomic neuropathy, hyperthyroidism, coronary artery disease, cardiac arrhythmias, congestive heart failure, hypertension, hiatal hernia associated with reflux esophagitis, hepatic or renal disease, ulcerative colitis, or patients over 40 because of increased incidence of glaucoma.
• Give 30 minutes to 1 hour before meals and at bedtime. Bedtime dose can be larger and should be given at least 2 hours after last meal of day.
• Administer smaller doses to the elderly.
• Use with caution in hot or humid environments. Drug-induced heat stroke can develop.
• Monitor patient's vital signs and urinary output carefully.
• Instruct patient to avoid driving and other hazardous activities if he is drowsy, dizzy, or has blurred vision; to drink plenty of fluids to help prevent constipation; to report any skin rash. Gum or sugarless hard candy may relieve mouth dryness.

---

clidinium bromide
Quarzan

INDICATIONS & DOSAGE
Adjunctive therapy for peptic ulcers—

Dosage should be individualized according to severity of symptoms and occurrence of side effects.
Adults: 2.5 to 5 mg P.O. t.i.d. or q.i.d. before meals and at bedtime.
Geriatric or debilitated patients: 2.5 mg P.O. t.i.d. before meals.

SIDE EFFECTS
CNS: headache, insomnia, drowsiness, dizziness, *confusion or excitement in elderly patients,* nervousness, weakness.
CV: *palpitations,* tachycardia.
EENT: *blurred vision,* mydriasis, increased ocular tension, cycloplegia, photophobia.
GI: *dry mouth,* dysphagia, heartburn, loss of taste, nausea, vomiting, *paralytic ileus, constipation.*
GU: *urinary hesitancy and retention,* impotence.
Skin: urticaria, decreased sweating or anhidrosis, other dermal manifestations.
Other: fever, allergic reactions. Overdosage may cause curare-like symptoms.

INTERACTIONS
None significant.

NURSING CONSIDERATIONS
• Contraindicated in narrow-angle glaucoma, obstructive uropathy, obstructive disease of GI tract, severe ulcerative colitis, myasthenia gravis, hypersensitivity to anticholinergics, paralytic ileus, intestinal atony, unstable cardiovascular status in acute hemorrhage, and toxic megacolon. Use cautiously in autonomic neuropathy, hyperthyroidism, coronary artery disease, cardiac arrhythmias, congestive heart failure, hypertension, hiatal hernia associated with reflux esophagitis, hepatic or renal disease, ulcerative colitis, or patients over 40 because of increased incidence of glaucoma.
• Give 30 minutes to 1 hour before

Italicized side effects are common or life-threatening.

meals and at bedtime. Bedtime dose can be larger and should be given at least 2 hours after last meal of day.
- Administer smaller doses to the elderly.
- Use with caution in hot or humid environments. Drug-induced heat stroke may develop.
- Monitor patient's vital signs and urinary output carefully.
- Instruct patient to avoid driving and other hazardous activities if he is drowsy, dizzy, or has blurred vision; to drink plenty of fluids to help prevent constipation; and to report any skin rash or local eruption. Gum or sugarless hard candy may relieve mouth dryness.

dicyclomine hydrochloride

Antispas, Bentyl, Bentylol♦♦, Cyclo-bec♦♦, Dibent, Dicen, Formulex♦♦, Menospasm♦♦, Nospaz, Or-Tyl, Rocyclo, Rotyl HCl, Stannitol, Viscerol♦♦

INDICATIONS & DOSAGE

Adjunctive therapy for peptic ulcers and other functional gastrointestinal disorders—
Adults: 10 to 20 mg P.O. t.i.d. or q.i.d.; 20 mg I.M. q 4 to 6 hours.
Children: 10 mg P.O. t.i.d. or q.i.d.
Infant colic—
Infants: 5 mg P.O. t.i.d. or q.i.d.
Always adjust dosage according to patient's needs and response.

SIDE EFFECTS

CNS: *headache,* insomnia, drowsiness, *dizziness.*
CV: *palpitations,* tachycardia.
GI: nausea, *constipation,* vomiting, *paralytic ileus.*
GU: urinary hesitancy and retention, impotence.
Skin: urticaria, decreased sweating or anhidrosis, other dermal manifestations.

Other: fever, allergic reactions. Overdosage may cause curare-like symptoms.

INTERACTIONS

None significant.

NURSING CONSIDERATIONS

- Contraindicated in obstructive uropathy, obstructive disease of GI tract, severe ulcerative colitis, myasthenia gravis, hypersensitivity to anticholinergics, paralytic ileus, intestinal atony, unstable cardiovascular status in acute hemorrhage, and toxic megacolon. Use cautiously in autonomic neuropathy, narrow-angle glaucoma, hyperthyroidism, coronary artery disease, cardiac arrhythmias, congestive heart failure, hypertension, hiatal hernia associated with reflux esophagitis, hepatic or renal disease, ulcerative colitis.
- Use with caution in hot or humid environments. Drug-induced heat stroke can develop.
- Give 30 minutes to 1 hour before meals and at bedtime. Bedtime dose can be larger and should be given at least 2 hours after last meal of day.
- Administer smaller doses to the elderly.
- Monitor patient's vital signs and urinary output carefully.
- Instruct patient to avoid driving and other hazardous activities if he is drowsy, dizzy, or has blurred vision; to drink plenty of fluids to help prevent constipation; and to report any skin rash. Gum or sugarless hard candy may relieve mouth dryness.
- A synthetic tertiary derivative that is relatively free of atropine-like side effects.

diphemanil methylsulfate
Prantal

INDICATIONS & DOSAGE

Adjunctive therapy in gastric hypersecretion associated with duodenal ulcer—
Adults: 100 to 200 mg P.O. q 4 to 6 hours, between meals (initial dose). Daily dosage should be adjusted according to response and tolerance. Maintenance dose: 50 to 100 mg q 4 to 6 hours.

SIDE EFFECTS

CNS: headache, insomnia, drowsiness, dizziness, *confusion or excitement in elderly patients,* nervousness, weakness.
CV: *palpitations,* tachycardia.
EENT: *blurred vision,* mydriasis, increased ocular tension, cycloplegia, photophobia.
GI: *dry mouth,* dysphagia, *constipation,* heartburn, loss of taste, nausea, vomiting, *paralytic ileus.*
GU: *urinary hesitancy and retention,* impotence.
Skin: urticaria, decreased sweating, anhidrosis, other dermal manifestations.
Other: fever, allergic reactions. Overdosage may cause curare-like symptoms.

INTERACTIONS

None significant.

NURSING CONSIDERATIONS

• Contraindicated in narrow-angle glaucoma, obstructive uropathy, obstructive disease of GI tract, severe ulcerative colitis, myasthenia gravis, hypersensitivity to anticholinergics, paralytic ileus, intestinal atony, unstable cardiovascular status in acute hemorrhage, and toxic megacolon. Use cautiously in autonomic neuropathy, hyperthyroidism, coronary artery disease, cardiac arrhythmias, congestive heart failure, hypertension, hiatal hernia associated with reflux esophagitis, hepatic or renal disease, ulcerative colitis, or patients over 40 because of increased incidence of glaucoma.
• Use with caution in hot or humid environments. Drug-induced heat stroke can develop.
• Give 30 minutes to 1 hour before meals and at bedtime. Bedtime dose can be larger and should be given at least 2 hours after last meal of day.
• Administer smaller doses to the elderly.
• Monitor patient's vital signs and urinary output carefully.
• Instruct patient to avoid driving and other hazardous activities if he is drowsy, dizzy, or has blurred vision; to drink plenty of fluids to help prevent constipation; and to report any skin rash. Gum or sugarless hard candy may relieve mouth dryness.

glycopyrrolate
Robinul♦, Robinul Forte♦

INDICATIONS & DOSAGE

Adjunctive therapy in peptic ulcers and other gastrointestinal disorders—
Adults: 1 to 2 mg P.O. t.i.d. or 0.1 mg I.M. t.i.d. or q.i.d. Dosage should be individualized.

SIDE EFFECTS

CNS: headache, insomnia, drowsiness, dizziness, *confusion or excitement in elderly patients,* nervousness, weakness.
CV: *palpitations,* tachycardia.
EENT: *blurred vision,* mydriasis, increased ocular tension, cycloplegia, photophobia.
GI: *dry mouth,* dysphagia, *constipation,* heartburn, loss of taste, nausea, vomiting, *paralytic ileus.*

GU: *urinary hesitancy and retention,* impotence.
Skin: urticaria, decreased sweating or anhidrosis, other dermal manifestations.
Other: fever, allergic reactions. Overdosage may cause curare-like symptoms.

INTERACTIONS
None significant.

NURSING CONSIDERATIONS
• Contraindicated in narrow-angle glaucoma, obstructive uropathy, obstructive disease of GI tract, severe ulcerative colitis, myasthenia gravis, hypersensitivity to anticholinergics, paralytic ileus, intestinal atony, unstable cardiovascular status in acute hemorrhage, and toxic megacolon. Use cautiously in autonomic neuropathy, hyperthyroidism, coronary artery disease, cardiac arrhythmias, congestive heart failure, hypertension, hiatal hernia associated with reflux esophagitis, hepatic or renal disease, ulcerative colitis, or patients over 40 because of increased incidence of glaucoma.
• Use with caution in hot or humid environments. Drug-induced heat stroke can develop.
• Administer 30 minutes to 1 hour before meals.
• Administer smaller doses to the elderly.
• Monitor patient's vital signs and urinary output carefully.
• Instruct patient to avoid driving and other hazardous activities if he is drowsy, dizzy, or has blurred vision; to drink plenty of fluids to help prevent constipation; to report any skin rash. Gum or sugarless hard candy may relieve mouth dryness.

hexocyclium methylsulfate
Tral

INDICATIONS & DOSAGE
Adjunctive therapy in peptic ulcer and other gastrointestinal disorders—
Adults: 25 mg q.i.d. before meals and h.s.

SIDE EFFECTS
CNS: headache, insomnia, drowsiness, dizziness, *confusion or excitement in elderly patients,* nervousness, weakness.
CV: *palpitations,* tachycardia.
EENT: *blurred vision,* mydriasis, increased ocular tension, cycloplegia, photophobia.
GI: *dry mouth,* dysphagia, heartburn, loss of taste, nausea, *constipation,* vomiting, *paralytic ileus.*
GU: *urinary hesitancy and retention,* impotence.
Skin: urticaria, decreased sweating or anhidrosis, other dermal manifestations.
Other: fever, allergic reactions. Overdosage may cause curare-like symptoms.

INTERACTIONS
None significant.

NURSING CONSIDERATIONS
• Contraindicated in narrow-angle glaucoma, obstructive uropathy, obstructive disease of GI tract, severe ulcerative colitis, myasthenia gravis, hypersensitivity to anticholinergics, paralytic ileus, intestinal atony, unstable cardiovascular status in acute hemorrhage, toxic megacolon. Use cautiously in autonomic neuropathy, hyperthyroidism, coronary artery disease, cardiac arrhythmias, congestive heart failure, hypertension, hiatal hernia associated with reflux esophagitis, hepatic or renal disease, ulcera-

tive colitis, or patients over 40 because of increased incidence of
glaucoma.
• Use with caution in hot or humid
environments. Drug-induced heat
stroke can develop.
• Give 30 minutes to 1 hour before
meals and at bedtime. Bedtime dose
can be larger and should be given at
least 2 hours after last meal of day.
• Administer smaller doses to the
elderly.
• Monitor patient's vital signs and
urinary output carefully.
• Instruct patient to avoid driving and
other hazardous activities if he is
drowsy, dizzy, or has blurred vision;
to drink plenty of fluids to help prevent constipation; and to report any
skin rash. Gum or sugarless hard
candy may relieve mouth dryness.
• Tablets contain tartrazine dye. May
cause allergy in susceptible patients.

---

homatropine methylbromide
Ru-Spas No. 2, Sed-Tens SE

INDICATIONS & DOSAGE
*Treatment of gastrointestinal spasm,
hyperchlorhydria, and other mild
spastic conditions of the bile ducts and
gallbladder—*
Adults: 2.5 to 5 mg t.i.d. to q.i.d. before meals and h.s.

SIDE EFFECTS
CNS: headache, insomnia, drowsiness, dizziness, *confusion or excitement in elderly patients,* nervousness,
weakness.
CV: *palpitations,* tachycardia.
EENT: *blurred vision,* mydriasis, increased ocular tension, cycloplegia,
photophobia.
GI: *dry mouth,* dysphagia, *constipation,* heartburn, loss of taste, nausea,
vomiting, *paralytic ileus.*
GU: *urinary hesitancy and retention,*
impotence.

Skin: urticaria, decreased sweating or
anhidrosis, other dermal manifestations.
Other: fever, allergic reactions.
Overdosage may cause curare-like
symptoms.

INTERACTIONS
None significant.

NURSING CONSIDERATIONS
• Contraindicated in narrow-angle
glaucoma, obstructive uropathy, obstructive disease of GI tract, severe
ulcerative colitis, myasthenia gravis,
hypersensitivity to anticholinergics,
paralytic ileus, intestinal atony, unstable cardiovascular status in acute
hemorrhage, and toxic megacolon.
Use cautiously in autonomic neuropathy, hyperthyroidism, coronary artery
disease, cardiac arrhythmias, congestive heart failure, hypertension, hiatal
hernia associated with reflux esophagitis, hepatic or renal disease, ulcerative colitis, or patients over 40 because of increased incidence of
glaucoma.
• Use with caution in hot or humid
environments. Drug-induced heat
stroke can develop.
• Give 30 minutes to 1 hour before
meals and at bedtime. Bedtime dose
can be larger and should be given at
least 2 hours after last meal of day.
• Administer smaller doses to the
elderly.
• Monitor patient's vital signs and
urinary output carefully.
• Instruct patient to avoid driving and
other hazardous activities if he is
drowsy, dizzy, or has blurred vision;
to drink plenty of fluids to help prevent constipation; and to report any
skin rash. Gum or sugarless hard
candy may relieve mouth dryness.

Italicized side effects are common or life-threatening.

isopropamide iodide
Darbid♦

INDICATIONS & DOSAGE
Adjunctive therapy for peptic ulcer, irritable bowel syndrome—
Adults, and children over 12 years: 5 mg P.O. q 12 hours. Some patients may require 10 mg or more b.i.d. Dose should be individualized to patient's need.

SIDE EFFECTS
CNS: headache, insomnia, drowsiness, dizziness, *confusion or excitement in elderly patients,* nervousness, weakness.
CV: *palpitations,* tachycardia.
EENT: *blurred vision,* mydriasis, increased ocular tension, cycloplegia, photophobia.
GI: *dry mouth,* dysphagia, heartburn, loss of taste, nausea, vomiting, *constipation, paralytic ileus.*
GU: *urinary hesitancy and retention,* impotence.
Skin: urticaria, decreased sweating or anhidrosis, other dermal manifestations, iodine skin rash.
Other: fever, allergic reactions. Overdosage may cause curare-like symptoms.

INTERACTIONS
None significant.

NURSING CONSIDERATIONS
• Contraindicated in narrow-angle glaucoma, obstructive uropathy, obstructive disease of GI tract, severe ulcerative colitis, myasthenia gravis, hypersensitivity to anticholinergics, paralytic ileus, intestinal atony, unstable cardiovascular status in acute hemorrhage, toxic megacolon. Use cautiously in autonomic neuropathy, hyperthyroidism, coronary artery disease, cardiac arrhythmias, congestive heart failure, hypertension, hiatal hernia associated with reflux esophagitis, hepatic or renal disease, ulcerative colitis, or patients over 40 because of increased incidence of glaucoma.
• Use with caution in hot or humid environments. Drug-induced heat stroke can develop.
• Give 30 minutes to 1 hour before meals and at bedtime. Bedtime dose can be larger and should be given at least 2 hours after the last meal of the day.
• Administer smaller doses to the elderly.
• Monitor patient's vital signs and urinary output carefully.
• Instruct patient to avoid driving and other hazardous activities if he is drowsy, dizzy, or has blurred vision; to drink plenty of fluids to help prevent constipation; and to report any skin rash. Gum or sugarless hard candy may relieve mouth dryness.
• Single dose produces 10- to 12-hour antisecretory effect and gastrointestinal antispasmodic effect.
• Discontinue 1 week before thyroid function tests.

levorotatory alkaloids of belladonna
(as maleate salts)
Bellafoline

INDICATIONS & DOSAGE
Adjunctive therapy for peptic ulcer, irritable bowel syndrome, and functional gastrointestinal disorders—
Adults: 0.25 to 0.5 P.O. t.i.d.; or 0.125 to 0.5 mg S.C. daily or b.i.d.
Children over 6 years: 0.125 to 0.25 mg P.O. t.i.d.

SIDE EFFECTS
CNS: headache, insomnia, drowsiness, dizziness, *confusion or excitement in elderly patients,* nervousness, weakness.

Unmarked trade names available in the United States only.
♦ Also available in Canada ♦♦ Available in Canada only.

CV: *palpitations,* tachycardia.
EENT: *blurred vision,* mydriasis, increased ocular tension, cycloplegia, photophobia.
GI: *dry mouth,* dysphagia, heartburn, loss of taste, *constipation, paralytic ileus.*
GU: *urinary hesitancy and retention,* impotence.
Skin: urticaria, decreased sweating or anhidrosis, other dermal manifestations.
Other: fever, allergic reactions. Overdosage may cause curare-like symptoms.

INTERACTIONS
None significant.

NURSING CONSIDERATIONS
• Contraindicated in narrow-angle glaucoma, obstructive uropathy, obstructive disease of GI tract, severe ulcerative colitis, myasthenia gravis, hypersensitivity to anticholinergics, paralytic ileus, intestinal atony, unstable cardiovascular status in acute hemorrhage, and toxic megacolon. Use cautiously in autonomic neuropathy, hyperthyroidism, coronary artery disease, cardiac arrhythmias, congestive heart failure, hypertension, hiatal hernia associated with reflux esophagitis, hepatic or renal disease, ulcerative colitis, or patients over 40 because of increased incidence of glaucoma.
• Use with caution in hot or humid environments. Drug-induced heat stroke can develop.
• Administer 30 minutes to 1 hour before meals.
• Administer smaller doses to the elderly.
• Monitor patient's vital signs and urinary output carefully.
• Instruct patient to avoid driving and other hazardous activities if he is drowsy, dizzy, or has blurred vision; to drink plenty of fluids to help prevent constipation; to report any skin rash. Gum or sugarless hard candy may relieve mouth dryness.

---

l-hyoscyamine sulfate
Anaspaz, Levsin♦, Levsinex, Levsinex Time Caps

INDICATIONS & DOSAGE
Treatment of gastrointestinal tract disorders due to spasm; adjunctive therapy for peptic ulcers—
Adults: 0.125 to 0.25 mg P.O. t.i.d. or q.i.d. before meals and at bedtime; sustained-release form 0.375 mg P.O. q 12 hours; or 0.25 to 0.5 mg (1 or 2 ml) I.M., I.V., or S.C. q 6 hours. (Substitute oral medication when symptoms are controlled.)
Children 2 to 10 years: ½ adult dose P.O.
Children under 2 years: ¼ adult dose P.O.

SIDE EFFECTS
CNS: headache, insomnia, drowsiness, dizziness, *confusion or excitement in elderly patients,* nervousness, weakness.
CV: *palpitations,* tachycardia.
EENT: *blurred vision,* mydriasis, increased ocular tension, cycloplegia, photophobia.
GI: *dry mouth,* dysphagia, *constipation,* heartburn, loss of taste, nausea, vomiting, *paralytic ileus.*
GU: *urinary hesitancy and retention,* impotence.
Skin: urticaria, decreased sweating or anhidrosis, other dermal manifestations.
Other: fever, allergic reactions. Overdosage may cause curare-like symptoms.

INTERACTIONS
None significant.

NURSING CONSIDERATIONS
• Contraindicated in narrow-angle

glaucoma, obstructive uropathy, obstructive disease of GI tract, severe ulcerative colitis, myasthenia gravis, hypersensitivity to anticholinergics, paralytic ileus, intestinal atony, unstable cardiovascular status in acute hemorrhage, toxic megacolon. Use cautiously in autonomic neuropathy, hyperthyroidism, coronary artery disease, cardiac arrhythmias, congestive heart failure, hypertension, hiatal hernia associated with reflux esophagitis, hepatic or renal disease, ulcerative colitis, or patients over 40 because of the increased incidence of glaucoma.

• Use with caution in hot or humid environments. Drug-induced heat stroke can develop.

• Give 30 minutes to 1 hour before meals and at bedtime. Bedtime dose can be larger and should be given at least 2 hours after the last meal of the day.

• Administer smaller doses to the elderly.

• Monitor patient's vital signs and urinary output carefully.

• Instruct patient to avoid driving and other hazardous activities if he is drowsy, dizzy, or has blurred vision; to drink plenty of fluids to help prevent constipation; and to report any skin rash. Gum or sugarless hard candy may relieve mouth dryness.

---

mepenzolate bromide
Cantil

INDICATIONS & DOSAGE
Adjunctive therapy in treating peptic ulcer, irritable bowel syndrome, and neurologic bowel disturbances—
Adults: 25 to 50 mg P.O. q.i.d. with meals and at bedtime. Adjust dosage to individual patient's needs.

SIDE EFFECTS
CNS: headache, insomnia, drowsiness, dizziness, *confusion or excitement in elderly patients,* nervousness, weakness.
CV: *palpitations,* tachycardia.
EENT: *blurred vision,* mydriasis, increased ocular tension, cycloplegia, photophobia.
GI: *dry mouth,* dysphagia, heartburn, loss of taste, nausea, *constipation,* vomiting, *paralytic ileus.*
GU: *urinary hesitancy and retention,* impotence.
Skin: urticaria, decreased sweating or anhidrosis, other dermal manifestations.
Other: fever, allergic reactions. Overdosage may cause curare-like symptoms.

INTERACTIONS
None significant.

NURSING CONSIDERATIONS
• Contraindicated in narrow-angle glaucoma, obstructive uropathy, obstructive disease of GI tract, severe ulcerative colitis, myasthenia gravis, hypersensitivity to anticholinergics, paralytic ileus, intestinal atony, unstable cardiovascular status in acute hemorrhage, toxic megacolon. Use cautiously in autonomic neuropathy, hyperthyroidism, coronary artery disease, cardiac arrhythmias, congestive heart failure, hypertension, hiatal hernia associated with reflux esophagitis, hepatic or renal disease, ulcerative colitis, or patients over 40 because of increased incidence of glaucoma.

• Use with caution in hot or humid environments. Drug-induced heat stroke can develop.

• Give with meals and at bedtime.

• Administer smaller doses to the elderly.

• Monitor patient's vital signs and urinary output carefully.

• Instruct patient to avoid driving and other hazardous activities if he is drowsy, dizzy, or has blurred vision;

Unmarked trade names available in the United States only.
♦ Also available in Canada   ♦ ♦ Available in Canada only.

to drink plenty of fluids to help prevent constipation; and to report any skin rash. Gum or sugarless hard candy may relieve mouth dryness.

methantheline bromide
Banthine

INDICATIONS & DOSAGE
Adjunctive therapy in peptic ulcer, pylorospasm, spastic colon, biliary dyskinesia, pancreatitis, and certain forms of gastritis—
Adults: 50 to 100 mg P.O. q 6 hours.
Children over 1 year: 12.5 to 50 mg q.i.d.
Children under 1 year: 12.5 to 25 mg q.i.d.

SIDE EFFECTS
CNS: headache, insomnia, drowsiness, dizziness, *confusion or excitement in elderly patients,* nervousness, weakness.
CV: *palpitations,* tachycardia.
EENT: *blurred vision,* mydriasis, increased ocular tension, cycloplegia, photophobia.
GI: *dry mouth,* dysphagia, *constipation,* heartburn, loss of taste, nausea, vomiting, *paralytic ileus.*
GU: *urinary hesitancy and retention,* impotence.
Skin: urticaria, decreased sweating or anhidrosis, other dermal manifestations.
Other: fever, allergic reactions.
Overdosage may cause curare-like symptoms.

INTERACTIONS
None significant.

NURSING CONSIDERATIONS
• Contraindicated in narrow-angle glaucoma, obstructive uropathy, obstructive disease of GI tract, severe ulcerative colitis, myasthenia gravis, hypersensitivity to anticholinergics, paralytic ileus, intestinal atony, unstable cardiovascular status in acute hemorrhage, toxic megacolon. Use cautiously in autonomic neuropathy, hyperthyroidism, coronary artery disease, cardiac arrhythmias, congestive heart failure, hypertension, hiatal hernia associated with reflux esophagitis, hepatic or renal disease, ulcerative colitis, or patients over 40 because of the increased incidence of glaucoma.
• Use with caution in hot or humid environments. Drug-induced heat stroke can develop.
• Give 30 minutes to 1 hour before meals and at bedtime. Bedtime dose can be larger and should be given at least 2 hours after the last meal of the day.
• Administer smaller doses to the elderly.
• If patient is also taking antihistamines, he may experience increased dryness of mouth.
• Monitor patient's vital signs and urinary output carefully.
• Instruct patient to avoid driving and other hazardous activities if he is drowsy, dizzy, or has blurred vision; to drink plenty of fluids to help prevent constipation; and to report any skin rash. Gum or sugarless hard candy may relieve mouth dryness.
• Therapeutic effects appear in 30 to 45 minutes; persist for 4 to 6 hours after oral administration.

methixene hydrochloride
Trest♦

INDICATIONS & DOSAGE
Adjunctive treatment of gastrointestinal disorders associated with hypermotility or spasm—
Adults: 1 or 2 mg P.O. t.i.d.

SIDE EFFECTS
CNS: *headache*, insomnia, drowsiness, *dizziness*.
CV: *palpitations*, tachycardia.
EENT: *blurred vision*, mydriasis, increased ocular tension, cycloplegia, photophobia.
GI: *constipation*, nausea, vomiting, *paralytic ileus*.
GU: urinary hesitancy and retention, impotence.
Skin: urticaria, decreased sweating or anhidrosis, other dermal manifestations.
Other: fever, allergic reactions. Overdosage may cause curare-like symptoms.

INTERACTIONS
None significant.

NURSING CONSIDERATIONS
• Contraindicated in narrow-angle glaucoma, obstructive uropathy, obstructive disease of GI tract, severe ulcerative colitis, myasthenia gravis, hypersensitivity to anticholinergics, paralytic ileus, intestinal atony, unstable cardiovascular status in acute hemorrhage, toxic megacolon. Use cautiously in autonomic neuropathy, hyperthyroidism, coronary artery disease, cardiac arrhythmias, congestive heart failure, hypertension, hiatal hernia associated with reflux esophagitis, hepatic or renal disease, ulcerative colitis, or patients over 40 because of the increased incidence of glaucoma.
• Use with caution in hot or humid environment. Drug-induced heat stroke could develop.
• Administer 30 minutes to 1 hour before meals.
• Administer smaller doses to the elderly.
• Monitor patient's vital signs and urinary output
• Instruct patient to avoid driving and other hazardous activities if he is drowsy, dizzy, or has blurred vision; to drink plenty of fluids to help prevent constipation; and to report any skin rash. Gum or sugarless hard candy may relieve mouth dryness.
• Synthetic tertiary derivative that is relatively free of atropine-like side effects.

---

methscopolamine bromide
Pamine♦, Scoline

INDICATIONS & DOSAGE
Adjunctive therapy in peptic ulcer—
Adults: 2.5 to 5 mg ½ hour before meals and h.s.

SIDE EFFECTS
CNS: headache, insomnia, dizziness, *confusion or excitement in elderly patients*, nervousness, weakness.
CV: *palpitations*, tachycardia.
EENT: *blurred vision*, mydriasis, increased ocular tension, cycloplegia, photophobia.
GI: *dry mouth*, dysphagia, *constipation*, heartburn, loss of taste, nausea, vomiting, *paralytic ileus*.
GU: *urinary hesitancy and retention*, impotence.
Skin: urticaria, decreased sweating or anhidrosis, other dermal manifestations.
Other: fever, allergic reactions. Overdosage may cause curare-like symptoms.

INTERACTIONS
None significant.

NURSING CONSIDERATIONS
• Contraindicated in narrow-angle glaucoma, obstructive uropathy, obstructive disease of GI tract, severe ulcerative colitis, myasthenia gravis, hypersensitivity to anticholinergics, paralytic ileus, intestinal atony, unstable cardiovascular status in acute hemorrhage, toxic megacolon. Use cautiously in autonomic neuropathy,

hyperthyroidism, coronary artery disease, cardiac arrhythmias, congestive heart failure, hypertension, hiatal hernia associated with reflux esophagitis, hepatic or renal disease, ulcerative colitis, or patients over 40 because of increased incidence of glaucoma.
• Use with caution in hot or humid environments. Drug-induced heat stroke can develop.
• Give 30 minutes to 1 hour before meals and at bedtime. Bedtime dose can be larger and should be given at least 2 hours after the last meal of the day.
• Administer smaller doses to the elderly.
• Monitor patient's vital signs and urinary output carefully.
• Instruct patient to avoid driving and other hazardous activities if he is drowsy, dizzy, or has blurred vision; to drink plenty of fluids to help prevent constipation; and to report any skin rash. Gum or sugarless hard candy may relieve mouth dryness.

---

oxyphencyclimine hydrochloride
Daricon◆

INDICATIONS & DOSAGE
Adjunctive treatment of peptic ulcer—
Adults: 10 mg b.i.d. in the morning and h.s., or 5 mg b.i.d. or t.i.d.

SIDE EFFECTS
CNS: *headache,* insomnia, drowsiness, *dizziness.*
CV: *palpitations,* tachycardia.
EENT: *blurred vision,* mydriasis, increased ocular tension, cycloplegia, photophobia.
GI: *constipation,* nausea, vomiting, *paralytic ileus.*
GU: urinary hesitancy and retention, impotence.
Skin: urticaria, decreased sweating or

Skin: urticaria, decreased sweating or anhidrosis, other dermal manifestations.
Other: fever, allergic reactions. Overdosage may cause curare-like symptoms.

INTERACTIONS
None significant.

NURSING CONSIDERATIONS
• Contraindicated in narrow-angle glaucoma, obstructive uropathy, obstructive disease of GI tract, severe ulcerative colitis, myasthenia gravis, hypersensitivity to anticholinergics, paralytic ileus, intestinal atony, unstable cardiovascular status in acute hemorrhage, toxic megacolon. Use cautiously in autonomic neuropathy, hyperthyroidism, coronary artery disease, cardiac arrhythmias, congestive heart failure, hypertension, hiatal hernia associated with reflux esophagitis, hepatic or renal disease, ulcerative colitis, or patients over 40 because of increased incidence of glaucoma.
• Use with caution in hot or humid environments. Drug-induced heat stroke can develop.
• Give 30 minutes to 1 hour before breakfast and at bedtime.
• Administer smaller doses to the elderly.
• Monitor patient's vital signs and urinary output carefully.
• Instruct patient to avoid driving and other hazardous activities if he is drowsy, dizzy, or has blurred vision; to drink plenty of fluids to help prevent constipation; and to report any skin rash. Gum or sugarless hard candy may relieve mouth dryness.
• Synthetic tertiary derivative that is relatively free of atropine-like side effects.

Italicized side effects are common or life-threatening.

oxyphenonium bromide
Antrenyl

INDICATIONS & DOSAGE
Adjunctive treatment of peptic ulcer—
Adults: 10 mg P.O. q.i.d. for several days, then reduced according to patient response.

SIDE EFFECTS
CNS: headache, insomnia, drowsiness, dizziness, *confusion or excitement in elderly patients,* nervousness, weakness.
CV: *palpitations,* tachycardia.
EENT: *blurred vision,* mydriasis, increased ocular tension, cycloplegia, photophobia.
GI: *dry mouth,* dysphagia, *constipation,* heartburn, loss of taste, nausea, vomiting, *paralytic ileus.*
GU: *urinary hesitancy and retention,* impotence.
Skin: urticaria, decreased sweating or anhidrosis, other dermal manifestations.
Other: fever, allergic reactions. Overdosage may cause curare-like symptoms.

INTERACTIONS
None significant.

NURSING CONSIDERATIONS
• Contraindicated in narrow-angle glaucoma, obstructive uropathy, obstructive disease of GI tract, severe ulcerative colitis, myasthenia gravis, hypersensitivity to anticholinergics, paralytic ileus, intestinal atony, unstable cardiovascular status in acute hemorrhage, toxic megacolon. Use cautiously in autonomic neuropathy, hyperthyroidism, coronary artery disease, cardiac arrhythmias, congestive heart failure, hypertension, hiatal hernia associated with reflux esophagitis, hepatic or renal disease, ulcera-
tive colitis, or patients over 40 because of increased incidence of glaucoma.
• Use with caution in hot or humid environments. Drug-induced heat stroke can develop.
• Give 30 minutes to 1 hour before meals and at bedtime. Bedtime dose can be larger and should be given at least 2 hours after the last meal of the day.
• Administer smaller doses to the elderly.
• Monitor patient's vital signs and urinary output.
• Instruct patient to avoid driving and other hazardous activities if he is drowsy, dizzy, or has blurred vision; to drink plenty of fluids to help prevent constipation; and to report any skin rash. Gum or sugarless hard candy may relieve mouth dryness.

propantheline bromide
Banlin♦♦, Norpanth, Pro-Banthine♦, Propanthel♦♦, Robantaline, Ropanth

INDICATIONS & DOSAGE
Adjunctive treatment of peptic ulcer and irritable bowel syndrome, and other gastrointestinal disorders—
Adults: 15 mg P.O. t.i.d. before meals, and 30 mg at bedtime up to 60 mg q.i.d. For elderly patients, 7.5 mg P.O. t.i.d. before meals.
When oral dosage not possible, 30 mg I.M. or I.V. q 6 hours, depending on individual response. Maintenance dose 15 mg I.M. q 6 hours.

SIDE EFFECTS
CNS: headache, insomnia, drowsiness, dizziness, *confusion or excitement in elderly patients,* nervousness, weakness.
CV: *palpitations,* tachycardia.
EENT: *blurred vision,* mydriasis, increased ocular tension, cycloplegia, photophobia.

GI: *dry mouth,* dysphagia, constipation, heartburn, loss of taste, nausea, vomiting, paralytic ileus.
GU: *urinary hesitancy and retention,* impotence.
Skin: urticaria, decreased sweating or anhidrosis, other dermal manifestations.
Other: fever, allergic reactions. Overdosage may cause curare-like symptoms.

INTERACTIONS
None significant.

NURSING CONSIDERATIONS
• Contraindicated in narrow-angle glaucoma, obstructive uropathy, obstructive disease of GI tract, severe ulcerative colitis, myasthenia gravis, hypersensitivity to anticholinergics, paralytic ileus, intestinal atony, unstable cardiovascular status in acute hemorrhage, toxic megacolon. Use cautiously in autonomic neuropathy, hyperthyroidism, coronary artery disease, cardiac arrhythmias, congestive heart failure, hypertension, hiatal hernia associated with reflux esophagitis, hepatic or renal disease, ulcerative colitis, or patients over 40 because of the increased incidence of glaucoma.
• Use with caution in hot or humid environments. Drug-induced heat stroke can develop.
• Give 30 minutes to 1 hour before meals and at bedtime. Bedtime dose can be larger and should be given at least 2 hours after the last meal of the day.
• Administer smaller doses to the elderly.
• Monitor patient's vital signs and urinary output carefully.
• Instruct patient to avoid driving and other hazardous activities if he is drowsy, dizzy, or has blurred vision; to drink plenty of fluids to help prevent constipation; and to report any skin rash. Gum or sugarless hard candy may relieve mouth dryness.

---

thiphenamil hydrochloride
Trocinate

INDICATIONS & DOSAGE
Hypermotility and spasm of the gastrointestinal tract—
Adults: initially, 400 mg P.O. repeated in 4 hours, usually to maximum of 4 doses. Maintenance dose may be given at a reduced frequency of dosage.

SIDE EFFECTS
CNS: headache, insomnia, drowsiness, dizziness, *confusion or excitement in elderly patients,* nervousness, weakness.
CV: *palpitations,* tachycardia.
EENT: *blurred vision,* mydriasis, increased ocular tension, cycloplegia, photophobia.
GI: *dry mouth,* dysphagia, *constipation,* heartburn, loss of taste, nausea, vomiting, *paralytic ileus.*
GU: *urinary hesitancy and retention,* impotence.
Skin: urticaria, decreased sweating or anhidrosis, other dermal manifestations.
Other: fever, allergic reactions. Overdosage may cause curare-like symptoms.

INTERACTIONS
None significant.

NURSING CONSIDERATIONS
• Contraindicated in narrow-angle glaucoma, obstructive uropathy, obstructive disease of GI tract, severe ulcerative colitis, myasthenia gravis, hypersensitivity to anticholinergics, paralytic ileus, intestinal atony, unstable cardiovascular status in acute hemorrhage, toxic megacolon. Use cautiously in autonomic neuropathy,

hyperthyroidism, coronary artery disease, cardiac arrhythmias, congestive heart failure, hypertension, hiatal hernia associated with reflux esophagitis, hepatic or renal disease, ulcerative colitis, or patients over 40 because of increased incidence of glaucoma.
• Use with caution in hot or humid environments. Drug-induced heat stroke can develop.
• Administer smaller doses to the elderly.
• Monitor patient's vital signs and urinary output carefully.
• Instruct patient to avoid driving and other hazardous activities if he is drowsy, dizzy, or has blurred vision; to drink plenty of fluids to help prevent constipation; and to report any skin rash. Gum or sugarless hard candy may relieve mouth dryness.

------

tridihexethyl chloride
Pathilon

INDICATIONS & DOSAGE
Adjunctive treatment of peptic ulcer, irritable bowel syndrome, and other gastrointestinal disorders—
Adults: initially, 25 to 50 mg P.O. t.i.d. before meals, and 50 mg h.s., increased to 75 mg q.i.d., if needed. With sustained-release capsules, 75 mg q 12 or q 6 hours. Maintenance dose usually half the therapeutic dose. Parenteral use: 10 to 20 mg I.V., I.M., or S.C. q 6 hours. Change to oral as soon as possible.

SIDE EFFECTS
CNS: headache, insomnia, drowsiness, dizziness, *confusion or excitement in elderly patients,* nervousness, weakness.
CV: *palpitations,* tachycardia.
EENT: *blurred vision,* mydriasis, increased ocular tension, cycloplegia, photophobia.

GI: *dry mouth,* dysphagia, *constipation,* heartburn, loss of taste, nausea, vomiting, *paralytic ileus.*
GU: *urinary hesitancy and retention,* impotence.
Skin: urticaria, decreased sweating or anhidrosis, other dermal manifestations.
Other: fever, allergic reactions. Overdosage may cause curare-like symptoms.

INTERACTIONS
None significant.

NURSING CONSIDERATIONS
• Contraindicated in narrow-angle glaucoma, obstructive uropathy, obstructive disease of GI tract, severe ulcerative colitis, myasthenia gravis, hypersensitivity to anticholinergics, paralytic ileus, intestinal atony, unstable cardiovascular status in acute hemorrhage, toxic megacolon. Use cautiously in autonomic neuropathy, hyperthyroidism, coronary artery disease, cardiac arrhythmias, congestive heart failure, hypertension, hiatal hernia associated with reflux esophagitis, hepatic or renal disease, ulcerative colitis, or patients over 40 because of increased incidence of glaucoma.
• Use with caution in hot or humid environments. Drug-induced heat stroke can develop.
• Give 30 minutes to 1 hour before meals and at bedtime. Bedtime dose can be larger and should be given at least 2 hours after the last meal of the day.
• Administer smaller doses to the elderly.
• Monitor patient's vital signs and urinary output carefully.

• Instruct patient to avoid driving and other hazardous activities if he is drowsy, dizzy, or has blurred vision; to drink plenty of fluids to help prevent constipation; and to report any skin rash. Gum or sugarless hard candy may relieve mouth dryness.

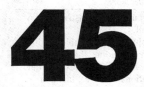

Miscellaneous gastrointestinals

choline
cimetidine
dexpanthenol
metoclopramide hydrochloride

---

choline

INDICATIONS & DOSAGE
Hepatic disorders and disturbed fat metabolism—
Adults and children: 650 to 750 mg P.O. daily.

SIDE EFFECTS
CNS: dizziness.
GI: irritation if taken on an empty stomach, nausea.
Metabolic: ketosis after excessive dosages.
Other: breath and body odor smelling like dead fish.

INTERACTIONS
None significant.

NURSING CONSIDERATIONS
• Foods supplying choline include egg yolk, beef liver, legumes, vegetables, and milk. Average diet contains from 500 to 900 mg per day.
• Lipotropic agent.
• Used in many multivitamin preparations, but no evidence supplemental choline intake is more beneficial for long periods than an adequate diet.
• Synthesized by the body from serine, with methionine acting as a methyl-donor in the reaction.
• Choline is no longer considered ef-

fective in treatment of hepatic disorders or disorders of lipid transport or metabolism.
• Investigative use in treatment of tardive dyskinesia: restores cholinergic tone and decreases choreic movements. Oral choline elevates brain choline and acetylcholine (the cholinergic neurotransmitter of the cholinergic nervous system) levels and restores cholinergic tone.
• Lecithin (available in health food stores) is a source of choline.

---

cimetidine
Tagamet♦

INDICATIONS & DOSAGE
Duodenal ulcer (short-term treatment)—
Adults, and children over 16 years: 300 mg P.O. q.i.d. with meals and h.s. for maximum therapy of 8 weeks. Once healing occurs, stop treatment or give bedtime dose only to control nocturnal hypersecretion. Parenteral: 300 mg diluted to 20 ml with 0.9% normal saline or other compatible I.V. solution by I.V. push over 1 to 2 minutes q 6 hours. Or 300 mg diluted in 100 ml 5% dextrose solution or other compatible I.V. solution by I.V. infusion over 15 to 20 minutes q 6 hours. Or 300 mg I.M. q 6 hours (no dilution necessary). To increase dose, give 300 mg doses more frequently to maximum daily dose of 2,400 mg.
Duodenal ulcer prophylaxis—

Adults, and children over 16 years:
400 mg P.O. h.s.
*Pathologic hypersecretory conditions
(such as Zollinger-Ellison syndrome,
systemic mastocytosis, and multiple
endocrine adenomas)—*
Adults, and children over 16 years:
300 mg P.O. q.i.d. with meals and
h.s.; adjust to individual needs. Maximum daily dose 2,400 mg.
Parenteral: 300 mg diluted to 20 ml
with 0.9% normal saline or other
compatible I.V. solutions by I.V. push
over 1 to 2 minutes q 6 hours. Or
300 mg diluted in 100 ml 5% dextrose solution or other compatible I.V.
solution by I.V. infusion over 15 to
20 minutes q 6 hours. To increase
dose, give 300 mg doses more frequently to maximum daily dose of
2,400 mg.

SIDE EFFECTS
Blood: *agranulocytosis,* neutropenia,
thrombocytopenia, aplastic anemia.
CNS: mental confusion, dizziness,
headaches.
CV: bradycardia.
GI: mild and transient diarrhea, perforation of chronic peptic ulcers after
abrupt cessation of drug.
GU: interstitial nephritis, *transient
elevations in BUN and serum creatinine.*
Hepatic: jaundice.
Skin: acne-like rash, urticaria, *exfoliative dermatitis.*
Other: hypersensitivity, muscle pain,
reduced sperm count; mild gynecomastia after use longer than 1 month
(but no change in endocrine function).

INTERACTIONS
Antacids: interfere with absorption of
cimetidine. Separate cimetidine and
antacids by at least 1 hour if possible.

NURSING CONSIDERATIONS
• Maintenance dosing for more than
12 months cannot be recommended.
Long-term effects are not known.

• I.M. route of administration may
be painful.
• I.V. solutions compatible for dilution with cimetidine: 0.9% sodium
chloride, 5% and 10% dextrose (and
combinations of these), lactated
Ringer's solution, and 5% sodium bicarbonate injection. Do not dilute
with sterile water for injection.
• Hemodialysis reduces blood levels
of cimetidine. Schedule cimetidine
dose at end of hemodialysis
treatment.
• Up to 10 g overdosage has been reported without untoward effects.
• Effectiveness in treatment of gastric ulcers not as great as in duodenal
ulcer. Cimetidine may prove useful
but is still unapproved in pancreatic
insufficiency, short-bowel syndrome,
psoriasis, prevention and treatment of
GI bleeding, relief of symptoms and
acid sensitivity in reflux esophagitis,
and to prevent gastric inactivation of
oral enzyme preparations by gastric
acid and pepsin.
• Best to administer with meals in
order to maintain blood levels.
• Large parenteral doses should be
avoided in asthmatics.
• Elderly patients more susceptible to
cimetidine-induced mental confusion.
Dose should be decreased in elderly
and in patients with renal insufficiency.
• I.V. cimetidine often used in critically ill patients prophylactically to
prevent GI bleeding.
• Available in liquid form
(300 mg/5 ml).
• Tablets available in two strengths:
200 mg (SKF T12) and 300 mg (SKF
T13). Both tablets are pale green.
Identify tablet when obtaining a drug
history.

Italicized side effects are common or life-threatening.

dexpanthenol
Ilopan♦, Intrapan, Motilyn♦♦,
Tonestat

INDICATIONS & DOSAGE
Postop abdominal distention (resulting from flatus retention)—
Adults and children: 250 to 500 mg I.M., repeat in 2 hours and again q 6 hours until distention is relieved. May require therapy for 48 to 72 hours or longer. Or, 500 mg infused slow I.V. drip in glucose or lactated Ringer's solution.
Treatment and postop prevention of paralytic ileus—
Adults and children: 500 mg I.M., repeat in 2 hours; then q 4 to 6 hours until distention is relieved. May require therapy for 48 to 72 hours or longer.

SIDE EFFECTS
Blood: prolonged bleeding time.
GI: excessive passage of flatus with increased doses or prolonged use, increased frequency of bowel movements, hyperperistalsis.

INTERACTIONS
None significant.

NURSING CONSIDERATIONS
• Contraindicated in hemophilia because bleeding time is prolonged.
• Don't administer full-strength solution I.V.; always dilute.
• Dexpanthenol use shouldn't delay treatment of mechanical ileus if present.
• A smooth-muscle stimulant; used postop against delayed resumption of intestinal motility. Also used as adjunctive treatment of peripheral neuritis and lupus erythematosus.
• Hypokalemia may cause a decreased response. If this occurs, potassium supplements should be started. Increased doses of dexpanthenol may be needed.
• May also be useful during laxative withdrawal after long-term use.
• Wait 12 hours after giving parasympathomimetics before starting dexpanthenol.

metoclopramide hydrochloride
Maxeran♦♦, Reglan♦

INDICATIONS & DOSAGE
To facilitate small-bowel intubation and to aid in radiologic examinations—
Adults: 10 mg (2 ml) I.V. as a single dose over 1 to 2 minutes.
Children 6 to 14 years: 2.5 to 5 mg (0.5 to 1 ml).
Children under 6 years: 0.1 mg/Kg.

SIDE EFFECTS
CNS: restlessness, *drowsiness,* fatigue, *lassitude,* insomnia, headache, dizziness.
GI: nausea, bowel disturbances.
Other: extrapyramidal symptoms.

INTERACTIONS
Anticholinergics, narcotic analgesics: antagonized effects of metoclopramide. Use together cautiously.

NURSING CONSIDERATIONS
• Contraindicated whenever stimulation of GI motility might be dangerous (hemorrhage, obstruction, perforation), pheochromocytoma, and epilepsy.
• Speeds gastric emptying by stimulating smooth muscle in upper GI tract.
• If I.V. injection is too rapid, a transient but intense feeling of anxiety and restlessness occurs, followed by drowsiness.

• Warn patient to avoid activities requiring alertness for 2 hours after taking each dose.
• Oral form available in Canada only. Give with meals.

• Injectable form may be useful as an antiemetic following chemotherapy.
• Used investigationally to treat diabetic gastric paresis.

46

Corticosteroids

beclomethasone dipropionate
Beclovent♦ Vanceril♦

INDICATIONS & DOSAGE
Steroid-dependent asthma—
Adults: 2 to 4 inhalations t.i.d. or
q.i.d. Maximum 20 inhalations daily.
Children 6 to 12 years: 1 to 2 inhalations t.i.d. or q.i.d. Maximum 10 inhalations daily.

SIDE EFFECTS
EENT: hoarseness, fungal infections
of mouth and throat.
GI: dry mouth.

INTERACTIONS
None significant.

NURSING CONSIDERATIONS
• Contraindicated in status asthmaticus. Not for asthma controlled by
bronchodilators or other noncortico-
steroids, or for nonasthmatic bronchial diseases.
• Oral therapy should be tapered
slowly. Acute adrenal insufficiency
and death have occurred in asthmatics
who changed abruptly from oral corticosteroids to beclomethasone.
• During times of stress (trauma, surgery, infection) systemic corticosteroids may be needed to prevent adrenal insufficiency in previously steroid-dependent patients.
• Instruct patient to carry a card indicating his need for supplemental systemic glucocorticoids during stress.

- Patient requiring bronchodilator should use it several minutes before beclomethasone.
- Don't store near heat or open flame.
- Glucocorticoid with potent anti-inflammatory action.
- Oral fungal infections can be prevented by following inhalations with glass of water.

betamethasone
Betnelan♦♦, Celestone♦
betamethasone acetate and betamethasone sodium phosphate
Celestone Soluspan♦
betamethasone disodium phosphate
Betnesol♦♦
betamethasone sodium phosphate
Celestone Phosphate

INDICATIONS & DOSAGE
Severe inflammation or immuno-suppression—
Adults: 0.6 to 7.2 mg P.O. daily; or 0.5 to 9 mg (sodium phosphate) I.M., I.V., or into joint or soft tissue daily; or 1.5 to 12 mg (sodium phosphate-acetate suspension) into joint or soft tissue q 1 to 2 weeks, p.r.n.

SIDE EFFECTS
Most side effects of corticosteroids are dose- or duration-dependent.
CNS: *euphoria, insomnia,* psychotic behavior, pseudotumor cerebri.
CV: *congestive heart failure,* hypertension, edema.
EENT: cataracts, glaucoma.
GI: *peptic ulcer,* gastrointestinal irritation, increased appetite.
Metabolic: *severe hypokalemia, hyperglycemia and carbohydrate intolerance,* growth suppression in children.
Skin: delayed wound healing, acne, various skin eruptions.
Other: muscle weakness, pancreatitis, hirsutism, susceptibility to infec-

tions. Acute adrenal insufficiency may follow increased stress (infection, surgery, trauma) or abrupt withdrawal after long-term therapy.
Withdrawal symptoms: rebound inflammation, fatigue, weakness, arthralgia, fever, dizziness, lethargy, depression, fainting, orthostatic hypotension, dyspnea, anorexia, hypoglycemia. *Sudden withdrawal may be fatal.*

INTERACTIONS
Barbiturates, phenytoin, rifampin: decreased corticosteroid effect. Corticosteroid dose may need to be increased.
Indomethacin, ASA: increased risk of GI distress and bleeding. Give together cautiously.

NURSING CONSIDERATIONS
- Contraindicated in systemic fungal infections. Use cautiously in GI ulceration or renal disease, hypertension, osteoporosis, varicella, vaccinia, exanthema, diabetes mellitus, Cushing's syndrome, thromboembolic disorders, seizures, myasthenia gravis, congestive heart failure, tuberculosis, ocular herpes simplex, hypoalbuminemia, emotional instability, or psychotic tendencies.
- Don't use for alternate-day therapy.
- Adrenal suppression may last up to 1 year after drug stopped. Gradually reduce drug dosage after long-term therapy. Tell patient not to stop drug abruptly or without doctor's consent.
- Always titrate to lowest effective dose.
- To prevent muscle atrophy, give by deep I.M. injection.
- Monitor serum electrolytes and blood sugar.
- Warn patients who are on long-term therapy about cushingoid symptoms.
- Observe for signs of infection, especially after steroid withdrawal.
- Instruct patient to carry a card indi-

Italicized side effects are common or life-threatening.

cating his need for supplemental glucocorticoids during stress.
• Give with milk or food to reduce gastric irritation.
• Glucocorticoid with little mineralocorticoid effect.
• Watch for additional potassium depletion from diuretics and amphotericin B.
• Immunizations may show decreased antibody response.
• Weigh patient daily; report any sudden weight gain to doctor.

cortisone acetate
Cortistan, Cortone Acetate♦

INDICATIONS & DOSAGE
Adrenal insufficiency, allergy, inflammation—
Adults: 25 to 300 mg P.O. or I.M. daily or on alternate days. Doses highly individualized, depending on severity of disease.

SIDE EFFECTS
Most side effects of corticosteroids are dose- or duration-dependent.
CNS: *euphoria, insomnia,* psychotic behavior, pseudotumor cerebri.
CV: *congestive heart failure,* hypertension, edema.
EENT: cataracts, glaucoma.
GI: *peptic ulcer,* gastrointestinal irritation, increased appetite.
Metabolic: *severe hypokalemia, hyperglycemia and carbohydrate intolerance,* growth suppression in children.
Skin: delayed wound healing, acne, various skin eruptions.
Local: atrophy at I.M. injection sites.
Other: muscle weakness, pancreatitis, hirsutism, susceptibility to infections. Acute adrenal insufficiency may follow increased stress (infection, surgery, trauma) or abrupt withdrawal after long-term therapy.
Withdrawal symptoms: rebound inflammation, fatigue, weakness, arthralgia, fever, dizziness, lethargy, depression, fainting, orthostatic hypotension, dyspnea, anorexia, hypoglycemia. *Sudden withdrawal may be fatal.*

INTERACTIONS
Barbiturates, phenytoin, rifampin: decreased corticosteroid effect. Corticosteroid dose may need to be increased.
Indomethacin, ASA: increased risk of GI distress and bleeding. Give together cautiously.

NURSING CONSIDERATIONS
• Contraindicated in systemic fungal infections. Use cautiously in GI ulceration or renal disease, hypertension, osteoporosis, varicella, vaccinia, exanthema, diabetes mellitus, Cushing's syndrome, thromboembolic disorders, seizures, myasthenia gravis, congestive heart failure, tuberculosis, ocular herpes simplex, hypoalbuminemia, emotional instability, or psychotic tendencies.
• Gradually reduce drug dosage after long-term therapy. Tell patient not to discontinue drug abruptly or without doctor's consent.
• Always titrate to lowest effective dose.
• Patient may need salt-restricted diet and potassium supplement.
• I.M. route causes slow onset of action. Don't use in acute conditions where rapid effect required.
• Glucocorticoid with potent mineralocorticoid effect; report sudden weight gain or edema to doctor.
• Observe for signs of infection, especially after steroid withdrawal.
• Drug of choice for replacement therapy in adrenal insufficiency.
• Not used for alternate-day therapy.
• Monitor serum electrolytes and blood sugar.
• Warn patients on long-term therapy about cushingoid symptoms.

• Give with milk or food to reduce gastric irritation.
• Instruct patient to carry a card indicating his need for supplemental glucocorticoids during stress.
• Not for I.V. use.
• Watch for additional potassium depletion from diuretics and amphotericin B.
• Immunizations may show decreased antibody response.

desoxycorticosterone acetate
Doca Acetate, Percorten Acetate
desoxycorticosterone pivalate
Percorten Pivalate

INDICATIONS & DOSAGE
Adrenal insufficiency (partial replacement), salt-losing adrenogenital syndrome—
Adults: 2 to 5 mg (acetate) I.M. daily; or 25 to 100 mg (pivalate) I.M. q 4 weeks. Or implant 1 pellet for each 0.5 mg of the daily injected maintenance dose. Pellets last for 8 to 12 months.

SIDE EFFECTS
CV: *sodium and water retention,* hypertension, cardiac hypertrophy, edema.
Metabolic: hypokalemia.

INTERACTIONS
None significant.

NURSING CONSIDERATIONS
• Contraindicated in hypertension, congestive heart failure, cardiac disease. Use cautiously in Addison's disease. Patients may have exaggerated side effects.
• Has no anti-inflammatory effect.
• Most potent mineralocorticoid. Has little glucocorticoid effect.
• Use with glucocorticoid for full treatment of adrenal insufficiency.

• Report significant weight gain, edema, hypertension, or cardiac symptoms to doctor. Drug may have to be stopped.
• Injection is sesame oil solution. Withdraw dose with 19-gauge needle, but give with 23-gauge needle. Inject in upper, outer quadrant of buttocks. Not for I.V. use.
• Monitor sodium and potassium levels, fluid intake. Patient may need salt-restricted diet, potassium supplement.
• Watch for additional potassium depletion from diuretics and amphotericin B.

dexamethasone
Decadron♦, Dexasone♦♦, Dexone, Dezone, Hexadrol, SK-Dexamethasone
dexamethasone acetate
Decadron-LA, Decameth-LA, Dexacen-LA, Dexasone-LA
dexamethasone sodium phosphate
Decadron Phosphate, Decaject, Decameth, Delladec, Dexacen-4, Dexasone, Dexon, Dexone, Dezone, Hexadrol Phosphate♦, Savacort-D, Solurex

INDICATIONS & DOSAGE
Cerebral edema—
Adults: initially, 10 mg (phosphate) I.V., then 4 to 6 mg I.M. q 6 hours for 2 to 4 days, then taper over 5 to 7 days.
Children: 0.2 mg/Kg P.O. daily in divided doses.
Inflammatory conditions, allergic reactions, neoplasias—
Adults: 0.25 to 4 mg P.O. b.i.d., t.i.d., or q.i.d.; or 4 to 16 mg (acetate) I.M. into joint or soft tissue q 1 to 3 weeks; or 0.8 to 1.6 mg (acetate) into lesions q 1 to 3 weeks.
Shock—
Adults: 1 to 6 mg/Kg (phosphate) I.V.

Italicized side effects are common or life-threatening.

single dose; or 40 mg I.V. q 2 to
6 hours, p.r.n.
Dexamethasone suppression test—
0.5 mg P.O. q 6 hours for 48 hours.

SIDE EFFECTS
Most side effects of corticosteroids
are dose- or duration-dependent.
CNS: *euphoria, insomnia,* psychotic
behavior, pseudotumor cerebri.
CV: *congestive heart failure,* hypertension, edema.
EENT: cataracts, glaucoma.
GI: *peptic ulcer,* gastrointestinal irritation, increased appetite.
Metabolic: *severe hypokalemia, hyperglycemia and carbohydrate intolerance,* growth suppression in children.
Skin: delayed wound healing, acne,
various skin eruptions.
Local: atrophy at I.M. injection sites.
Other: muscle weakness, pancreatitis, hirsutism, susceptibility to infections. Acute adrenal insufficiency
may follow increased stress (infection, surgery, trauma) or abrupt withdrawal after long-term therapy.
Withdrawal symptoms: rebound inflammation, fatigue, weakness, arthralgia, fever, dizziness, lethargy,
depression, fainting, orthostatic
hypotension, dyspnea, anorexia,
hypoglycemia. *Sudden withdrawal
may be fatal.*

INTERACTIONS
Barbiturates, phenytoin, rifampin: decreased corticosteroid effect. Corticosteroid dose may need to be increased.
Indomethacin, ASA: increased risk of
GI distress and bleeding. Give together cautiously.

NURSING CONSIDERATIONS
• Contraindicated in systemic fungal
infections and for alternate-day therapy. Use cautiously in GI ulceration or
renal disease, hypertension, osteoporosis, varicella, vaccinia, exanthema,
diabetes mellitus, Cushing's syn-

drome, thromboembolic disorders,
seizures, myasthenia gravis, metastatic cancer, congestive heart failure,
tuberculosis, ocular herpes simplex,
hypoalbuminemia, emotional instability or psychotic tendencies, and in
children.
• Gradually reduce drug dosage after
long-term therapy. Tell patient not to
discontinue drug abruptly or without
doctor's consent.
• Always titrate to lowest effective
dose.
• Monitor patient's weight, blood
pressure, serum electrolytes.
• Instruct patient to carry a card indicating his need for supplemental systemic glucocorticoids during stress,
especially as dose is decreased.
• Teach patient signs of early adrenal
insufficiency: fatigue, muscular
weakness, joint pain, fever, anorexia,
nausea, dyspnea, dizziness, fainting.
• May mask or exacerbate infections.
• Watch for depression or psychotic
episodes, especially in high-dose
therapy.
• Inspect patient's skin for petechiae.
Warn patient about easy bruising.
• Diabetics may need increased insulin; monitor urine for sugar.
• Monitor growth in infants and children on long-term therapy.
• Give I.M. injection deep into gluteal muscle. Avoid S.C. injection, as
atrophy and sterile abscesses may
occur.
• Give P.O. dose with food when
possible.
• Warn patients on long-term therapy
about cushingoid symptoms.
• Watch for additional potassium
depletion from diuretics and amphotericin B.
• Immunizations may show decreased antibody response.
• When performing dexamethasone
suppression test, obtain a baseline
24-hour urine specimen for 17-keto-
steroids.

fludrocortisone acetate
Florinef♦

INDICATIONS & DOSAGE
Adrenal insufficiency (partial replacement), salt-losing adrenogenital syndrome—
Adults: 0.1 to 0.2 mg P.O. daily.

SIDE EFFECTS
CV: *sodium and water retention,* hypertension, cardiac hypertrophy, edema.
Metabolic: hypokalemia.

INTERACTIONS
None significant.

NURSING CONSIDERATIONS
• Contraindicated in hypertension, congestive heart failure, cardiac disease. Use cautiously in Addison's disease.
• Monitor patient's blood pressure, serum electrolytes. Weigh patient daily; report sudden weight gain to doctor.
• Warn patient that mild peripheral edema is common.
• Unless contraindicated, give salt-restricted diet rich in potassium and protein. Potassium supplement may be needed.
• Has potent mineralocorticoid effects. Little glucocorticoid effect with usual doses.
• Used with cortisone or hydrocortisone in adrenal insufficiency.
• Watch for additional potassium depletion from diuretics and amphotericin B.

fluprednisolone
Alphadrol

INDICATIONS & DOSAGE
Severe inflammation—
Adults: 2.5 to 30 mg P.O. daily divided t.i.d. or q.i.d.
Children: 0.07 to 1 mg/Kg P.O. daily divided t.i.d. or q.i.d., or 2.5 to 30 mg/m^2 divided t.i.d. or q.i.d.

SIDE EFFECTS
Most side effects of corticosteroids are dose- or duration-dependent.
CNS: *euphoria, insomnia,* psychotic behavior, pseudotumor cerebri.
CV: *congestive heart failure,* hypertension, edema.
EENT: cataracts, glaucoma.
GI: *peptic ulcer,* gastrointestinal irritation, increased appetite.
Metabolic: *severe hypokalemia, hyperglycemia and carbohydrate intolerance,* growth suppression in children.
Skin: delayed wound healing, acne, various skin eruptions.
Other: muscle weakness, pancreatitis, hirsutism, susceptibility to infections. Acute adrenal insufficiency may follow increased stress (infection, surgery, trauma) or abrupt withdrawal after long-term therapy.
Withdrawal symptoms: rebound inflammation, fatigue, weakness, arthralgia, fever, dizziness, lethargy, depression, fainting, orthostatic hypotension, dyspnea, anorexia, hypoglycemia. *Sudden withdrawal may be fatal.*

INTERACTIONS
Barbiturates, phenytoin, rifampin: decreased corticosteroid effect. Corticosteroid dose may need to be increased.
Indomethacin, ASA: increased risk of GI distress and bleeding. Give together cautiously.

NURSING CONSIDERATIONS
• Contraindicated in systemic fungal infections. Use cautiously in GI ulceration or renal disease, hypertension, osteoporosis, varicella, vaccinia, exanthema, diabetes mellitus, Cushing's syndrome, thromboembolic disorders,

Italicized side effects are common or life-threatening.

seizures, myasthenia gravis, metastatic cancer, congestive heart failure, tuberculosis, ocular herpes simplex, hypoalbuminemia, emotional instability or psychotic tendencies, and in children.

• Gradually reduce drug dosage after long-term therapy. Tell patient not to discontinue drug abruptly or without doctor's consent.

• Always titrate to lowest effective dose.

• Glucocorticoid with little mineralocorticoid effect.

• Monitor patient's weight, blood pressure, serum electrolytes.

• May mask or exacerbate infections.

• Instruct patient to carry a card identifying his need for supplemental systemic glucocorticoids during stress.

• Teach patient signs of early adrenal insufficiency: fatigue, muscular weakness, joint pain, fever, anorexia, nausea, dyspnea, dizziness, fainting.

• Watch for depression or psychotic episodes, especially in high-dose therapy.

• Inspect patient's skin for petechiae. Warn patient about easy bruising.

• Diabetics may need increased insulin dose; monitor urine for sugar.

• Monitor growth in infants and children on long-term therapy.

• Unless contraindicated, give salt-restricted diet rich in potassium and protein. Potassium supplement may be needed.

• Give P.O. dose with food when possible.

• Warn patients on long-term therapy about cushingoid symptoms.

• Watch for additional potassium depletion from diuretics and amphotericin B.

• Immunizations may show decreased antibody response.

• Not for alternate-day therapy.

hydrocortisone
Cortef♦, Hydrocortone♦
hydrocortisone acetate
Cortril Acetate, Hydrocortone Acetate, Cortef Acetate
hydrocortisone sodium phosphate
Hydrocortone Phosphate
hydrocortisone sodium succinate
A-Hydrocort, S-Cortilean♦♦, Solu-Cortef♦, Solu-Ject♦♦
hydrocortisone retention enema
Cortenema, Rectoid

INDICATIONS & DOSAGE

Severe inflammation, adrenal insufficiency—
Adults: 5 to 30 mg P.O. b.i.d., t.i.d., or q.i.d. (as much as 80 mg P.O. q.i.d. may be given in acute situations); or initially, 100 to 250 mg (succinate) I.M. or I.V., then 50 to 100 mg I.M., as indicated; or 15 to 240 mg (phosphate) I.M. or I.V. q 12 hours; or 5 to 75 mg (acetate) into joints and soft tissue. Dose varies with size of joint. Often local anesthetics are injected with dose.
Shock—
Adults: 500 mg to 2 g (succinate) q 2 to 6 hours.
Children: 0.16 to 1 mg/Kg (phosphate or succinate) I.M. or I.V. b.i.d. or t.i.d.
Adjunctive treatment of ulcerative colitis and proctitis—
Adults: 1 enema (100 mg) nightly for 21 days.

SIDE EFFECTS

Most side effects of corticosteroids are dose- or duration-dependent.
CNS: *euphoria, insomnia,* psychotic behavior, pseudotumor cerebri.
CV: *congestive heart failure,* hypertension, edema.
EENT: cataracts, glaucoma.

GI: *peptic ulcer,* gastrointestinal irritation, increased appetite.
Metabolic: *severe hypokalemia, hyperglycemia and carbohydrate intolerance,* growth suppression in children.
Skin: delayed wound healing, acne, various skin eruptions.
Other: muscle weakness, pancreatitis, hirsutism, susceptibility to infections. Acute adrenal insufficiency may occur with increased stress (infection, surgery, trauma) or abrupt withdrawal after long-term therapy.
Withdrawal symptoms: rebound inflammation, fatigue, weakness, arthralgia, fever, dizziness, lethargy, depression, fainting, orthostatic hypotension, dyspnea, anorexia, hypoglycemia. *Sudden withdrawal may be fatal.*

INTERACTIONS
Barbiturates, phenytoin, rifampin: decreased corticosteroid effect. Corticosteroid dose may need to be increased.
Indomethacin, ASA: increased risk of GI distress and bleeding. Give together cautiously.

NURSING CONSIDERATIONS
• Contraindicated in systemic fungal infections. Use cautiously in GI ulceration or renal disease, hypertension, osteoporosis, varicella, vaccinia, exanthema, diabetes mellitus, Cushing's syndrome, thromboembolic disorders, seizures, myasthenia gravis, metastatic cancer, congestive heart failure, tuberculosis, ocular herpes simplex, hypoalbuminemia, emotional instability or psychotic tendencies, and in children.
• Gradually reduce drug dosage after long-term therapy. Tell patient not to discontinue drug abruptly or without doctor's consent.
• Always titrate to lowest effective dose.
• Glucocorticoid and mineralocorticoid effect.

• Monitor patient's weight, blood pressure, serum electrolytes.
• May mask or exacerbate infections.
• Stress (fever, trauma, surgery, emotional problems) may increase adrenal insufficiency. Dose may have to be increased.
• Instruct patient to carry a card identifying his need for supplemental systemic glucocorticoids during stress.
• Teach patient signs of early adrenal insufficiency: fatigue, muscular weakness, joint pain, fever, anorexia, nausea, dyspnea, dizziness, fainting.
• Watch for depression or psychotic episodes, especially in high-dose therapy.
• Inspect patient's skin for petechiae. Warn patient about easy bruising.
• Diabetics may need increased insulin; monitor urine for sugar.
• Monitor growth in infants and children on long-term therapy.
• Give I.M. injection deep into gluteal muscle. Avoid S.C. injection as atrophy and sterile abscesses may occur.
• Unless contraindicated, give salt-restricted diet rich in potassium and protein. Potassium supplement may be needed. Watch for additional potassium depletion from diuretics and amphotericin B.
• Give P.O. dose with food when possible.
• Warn patients on long-term therapy about cushingoid symptoms.
• Acetate form for I.M. use only.
• Enema may produce same systemic effects as other forms of hydrocortisone. If enema therapy must exceed 21 days, discontinue gradually by reducing administration to every other night for 2 or 3 weeks.
• Immunizations may show decreased antibody response.
• Do not confuse Solu-Cortef with Solu-Medrol.
• Not for alternate-day therapy.

Italicized side effects are common or life-threatening.

meprednisone
Betapar

INDICATIONS & DOSAGE
Severe inflammation—
Adults: 4 to 15 mg P.O. b.i.d., t.i.d., or q.i.d.

SIDE EFFECTS
Most side effects of corticosteroids are dose- or duration-dependent.
CNS: *euphoria, insomnia,* psychotic behavior, pseudotumor cerebri.
CV: *congestive heart failure,* hypertension, edema.
EENT: cataracts, glaucoma.
GI: *peptic ulcer,* gastrointestinal irritation, increased appetite.
Metabolic: *severe hypokalemia, hyperglycemia and carbohydrate intolerance,* growth suppression in children.
Skin: delayed wound healing, acne, various skin eruptions.
Other: muscle weakness, pancreatitis, hirsutism, susceptibility to infections. Acute adrenal insufficiency may occur with increased stress (infection, surgery, trauma) or abrupt withdrawal after long-term therapy.
Withdrawal symptoms: rebound inflammation, fatigue, weakness, arthralgia, fever, dizziness, lethargy, depression, fainting, orthostatic hypotension, dyspnea, anorexia, hypoglycemia. *Sudden withdrawal may be fatal.*

INTERACTIONS
Barbiturates, phenytoin, rifampin: decreased corticosteroid effect. Corticosteroid dose may need to be increased.
Indomethacin, ASA: increased risk of GI distress and bleeding. Give together cautiously.

NURSING CONSIDERATIONS
• Contraindicated in systemic fungal infections. Use cautiously in GI ulceration or renal disease, hypertension, osteoporosis, varicella, vaccinia, exanthema, diabetes mellitus, Cushing's syndrome, thromboembolic disorders, seizures, myasthenia gravis, metastatic cancer, congestive heart failure, tuberculosis, ocular herpes simplex, hypoalbuminemia, emotional instability or psychotic tendencies.
• Gradually reduce drug dosage after long-term therapy. Tell patient not to discontinue drug abruptly or without doctor's consent.
• Always titrate to lowest effective dose.
• Glucocorticoid with little mineralocorticoid effect.
• Monitor patient's weight, blood pressure, serum electrolytes.
• May mask or exacerbate infections.
• Instruct patient to carry a card identifying his need for supplemental systemic glucocorticoids during stress.
• Useful in rheumatoid and collagen diseases.
• Teach patient signs of early adrenal insufficiency: fatigue, muscular weakness, joint pain, fever, anorexia, nausea, dyspnea, dizziness, fainting.
• Watch for depression or psychotic episodes, especially in high-dose therapy.
• Diabetics may need increased insulin; monitor urine for sugar.
• Monitor growth in infants and children on long-term therapy.
• Unless contraindicated, give salt-restricted diet rich in potassium and protein. Potassium supplement may be needed. Watch for additional potassium depletion from diuretics and amphotericin B.
• Give P.O. dose with food when possible.
• Warn patients on long-term therapy about cushingoid symptoms.
• Immunizations may show decreased antibody response.
• Not for alternate-day therapy.

methylprednisolone
Medrol♦
methylprednisolone acetate
Depo-Medrol♦, D-Med, Medralone,
Methydrol-40, Pre-Dep, Rep-Pred
methylprednisolone sodium succinate
A-Methapred, Solu-Medrol♦

INDICATIONS & DOSAGE
Severe inflammation or immuno-suppression—
Adults: 2 to 60 mg P.O. in 4 divided doses; or 40 to 80 mg (acetate) daily, I.M. or 10 to 250 mg (succinate) I.M. or I.V. q 4 hours; or 4 to 30 mg (acetate) into joints and soft tissue, p.r.n.
Children: 117 mcg to 1.66 mg/Kg (succinate) I.V. in 3 or 4 divided doses.
Shock—100 to 250 mg (succinate) I.V. at 2- to 6-hour intervals.

SIDE EFFECTS
Most side effects of corticosteroids are dose- or duration-dependent.
CNS: *euphoria, insomnia,* psychotic behavior, pseudotumor cerebri.
CV: *congestive heart failure,* hypertension, edema.
EENT: cataracts, glaucoma.
GI: *peptic ulcer,* gastrointestinal irritation, increased appetite.
Metabolic: *severe hypokalemia, hyperglycemia and carbohydrate intolerance,* growth suppression in children.
Skin: delayed wound healing, acne, various skin eruptions.
Other: muscle weakness, pancreatitis, hirsutism, susceptibility to infections. Acute adrenal insufficiency may occur with increased stress (infection, surgery, trauma) or abrupt withdrawal after long-term therapy.
Withdrawal symptoms: rebound inflammation, fatigue, weakness, arthralgia, fever, dizziness, lethargy, depression, fainting, orthostatic hypotension, dyspnea, anorexia,
hypoglycemia. *Sudden withdrawal may be fatal.*

INTERACTIONS
Barbiturates, phenytoin, rifampin: decreased corticosteroid effect. Corticosteroid dose may need to be increased.
Indomethacin, ASA: increased risk of GI distress and bleeding. Give together cautiously.

NURSING CONSIDERATIONS
• Contraindicated in systemic fungal infections. Use cautiously in GI ulceration or renal disease, hypertension, osteoporosis, varicella, vaccinia, exanthema, diabetes mellitus, Cushing's syndrome, thromboembolic disorders, seizures, myasthenia gravis, metastatic cancer, congestive heart failure, tuberculosis, ocular herpes simplex, hypoalbuminemia, emotional instability or psychotic tendencies.
• Gradually reduce drug dosage after long-term therapy. Tell patient not to discontinue drug abruptly or without doctor's consent.
• Always titrate to lowest effective dose.
• Glucocorticoid with little mineralocorticoid effect.
• Discard reconstituted solutions after 48 hours.
• Don't use acetate salt when immediate onset of action needed.
• Dermal atrophy may occur with large doses of acetate salt. Use multiple small injections into lesions.
• Monitor weight, blood pressure, sleep patterns, serum electrolytes.
• May mask or exacerbate infections.
• Instruct patient to carry a card identifying his need for supplemental systemic glucocorticoids during stress.
• Teach patient signs of early adrenal insufficiency: fatigue, muscular weakness, joint pain, fever, anorexia, nausea, dyspnea, dizziness, fainting.

Italicized side effects are common or life-threatening.

- Watch for depression or psychotic episodes, especially in high-dose therapy.
- Diabetics may need increased insulin; monitor urine for sugar.
- Give I.M. injection deep into gluteal muscle. Avoid S.C. injection as atrophy and sterile abscesses may occur.
- Unless contraindicated, give salt-restricted diet rich in potassium and protein. Potassium supplement may be needed. Watch for additional potassium depletion from diuretics and amphotericin B.
- Give P.O. dose with food when possible.
- Give I.V. dose slowly over 1 minute; in shock, give massive I.V. doses over 3 to 15 minutes to prevent cardiac arrhythmias and circulatory collapse.
- Warn patients on long-term therapy about cushingoid symptoms.
- Acetate form not for I.V. use.
- Do not confuse Solu-Medrol with Solu-Cortef.
- Immunizations may show decreased antibody response.
- May be used for alternate-day therapy.

---

paramethasone acetate
Haldrone

INDICATIONS & DOSAGE

Inflammatory conditions—
Adults: 0.5 to 6 mg P.O. t.i.d. or q.i.d.
Children: 58 to 800 mcg/Kg daily divided t.i.d. or q.i.d.

SIDE EFFECTS

Most side effects of corticosteroids are dose- or duration-dependent.
CNS: *euphoria, insomnia,* psychotic behavior, pseudotumor cerebri.
CV: *congestive heart failure,* hypertension, edema.

EENT: cataracts, glaucoma.
GI: *peptic ulcer,* gastrointestinal irritation, increased appetite.
Metabolic: *severe hypokalemia, hyperglycemia and carbohydrate intolerance,* growth suppression in children.
Skin: delayed wound healing, acne, various skin eruptions.
Other: muscle weakness, pancreatitis, hirsutism, susceptibility to infections. Acute adrenal insufficiency may occur with increased stress (infection, surgery, trauma) or abrupt withdrawal after long-term therapy.
Withdrawal symptoms: rebound inflammation, fatigue, weakness, arthralgia, fever, dizziness, lethargy, depression, fainting, orthostatic hypotension, dyspnea, anorexia, hypoglycemia. *Sudden withdrawal may be fatal.*

INTERACTIONS

Barbiturates, phenytoin, rifampin: decreased corticosteroid effect. Corticosteroid dose may need to be increased.
Indomethacin, ASA: increased risk of GI distress and bleeding. Give together cautiously.

NURSING CONSIDERATIONS

- Contraindicated in systemic fungal infections and alternate-day therapy. Use cautiously in GI ulceration or renal disease, hypertension, osteoporosis, varicella, vaccinia, exanthema, diabetes mellitus, Cushing's syndrome, thromboembolic disorders, seizures, myasthenia gravis, metastatic cancer, congestive heart failure, tuberculosis, ocular herpes simplex, hypoalbuminemia, emotional instability or psychotic tendencies.
- Gradually reduce drug dosage after long-term therapy. Tell patient not to discontinue drug abruptly or without doctor's consent.
- Always titrate to lowest effective dose.

- Glucocorticoid with little mineralocorticoid effect.
- Monitor patient's weight, blood pressure, serum electrolytes.
- May mask or exacerbate infections.
- Instruct patient to carry a card identifying his need for supplemental systemic glucocorticoids during stress.
- Teach patient signs of early adrenal insufficiency: fatigue, muscular weakness, joint pain, fever, anorexia, nausea, dyspnea, dizziness, fainting.
- Watch for depression or psychotic episodes, especially in high-dose therapy.
- Diabetics may need increased insulin; monitor urine for sugar.
- Monitor growth in infants and children on long-term therapy.
- Unless contraindicated, give salt-restricted diet rich in potassium and protein. Potassium supplement may be needed. Watch for additional potassium depletion from diuretics and amphotericin B.
- Give P.O. dose with food when possible.
- Warn patients on long-term therapy about cushingoid symptoms.
- Immunizations may show decreased antibody response.

---

prednisolone
Cordrol, Delta-Cortef♦, Predoxine, Ropredlone, Ster 5, Sterane
prednisolone acetate

prednisolone sodium phosphate

prednisolone tebutate
Hydeltra-TBA, Metalone-TBA

INDICATIONS & DOSAGE
Severe inflammation or immunosuppression—
Adults: 2.5 to 15 mg P.O. b.i.d., t.i.d., or q.i.d.; 2 to 30 mg I.M. (acetate, phosphate), or I.V. (phosphate) q

12 hours; or 2 to 30 mg (phosphate) into joints, lesions, and soft tissue; or 4 to 40 mg (tebutate) into joints and lesions; or 0.25 to 1 ml (acetate-phosphate suspension) into joints weekly, p.r.n.

SIDE EFFECTS
Most side effects of corticosteroids are dose- or duration-dependent.
CNS: *euphoria, insomnia*, psychotic behavior, pseudotumor cerebri.
CV: *congestive heart failure*, hypertension, edema.
EENT: cataracts, glaucoma.
GI: *peptic ulcer*, gastrointestinal irritation, increased appetite.
Metabolic: *severe hypokalemia, hyperglycemia and carbohydrate intolerance*, growth suppression in children.
Skin: delayed wound healing, acne, various skin eruptions.
Other: muscle weakness, pancreatitis, hirsutism, susceptibility to infections. Acute adrenal insufficiency may occur with increased stress (infection, surgery, trauma) or abrupt withdrawal after long-term therapy.
Withdrawal symptoms: rebound inflammation, fatigue, weakness, arthralgia, fever, dizziness, lethargy, depression, fainting, orthostatic hypotension, dyspnea, anorexia, hypoglycemia. *Sudden withdrawal may be fatal.*

INTERACTIONS
Barbiturates, phenytoin, rifampin: decreased corticosteroid effect. Corticosteroid dose may need to be increased.
Indomethacin, ASA: increased risk of GI distress and bleeding. Give together cautiously.

NURSING CONSIDERATIONS
- Contraindicated in systemic fungal infections. Use cautiously in GI ulceration or renal disease, hypertension, osteoporosis, varicella, vaccinia, exanthema, diabetes mellitus, Cushing's

---

Italicized side effects are common or life-threatening.

syndrome, thromboembolic disorders, seizures, myasthenia gravis, metastatic cancer, congestive heart failure, tuberculosis, ocular herpes simplex, hypoalbuminemia, emotional instability or psychotic tendencies.

• Gradually reduce drug dosage after long-term therapy. Tell patient not to discontinue drug abruptly or without doctor's consent.

• Always titrate to lowest effective dose.

• Glucocorticoid with slight mineralocorticoid action.

• Prednisolone salts (acetate, sodium phosphate, and tebutate) are used parenterally less often than other corticosteroids that have more potent anti-inflammatory action.

• May use for alternate-day therapy.

• Monitor patient's weight, blood pressure, serum electrolytes.

• May mask or exacerbate infections.

• Instruct patient to carry a card identifying his need for supplemental systemic glucocorticoids during stress.

• Teach patient signs of early adrenal insufficiency: fatigue, muscular weakness, joint pain, fever, anorexia, nausea, dyspnea, dizziness, fainting.

• Watch for depression or psychotic episodes, especially in high-dose therapy.

• Diabetics may need increased insulin; monitor urine for sugar.

• Give I.M. injection deep into gluteal muscle. Avoid S.C. injection, as atrophy and sterile abscesses may occur.

• Unless contraindicated, give salt-restricted diet rich in potassium and protein. Potassium supplement may be needed. Watch for additional potassium depletion from diuretics and amphotericin B.

• Give P.O. dose with food when possible.

• Warn patients on long-term therapy about cushingoid symptoms.

• Acetate form not for I.V. use.

• Immunizations may show decreased antibody response.

prednisone
Colisone♦♦, Deltasone♦, Fernisone, Meticorten, Orasone, Paracort♦, Prednicen-M, SK-Prednisone, Sterapred

INDICATIONS & DOSAGE
Severe inflammation or immunosuppression—
Adults: 2.5 to 15 mg P.O. b.i.d., t.i.d., or q.i.d. Maintenance dose given once daily or every other day.
Children: 0.14 to 2 mg/Kg daily P.O. divided q.i.d.

SIDE EFFECTS
Most side effects of corticosteroids are dose- or duration-dependent.
CNS: *euphoria, insomnia,* psychotic behavior, pseudotumor cerebri.
CV: *congestive heart failure,* hypertension, edema.
EENT: cataracts, glaucoma.
GI: *peptic ulcer,* gastrointestinal irritation, increased appetite.
Metabolic: *severe hypokalemia, hyperglycemia and carbohydrate intolerance,* growth suppression in children.
Skin: delayed wound healing, acne, various skin eruptions.
Other: muscle weakness, pancreatitis, hirsutism, susceptibility to infections. Acute adrenal insufficiency may occur with increased stress (infection, surgery, trauma) or abrupt withdrawal after long-term therapy.
Withdrawal symptoms: rebound inflammation, fatigue, weakness, arthralgia, fever, dizziness, lethargy, depression, fainting, orthostatic hypotension, dyspnea, anorexia, hypoglycemia. *Sudden withdrawal may be fatal.*

INTERACTIONS
Barbiturates, phenytoin, rifampin: de-

creased corticosteroid effect. Corticosteroid dose may need to be increased.
Indomethacin, ASA: increased risk of GI distress and bleeding. Give together cautiously.

NURSING CONSIDERATIONS
• Contraindicated in systemic fungal infections. Use cautiously in GI ulceration or renal disease, hypertension, osteoporosis, varicella, vaccinia, exanthema, diabetes mellitus, Cushing's syndrome, thromboembolic disorders, seizures, myasthenia gravis, metastatic cancer, congestive heart failure, tuberculosis, ocular herpes simplex, hypoalbuminemia, emotional instability or psychotic tendencies
• Gradually reduce drug dosage after long-term therapy. Tell patient not to discontinue drug abruptly or without doctor's consent.
• Always titrate to lowest effective dose.
• Monitor patient's blood pressure, sleep patterns, serum potassium levels.
• Weigh patient daily; report sudden weight gain to doctor.
• May mask or exacerbate infections.
• Instruct patient to carry a card identifying his need for supplementai systemic glucocorticoids during stress.
• Teach patient signs of early adrenal insufficiency: fatigue, muscular weakness, joint pain, fever, anorexia, nausea, dyspnea, dizziness, fainting.
• Watch for depression or psychotic episodes, especially in high-dose therapy.
• Diabetics may need increased insulin; monitor urine for sugar.
• Monitor growth in infants and children on long-term therapy.
• Give salt-restricted diet rich in potassium and protein. Potassium supplement may be needed. Watch for additional potassium depletion from diuretics and amphotericin B.

• Unless contraindicated, give P.O. dose with food when possible.
• May use for alternate-day therapy.
• Warn patients on long-term therapy about cushingoid symptoms.
• Immunizations may show decreased antibody response.

---

triamcinolone
Aristocort♦, Cino, Kenacort♦, Spencort, Tricilone.
triamcinolone acetonide
Kenalog♦
triamcinolone diacetate
Amcort, Aristocort Parenteral Forte, Cenocort Forte, Cino-40, Tracilon, Triam-Forte, Tristoject
triamcinolone hexacetonide
Aristospan♦

INDICATIONS & DOSAGE
Severe inflammation or immunosuppression—
Adults: 4 to 48 mg P.O. daily divided b.i.d., t.i.d., or q.i.d., or 40 mg I.M. (diacetate or acetonide) weekly; or 5 to 48 mg (diacetate or acetonide) into lesions; or 2 to 40 mg (diacetate or acetonide) into joints and soft tissue; or up to 0.5 mg (hexacetonide) per square inch of affected skin intralesional; or 2 to 20 mg (hexacetonide) intra-articular or intrasynovial into soft tissue or into joint or lesion. Often, a local anesthetic is injected into the joint with triamcinolone.

SIDE EFFECTS
Most side effects of corticosteroids are dose- or duration-dependent.
CNS: *euphoria, insomnia,* psychotic behavior, pseudotumor cerebri.
CV: *congestive heart failure,* hypertension, edema.
EENT: cataracts, glaucoma.
GI: *peptic ulcer,* gastrointestinal irritation, increased appetite.
Metabolic: *severe hypokalemia, hy-*

Italicized side effects are common or life-threatening.

perglycemia and carbohydrate intolerance, growth suppression in children.
Skin: delayed wound healing, acne, various skin eruptions.
Other: muscle weakness, pancreatitis, hirsutism, susceptibility to infections. Acute adrenal insufficiency may occur with increased stress (infection, surgery, trauma) or abrupt withdrawal after long-term therapy.
Withdrawal symptoms: rebound inflammation, fatigue, weakness, arthralgia, fever, dizziness, lethargy, depression, fainting, orthostatic hypotension, dyspnea, anorexia, hypoglycemia. *Sudden withdrawal may be fatal.*

INTERACTIONS
Barbiturates, phenytoin, rifampin: decreased corticosteroid effect. Corticosteroid dose may need to be increased.
Indomethacin, ASA: increased risk of GI distress and bleeding. Give together cautiously.

NURSING CONSIDERATIONS
• Contraindicated in systemic fungal infections. Use cautiously in GI ulceration or renal disease, hypertension, osteoporosis, varicella, vaccinia, exanthema, diabetes mellitus, Cushing's syndrome, thromboembolic disorders, seizures, myasthenia gravis, metastatic cancer, congestive heart failure, tuberculosis, ocular herpes simplex, hypoalbuminemia, emotional instability or psychotic tendencies.
• Gradually reduce drug dosage after long-term therapy. Tell patient not to discontinue drug abruptly or without doctor's consent.

• Always titrate to lowest effective dose.
• Monitor patient's weight, blood pressure, serum electrolytes.
• May mask or exacerbate infections.
• Instruct patient to carry a card identifying his need for supplemental systemic glucocorticoids during stress.
• Teach patient signs of early adrenal insufficiency: fatigue, muscular weakness, joint pain, fever, anorexia, nausea, dyspnea, dizziness, fainting.
• Watch for depression or psychotic episodes, especially in high-dose therapy.
• Diabetics may need increased insulin; monitor urine for sugar.
• Give I.M. injection deep into gluteal muscle. Avoid S.C. injection, as atrophy and sterile abscesses may occur.
• Unless contraindicated, give salt-restricted diet rich in potassium and protein. Potassium supplement may be needed. Watch for additional potassium depletion from diuretics and amphotericin B.
• Give P.O. dose with food when possible.
• Glucocorticoid with very little mineralocorticoid effect.
• Discard unused diluted suspension within 7 days.
• Don't use diluents that contain preservatives. Flocculation may occur.
• Warn patients on long-term therapy about cushingoid symptoms.
• Immunizations may show decreased antibody response.
• Not for alternate-day therapy.
• No forms for I.V. use. Hexacetonide not for I.V. or I.M. use.

47

Androgens

danazol
ethylestrenol
fluoxymesterone
methandrostenolone
methyltestosterone
nandrolone decanoate
nandrolone phenpropionate
oxandrolone
oxymetholone
stanozolol
testosterone
testosterone cypionate
testosterone enanthate
testosterone propionate

---

danazol
Cyclomen♦♦, Danocrine

INDICATIONS & DOSAGE
Endometriosis—
Women: 400 mg P.O. b.i.d. uninterrupted for 3 to 6 months; may continue for 9 months.
Fibrocystic breast disease—
Women: 100 to 400 mg P.O. daily uninterrupted for 2 to 6 months.

SIDE EFFECTS
Androgenic: acne, edema, *weight gain, hirsutism,* hoarseness, clitoral enlargement, *decrease in breast size,* changes in libido, male pattern baldness, *oiliness of skin or hair.*
CNS: dizziness, headache, sleep disorders, fatigue, tremor, irritability, excitation, lethargy, mental depression, chills, paresthesias.
CV: elevated blood pressure.
EENT: visual disturbances.

GI: gastric irritation, nausea, vomiting, diarrhea, constipation, change in appetite.
GU: hematuria.
Hepatic: jaundice.
Hypoestrogenic: flushing; sweating; vaginitis, including itching, dryness, burning, and vaginal bleeding; nervousness, emotional lability.
Other: muscle cramps or spasms.

INTERACTIONS
None significant.

NURSING CONSIDERATIONS
• Contraindicated in undiagnosed abnormal genital bleeding; impaired renal, cardiac, or hepatic function. Use cautiously in epilepsy or migraines.
• Use with diet high in calories and protein unless contraindicated.
• Monitor closely for signs of virilization. Some androgenic effects may not be reversible upon discontinuation of drug.

---

ethylestrenol
Maxibolin♦

INDICATIONS & DOSAGE
Promote weight gain and combat tissue depletion, refractory anemias, catabolic effects of corticosteroid therapy, osteoporosis, prolonged immobilization, and debilitated states—
Adults: 4 to 8 mg P.O. daily, reduced to minimum levels at first evidence of clinical response.

Children: 1 to 3 mg P.O. daily; highly individualized.
A single course of therapy in both adults and children should not exceed 6 weeks; may be reinstituted after 4-week interval.

SIDE EFFECTS
Androgenic: in females—*acne, edema, oily skin, weight gain, hirsutism, hoarseness,* clitoral enlargement, changes in libido. In males—prepubertal: premature epiphyseal closure, acne, priapism, growth of body and facial hair, phallic enlargement; postpubertal: testicular atrophy, oligospermia, decreased ejaculatory volume, impotence, gynecomastia, epididymitis.
CV: edema.
GI: gastroenteritis, nausea, vomiting, diarrhea, constipation, change in appetite.
GU: bladder irritability.
Hepatic: jaundice.
Hypoestrogenic: in females—flushing; sweating; vaginitis with itching, drying, burning, or bleeding; menstrual irregularities.
Other: hypercalcemia.

INTERACTIONS
None significant.

NURSING CONSIDERATIONS
• Contraindicated in prostatic hypertrophy with obstruction; carcinoma of male breast; hypercalcemia; prostatic cancer; cardiac, hepatic, or renal decompensation; nephrosis; premature infants. Use cautiously in prepubertal males; patients with diabetes or coronary disease; patients taking ACTH, corticosteroids, or anticoagulants.
• Hypercalcemic symptoms may be difficult to distinguish from symptoms of condition being treated unless anticipated and thought of as a symptom cluster. Hypercalcemia is particularly likely to occur in patients with

metastatic breast cancer and may indicate bone metastases.
• Tell females to report menstrual irregularities; therapy should be discontinued pending etiologic determination.
• Watch for virilizing effects; may be irreversible despite prompt stopping of therapy. Doctor must decide if benefits outweigh effects.
• Closely monitor boys under 7 for precocious development of male sexual characteristics.
• In children: therapy should be preceded by X-ray of wrist bones to establish level of bone maturation. During treatment, bone maturation may proceed more rapidly than linear growth; dosage should be intermittent.
• Edema is generally controllable with salt restriction and/or diuretics.
• Watch for symptoms of jaundice. Dose adjustment may reverse condition. If liver function tests are abnormal, discontinue therapy.
• Observe patient on concomitant anticoagulant therapy for ecchymotic areas, petechiae, or abnormal bleeding. Monitor prothrombin time.
• Watch for symptoms of hypoglycemia in diabetics. Dosage of antidiabetic drug may need adjustment.
• Use with diet high in calories and protein unless contraindicated.

---

fluoxymesterone
Android-F, Halotestin♦, Oratestin♦♦, Oratestryl

INDICATIONS & DOSAGE
Hypogonadism and impotence due to testicular deficiency—
Adults: 2 to 10 mg P.O. daily.
Palliation of breast cancer in women—
15 to 30 mg P.O. daily in divided dosages. All dosage should be individualized and reduced to minimum when effect is noted.

Postpartum breast engorgement—
2.5 mg P.O. followed by 5 to 10 mg
daily for 5 days.

SIDE EFFECTS
Androgenic: in females—*acne,
edema, oily skin, weight gain, hirsutism, hoarseness,* clitoral enlargement,
change in libido. In males—prepubertal: premature epiphyseal closure,
acne, priapism, growth of body and
facial hair, phallic enlargement; postpubertal: testicular atrophy, oligospermia, decreased ejaculatory volume, impotence, gynecomastia, epididymitis.
CV: edema.
GI: gastroenteritis, nausea, vomiting,
constipation, change in appetite,
diarrhea.
GU: bladder irritability.
Hepatic: jaundice.
Hypoestrogenic: in females—*flushing; sweating; vaginitis with itching,
drying, burning, or bleeding; menstrual irregularities;* emotional
lability.
Other: hypercalcemia.

INTERACTIONS
None significant.

NURSING CONSIDERATIONS
• Contraindicated in prostatic hypertrophy with obstruction; carcinoma of
male breast; prostatic cancer; cardiac,
hepatic, or renal decompensation; nephrosis; hypercalcemia. Use cautiously in prepubertal males; patients
with diabetes or coronary disease;
and patients taking ACTH, corticosteroids, or anticoagulants.
• Hypercalcemic symptoms may be
difficult to distinguish from symptoms associated with condition being
treated unless anticipated and thought
of as a symptom cluster. Hypercalcemia is particularly likely to occur in
patients with metastatic breast cancer
and may indicate bone metastases.
• Explain to patient on drug for pal-

liation of breast cancer that virilization usually occurs at dosage used.
Give emotional support. Tell patient
to report androgenic effects immediately. Stopping drug will prevent further androgenic changes but will
probably not reverse those already
existing.
• When used in breast cancer, subjective effects may not be seen for about
1 month; objective symptoms not for
3 months.
• Tell females to report menstrual
irregularities; therapy should be discontinued pending etiologic determination.
• Edema is generally controllable
with salt restriction and/or diuretics.
• Watch for symptoms of jaundice.
Dose adjustment may reverse condition. If liver function tests are abnormal, therapy should be discontinued.
• Observe patient on concomitant anticoagulant therapy for ecchymotic
areas, petechiae, or abnormal bleeding. Monitor prothrombin time.
• Watch for symptoms of hypoglycemia in diabetics. Dosage of antidiabetic drug may need adjustment.
• Use with diet high in calories and
protein unless contraindicated.

---

methandrostenolone
Danabol♦♦, Dianabol

INDICATIONS & DOSAGE
*Senile and postmenopausal osteo-
porosis*—
Adults: initially 5 mg P.O. daily.
Maintenance 2.5 to 5 mg P.O. daily.
Anabolic effect—
Adults: 5 to 10 mg P.O. daily.
Severe debilitation—
Adults: 10 to 20 mg P.O. daily for
3 weeks, reduced to 5 to 10 mg P.O.
daily for maintenance.
*Severe maturational delay when
growth hormone is unavailable*—

Children: (postpubertal) up to
0.05 mg/Kg P.O. daily.
Intermittent therapy is recommended
in prolonged use.

SIDE EFFECTS
Androgenic: in females—*acne,
edema, oily skin, weight gain, hirsutism, hoarseness,* clitoral enlargement,
changes in libido. In males—prepubertal: premature epiphyseal closure,
acne, priapism, growth of body and
facial hair, phallic enlargement; postpubertal: testicular atrophy, oligospermia, decreased ejaculatory volume, impotence, gynecomastia, epididymitis.
CV: edema.
EENT: burning of tongue.
GI: gastroenteritis, nausea, vomiting,
change in appetite, diarrhea, anorexia, constipation.
GU: bladder irritability.
Hepatic: jaundice.
Hypoestrogenic: in females—flushing; sweating; vaginitis with itching,
drying, burning, or bleeding; menstrual irregularities.
Other: hypercalcemia.

INTERACTIONS
None significant.

NURSING CONSIDERATIONS
• Contraindicated in prostatic hypertrophy with obstruction, carcinoma of
male breast, prostatic cancer; cardiac,
hepatic, or renal decompensation; nephrosis. Use cautiously in prepubertal
males; patients with diabetes or coronary disease; patients taking ACTH,
corticosteroids, or anticoagulants.
• Hypercalcemic symptoms may be
difficult to distinguish from symptoms of condition being treated unless
anticipated and thought of as a cluster. Hypercalcemia is particularly
likely to occur with metastatic breast
cancer and may indicate bone metastases. Therapy should be discontinued.

• Tell females to report menstrual
irregularities; therapy should be discontinued pending etiologic determination.
• Watch closely for virilizing effects;
they may be irreversible despite
prompt discontinuation of therapy.
• In children, therapy should be preceded by X-ray of wrist bones to establish level of bone maturation. During treatment, bone maturation may
proceed more rapidly than linear
growth; dosage should be intermittent.
• Edema is generally controllable
with salt restriction and/or diuretics.
• Watch for symptoms of jaundice.
Dose adjustment may reverse condition. If liver function tests are abnormal, therapy should be discontinued.
• Watch for ecchymotic areas, petechiae, or abnormal bleeding in patients on concomitant anticoagulant
therapy. Monitor prothrombin time.
• Watch for symptoms of hypoglycemia in diabetics. Dosage of antidiabetic drug may need adjustment.
• May lower fasting blood sugar in
both diabetic and nondiabetic
patients.
• Erroneously thought to enhance
athletic ability.

methyltestosterone
Android-5, Android-10, Metandren♦,
Oreton-Methyl, Testred, Virilon

INDICATIONS & DOSAGE
Adults:
*Breast engorgement of nonnursing
mothers*—80 mg P.O. daily, or 40 mg
buccal daily for 3 to 5 days.
*Breast cancer in women 1 to 5 years
postmenopausal*—200 mg P.O. daily;
or 100 mg buccal daily.
*Eunuchoidism and eunuchism, male
climacteric symptoms*—10 to 40 mg
P.O. daily; or 5 to 20 mg buccal daily.

Postpubertal cryptorchidism—30 mg
P.O. daily; or 15 mg buccal daily.

SIDE EFFECTS
Androgenic: in females—*acne,
edema, oily skin, weight gain, hirsutism, hoarseness,* clitoral enlargement,
changes in libido. In males—prepubertal: premature epiphyseal closure,
acne, priapism, growth of body and
facial hair, phallic enlargement; postpubertal: testicular atrophy, oligospermia, decreased ejaculatory volume, impotence, gynecomastia, epididymitis.
CV: edema.
GI: gastroenteritis, constipation, nausea, vomiting, diarrhea, change in
appetite.
GU: bladder irritability.
Hepatic: jaundice.
Hypoestrogenic: in females—flushing; sweating; vaginitis with itching,
drying, burning, or bleeding; menstrual irregularities.
Local: irritation of oral mucosa with
buccal administration.
Other: hypercalcemia.

INTERACTIONS
None significant.

NURSING CONSIDERATIONS
• Contraindicated in women of childbearing potential (possible masculinization of female infant); hypercalcemia; cardiac, hepatic, or renal decompensation; prostatic or breast cancer
in males; benign prostatic hypertrophy with obstruction; elderly, asthenic
males who may react adversely to androgen overstimulation; conditions
aggravated by fluid retention; hypertension. Use cautiously in myocardial
infarction or coronary artery disease.
• Treatment of breast cancer usually
restricted to patients 1 to 5 years postmenopausal.
• Edema is generally controllable
with salt restriction and/or diuretics.
• Periodic serum cholesterol and cal-

cium determinations, and cardiac and
liver function tests recommended.
Watch closely for jaundice.
• In metastatic breast cancer, hypercalcemia may indicate progression of
bone metastases. Report signs of
hypercalcemia.
• Therapeutic response in breast cancer is usually apparent within
3 months. Therapy should be stopped
if signs of disease progression appear.
• Enhances hypoglycemia; tell
patient to report signs of hyperinsulinism.
• Watch for ecchymoses, petechiae,
and abnormal bleeding in patients receiving concomitant anticoagulants.
• Promptly report signs of virilization in females.
• Use with diet high in calories and
protein unless contraindicated.
• Buccal tablets twice as potent as
oral tablets. Tell patient to avoid eating, drinking, chewing, or smoking
while buccal tablet is in place, and
that tablet is not to be swallowed.
• Erroneously thought to enhance
athletic ability.

nandrolone decanoate
Deca-Durabolin♦, Deca-Hybolin
nandrolone phenpropionate
Anabolin, Anorolone, Durabolin♦,
Nandrolin

INDICATIONS & DOSAGE
Severe debility or disease states (decanoate)—
Adults: 100 to 200 mg I.M. weekly.
Therapy should be intermittent.
Tissue-building (decanoate)—
Adults: 50 to 100 mg I.M. q 3 to 4
weeks.
Children 2 to 13 years: 25 to 50 mg
I.M. q 3 to 4 weeks.

Severe debility or disease states (phenpropionate)—
Adults: 50 to 100 mg I.M. weekly.

Italicized side effects are common or life-threatening.

Children 2 to 13 years: 12.5 to
25 mg I.M. q 2 to 4 weeks.
Children under 2 years: 12.5 mg
I.M. q 2 to 4 weeks.
Therapy should be intermittent, based
on therapeutic response.
*Tissue building and/or erythropoietic
effects (phenpropionate)—*
Adults: 25 to 50 mg I.M. weekly.

SIDE EFFECTS
Androgenic: in females—*acne,
edema, oily skin, weight gain, hirsutism, hoarseness,* clitoral enlargement,
decreased or increased libido. In
males—prepubertal: premature
epiphyseal closure, acne, priapism,
growth of body and facial hair, phallic enlargement; postpubertal: testicular atrophy, oligospermia, decreased
ejaculatory volume, impotence, gynecomastia, epididymitis.
CV: edema.
GI: gastroenteritis, nausea, vomiting,
diarrhea, change in appetite.
GU: bladder irritability.
Hepatic: jaundice.
Hypoestrogenic: in females—flushing; sweating; vaginitis with itching,
drying, burning, or bleeding; menstrual irregularities with large doses.
Local: pain at injection site,
induration.
Other: hypercalcemia, hypercalciuria.

INTERACTIONS
None significant.

NURSING CONSIDERATIONS
• Contraindicated in prostatic hypertrophy with obstruction; male breast
and prostatic cancer; cardiac, hepatic,
or renal decompensation; nephrosis.
Use cautiously in prepubertal males;
patients with diabetes or coronary
disease; patients taking ACTH, corticosteroids, or anticoagulants.
• Inject drug deep I.M., preferably
into upper outer quadrant of gluteal
muscle in adults.

• Monitor serum cholesterol in cardiac patients.
• Hypercalcemia is most likely to occur in patients with mammary carcinoma; these patients should have
quantitative urinary and serum calcium level determinations.
• Tell females to report menstrual irregularities; therapy should be discontinued pending etiologic determination.
• Watch for virilizing effects; they
may be irreversible despite prompt
discontinuation of therapy.
• Closely observe boys under 7 for
precocious development of male sexual characteristics.
• In children, therapy should be preceded by X-ray of wrist bones to establish level of bone maturation. During treatment, bone maturation may
proceed more rapidly than linear
growth; dosage should be intermittent.
• Edema is generally controllable
with salt restrictions and/or diuretics.
• Watch for symptoms of jaundice.
Dose adjustment may reverse condition. If liver function tests are abnormal, therapy should be discontinued.
• Observe patients receiving concomitant anticoagulant therapy for ecchymotic areas, petechiae, or abnormal
bleeding. Monitor prothrombin time.
• Watch for symptoms of hypoglycemia in diabetics. Dosage of antidiabetic drug may need adjustment.
• Use with diet high in calories and
protein unless contraindicated.
• Erroneously thought to enhance
athletic ability.
• Considered an adjunctive therapy.

oxandrolone
Anavar

INDICATIONS & DOSAGE
*To combat catabolic effects of cortico-
steroid therapy, osteoporosis, pro-*

longed immobilization and debilitated states—
Adults: 2.5 mg P.O. b.i.d., t.i.d., or q.i.d.; up to 20 mg daily for 2 to 4 weeks.
Children: 0.25 mg/Kg daily P.O. for 2 to 4 weeks.
Continuous therapy should not exceed 3 months.

SIDE EFFECTS
Androgenic: in females—*acne, edema, oily skin, weight gain, hirsutism, hoarseness,* clitoral enlargement, decreased or increased libido. In males—prepubertal: premature epiphyseal closure, acne, priapism, growth of body and facial hair, phallic enlargement; postpubertal: testicular atrophy, oligospermia, decreased ejaculatory volume, impotence, gynecomastia, epididymitis.
CV: edema.
GI: gastroenteritis, nausea, vomiting, constipation or diarrhea, change in appetite.
GU: bladder irritability.
Hepatic: jaundice.
Hypoestrogenic: in females—flushing; sweating; vaginitis with itching, drying, burning, or bleeding; menstrual irregularities.
Other: hypercalcemia.

INTERACTIONS
None significant.

NURSING CONSIDERATIONS
• Contraindicated in prostatic hypertrophy with obstruction; prostatic and male breast cancer; cardiac, hepatic, or renal decompensation; nephrosis; premature infants. Use cautiously in prepubertal males; patients with diabetes or coronary disease; patients taking ACTH, corticosteroids, or anticoagulants.
• Hypercalcemia symptoms may be difficult to distinguish from symptoms of condition being treated unless anticipated and thought of as a cluster. Hypercalcemia most likely to occur with metastatic breast cancer and may indicate bone metastases.
• Tell females to report menstrual irregularities; therapy should be discontinued pending etiologic determination.
• Watch for virilizing effects; may be irreversible despite prompt stopping of therapy. Doctor must decide if benefits outweigh effects.
• Boys under 7 should be closely observed for precocious development of male sexual characteristics.
• In children, therapy should be preceded by X-ray of wrist bones to establish level of bone maturation. During treatment, bone maturation may proceed more rapidly than linear growth; dosage should be intermittent.
• Edema is generally controllable with salt restriction and/or diuretics.
• Watch for symptoms of jaundice. Dose adjustment may reverse condition. Periodic liver function tests are recommended.
• Observe patient on concomitant anticoagulant therapy for ecchymotic areas, petechiae, or abnormal bleeding. Monitor prothrombin time.
• Watch for symptoms of hypoglycemia in diabetics. Change of dosage in antidiabetic drug may be required.
• Use with diet high in calories and protein unless contraindicated.
• Erroneously thought to enhance athletic ability.

oxymetholone
Adroyd♦, Anadrol-50, Anapolon 50♦♦

INDICATIONS & DOSAGE
Aplastic anemia—
Adults and children: 1 to 5 mg/Kg P.O. daily. Dose highly individualized; response not immediate. Trial of 3 to 6 months required.

Osteoporosis, catabolic conditions—
Adults: 5 to 15 mg P.O. daily, or up to 30 mg P.O. daily.
Children over 6 years: up to 10 mg P.O. daily.
Children under 6 years: 1.25 mg P.O. daily or up to q.i.d. Continuous therapy should not exceed 30 days in children; 90 days in any patient.

SIDE EFFECTS
Androgenic: in females—*acne, edema, oily skin, weight gain, hirsutism, hoarseness,* clitoral enlargement, decreased or increased libido, male pattern hair loss. In males—prepubertal: premature epiphyseal closure, acne, priapism, growth of body and facial hair, phallic enlargement; postpubertal: testicular atrophy, oligospermia, decreased ejaculatory volume, impotence, gynecomastia, epididymitis.
CV: edema.
GI: gastroenteritis, nausea, vomiting, constipation, diarrhea, change in appetite.
GU: bladder irritability.
Hepatic: jaundice.
Hypoestrogenic: in females—flushing; sweating; vaginitis with itching, drying, burning or bleeding; menstrual irregularities.
Other: hypercalcemia.

INTERACTIONS
None significant.

NURSING CONSIDERATIONS
• Contraindicated in prostatic hypertrophy with obstruction; prostatic and male breast cancer; cardiac, hepatic, or renal decompensation; nephrosis; premature infants. Use cautiously in prepubertal males; patients with diabetes or coronary diseases; patients taking ACTH, corticosteroids, or anticoagulants.
• Hypercalcemia symptoms may be difficult to distinguish from symptoms of condition being treated unless

anticipated and thought of as a cluster. Hypercalcemia most likely to occur in metastatic breast cancer and may indicate bone metastases.
• Supportive treatment of anemias (transfusions, correction of iron, folic acid, vitamin B_{12}, or pyroxidine deficiency). Give 3 to 6 months for response.
• Effects in osteoporosis usually seen in 4 to 6 weeks.
• Tell females to report menstrual irregularities; therapy should be discontinued pending etiologic determination.
• Watch for virilizing effects; may be irreversible despite prompt stopping of therapy. Doctor must decide if benefits outweigh effects.
• Boys under 7 should be closely observed for precocious development of male sexual characteristics.
• In children, therapy should be preceded by X-ray of wrist bones to establish level of bone maturation. During treatment, bone maturation may proceed more rapidly than linear growth; dosage should be intermittent. Epiphyseal development may continue 6 months after stopping therapy.
• Edema is generally controllable with salt restriction and/or diuretics.
• Watch for symptoms of jaundice. Dose adjustment may reverse condition; if liver function tests are abnormal, therapy should be discontinued.
• Observe patient on concomitant anticoagulant therapy for ecchymotic areas, petechiae, or abnormal bleeding. Monitor prothrombin time.
• Watch for symptoms of hypoglycemia in diabetics. Change of dosage in antidiabetic drug may be required.
• Use with diet high in calories and protein unless contraindicated.
• Erroneously thought to enhance athletic ability.

stanozolol
Winstrol ♦

INDICATIONS & DOSAGE

To increase hemoglobin in some cases of aplastic anemia—
Adults: 2 mg P.O. t.i.d.
Children 6 to 12 years: up to 2 mg P.O. t.i.d.
Children under 6 years: 1 mg P.O. b.i.d.
Therapy should be intermittent.

SIDE EFFECTS

Androgenic: in females—*acne, edema, oily skin, weight gain, hirsutism, hoarseness,* clitoral enlargement, decreased or increased libido. In males— prepubertal: premature epiphyseal closure, acne, priapism, growth of body and facial hair, phallic enlargement; postpubertal: testicular atrophy, oligospermia, decreased ejaculatory volume, impotence, gynecomastia, epididymitis.
CV: edema.
GI: gastroenteritis, nausea, vomiting, constipation, diarrhea, change in appetite.
GU: bladder irritability.
Hypoestrogenic: in females—flushing; sweating; vaginitis with itching, drying, burning or bleeding; menstrual irregularities.
Other: hypercalcemia.

INTERACTIONS

None significant.

NURSING CONSIDERATIONS

• Contraindicated in prostatic hypertrophy with obstruction; prostatic and male breast cancer; cardiac, hepatic, or renal decompensation; nephrosis; premature infants. Use cautiously in prepubertal males; patients with diabetes or coronary disease; patients taking ACTH, corticosteroids, or anticoagulants.

• Hypercalcemia symptoms may be difficult to distinguish from symptoms of condition being treated unless anticipated and thought of as a cluster. Hypercalcemia most likely to occur in metastatic breast cancer and may indicate bone metastases.

• Tell females to report menstrual irregularities; therapy should be discontinued pending etiologic determination.

• Smaller dose (2 mg b.i.d.) is used in females to avoid virilizing effects. Watch for virilizing effects; may be irreversible despite prompt stopping of therapy. Doctor must decide if benefits outweigh effects.

• Boys under 7 should be closely observed for precocious development of male sexual characteristics.

• In children, therapy should be preceded by X-ray of wrist bones to establish level of bone maturation. During treatment, bone maturation may proceed more rapidly than linear growth; dosage should be intermittent.

• Edema is generally controllable with salt restriction and/or diuretics.

• Watch for symptoms of jaundice. Dose adjustment may reverse condition; check liver function tests regularly. If abnormal, therapy should be discontinued.

• Observe patient on concomitant anticoagulant therapy for ecchymotic areas, petechiae, or abnormal bleeding. Monitor prothrombin time.

• Watch for symptoms of hypoglycemia in diabetics. Change of dosage in antidiabetic drug may be required.

• Use with diet high in calories and protein unless contraindicated.

• Administer before or with meals to minimize GI distress.

• Monitor serum cholesterol in cardiac patients.

• Erroneously thought to enhance athletic ability.

Italicized side effects are common or life-threatening.

testosterone

Android-T, Andronaq, Histerone,
Malogen♦, Oreton, Testaqua,
Testoject.

INDICATIONS & DOSAGE

Eunuchoidism, eunuchism, male climacteric symptoms—
Adults: 10 to 25 mg I.M. 2 to 5 times
weekly; or 2 to 6 pellets (75 mg each)
implanted subcutaneously q 3 to
6 months.
*Breast engorgement of nonnursing
mothers—*25 to 50 mg I.M. daily for 3
to 4 days, starting at delivery.
*Breast cancer in women 1 to 5 years
postmenopausal—*100 mg I.M.
3 times weekly as long as improvement maintained.

SIDE EFFECTS

Androgenic: in females—*acne,
edema, oily skin, weight gain, hirsutism, hoarseness,* clitoral enlargement,
decreased or increased libido. In
males—prepubertal: premature
epiphyseal closure, acne, priapism,
growth of body and facial hair, phallic enlargement; postpubertal: testicular atrophy, oligospermia, decreased
ejaculatory volume, impotence, gynecomastia, epididymitis.
CV: edema.
GI: gastroenteritis, nausea, vomiting,
constipation, diarrhea, change in
appetite.
GU: bladder irritability.
Hepatic: jaundice.
Hypoestrogenic: in females—flushing; sweating; vaginitis with itching,
drying, burning, or bleeding; menstrual irregularities.
Local: pain at injection site, induration, irritation and sloughing with pellet implantation, edema.
Other: hypercalcemia.

INTERACTIONS

None significant.

NURSING CONSIDERATIONS

• Contraindicated in women of childbearing potential (possible masculinization of female infant); hypercalcemia; cardiac, hepatic, or renal decompensation; prostatic or breast cancer
in males; benign prostatic hypertrophy with obstruction; elderly, asthenic
males who may react adversely to androgen overstimulation; conditions
aggravated by fluid retention; hypertension. Use cautiously in myocardial
infarction or coronary artery disease,
prepubertal males.
• Periodic liver function tests should
be performed.
• In metastatic breast cancer, hypercalcemia usually indicates progression
of bone metastases. Report signs of
hypercalcemia.
• Therapeutic response in breast cancer is usually apparent within
3 months. Stop therapy if signs of disease progression appear.
• Enhances hypoglycemia; tell patient to report signs of hyperinsulinism.
• Instruct males to report priapism,
reduced ejaculatory volume, and
gynecomastia. Withdraw drug.
• Watch for signs of ecchymoses, petechiae with concomitant anticoagulants. Monitor prothrombin time.
• Report signs of virilization in females; reevaluate treatment.
• Monitor prepubertal males by
X-ray for rate of bone maturation.
• Edema is generally controllable
with salt restriction and/or diuretics.
• Use with diet high in calories and
protein unless contraindicated.
• Inject deep into upper outer quadrant of gluteal muscle.
• Watch for irritation and sloughing
with pellet implantation.
• Watch for ecchymotic areas, petechiae, or abnormal bleeding in patients on concomitant anticoagulant
therapy. Monitor prothrombin time.
• Implantation of pellets may take
place in physician's office in a minor

surgical procedure with aseptic precautions observed.

testosterone cypionate
Andro-Cyp, Androgen-860, D-Test, Depotest, Depo-Test, Depo-Testosterone♦, Durandro, Duratest, Jactatest, Malogen Cyp
testosterone enanthate
Android-T, Andryl, Arderone, Delatestryl♦, Everone, Malogen LA, Malogex♦♦, Span-Test, Testate, Testone LA, Testostroval-P.A.
testosterone propionate
Androlan, Androlin, Malogen in Oil♦♦, Oreton Propionate, Testex, Vulvan

INDICATIONS & DOSAGE
Eunuchism, eunuchoidism, deficiency after castration and male climacteric—
Adults: 200 to 400 mg (cypionate or enanthate) I.M. q 4 weeks.
Oligospermia—
Adults: 100 to 200 mg (cypionate or enanthate) I.M. q 4 to 6 weeks for development and maintenance of testicular function.
Eunuchism and eunuchoidism, male climacteric, impotency—
Adults: 10 to 25 mg (propionate) I.M. 2 to 4 times weekly; or 5 to 20 mg buccal daily (strictly individualized).
*Breast engorgement of nonnursing mothers—*40 mg (propionate) buccal daily, for 3 to 5 days starting at delivery.
*Metastatic breast cancer in women—*50 to 100 mg (propionate) I.M. 3 times weekly; or 100 mg buccal daily as long as improvement maintained.
*Postpubertal cryptorchidism—*15 mg (propionate) buccal daily.

SIDE EFFECTS
Androgenic: in females—*acne,*
edema, oily skin, weight gain, hirsutism, hoarseness, clitoral enlargement, changes in libido. In males—prepubertal: premature epiphyseal closure, acne, priapism, growth of body and facial hair, phallic enlargement; postpubertal: testicular atrophy, oligospermia, decreased ejaculatory volume, impotence, gynecomastia, epididymitis.
CV: edema.
GI: gastroenteritis, nausea, vomiting, constipation, diarrhea, change in appetite.
GU: bladder irritability.
Hepatic: jaundice.
Local: pain at injection site, induration, postinjection furunculosis.
Other: hypercalcemia.

INTERACTIONS
None significant.

NURSING CONSIDERATIONS
• Contraindicated in women of childbearing potential (possible masculinization of female infant); hypercalcemia; cardiac, hepatic, or renal decompensation; prostatic or breast cancer in males; benign prostatic hypertrophy with obstruction; elderly, asthenic males who may react adversely to androgen overstimulation; conditions aggravated by fluid retention; hypertension. Use cautiously in myocardial infarction or coronary artery disease, prepubertal males.
• Periodic liver function tests should be performed.
• In metastatic breast cancer, hypercalcemia usually indicates progression of bone metastases. Report signs of hypercalcemia.
• Response in breast cancer is usually apparent within 3 months. Stop therapy if signs of disease progression appear.
• Enhances hypoglycemia; tell patient to report signs of hyperinsulinism.
• Instruct males to report priapism,

reduced ejaculatory volume, and gynecomastia. Withdraw drug.
- Watch for signs of ecchymoses, petechiae with concomitant anticoagulants. Monitor prothrombin time.
- Inject deep into upper outer quadrant of gluteal muscle. Report soreness at site; possibility of postinjection furunculosis.
- Report signs of virilization in females; reevaluate treatment.

- Monitor prepubertal males by X-ray for rate of bone maturation.
- Edema is generally controllable with salt restriction and/or diuretics.
- Use with diet high in calories and protein unless contraindicated.
- Good oral hygiene decreases possibility of irritation from buccal tablet. Patient shouldn't eat, drink, chew, or smoke while tablet is in place.
- Daily requirements best administered in divided doses.

48

Oral contraceptives

estrogen with progestogen

estrogen with progestogen

Brevicon, Demulen♦, Enovid, Enovid-E, Loestrin 1/20, Loestrin 1.5/30♦, Lo/Ovral, Min-Ovral♦♦, Modicon, Norinyl 1 + 50♦, Norinyl 1 + 80♦, Norinyl 2 mg♦, Norlestrin♦, Ortho-Novum 1/50♦, Ortho-Novum 1/80♦, Ortho-Novum 2 mg♦, Ortho-Novum 10 mg, Ovcon 35, Ovcon 50, Ovral, Ovulen♦.

INDICATIONS & DOSAGE

Contraception—
Women: 1 tablet P.O. daily, beginning on day 5 of menstrual cycle (first day of menstrual flow is day 1). With 20- and 21-tablet packages, new dosing cycle begins 7 days after last tablet taken. With 28-tablet packages, dosage is 1 tablet daily without interruption; extra tablets are placebos or contain iron.

If only 1 or 2 doses are missed, dosage may continue on schedule. If 3 or more doses are missed, remaining tablets in monthly package must be discarded and another contraceptive method substituted. If next menstrual period doesn't begin on schedule, rule out pregnancy before starting new dosing cycle. If menstrual period begins, start new dosing cycle 7 days after last tablet was taken. If all doses have been taken on schedule and 1 menstrual period is missed, continue dosing cycle. If 2 consecutive menstrual periods are missed, pregnancy test is required before new dosing cycle.

Hypermenorrhea—
Women: use high-dose combinations only. Dose same as for contraception.

Endometriosis—
Women: Cyclic therapy: 1 tablet Ortho-Novum 10 mg P.O. daily for 20 days from day 5 to day 24 of menstrual cycle.

Suppressive therapy: 1 tablet Ortho-Novum 10 mg P.O. daily for 3 to 9 months. May increase to 20 to 30 mg daily if breakthrough bleeding occurs.

Enovid 5 mg or 10 mg—1 tablet P.O. daily for 2 weeks starting on day 5 of menstrual cycle. Continue without interruption for 6 to 9 months, increasing dose by 5 to 10 mg q 2 weeks, up to 20 mg daily. Up to 40 mg daily may be needed if breakthrough bleeding occurs.

SIDE EFFECTS

CNS: *headache, dizziness,* depression, libido changes, lethargy.
CV: *thromboembolism,* hypertension.
EENT: worsening of myopia or astigmatism, intolerance to contact lenses.
GI: *nausea,* vomiting, abdominal cramps, bloating, diarrhea, constipation, anorexia, increased appetite, weight changes, *bowel ischemia.*
GU: *breakthrough bleeding,* dysmenorrhea, amenorrhea, cervical erosion or abnormal secretions, enlargement of uterine fibromas, vaginal candidiasis.
Hepatic: gallbladder disease, cholestatic jaundice, liver tumors.

Metabolic: hyperglycemia, hypercalcemia, folic acid deficiency.
Skin: rash, acne, seborrhea, oily skin.
Other: edema, migraine, *breast tenderness,* enlargement, secretion. Adverse effects may be more serious, frequent, and rapid in onset with high-dose than with low-dose combinations.

INTERACTIONS
Ampicillin, tetracycline, barbiturates, anticonvulsants, rifampin: may diminish contraceptive effectiveness. Use supplemental form of contraception.

NURSING CONSIDERATIONS
• Contraindicated in thromboembolic disorders, cerebrovascular or coronary artery disease, myocardial infarction, known or suspected cancer of breasts or reproductive organs, benign or malignant liver tumors, undiagnosed abnormal vaginal bleeding, known or suspected pregnancy, lactation. Also contraindicated in women 35 years or older who smoke over 15 cigarettes a day, and in all women over 40. Use cautiously in hypertension, mental depression, migraine, epilepsy, diabetes mellitus, amenorrhea. Report development or worsening of these conditions to doctor.

• If 1 menstrual period is missed and tablets have been taken on schedule, tell patient to continue taking them. If 2 consecutive menstrual periods are missed, tell patient to stop drug and to have pregnancy test. Progestogens may cause birth defects if taken early in pregnancy.
• Missed doses in midcycle greatly increase likelihood of pregnancy.
• Warn patient that headache, nausea, dizziness, breast tenderness, spotting, and breakthrough bleeding are common at first. These should diminish after 3 to 6 dosing cycles. However, breakthrough bleeding in patients taking high-dose estrogen-progestogen combinations for menstrual disorders may require dosage adjustment.
• Warn patient to immediately report abdominal pain; numbness, stiffness or pain in legs or buttocks; pressure or pain in chest; shortness of breath; severe headache; visual disturbances, such as blind spots, blurriness, or flashing lights; undiagnosed vaginal bleeding or discharge; 2 consecutive missed menstrual periods; lumps in the breast; swelling of hands or feet.
• Tell patient to take tablets at same time each day; nighttime dosing may reduce nausea and headaches.
• Stress importance of semiannual Pap smears and annual gynecologic exams while taking estrogen-progestogen combinations.

49

Estrogens

chlorotrianisene
dienestrol
diethylstilbestrol
diethylstilbestrol diphosphate
esterified estrogens
estradiol
estradiol cypionate
estradiol valerate
estrogenic substances, conjugated
estrone
ethinyl estradiol
quinestrol

chlorotrianisene
Tace ♦

INDICATIONS & DOSAGE
Men:
Prostatic cancer—12 to 25 mg P.O.
daily.
Nonnursing mothers:
Postpartum breast engorgement—
72 mg P.O. b.i.d. for 2 days; or 50 mg
q 6 hours for 6 doses; or 12 mg q.i.d.
for 7 days. Start dosing within 8 hours
after delivery.
Women:
Menopausal symptoms—12 to 25 mg
P.O. daily for 30 days or cyclic
(3 weeks on, 1 week off).
Female hypogonadism—12 to 25 mg
P.O. for 21 days, followed by 1 dose
of progesterone 100 mg I.M. or
5 days of oral progestogen given concurrently with last 5 days of chlorotrianisene (i.e., medroxyprogesterone
5 to 10 mg).
Atrophic vaginitis—12 to 25 mg P.O.
daily for 30 to 60 days.

SIDE EFFECTS
CNS: headache, dizziness, chorea,
migraine, depression, libido changes.
CV: thrombophlebitis; *thromboembolism;* hypertension; edema; *increased risk of stroke, pulmonary embolism, and myocardial infarction.*
EENT: worsening of myopia or astigmatism, intolerance to contact lenses.
GI: *nausea,* vomiting, abdominal
cramps, bloating, diarrhea, constipation, anorexia, increased appetite, excessive thirst, weight changes.
GU: breakthrough bleeding, altered
menstrual flow, dysmenorrhea, amenorrhea, cervical erosion or abnormal
secretions, enlargement of uterine fibromas, vaginal candidiasis; *in males:
gynecomastia, testicular atrophy, impotence.*
Metabolic: hyperglycemia, hypercalcemia, folic acid deficiency.
Skin: melasma, urticaria, acne, seborrhea, oily skin, hirsutism or loss of
hair.
Other: cholestatic jaundice, leg
cramps, purpura, breast changes (tenderness, enlargement, secretion).

INTERACTIONS
None significant.

NURSING CONSIDERATIONS
• Contraindicated in thrombophlebitis or thromboembolic disorders; cancer of breast, reproductive organs, or
genital tract; undiagnosed abnormal
genital bleeding. Use cautiously in
hypertension, asthma, mental depression, bone diseases, blood dyscrasias,
gallbladder disease, migraine, sei-

zures, diabetes mellitus, amenorrhea, cardiac failure, hepatic or renal dysfunction. Development or worsening of these conditions may require stopping drug.

- Long-term therapy contraindicated in menopause.
- FDA regulations require that female patients receive package insert explaining possible estrogen side effects before first dose.
- Warn patient to report immediately: abdominal pain; pain, numbness, or stiffness in legs or buttocks; pressure or pain in chest; shortness of breath; severe headaches; visual disturbances, such as blind spots, flashing lights, blurriness; undiagnosed vaginal bleeding or discharge; breast lumps; swelling of hands or feet.
- Tell male patients on long-term therapy about possible gynecomastia and impotence.
- Not used for menstrual disorders because duration of action is very long.
- Pathologist should be advised of estrogen therapy when specimen sent.
- Diabetics should report positive urine tests so diabetic medication dose can be adjusted.

---

dienestrol

Dienestrol cream♦
Available in combination with sulfanilamide and aminacrine as AVC/Dienestrol, cream or suppositories

---

INDICATIONS & DOSAGE
Postmenopausal women:
Atrophic vaginitis and kraurosis vulvae—1 to 2 applicatorfuls of cream daily for 2 weeks, then half that dose for 2 more weeks; or 1 to 2 vaginal suppositories daily through 1 complete menstrual cycle.
Atrophic and senile vaginitis and kraurosis vulvae when complicated by infection—1 applicatorful AVC/Dienestrol cream intravaginally daily or b.i.d. for 1 to 2 weeks, then every other day for 1 to 2 weeks.

SIDE EFFECTS
GU: vaginal discharge; with excessive use, uterine bleeding.
Local: increased discomfort, burning sensation. Systemic effects possible.
Other: breast tenderness.

INTERACTIONS
None significant.

NURSING CONSIDERATIONS
- Contraindicated in thrombophlebitis or thromboembolic disorders; cancer of breast, reproductive organs, or genital tract; undiagnosed abnormal genital bleeding. Use cautiously in menstrual irregularities or endometriosis.
- Prolonged therapy with estrogen-containing products is contraindicated.
- FDA regulations require that female patients receive package insert explaining possible estrogen side effects before first dose.
- Systemic reactions possible with normal intravaginal use. Monitor closely.
- Warn patient not to exceed dose.
- Withdrawal bleeding may be precipitated if estrogen is suddenly stopped.

---

diethylstilbestrol
DES, Stilbestrol, Stibilium♦♦,
diethylstilbestrol diphosphate
Honvol♦♦, Stilphostrol

INDICATIONS & DOSAGE
Women:
Atrophic vaginitis or kraurosis vulvae—0.1 to 1 mg as suppository daily for 10 to 14 days concurrently with oral therapy; or up to 5 mg weekly as suppository.

Hypogonadism, castration, primary ovarian failure—0.2 to 0.5 mg P.O. daily.

Menopausal symptoms—0.1 to 2 mg P.O. daily in cycles of 3 weeks on and 1 week off.

Postcoital contraception ("morning-after pill")—25 mg P.O. b.i.d. for 5 days, starting within 72 hours after coitus.

Postpartum breast engorgement— 5 mg P.O. daily or t.i.d. up to total dose of 30 mg.

Men:

Prostatic cancer—1 to 3 mg P.O. daily, initially; may be reduced to 1 mg P.O. daily, or 5 mg I.M. twice weekly initially, followed by up to 4 mg I.M. twice weekly. Or 50 to 200 mg (diphosphate) P.O. t.i.d.; or 0.25 to 1 g I.V. daily for 5 days, then once or twice weekly.

Men and postmenopausal women:

Breast cancer—15 mg P.O. daily.

SIDE EFFECTS

CNS: headache, dizziness, chorea, depression, lethargy.

CV: *thrombophlebitis; thromboembolism;* hypertension; edema; *increased risk of stroke, pulmonary embolism, and mycardial infarction.*

EENT: worsening of myopia or astigmatism, intolerance to contact lenses.

GI: *nausea,* vomiting, abdominal cramps, bloating, diarrhea, constipation, anorexia, increased appetite, excessive thirst, weight changes.

GU: breakthrough bleeding, altered menstrual flow, dysmenorrhea, amenorrhea, cervical erosion, altered cervical secretions, enlargement of uterine fibromas, vaginal candidiasis, loss of libido; *in males:* gynecomastia, testicular atrophy, impotence.

Metabolic: hyperglycemia, hypercalcemia, folic acid deficiency.

Skin: melasma, urticaria, acne, seborrhea, oily skin, hirsutism or loss of hair.

Other: cholestatic jaundice, leg cramps, breast tenderness or enlargement.

INTERACTIONS

None significant.

NURSING CONSIDERATIONS

• Contraindicated in thrombophlebitis or thromboembolic disorders; undiagnosed abnormal genital bleeding. Use cautiously in hypertension, asthma, mental depression, bone disease, migraine, seizures, blood dyscrasias, diabetes mellitus, gallbladder disease, amenorrhea, cardiac failure, hepatic or renal dysfunction. Development or worsening of these conditions may require stopping drug.

• Long-term therapy contraindicated in menopause; linked with increased risk of endometrial cancer in premenopausal women.

• FDA regulations require that all female patients receive package insert explaining possible estrogen side effects before first dose.

• Only 25 mg tablet approved by FDA as the "morning-after pill." To be effective, it must be taken within 72 hours after coitus.

• Warn patient to stop taking drug immediately if she becomes pregnant, since it can affect the fetus adversely.

• Warn patient to report immediately: abdominal pain; pain, numbness, or stiffness in legs or buttocks; pressure or pain in chest; shortness of breath; severe headache; visual disturbances, such as blind spots, flashing lights, or blurriness; undiagnosed vaginal bleeding or discharge; breast lumps; swelling of hands or feet.

• Pathologist should be advised of estrogen therapy when specimen sent.

• Diabetics should report positive urine tests so diabetic medication dose can be adjusted.

• High incidence of gross nonmalignant genital changes in offspring of women taking drug during pregnancy. Female offspring also have higher

Italicized side effects are common or life-threatening.

than normal risk of developing cervical and vaginal adenocarcinoma.

• Increased number of cardiovascular deaths reported in men taking diethylstilbestrol tablet (5 mg daily) for prostatic cancer over long period of time. This effect not associated with 1 mg daily dose.

---

esterified estrogens
Amnestrogen, Climestrone♦♦, Estabs, Estratab, Evex, Femogen, Menest, Menotrol♦♦, Ms-Med, Neo-Estrone♦♦

INDICATIONS & DOSAGE
Men:
Prostatic cancer—1.25 to 2.5 mg P.O. t.i.d.
Men and postmenopausal women:
Breast cancer—10 mg P.O. t.i.d. for 3 or more months.
Women:
Hypogonadism, castration, primary ovarian failure—2.5 mg 1 to t.i.d. in cycles of 3 weeks on, 1 week off.
Menopausal symptoms—average 0.3 to 3.75 mg P.O. daily in cycles of 3 weeks on, 1 week off.

SIDE EFFECTS
CNS: headache, dizziness, chorea, depression, libido changes, lethargy.
CV: thrombophlebitis; *thromboembolism;* hypertension; edema; *increased risk of stroke, pulmonary embolism, and myocardial infarction.*
EENT: worsening of myopia or astigmatism, intolerance to contact lenses.
GI: *nausea,* vomiting, abdominal cramps, bloating, diarrhea, constipation, anorexia, increased appetite, weight changes.
GU: breakthrough bleeding, altered menstrual flow, dysmenorrhea, amenorrhea, cervical erosion, altered cervical secretions, enlargement of uterine fibromas, vaginal candidiasis; *in*

males: gynecomastia, testicular atrophy, impotence.
Metabolic: hyperglycemia, hypercalcemia, folic acid deficiency.
Skin: melasma, rash, acne, hirsutism or hair loss, seborrhea, oily skin.
Other: breast changes (tenderness, enlargement, secretion), cholestatic jaundice.

INTERACTIONS
None significant.

NURSING CONSIDERATIONS
• Contraindicated in thrombophlebitis or thromboembolic disorders; undiagnosed abnormal genital bleeding. Use cautiously in history of hypertension, mental depression, gallbladder disease, migraine, seizure, diabetes mellitus, or amenorrhea. Development or worsening of these conditions may necessitate discontinuing drug.
• Long-term therapy contraindicated in menopause.
• FDA regulations require that female patients receive package insert explaining possible estrogen side effects before first dose.
• Warn patient to report immediately: abdominal pain; pain, numbness, or stiffness in legs or buttocks; pressure or pain in chest; shortness of breath; severe headaches; visual disturbances, such as blind spots, flashing lights, or blurriness; undiagnosed vaginal bleeding or discharge; breast lumps; swelling of hands or feet.
• Pathologist should be advised of estrogen therapy when specimen sent.
• Diabetics should report positive urine tests so diabetic medication dose can be adjusted.

Unmarked trade names available in the United States only.
♦ Also available in Canada ♦♦ Available in Canada only.

estradiol
Estrace♦, Progynon
estradiol cypionate
D-Est 5, Depo-Estradiol Cypionate,
Depogen, Duraestrin, E-Ionate P.A.,
Estro-Cyp, Estroject-L.A.
estradiol valerate
Ardefem, Delestrogen♦♦, Dioval♦,
Duragen, Estate, Estradiol L.A., Es-
traval, Rep Estra, Repo-Estro Med,
Reposo-E, Retestrin, Valergen

INDICATIONS & DOSAGE
Women:
*Menopausal symptoms, hypogonad-
ism, castration, primary ovarian failure*—1 to 2 mg P.O. daily, in cycles of
21 days on and 7 days off, or cycles of
5 days on and 2 days off; or 0.2 to
1 mg I.M. weekly.
Kraurosis vulvae—1 to 1.5 mg I.M.
once or more per week.
Menopausal symptoms—1 to 5 mg
(cypionate) I.M. q 3 to 4 weeks. Or 5
to 20 mg (valerate) I.M., repeated
once after 2 to 3 weeks
Postpartum breast engorgement—10
to 25 mg (valerate) I.M. at end of first
stage of labor.
Men:
Prostatic cancer—25 mg S.C. pellet
implants (Progynon) q 3 to 4 months,
or 50 mg q 4 to 6 months. Or 30 mg
(valerate) I.M. q 1 to 2 weeks.

SIDE EFFECTS
CNS: headache, dizziness, chorea,
depression, libido changes, lethargy.
CV: thrombophlebitis, *thromboembolism,* hypertension, edema.
EENT: worsening of myopia or astigmatism, intolerance to contact lenses.
GI: *nausea,* vomiting, abdominal
cramps, bloating, diarrhea, constipation, anorexia, increased appetite,
weight changes.
GU: breakthrough bleeding, altered
menstrual flow, dysmenorrhea, amenorrhea, cervical erosion, altered cer-

vical secretions, enlargement of uterine fibromas, vaginal candidiasis; *in
males:* gynecomastia, testicular atrophy, impotence.
Metabolic: hyperglycemia, hypercalcemia, folic acid deficiency.
Skin: melasma, urticaria, acne, seborrhea, oily skin, hirsutism or hair
loss.
Other: breast changes (tenderness,
enlargement, secretion), cholestatic
jaundice, leg cramps.

INTERACTIONS
None significant.

NURSING CONSIDERATIONS
• Contraindicated in thrombophlebitis or thromboembolic disorders; cancer of breast, reproductive organs;
undiagnosed abnormal genital bleeding. Use cautiously in hypertension,
mental depression, bone diseases,
blood dyscrasias, migraine, seizures,
diabetes mellitus, amenorrhea, cardiac failure, hepatic or renal dysfunction. Development or worsening of
these conditions may require stopping
drug.
• FDA regulations require that female
patients receive package insert explaining possible estrogen side effects
before first dose.
• Warn patient to report immediately:
abdominal pain; pain, numbness, or
stiffness in legs or buttocks; pressure
or pain in chest; shortness of breath;
severe headaches; visual disturbances, such as blind spots, flashing
lights, or blurriness; undiagnosed
vaginal bleeding or discharge; breast
lumps; swelling of hands or feet.
• Risk of endometrial cancer is increased in postmenopausal women
who take estrogens for more than
1 year.
• Diabetics should report positive
urine tests so diabetic medication
dose can be adjusted.
• Pathologist should be advised of estrogen therapy when specimen sent.

Italicized side effects are common or life-threatening.

- Estradiol available as aqueous suspension or solution in peanut oil.
- Estradiol cypionate available as solution in cottonseed oil or vegetable oil.
- Estradiol valerate available as solution in castor oil, sesame oil, and vegetable oil. Check for allergy.
- Before injection, make sure drug is well dispersed in solution by rolling vial between palms.

---

estrogenic substances, conjugated
Estrocon, Menotab, Ovest, Premarin♦, Sodestrin-H

INDICATIONS & DOSAGE
Women:
Abnormal uterine bleeding (hormonal imbalance)—25 mg I.V. or I.M. Repeat in 6 to 12 hours.
Breast cancer (at least 5 years after menopause)—10 mg P.O. t.i.d. for 3 months or more.
Castration, primary ovarian failure, and osteoporosis—1.25 mg P.O. daily in cycles of 3 weeks on, 1 week off.
Hypogonadism—2.5 mg P.O. b.i.d. or t.i.d. for 20 consecutive days each month.
Menopausal symptoms—0.3 to 1.25 mg P.O. daily in cycles of 3 weeks on, 1 week off.
Postpartum breast engorgement—3.75 mg P.O. q 4 hours for 5 doses or 1.25 mg q 4 hours for 5 days.
Men:
Prostatic cancer—1.25 to 2.5 mg P.O. t.i.d.

SIDE EFFECTS
CNS: headache, dizziness, chorea, depression, libido changes, lethargy.
CV: thrombophlebitis; *thromboembolism;* hypertension; edema; *increased risk of stroke, pulmonary embolism, and myocardial infarction.*

EENT: worsening of myopia or astigmatism, intolerance to contact lenses.
GI: *nausea,* vomiting, abdominal cramps, bloating, diarrhea, constipation, anorexia, increased appetite, weight changes.
GU: breakthrough bleeding, altered menstrual flow, dysmenorrhea, amenorrhea, cervical erosion, altered cervical secretions, enlargement of uterine fibromas, vaginal candidiasis; *in males:* gynecomastia, testicular atrophy, impotence.
Metabolic: hyperglycemia, hypercalcemia, folic acid deficiency.
Skin: melasma, urticaria, acne, seborrhea, oily skin, flushing (when given rapidly I.V.), hirsutism or loss of hair.
Other: breast changes (tenderness, enlargement, secretion), cholestatic jaundice, leg cramps.

INTERACTIONS
None significant.

NURSING CONSIDERATIONS
- Contraindicated in thrombophlebitis or thromboembolic disorders; undiagnosed abnormal genital bleeding. Use cautiously in hypertension, gallbladder disease, bone diseases, blood dyscrasias, migraine, seizures, diabetes mellitus, amenorrhea, cardiac failure, hepatic or renal dysfunction. Development or worsening of these conditions may require stopping drug.
- Long-term therapy contraindicated in menopause.
- FDA regulations require that female patients receive package insert explaining possible estrogen side effects before first dose.
- Warn patient to report any unusual symptoms immediately, especially abdominal pain; pain, numbness, or stiffness in legs or buttocks; pressure or pain in chest; shortness of breath; severe headaches; visual disturbances, such as blind spots, flashing lights, or blurriness; undiagnosed

vaginal bleeding or discharge; breast lumps; swelling of hands or feet.
- I.M. or I.V. use preferred for rapid treatment of dysfunctional uterine bleeding or reduction of surgical bleeding.
- Refrigerate before reconstituting. Agitate gently after adding diluent.
- Pathologist should be advised of estrogen therapy when specimen sent.
- Diabetics should report positive urine tests so diabetic medication dose can be adjusted.
- Use associated with increased risk of endometrial cancer.

---

estrone
Foygen, Gravigen, Ogen♦, Theelin

INDICATIONS & DOSAGE
Women:
Atrophic vaginitis—0.2 mg intravaginal suppository daily or apply cream to vagina once nightly.
Hypogonadism, castration, ovarian failure—1.25 to 7.5 mg P.O. daily for 20 consecutive days each month; or 0.1 to 2 mg I.M. weekly.
Menopausal symptoms—0.625 to 5 mg P.O. daily in cycle of 3 weeks on, 1 week off; or 0.1 to 0.5 mg I.M. 2 to 3 times weekly.
Men:
Prostatic cancer—2 to 4 mg I.M. 2 to 3 times weekly.

SIDE EFFECTS
CNS: headache, dizziness, chorea, depression, libido changes, lethargy.
CV: thrombophlebitis, *thromboembolism,* hypertension, edema.
EENT: worsening of myopia or astigmatism, intolerance to contact lenses.
GI: *nausea,* vomiting, abdominal cramps, bloating, diarrhea, constipation, anorexia, increased appetite, weight changes.
GU: breakthrough bleeding, altered menstrual flow, dysmenorrhea, amen-orrhea, cervical erosion, altered cervical secretions, enlargement of uterine fibromas, vaginal candidiasis; *in males:* gynecomastia, testicular atrophy, impotence.
Metabolic: hyperglycemia, hypercalcemia, folic acid deficiency.
Skin: melasma, urticaria, acne, seborrhea, oily skin, hirsutism or hair loss.
Other: breast changes (tenderness, enlargement, secretion), cholestatic jaundice, leg cramps.

INTERACTIONS
None significant.

NURSING CONSIDERATIONS
- Contraindicated in thrombophlebitis or thromboembolic disorders; cancer of breast or reproductive organs; undiagnosed abnormal genital bleeding. Use cautiously in hypertension, mental depression, migraine, seizures, diabetes mellitus, amenorrhea, hepatic or renal dysfunction. Development or worsening of these may require stopping drug.
- I.V. use contraindicated.
- Long-term therapy contraindicated in menopause.
- FDA regulations require that female patients receive package insert explaining possible estrogen side effects before first dose.
- Warn patient to report any unusual symptoms immediately, especially abdominal pain; pain, numbness, or stiffness in legs or buttocks; pressure or pain in chest; shortness of breath; severe headaches; visual disturbances, such as blind spots, flashing lights, or blurriness; undiagnosed vaginal bleeding or discharge; breast lumps; swelling of hands or feet.
- Oil preparation may become cloudy if chilled. Warm solution until clear before use. Also available in aqueous suspension.
- Pathologist should be advised of estrogen therapy when specimen sent.

Italicized side effects are common or life-threatening.

• Diabetics should report positive urine test so diabetic medication dose can be adjusted.

ethinyl estradiol
Estinyl♦, Feminone

INDICATIONS & DOSAGE
Women:
Breast cancer (at least 5 years after menopause)—1 mg P.O. t.i.d.
Hypogonadism—0.05 mg daily to t.i.d. for 2 weeks a month, followed by 2 weeks progesterone therapy; continue for 3 to 6 monthly dosing cycles, followed by 2 months off.
Menopausal symptoms—0.02 to 0.05 mg P.O. daily for cycles of 3 weeks on, 1 week off.
Postpartum breast engorgement—0.5 to 1 mg P.O. daily for 3 days, then taper over 7 days to 0.1 mg and discontinue.
Men:
Prostatic cancer—0.15 to 2 mg P.O. daily.

SIDE EFFECTS
CNS: headache, dizziness, chorea, depression, libido changes, lethargy.
CV: thrombophlebitis, *thromboembolism,* hypertension, edema.
EENT: worsening of myopia or astigmatism, intolerance to contact lenses.
GI: *nausea,* vomiting, abdominal cramps, bloating, diarrhea, constipation, anorexia, increased appetite, weight changes.
GU: breakthrough bleeding, altered menstrual flow, dysmenorrhea, amenorrhea, cervical erosion, altered cervical secretions, enlargement of uterine fibromas, vaginal candidiasis; *in males:* gynecomastia, testicular atrophy, impotence.
Metabolic: hyperglycemia, hypercalcemia, folic acid deficiency.
Skin: melasma, urticaria, acne, seb-

orrhea, oily skin, hirsutism or hair loss.
Other: breast changes (tenderness, enlargement, secretion), cholestatic jaundice, leg cramps.

INTERACTIONS
None significant.

NURSING CONSIDERATIONS
• Contraindicated in thrombophlebitis or thromboembolic disorders; undiagnosed abnormal genital bleeding. Use cautiously in hypertension, mental depression, bone diseases, migraine, seizures, blood dyscrasias, diabetes mellitus, amenorrhea, cardiac failure, hepatic or renal dysfunction. Development or worsening of these conditions may require stopping drug.
• FDA regulations require that female patients receive package insert explaining possible estrogen side effects before first dose.
• Warn patient to report any unusual symptoms immediately, especially abdominal pain; pain, numbness, or stiffness in legs or buttocks; pressure or pain in chest; shortness of breath; severe headaches; visual disturbances, such as blind spots, flashing lights, or blurriness; undiagnosed vaginal bleeding or discharge; breast lumps; swelling of hands or feet.
• Pathologist should be advised of estrogen therapy when specimen sent.
• Diabetics should report positive urine test so diabetic medication dose can be adjusted.

quinestrol
Estrovis

INDICATIONS & DOSAGE
Women:
Moderate to severe vasomotor symptoms associated with menopause, and for atrophic vaginitis, kraurosis vul-

vae, female hypogonadism, female castration and primary ovarian failure—
100 mcg tablet once daily for 7 days, followed by 100 mcg weekly as maintenance dose beginning 2 weeks after start of treatment. Dosage may be increased to 200 mcg weekly.

SIDE EFFECTS
CNS: headache, dizziness, chorea, migraine, depression, libido changes.
CV: thrombophlebitis; *thromboembolism;* hypertension; edema; *increased risk of stroke, pulmonary embolism, and myocardial infarction.*
EENT: worsening of myopia or astigmatism, intolerance to contact lenses.
GI: *nausea,* vomiting, abdominal cramps, bloating, diarrhea, constipation, anorexia, increased appetite, excessive thirst, weight changes.
GU: breakthrough bleeding, altered menstrual flow, dysmenorrhea, amenorrhea, cervical erosion or abnormal secretions, enlargement of uterine fibromas, vaginal candidiasis.
Metabolic: hyperglycemia, hypercalcemia, folic acid deficiency.
Skin: melasma, urticaria, acne, seborrhea, oily skin, hirsutism or loss of hair.
Other: cholestatic jaundice, leg cramps, purpura, breast changes (tenderness, enlargement, secretion).

INTERACTIONS
None significant.

NURSING CONSIDERATIONS
• Contraindicated in thrombophlebitis or thromboembolic disorders; cancer of breast or reproductive organs; undiagnosed abnormal gential bleeding. Use cautiously in hypertension, mental depression, migraine, seizures, diabetes melitus, amenorrhea, hepatic or renal dysfunction. Development or worsening of these may require stopping drug.
• Long-term therapy contraindicated in menopause.
• FDA regulations require that female patients receive package insert explaining possible estrogen side effects before first dose.
• Warn patient to report any unusual symptoms immediately, especially abdominal pain; pain, numbness, or stiffness in legs or buttocks; pressure or pain in chest; shortness of breath; severe headaches; visual disturbances, such as blind spots, flashing lights, or blurriness; undiagnosed vaginal bleeding or discharge; breast lumps; swelling of hands or feet.
• Pathologist should be advised of estrogen therapy when specimen sent.
• Diabetics should report positive urine test so diabetic medication dose can be adjusted.
• Attempts to discontinue medication should be made at 3- to 6-month intervals.
• Similar in effectiveness to conjugated estrogens in treatment of postmenopausal symptoms. Biggest advantage is quinestrol can be taken once a week.

Italicized side effects are common or life-threatening.

50

Progestogens

dydrogesterone
hydroxyprogesterone caproate
medroxyprogesterone acetate
norethindrone
norethindrone acetate
norgestrel
progesterone

---

dydrogesterone
Duphaston◆

INDICATIONS & DOSAGE
Women:
Primary and secondary amenorrhea—
5 mg P.O. b.i.d. or q.i.d. from day 15
to day 25 of menstrual cycle.
Oligomenorrhea—5 mg P.O. b.i.d.
for 5 days.
Abnormal uterine bleeding—
5 mg P.O. b.i.d. or q.i.d. for 5 to
10 days before usual menses. Thereafter, 5 mg P.O. b.i.d. to q.i.d. for 5
days on the 21st to 25th day of cycle.

SIDE EFFECTS
CNS: dizziness, migraine headache,
lethargy, depression, decreased libido, cerebral thrombosis.
CV: hypertension, thrombophlebitis,
pulmonary embolism.
GI: nausea, vomiting, abdominal
cramps.
GU: breakthrough bleeding, dysmenorrhea, amenorrhea; cervical erosion
and abnormal secretions; uterine fibromas; vaginal candidiasis.
Metabolic: hyperglycemia.
Skin: melasma, rash, pruritus.

Other: breast tenderness, enlargement, or secretion; edema; jaundice.

INTERACTIONS
None significant.

NURSING CONSIDERATIONS
• Contraindicated in thromboembolic
disorders, breast cancer, undiagnosed
abnormal vaginal bleeding, missed
abortion, pregnancy, liver dysfunction
Use cautiously in diabetes mellitus,
seizure disorder, migraine, cardiac or
renal disease, asthma, or mental illness.
• FDA regulations require that patients receive before first dose package insert explaining possible progestogen side effects. Patient should report any unusual symptoms immediately and should stop drug and call
doctor if visual disturbances or migraine occurs.
• Don't use as test for pregnancy;
drug may cause birth defects.
• Preliminary estrogen treatment
usually needed in menstrual
disorders.
• Not approved by FDA for use as
contraceptive in U.S.A.

---

hydroxyprogesterone caproate
Curretab, Delalutin◆, Dura-Lutin

INDICATIONS & DOSAGE
Women:
Menstrual disorders—125 to 375 mg
I.M. q 4 weeks. Stop after 4 cycles.
Uterine cancer—1 to 5 g I.M. weekly.

SIDE EFFECTS

CNS: dizziness, migraine headache, lethargy, depression, decreased libido.
CV: hypertension, thrombophlebitis, *pulmonary embolism, edema*.
GI: nausea, vomiting, abdominal cramps.
GU: breakthrough bleeding, dysmenorrhea, amenorrhea; cervical erosion or abnormal secretions; uterine fibromas; vaginal candidiasis.
Local: irritation, pain.
Metabolic: hyperglycemia.
Skin: melasma, rash.
Other: breast tenderness, enlargement, or secretion; cholestatic jaundice.

INTERACTIONS

None significant.

NURSING CONSIDERATIONS

• Contraindicated in thromboembolic disorders, breast cancer, undiagnosed abnormal vaginal bleeding, severe hepatic disease, missed abortion, or pregnancy. Use cautiously in diabetes mellitus, seizure disorder, migraine, cardiac or renal disease, asthma, or mental illness.
• FDA regulations require that patients receive before first dose package insert explaining possible progestogen side effects. Patient should report any unusual symptoms immediately and should stop drug and call doctor if visual disturbances or migraine occurs.
• 'Don't use as test for pregnancy; drug may cause birth defects.
• Warn patient that edema and weight gain are likely.
• Give oil solutions (sesame oil and castor oil) deep I.M. in gluteal muscle.
• Preliminary estrogen treatment usually needed in menstrual disorders.
• Effect lasts 7 to 14 days.
• For I.M. use only.

---

medroxyprogesterone acetate
Amen, Depo-Provera♦, Provera♦

INDICATIONS & DOSAGE

Women:
Abnormal uterine bleeding due to hormonal imbalance—5 to 10 mg P.O. daily for 5 to 10 days beginning on the 16th day of cycle. If patient has received estrogen—10 mg P.O. daily for 10 days beginning on 16th day of cycle.
Secondary amenorrhea—5 to 10 mg P.O. daily for 5 to 10 days.

SIDE EFFECTS

CNS: dizziness, migraine headache, lethargy, depression, decreased libido.
CV: hypertension, thrombophlebitis, *pulmonary embolism, edema*.
GI: nausea, vomiting, abdominal cramps.
GU: breakthrough bleeding, dysmenorrhea, amenorrhea; cervical erosion or abnormal secretions; uterine fibromas, vaginal candidiasis.
Metabolic: hyperglycemia.
Skin: melasma, rash.
Other: breast tenderness, enlargement, or secretion; cholestatic jaundice.

INTERACTIONS

None significant.

NURSING CONSIDERATIONS

• Contraindicated in thromboembolic disorders, breast cancer, undiagnosed abnormal vaginal bleeding, pregnancy, missed abortion, hepatic dysfunction. Use cautiously in diabetes mellitus, seizure disorder, migraine, cardiac or renal disease, asthma, or mental illness.
• FDA regulations require that patients receive before first dose package insert explaining possible progestogen side effects. Patient should re-

port any unusual symptoms immediately and should stop drug and call doctor if visual disturbances or migraine occurs.
• Don't use as test for pregnancy; drug may cause birth defects.

---

norethindrone
Norlutin♦, Nor-Q.D.

INDICATIONS & DOSAGE
Women:
Amenorrhea; abnormal uterine bleeding—5 to 20 mg P.O. daily on days 5 to 25 of menstrual cycle.
Endometriosis—10 mg P.O. daily for 14 days, then increase by 5 mg P.O. daily q 2 weeks up to 30 mg daily.

SIDE EFFECTS
CNS: dizziness, migraine headache, lethargy, depression, decreased libido.
CV: hypertension, thrombophlebitis, *pulmonary embolism, edema.*
GI: nausea, vomiting, abdominal cramps.
GU: breakthrough bleeding, dysmenorrhea, amenorrhea; cervical erosion or abnormal secretions; uterine fibromas; vaginal candidiasis.
Metabolic: hyperglycemia.
Skin: melasma, rash.
Other: breast tenderness, enlargement, or secretion; cholestatic jaundice.

INTERACTIONS
None significant.

NURSING CONSIDERATIONS
• Contraindicated in thromboembolic disorders, breast cancer, undiagnosed abnormal vaginal bleeding, severe hepatic disease, missed abortion, or pregnancy. Use cautiously in diabetes mellitus, seizure disorder, migraine, cardiac or renal disease, asthma, or mental illness.

• Don't use as test for pregnancy; drug may cause birth defects.
• FDA regulations require that patients receive before first dose package insert explaining possible progestogen side effects. Patient should report any unusual symptoms immediately and should stop drug and call doctor if visual disturbances or migraine occurs.
• Watch patient carefully for signs of edema.
• Preliminary estrogen treatment usually needed in menstrual disorders.

---

norethindrone acetate
Norlutate♦

INDICATIONS & DOSAGE
Women:
Amenorrhea, abnormal uterine bleeding—2.5 to 10 mg P.O. daily on days 5 to 25 of menstrual cycle.
Endometriosis—5 mg P.O. daily for 14 days, then increase by 2.5 mg daily q 2 weeks up to 15 mg daily.

SIDE EFFECTS
CNS: dizziness, migraine headache, lethargy, depression, decreased libido.
CV: hypertension, thrombophlebitis, *pulmonary embolism, edema.*
GI: nausea, vomiting, abdominal cramps.
GU: breakthrough bleeding, dysmenorrhea, amenorrhea; cervical erosion or abnormal secretions; uterine fibromas; vaginal candidiasis.
Metabolic: hyperglycemia.
Skin: melasma, rash.
Other: breast tenderness, enlargement, or secretion; cholestatic jaundice.

INTERACTIONS
None significant.

Unmarked trade names available in the United States only.
♦ Also available in Canada   ♦♦ Available in Canada only.

NURSING CONSIDERATIONS
• Contraindicated in thromboembolic disorders, breast cancer, undiagnosed abnormal vaginal bleeding, severe hepatic disease, missed abortion, or pregnancy. Use cautiously in diabetes mellitus, seizure disorder, migraine, cardiac or renal disease, asthma, or mental illness.
• FDA regulations require that patients receive before first dose package insert explaining possible progestogen effects. Patient should report any unusual symptoms immediately and should stop drug and call doctor if visual disturbances or migraine occurs.
• Don't use as test for pregnancy; drug may cause birth defects.
• Preliminary estrogen treatment usually needed in menstrual disorders.
• Twice as potent as norethindrone.

norgestrel
Ovrette

INDICATIONS & DOSAGE
Women:
Contraception—1 tablet P.O. daily.

SIDE EFFECTS
CNS: cerebral thrombosis or hemorrhage, migraine headache, lethargy, depression.
CV: hypertension, thrombophlebitis, *pulmonary embolism, edema.*
GI: nausea, vomiting, abdominal cramps, gallbladder disease.
GU: *breakthrough bleeding, change in menstrual flow,* dysmenorrhea, spotting, amenorrhea; cervical erosion, vaginal candidiasis.
Skin: melasma, rash.
Other: breast tenderness, enlargement, or secretions; cholestatic jaundice.

INTERACTIONS
None significant.

NURSING CONSIDERATIONS
• Contraindicated in thromboembolic disorders, breast cancer, undiagnosed abnormal vaginal bleeding, severe hepatic disease, missed abortion, or pregnancy. Use cautiously in diabetes mellitus, seizure disorder, migraine, cardiac or renal disease, asthma, or mental illness.
• FDA regulations require that before first dose patients receive package insert explaining possible progestogen effects. Patient should report any unusual symptoms immediately and should stop drug and call doctor if visual disturbances or migraine occurs.
• Tell patient to take pill every day even if menstruating.
• Progestogen—only oral contraceptive known as "mini-pill."

progesterone
Profac-O, Progelan, Progestasert♦, Progestilin♦♦, Progestin

INDICATIONS & DOSAGE
Women:
Amenorrhea—5 to 10 mg I.M. daily for 6 to 8 days.
Functional uterine bleeding—5 to 10 mg I.M. daily for 6 doses.

SIDE EFFECTS
CNS: dizziness, migraine headache, lethargy, depression, decreased libido.
CV: hypertension, thrombophlebitis, *pulmonary embolism, edema.*
GI: nausea, vomiting, abdominal cramps.
GU: breakthrough bleeding, dysmenorrhea, amenorrhea; cervical erosion or abnormal secretions; uterine fibromas; vaginal candidiasis.
Local: pain at injection site.
Metabolic: hyperglycemia.

Italicized side effects are common or life-threatening.

Skin: melasma, rash.
Other: breast tenderness, enlargement or secretion; cholestatic jaundice.

INTERACTIONS
None significant.

NURSING CONSIDERATIONS
• Contraindicated in thromboembolic disorders, breast cancer, undiagnosed abnormal vaginal bleeding, severe hepatic disease, or missed abortion. Use cautiously in diabetes mellitus, seizure disorder, migraine, cardiac or renal disease, asthma, or mental illness.

• FDA regulations require that patients receive before first dose package insert explaining possible progestogen side effects. Patient should report any unusual symptoms immediately.
• Give oil solutions (peanut oil or sesame oil) deep I.M.
• A progesterone-containing IUD (Progestasert) available which releases 65 mcg progesterone daily for 1 year.
• Preliminary estrogen treatment usually needed in menstrual disorders.

51

Gonadotropins

**chorionic gonadotropin, human
menotropins**

chorionic gonadotropin, human
Android HCG, Antuitrin-S♦,
A.P.L. ♦, Chorex, Follutein, Gona-
dex, Libigen, Pregnyl, Stemultrolin,
Glukor

INDICATIONS & DOSAGE
Anovulation and infertility—
Women: 10,000 units I.M. 1 day
after last dose of menotropins.
Hypogonadism—
Men: 500 to 1,000 units I.M. 3 times
weekly for 3 weeks, then twice
weekly for 3 weeks; or 4,000 units
I.M. 3 times weekly for 6 to
9 months, then 2,000 units 3 times
weekly for 3 more months.
Nonobstructive cryptorchism—
Boys 4 to 9 years: 5,000 units I.M.
every other day for 4 doses.

SIDE EFFECTS
CNS: headache, fatigue, irritability,
restlessness, depression.
GU: early puberty (growth of testes,
penis, pubic and axillary hair; voice
change; down on upper lip; growth of
body hair).
Local: *pain at injection site.*
Other: gynecomastia, edema.

INTERACTIONS
None significant.

NURSING CONSIDERATIONS
• Contraindicated in pituitary hypertrophy or tumor, prostatic cancer, and
early puberty (usual onset between 10
and 13 years of age). Use cautiously
in epilepsy, migraine, asthma, cardiac
or renal disease.
• Not for obesity control.
• When used with menotropins to
induce ovulation, multiple births
possible.
• In infertility, encourage daily
intercourse from day before chorionic
gonadotropin is given until ovulation
occurs.
• Inspect genitalia of boys for signs
of early puberty. Notify doctor, who
may discontinue drug if early puberty
occurs.

menotropins
Pergonal

INDICATIONS & DOSAGE
Anovulation—
Women: 75 IU (international units)
each FSH (follicle-stimulating hormone) and LH (luteinizing hormone)
I.M. daily for 9 to 12 days, followed
by 10,000 units chorionic gonadotropin I.M. 1 day after last dose of
menotropins. Repeat for 1 to 3 menstrual cycles until ovulation occurs.
Infertility with ovulation—
75 IU each of FSH and LH I.M. daily
for 9 to 12 days, followed by 10,000
units chorionic gonadotropin I.M.
1 day after last dose of menotropins.
Repeat for 2 menstrual cycles and
then increase to 150 IU each FSH and
LH I.M. daily for 9 to 12 days, fol-

lowed by 10,000 units chorionic gonadotropin I.M. 1 day after last dose
of menotropins. Repeat for
2 menstrual cycles.
Menotropins available in ampuls containing 75 IU each FSH and LH.

SIDE EFFECTS
Blood: hemoconcentration with fluid
loss into abdomen.
GI: nausea, vomiting, diarrhea.
GU: *ovarian enlargement with pain
and abdominal distention,* multiple
births, ovarian hyperstimulation syndrome (sudden ovarian enlargement,
ascites with or without pain, or
pleural effusion).
Other: fever.

INTERACTIONS
None significant.

NURSING CONSIDERATIONS
- Contraindicated in high urinary gonadotropin levels, thyroid or adrenal
dysfunction, pituitary tumor, abnormal uterine bleeding, ovarian cysts or
enlargement, and pregnancy.
- Tell patient that there is a possibility of multiple births.
- In infertility, encourage daily intercourse from day before chorionic gonadotropin is given until ovulation
occurs.
- Reconstitute with 1 to 2 ml sterile
saline injection. Use immediately.

52

Antidiabetic agents

acetohexamide
chlorpropamide
glucagon
insulins
tolazamide
tolbutamide

---

acetohexamide
Dimelor♦♦, Dymelor

INDICATIONS & DOSAGE
Stable, maturity-onset nonketotic diabetes mellitus uncontrolled by diet alone and previously untreated—
Adults: initially, 250 mg P.O. daily before breakfast; may increase dose q 5 to 7 days (by 250 to 500 mg) as needed to maximum 1.5 g daily, divided b.i.d. to t.i.d. before meals.
*To replace insulin therapy—*if insulin dose is less than 20 units daily, insulin may be stopped and oral therapy started with 250 mg P.O. daily, before breakfast, increased as above if needed. If insulin dose is 20 to 40 units daily, start oral therapy with 250 mg P.O. daily, before breakfast, while reducing insulin dose 25% to 30% daily or every other day, depending on response to oral therapy.

SIDE EFFECTS
Blood: *bone marrow aplasia.*
GI: nausea, heartburn, vomiting.
Metabolic: sodium loss, *hypoglycemia.*
Skin: rash, pruritus, facial flushing.
Other: hypersensitivity reactions.

INTERACTIONS
Alcohol, corticosteroids, dextrothyroxine, estrogens, glucagon, rifampin, thiazide diuretics, thyroxine: decreased hypoglycemic response. Monitor blood glucose.
Anabolic steroids, clofibrate, guanethidine, halofenate, MAO inhibitors, phenylbutazone, salicylates, sulfonamides, oral anticoagulants: increased hypoglycemic activity. Monitor blood glucose.
Metoprolol, propranolol, clonidine: prolonged hypoglycemic effect and masked symptoms of hypoglycemia. Use together cautiously.

NURSING CONSIDERATIONS
• Contraindicated in treatment of juvenile, growth-onset, brittle, and severe diabetes; in diabetes mellitus adequately controlled by diet and in maturity-onset diabetes complicated by ketosis, acidosis, diabetic coma, Raynaud's gangrene, renal or hepatic impairment, thyroid or other endocrine dysfunction. Use cautiously in sulfonamide hypersensitivity.
• Instruct patient about nature of disease; importance of following therapeutic regimen and adhering to specific diet, weight reduction, exercise, personal hygiene, and avoiding infection; how and when to test for glycosuria and ketonuria; recognition of hypoglycemia.
• Be sure patient knows that therapy relieves symptoms but doesn't cure disease.
• Patient transferring from another

oral sulfonylurea antidiabetic drug usually needs no transition period.

• Monitor patient transferring from insulin therapy to an oral antidiabetic for urinary glucose and ketones at least t.i.d.; patient may require hospitalization during transition.

• During periods of increased stress, such as infection, fever, surgery, or trauma, patient may require insulin therapy. Monitor patient closely for hyperglycemia in these situations.

• Advise patient to avoid moderate to large intake of alcohol; Antabuse reaction possible.

chlorpropamide

Chloromide♦♦, Chloronase♦♦, Diabinese♦, Novopropamide♦♦, Stabinol♦♦

INDICATIONS & DOSAGE

Stable, maturity-onset nonketotic diabetes mellitus uncontrolled by diet alone and previously untreated—
Adults: 250 mg P.O. daily with breakfast or in divided doses if GI disturbances occur. First dosage increase may be made after 5 to 7 days, then dose may be increased q 3 to 5 days by 50 to 125 mg, if needed, to maximum 750 mg daily. Start with dose of 100 to 125 mg in older patients.
*To change from insulin to oral therapy—*If insulin dose less than 40 units daily, insulin may be stopped and oral therapy started as above. If insulin dose is 40 units or more daily, start oral therapy as above with insulin dose reduced 50%. Further insulin reductions should be made according to patient response.

SIDE EFFECTS

Blood: *bone marrow aplasia.*
GI: nausea, heartburn, vomiting,
GU: tea-colored urine.

Metabolic: prolonged hypoglycemia, *dilutional hyponatremia.*
Skin: rash, pruritus, facial flushing.
Other: *hypersensitivity reactions.*

INTERACTIONS

Alcohol, corticosteroids, dextrothyroxine, glucagon, rifampin, thiazide diuretics: decreased hypoglycemic response. Monitor blood glucose.
Anabolic steroids, chloramphenicol, clofibrate, guanethidine, halofenate, MAO inhibitors, phenylbutazone, salicylates, sulfonamides, oral anticoagulants: increased hypoglycemic activity. Monitor blood glucose.
Metoprolol, propranolol, clonidine: prolonged hypoglycemic effect and masked symptoms of hypoglycemia. Use together cautiously.

NURSING CONSIDERATIONS

• Contraindicated in the treatment of juvenile, growth-onset, brittle, and severe diabetes.

• Contraindicated in diabetes mellitus adequately controlled by diet and in maturity-onset diabetes complicated by fever, ketosis, acidosis, diabetic coma, major surgery, severe trauma, Raynaud's gangrene, renal or hepatic impairment, thyroid or other endocrine dysfunction.

• Use cautiously in sulfonamide hypersensitivity.

• Instruct patient about nature of the disease; importance of following therapeutic regimen and adhering to specific diet, weight reduction, exercise, personal hygiene, avoiding infection; how and when to test for glycosuria and ketonuria; and recognition of hypoglycemia.

• Make sure patient understands that therapy relieves symptoms but does not cure the disease.

• Side effects, especially hypoglycemia, may be more frequent or severe than with some other sulfonylurea drugs (acetohexamide, tolazamide,

and tolbutamide) because of its long
duration of effect (36 hours).
• If hypoglycemia occurs, patient
should be monitored closely for a
minimum of 3 to 5 days.
• Patient transferring from another
oral sulfonylurea antidiabetic drug
usually needs no transition period.
• Monitor patient transferring from
insulin therapy to an oral antidiabetic
for urinary glucose and ketones at
least t.i.d.; patient may require hospitalization during transition.
• May accumulate in renal insufficiency.
• Advise patient to avoid moderate to
large intake of alcohol; Antabuse reaction possible.

---

glucagon

INDICATIONS & DOSAGE
Coma of insulin-shock therapy—
Adults: 0.5 to 1 mg S.C., I.M., or
I.V. 1 hour after coma develops; may
repeat within 25 minutes, if necessary. In very deep coma, also give
glucose 10% to 50% I.V. for faster response. When patient responds, give
additional carbohydrate immediately.
*Severe insulin-induced hypoglycemia
during diabetic therapy—*
Adults and children: 0.5 to 1 mg
S.C., I.M., or I.V.; may repeat q
20 minutes for 2 doses, if necessary.
If coma persists, give glucose 10% to
50% I.V.

SIDE EFFECTS
GI: nausea, vomiting.
Other: hypersensitivity.

INTERACTIONS
Phenytoin: inhibited glucagon-in-
duced insulin release. Use cautiously.

NURSING CONSIDERATIONS
• Use glucagon only under medical
supervision.
• Hypoglycemic juvenile or unstable
diabetics usually do not respond to
glucagon. Give dextrose I.V. instead.
• It is vital to arouse the patient from
coma as quickly as possible and to
give additional carbohydrates to
prevent secondary hypoglycemic
reactions.
• For I.V. drip infusion, glucagon
compatible with dextrose solution
but forms a precipitate in chloride
solutions.
• Instruct patient and family in
proper glucagon use, recognition of
hypoglycemia, and urgency of calling
doctor immediately in emergencies.
• May be used as diagnostic aid in
radiologic examination of stomach,
duodenum, small bowel, and colon
when hypotonic state would be advan-
tageous.
• May be stored for 3 months at 2° to
15° C. (35.6° to 59° F.) after reconstitution.

---

insulins

regular insulin
Actrapid, Beef Regular Iletin II (acid neutral CZI), Insulin-Toronto (beef or pork)♦♦, Pork Regular Iletin II
regular insulin concentrated
Regular (concentrated) Iletin
prompt insulin zinc suspension
Semilente Iletin, Semilente Insulin♦, Semitard
isophane insulin suspension (NPH)
Beef NPH Iletin II, Lentard, NPH Iletin, NPH Insulin♦♦, Pork NPH Iletin II
insulin zinc suspension
Beef Lente Iletin, Lente Iletin, Lente Insulin♦, Pork Lente Iletin II
globin zinc insulin
protamine zinc insulin suspension (PZI)
Beef Protamine Zinc Iletin II, Pork Protamine Zinc Iletin II, Protamine Zinc Iletin
extended insulin zinc suspension
Ultralente Iletin, Ultralente Insulin♦, Ultratard

INDICATIONS & DOSAGE
Diabetic ketoacidosis (use regular insulin only)—
Adults: 25 to 150 units I.V. stat, then additional doses may be given q 1 hour based on blood sugar levels until patient is out of acidosis; then give S.C. q 6 hours thereafter. Alternative dosage schedule: 50 to 100 units I.V. and 50 to 100 units S.C. stat; additional doses may be given q 2 to 6 hours based on blood sugar levels; or 0.33 units/Kg I.V. bolus, followed by 7 to 10 units/hour I.V. by continuous infusion. Continue infusion until blood sugar drops to 250 mg%, then start S.C. insulin q 6 hours.
Children: 0.5 to 1 unit/Kg divided into 2 doses, 1 given I.V. and the other S.C., followed by 0.5 to 1 unit/Kg I.V. q 1 to 2 hours; or 0.1 unit/Kg I.V. bolus, then 0.1 unit/Kg/hour continuous I.V. infusion until blood sugar drops to 250 mg%, then start S.C. insulin.
Preparation of infusion: add 100 units regular insulin and 1 g albumin to 100 ml 0.9% saline solution. Insulin concentration will be 1 unit/ml.
Ketosis-prone and juvenile-onset diabetes mellitus, diabetes mellitus inadequately controlled by diet and oral hypoglycemics—
Adults and children: therapeutic regimen prescribed by doctor and adjusted according to patient's blood and urine glucose concentrations.

SIDE EFFECTS
Metabolic: *hypoglycemia, hyperglycemia (rebound, or Somogyi, effect).*
Skin: *urticaria.*
Local: *lipoatrophy, lipohypertrophy, itching, swelling, redness, stinging, warmth at site of injection.*
Other: *anaphylaxis.*

INTERACTIONS
Metoprolol, propranolol: hyperglycemia or hypoglycemia may occur. Symptoms of hypoglycemia may be masked. Use together cautiously.
Alcohol, corticosteroids, dextrothyroxine, estrogens, glucagon, rifampin, thiazide diuretics, thyroxine: decreased insulin response. Monitor blood glucose.
Anabolic steroids, clofibrate, guanethidine, halofenate, MAO inhibitors, phenylbutazone, salicylates, sulfonamides, oral anticoagulants: increased insulin response. Monitor for blood glucose.

NURSING CONSIDERATIONS
• Use only regular insulin in patients with circulatory collapse, diabetic ketoacidosis, or hyperkalemia. Do not use regular insulin concentrated, I.V.

Do not use intermediate or long-acting insulins for coma or other emergency requiring rapid drug action.

• During 1980, more purified forms of insulin became available. These new, highly purified forms may require dosage adjustment in patients previously stabilized on insulin. Observe closely until dosage is established.

• Accuracy of measurement is very important, especially with regular insulin concentrated.

• With regular insulin concentrated, a deep secondary hypoglycemic reaction may occur 18 to 24 hours after injection.

• Dosage is always expressed in USP units.

• Regular, intermediate, and long-acting insulin may be mixed to meet patient's needs. All components should have same concentration.

• Store insulin in cool area. Refrigeration desirable but not essential, except with regular insulin concentrated.

• Don't use insulin that has changed color.

• Check expiration date on vial before using contents.

• Administration route is S.C. because absorption rate and pain are less than with I.M. injections. Ketosis-prone juvenile-onset, severely ill, and newly diagnosed diabetics with very high blood sugar levels may require hospitalization and I.V. treatment with regular fast-acting insulin. Ketosis-resistant diabetics may be treated as outpatients with intermediate-acting insulin and instructions on how to alter dosage according to self-performed urine glucose determinations.

• Press but do not rub site after injection. Rotate injection sites. Chart sites to avoid overuse of one area. However, unstable diabetics may achieve better control if injection site is rotated within same anatomic region.

• To mix insulin suspension, swirl vial gently or rotate between palms. Don't shake vigorously.

• Insulin requirements increase, sometimes drastically, in pregnant diabetics, then decline immediately postpartum.

• Be sure patient knows that therapy relieves symptoms but doesn't cure disease.

• Tell patient about nature of disease, importance of following therapeutic regimen and specific diet, weight reduction, exercise, personal hygiene, avoiding infection, and timing of injection and eating. Teach that urine tests are essential guides to dosage and success of therapy; important to recognize hypoglycemic symptoms because insulin-induced hypoglycemia is hazardous and may cause brain damage if prolonged; most side effects are self-limiting and temporary.

• Advise patient to wear medical I.D. always; to carry ample insulin supply and syringes on trips; to have carbohydrates (lump of sugar or candy) on hand for emergency; to take note of time zone changes for dose schedule when traveling.

• Marijuana may increase insulin requirements.

• U-80 strength no longer certified by Food and Drug Administration. Instruct patient in use of U-100 strength.

---

tolazamide
Tolinase

INDICATIONS & DOSAGE

Stable, maturity-onset nonketotic diabetes mellitus uncontrolled by diet alone and previously untreated—
Adults: initially, 100 mg P.O. daily with breakfast if fasting blood sugar (FBS) under 200 mg%; or 250 mg if FBS is over 200 mg%. May adjust dose at weekly intervals by 100 to

---

Italicized side effects are common or life-threatening.

250 mg. Maximum dose 500 mg
b.i.d.
Elderly or debilitated patients: increase dose by 50 to 125 mg at weekly intervals.
To change from insulin to oral therapy—if insulin dose under 20 units daily, insulin may be stopped and oral therapy started at 100 mg P.O. daily with breakfast. If insulin dose is 20 to 40 units daily, insulin may be stopped and oral therapy started at 250 mg P.O. daily with breakfast. If insulin dose is over 40 units daily, decrease insulin dose 50% and start oral therapy at 250 mg P.O. daily with breakfast. Increase doses as above.

SIDE EFFECTS
Blood: *bone marrow aplasia.*
GI: nausea, vomiting.
Metabolic: hypoglycemia.
Skin: rash, urticaria, facial flushing.
Other: hypersensitivity reactions.

INTERACTIONS
Alcohol, corticosteroids, dextrothyroxine, estrogens, glucagon, rifampin, thiazide diuretics, thyroxine: decreased hypoglycemic response. Monitor blood glucose.
Anabolic steroids, clofibrate, guanethidine, halofenate, MAO inhibitors, phenylbutazone, salicylates, sulfonamides, oral anticoagulants: increased hypoglycemic activity. Monitor blood glucose.
Metoprolol, propranolol, clonidine: prolonged hypoglycemic effect and masked symptoms of hypoglycemia. Use together cautiously.

NURSING CONSIDERATIONS
• Contraindicated in juvenile, growth-onset, and severe diabetes mellitus; diabetes mellitus adequately controlled by diet or in maturity-onset diabetes mellitus complicated by fever, ketosis, acidosis, or coma; major surgery; severe trauma; Raynaud's gangrene; renal or hepatic impair-

ment; thyroid or other endocrine dysfunction. Use cautiously in sulfonamide hypersensitivity and in elderly, debilitated, or malnourished patients.
• Instruct patient about nature of disease; importance of following therapeutic regimen and specific diet, weight reduction, exercise, personal hygiene, avoiding infection; how and when to test for glycosuria and ketonuria; and recognition of hypoglycemia.
• Be sure patient knows that therapy relieves symptoms but doesn't cure disease.
• Patient transferring from another oral sulfonylurea antidiabetic drug usually needs no transition period.
• Patient transferring from insulin therapy to an oral hypoglycemic should test urine for glucose and ketones at least t.i.d.; hospitalization may be required during the transition.
• Advise patient to avoid moderate to large intake of alcohol; Antabuse reaction possible.

tolbutamide
Mellitol♦♦, Mobenol♦♦, Neo-Diabetic♦♦, Novobutamide♦♦, Oramide♦♦, Orinase♦, SK-Tolbutamide, Tolbutone♦♦

INDICATIONS & DOSAGE
Stable, maturity-onset nonketotic diabetes mellitus uncontrolled by diet alone and previously untreated—
Adults: initially, 1 to 2 g P.O. daily as single dose or divided b.i.d. to t.i.d. May adjust dose to maximum 3 g daily.
To change from insulin to oral therapy—if insulin dose is under 20 units daily, insulin may be stopped and oral therapy started at 1 to 2 g daily. If insulin dose is 20 to 40 units daily, insulin dose is reduced 30% to 50% and oral therapy started as above. If insulin dose is over 40 units daily, insulin

dose is decreased 20% and oral therapy started as above. Further reductions in insulin dose are based on patient's response to oral therapy.

SIDE EFFECTS
Blood: *bone marrow aplasia.*
GI: nausea, heartburn.
Metabolic: hypoglycemia.
Skin: rash, pruritus, facial flushing.
Other: hypersensitivity reactions.

INTERACTIONS
*Alcohol, corticosteroids, dextrothy-
roxine, estrogens, glucagon, rifampin,
thiazide diuretics, thyroxine:* decreased hypoglycemic response. Monitor blood glucose.
*Anabolic steroids, chloramphenicol,
clofibrate, guanethidine, halofenate,
MAO inhibitors, phenylbutazone,
salicylates, sulfonamides, oral anticoagulants:* increased hypoglycemic
activity. Monitor blood glucose.
Metoprolol, propranolol, clonidine:
prolonged hypoglycemic effect and
masked symptoms of hypoglycemia.
Use together cautiously.

NURSING CONSIDERATIONS
• Contraindicated in juvenile,
growth-onset, brittle, and severe diabetes; diabetes mellitus adequately
controlled by diet or in maturity-onset
diabetes mellitus complicated by fever, ketosis, acidosis, or coma; major
surgery; severe trauma; Raynaud's
gangrene; renal or hepatic impairment; thyroid or other endocrine dysfunction; pregnancy. Use cautiously in
sulfonamide hypersensitivity.
• Instruct patient about nature of disease; importance of following therapeutic regimen and specific diet,
weight reduction, exercise, personal
hygiene, and avoiding infection; how
and when to test for glycosuria and
ketonuria; and recognition of hypoglycemia.
• Be sure patient knows that therapy
relieves symptoms but doesn't cure
disease.
• Patient transferring from another
oral sulfonylurea antidiabetic drug
usually needs no transition period.
• Patient transferring from insulin
therapy to an oral hypoglycemic
should test urine for glucose and ketones at least t.i.d.; hospitalization
may be required during the transition.
• Advise patient to avoid moderate to
large intake of alcohol: Antabuse reaction possible.

Italicized side effects are common or life-threatening.

53

Thyroid hormones

levothyroxine sodium (T$_4$)
liothyronine sodium (T$_3$)
liotrix
thyroglobulin
thyroid USP (desiccated)
thyrotropin

---

levothyroxine sodium (T$_4$)
Eltroxin♦ ♦, Levoid, Levothroid,
LTS, Noroxine, Synthroid♦

INDICATIONS & DOSAGE
*Cretinism in children younger than
1 year*— initially, 0.025 to 0.05 mg
P.O. daily, increased by 0.05 mg P.O.
q 2 to 3 weeks to total daily dose 0.1
to 0.4 mg P.O.
Myxedematous coma—
Adults: 0.2 to 0.5 mg I.V. If no response in 24 hours, additional 0.1 to
0.3 mg I.V. After condition stabilized, oral maintenance.
Thyroid hormone replacement—
Adults: initially, 0.025 mg to 0.1 mg
P.O. daily, increased by 0.05 to
0.1 mg P.O. q 1 to 4 weeks until desired response. Maintenance dose 0.1
to 0.4 mg daily.
Children: initially, maximum
0.05 mg P.O. daily, gradually increased by 0.025 to 0.05 mg P.O.
q 1 to 4 weeks until desired response.

SIDE EFFECTS
Side effects of thyroid hormones are
extensions of their pharmacologic
properties and reflect patient sensitivity to them.
Signs of overdosage:

CNS: *nervousness, insomnia, tremor*.
CV: *tachycardia, palpitations, angina
pectoris*, hypertension.
GI: change in appetite, nausea, diarrhea.
Other: headache, leg cramps, weight
loss, sweating, heat intolerance, fever,
menstrual irregularities.

INTERACTIONS
Cholestyramine: levothyroxine ab-
sorption impaired. Separate doses by
4 to 5 hours.
I.V. phenytoin: free thyroid released.
Monitor for tachycardia.

NURSING CONSIDERATIONS
• Contraindicated in myocardial infarction, thyrotoxicosis (except with
antithyroid drugs), or uncorrected adrenal insufficiency (thyroid hormones
increase tissue demand for adrenocortical hormone and may cause acute
adrenal crisis). Use with extreme caution in angina pectoris, hypertension,
or other cardiovascular disorders;
renal insufficiency; or ischemic states.
• Use carefully in myxedema; patients unusually sensitive to thyroid
hormone.
• Rapid replacement in patients with
arteriosclerosis may precipitate angina, coronary occlusion, or stroke.
Use cautiously in such patients.
• In patients with coronary artery
disease who must receive thyroid, observe carefully for possible coronary
insufficiency if catecholamines must
be given.
• Potentially dangerous; not indicated to relieve vague symptoms, such

as physical and mental sluggishness, irritability, depression, nervousness, ill-defined pains; to treat obesity in euthyroid persons; to treat metabolic insufficiency not associated with thyroid insufficiency; or to treat menstrual disorders or male infertility, unless associated with hypothyroidism.

• When changing from levothyroxine to liothyronine, stop levothyroxine and begin liothyronine. Increase in small increments after residual effects of levothyroxine have disappeared. When changing from liothyronine to levothyroxine, start levothyroxine several days before withdrawing liothyronine to avoid relapse.

• Warn patient to tell doctor at once if chest pain (especially in elderly), palpitations, sweating, nervousness, or other overdosage signs occur. Also notify doctor immediately if any signs of aggravated cardiovascular disease develop (chest pain, dyspnea, tachycardia).

• Tell patient to take thyroid hormones regularly, at the same time each day, to maintain constant hormone levels.

• Suggest morning dosage to prevent insomnia.

• Monitor pulse rate, blood pressure.

• Protect from moisture and light. Prepare I.V. dose immediately before injection.

---

liothyronine sodium (T₃)

Cytomel♦, Cytomine

INDICATIONS & DOSAGE

Cretinism—
Children 3 years and older: 50 to 100 mcg P.O. daily.
Children under 3 years: 5 mcg P.O. daily, increased by 5 mcg q 3 to 4 days until desired response.
Myxedema—
Adults: initially 5 mcg daily, in-

creased by 5 to 10 mcg q 1 or 2 weeks. Maintenance dose 50 to 100 mcg daily.
Nontoxic goiter—
Adults: initially, 5 mcg P.O. daily; may be increased by 12.5 to 25 mcg daily q 1 to 2 weeks. Usual maintenance dose 75 mcg daily.
Elderly: initially, 5 mcg P.O. daily, increased by 5 mcg increments at weekly intervals until desired response.
Children: initially, 5 mcg P.O. daily, increased by 5 mcg increments at weekly intervals until desired response.
Thyroid hormone replacement—
Adults: initially, 25 mcg P.O. daily, increased by 12.5 to 25 mcg q 1 to 2 weeks until satisfactory response. Usual maintenance dose 25 to 75 mcg daily.

SIDE EFFECTS

Side effects of thyroid hormones are extensions of their pharmacologic properties and reflect patient sensitivity to them.
CNS: hyperirritability, *nervousness, insomnia,* twitching, *tremors,* headache.
CV: increased cardiac output, *tachycardia,* cardiac arrhythmias, *angina pectoris,* increased blood pressure, *cardiac decompensation and collapse.*
GI: diarrhea, abdominal cramps, vomiting.
Other: weight loss, heat intolerance, hyperhidrosis, menstrual irregularities; in infants and children—accelerated rate of bone maturation.

INTERACTIONS

Cholestyramine: liothyronine absorption impaired. Separate doses by 4 to 5 hours.
I.V. phenytoin: free thyroid released. Monitor for tachycardia.

NURSING CONSIDERATIONS

• Contraindicated in myocardial in-

Italicized side effects are common or life-threatening.

farction, thyrotoxicosis (except with antithyroid drugs), or uncorrected adrenal insufficiency (thyroid hormones increase tissue demand for adrenocortical hormone and may cause acute adrenal crisis). Use with extreme caution in angina pectoris, hypertension, or other cardiovascular disorders; renal insufficiency; or ischemic states.

• Rapid replacement in patients with arteriosclerosis may precipitate angina, coronary occlusion, or stroke. Use cautiously in such patients.

• In patients with coronary artery disease who must receive thyroid, observe carefully for possible coronary insufficiency if catecholamines must be given.

• Use carefully in myxedema; patients unusually sensitive to thyroid hormone.

• Potentially dangerous; not indicated to relieve vague symptoms, such as physical and mental sluggishness, irritability, depression, nervousness, and ill-defined aches and pains; to treat obesity in euthyroid persons; to treat metabolic insufficiency; or to treat menstrual disorders or male infertility, unless associated with hypothyroidism.

• When changing from levothyroxine to liothyronine, stop levothyroxine and begin liothyronine. Increase in small increments after residual effects of levothyroxine have disappeared. When changing from liothyronine to levothyroxine, start levothyroxine several days before withdrawing liothyronine to avoid relapse.

• Warn patient to tell doctor at once if chest pain (especially in elderly), palpitations, sweating, nervousness, or other overdosage signs occur. Also notify doctor immediately if any signs of aggravated cardiovascular disease develop (chest pain, dyspnea, tachycardia).

• Tell patient to take thyroid hormones regularly, at the same time each day, to maintain constant hormone levels.

• Suggest morning dosage to prevent insomnia.

• Monitor pulse rate, blood pressure.

---

liotrix
Euthroid, Thyrolar♦

INDICATIONS & DOSAGE
Hypothyroidism— dosages must be individualized to approximate the deficit in the patient's thyroid secretion.
Adults and children: initially, 15 mg to 30 mg P.O. daily, increasing by 15 mg to 30 mg q 1 to 2 weeks to desired response; increments in children's dose q 2 weeks.
Elderly: initially, 15 mg to 30 mg. Usual adult dose doubled q 6 to 8 weeks to desired response.

SIDE EFFECTS
Side effects of thyroid hormones are extensions of their pharmacologic properties and reflect patient sensitivity to them.
CNS: hyperirritability, *nervousness, insomnia,* twitching, *tremors.*
CV: increased cardiac output, *tachycardia,* cardiac arrhythmia, *angina pectoris,* increased blood pressure, *cardiac decompensation and collapse.*
GI: diarrhea, abdominal cramps, vomiting.
Other: weight loss, menstrual irregularities, heat intolerance, hyperhidrosis; infants and children—accelerated rate of bone maturation.

INTERACTIONS
Cholestyramine: liotrix absorption impaired. Separate doses by 4 to 5 hours.
I.V. phenytoin: free thyroid released. Monitor for tachycardia.

NURSING CONSIDERATIONS
• Contraindicated in myocardial in-

farction, thyrotoxicosis (except with antithyroid drugs), or uncorrected adrenal insufficiency (thyroid hormones increase tissue demand for adrenocortical hormone and may cause acute adrenal crisis). Use with extreme caution in angina pectoris, hypertension, or other cardiovascular disorders; renal insufficiency; or ischemic states.

• Rapid replacement in patients with arteriosclerosis may precipitate angina, coronary occlusion, or stroke. Use cautiously in such patients.

• Use carefully in myxedema; patients are unusually sensitive to thyroid hormone.

• In patients with coronary artery disease who must receive thyroid, observe carefully for possible coronary insufficiency if catecholamines must be given. Also observe carefully during surgery, since cardiac arrhythmias can be precipitated.

• Potentially dangerous; not indicated to relieve vague symptoms, such as physical and mental sluggishness, irritability, depression, nervousness, ill-defined pains; to treat obesity in euthyroid persons; to treat metabolic insufficiency not associated with thyroid insufficiency; or to treat menstrual disorders or male infertility, unless associated with hypothyroidism.

• Tell patient to take thyroid hormones regularly, at the same time each day, preferably before breakfast, to maintain constant hormone levels.

• Warn patient to tell doctor at once if chest pain (especially in elderly), palpitations, sweating, nervousness, or other overdosage signs occur. Also notify doctor immediately if any signs of aggravated cardiovascular disease develop (chest pain, dyspnea, tachycardia).

• The two commercially prepared liotrix drugs contain different amounts of each ingredient; do not change from one brand to the other without considering the differences in

potency: Thyrolar-½ contains 25 mcg T_4 and 6.25 mcg T_3; Euthroid-½ contains 30 mcg T_4 and 7.5 mcg T_3.

• Monitor pulse rate, blood pressure.

• Protect from heat, light, moisture.

---

thyroglobulin
Proloid♦

INDICATIONS & DOSAGE
Cretinism and juvenile hypothyroidism—
Children 1 year and older: dosage may approach adult dose (60 to 180 mg P.O. daily), depending on response.
Children 4 to 12 months: 60 to 80 mg P.O. daily.
Children 1 to 4 months: initially, 15 to 30 mg P.O. daily, increased at 2-week intervals. Usual maintenance dose 30 to 45 mg P.O. daily.
Hypothyroidism or myxedema—
Adults: initially, 15 to 30 mg P.O. daily, increased by 15 to 30 mg at 2-week intervals until desired response. Usual maintenance dose 60 to 180 mg P.O. daily, as a single dose.
Elderly: initially 7.5 to 15 mg P.O. daily; the dose is doubled at 6- to 8-week intervals until desired response is obtained.

SIDE EFFECTS
Side effects of thyroid hormones are extensions of their pharmacologic properties and reflect patient sensitivity to them.
CNS: hyperirritability, *nervousness, insomnia,* twitching, *tremors,* headache.
CV: increased cardiac output, *tachycardia,* cardiac arrhythmias, *angina pectoris,* increased blood pressure, *cardiac decompensation and collapse.*
GI: diarrhea, abdominal cramps, vomiting.
Other: weight loss, heat intolerance, hyperhidrosis, menstrual irregulari-

---

Italicized side effects are common or life-threatening.

ties; in infants and children—accelerated rate of bone maturation.

INTERACTIONS

Cholestyramine: thyroglobulin absorption impaired. Separate doses by 4 to 5 hours.
I.V. phenytoin: free thyroid released. Monitor for tachycardia.

NURSING CONSIDERATIONS

• Contraindicated in myocardial infarction, thyrotoxicosis (except with antithyroid drugs), or uncorrected adrenal insufficiency (thyroid hormones increase tissue demand for adrenocortical hormone and may cause acute adrenal crisis). Use with extreme caution in angina pectoris, hypertension, or other cardiovascular disorders; renal insufficiency; or ischemic states.
• In patients with coronary artery disease who must receive thyroid, observe carefully for possible coronary insufficiency if catecholamines must be given.
• Use carefully in myxedema; patients unusually sensitive to thyroid hormone.
• Potentially dangerous; not indicated to relieve vague symptoms, such as physical and mental sluggishness, irritability, depression, nervousness, and ill-defined pains; to treat obesity in euthyroid persons; to treat metabolic insufficiency not associated with thyroid insufficiency; or to treat menstrual disorders or male infertility, unless associated with hypothyroidism.
• Tell patient to take thyroid hormones regularly, at the same time each day, to maintain constant hormone levels.
• Warn patient to tell doctor at once if chest pain (especially in elderly), palpitations, sweating, nervousness, or other signs of overdosage occur. Also notify doctor immediately if any signs of aggravated cardiovascular

disease develop (chest pain, dyspnea, tachycardia).
• Suggest morning dosage to prevent insomnia.
• Monitor pulse rate, blood pressure.

---

thyroid USP (desiccated)
Dathroid, Delcoid, S-P-T, Thyrar, Thyro-Teric

INDICATIONS & DOSAGE

Adult hypothyroidism—
Adults: initially, 60 mg P.O. daily, increased by 60 mg q 30 days until desired response. Usual maintenance dose 60 to 180 mg P.O. daily, as a single dose.
Elderly: 7.5 to 15 mg P.O. daily; dose is doubled at 6- to 8-week intervals.
Adult myxedema—
Adults: 16 mg P.O. daily. May double dose q 2 weeks to maximum 120 mg.
Cretinism and juvenile hypothyroidism—
Children 1 year and older: dosage may approach adult dose (60 to 180 mg) daily, depending on response.
Children 4 to 12 months: 30 to 60 mg P.O. daily.
Children 1 to 4 months: initially, 15 to 30 mg P.O. daily, increased at 2-week intervals. Usual maintenance dose 30 to 45 mg P.O. daily.

SIDE EFFECTS

Side effects of thyroid hormones are extensions of their pharmacologic properties and reflect patient sensitivity to them.
CNS: *hyperirritability, nervousness, insomnia,* twitching, tremors, headache.
CV: increased cardiac output, *tachycardia,* cardiac arrhythmias, *angina pectoris,* increased blood pressure, *cardiac decompensation and collapse.*

GI: diarrhea, abdominal cramps, vomiting.
Other: weight loss, heat intolerance, hyperhidrosis, menstrual irregularities; in infants and children—accelerated rate of bone maturation.

INTERACTIONS
Cholestyramine: thyroid absorption impaired. Separate doses by 4 to 5 hours.
I.V. phenytoin: free thyroid released. Monitor for tachycardia.

NURSING CONSIDERATIONS
• Contraindicated in myocardial infarction, thyrotoxicosis (except with antithyroid drugs), or uncorrected adrenal insufficiency (thyroid hormones increase tissue demand for adrenocortical hormone and may cause acute adrenal crisis). Use with extreme caution in angina pectoris, hypertension, or other cardiovascular disorders; renal insufficiency; or ischemic states.
• In patients with coronary artery disease who must receive thyroid, observe carefully for possible coronary insufficiency if catecholamines must be given.
• Potentially dangerous; not indicated to relieve vague symptoms, such as physical and mental sluggishness, irritability, depression, nervousness, ill-defined pains; to treat obesity in euthyroid persons; to treat metabolic insufficiency not associated with thyroid insufficiency; or to treat menstrual disorders or male infertility, unless associated with hypothyroidism.
• Tell patient to take thyroid hormones regularly, at the same time each day, to maintain constant hormone levels.
• Warn patient to tell doctor at once if chest pain (especially in elderly), palpitations, sweating, nervousness, or other signs of overdosage occur. Also notify doctor immediately if any signs of aggravated cardiovascular

disease develop (chest pain, dyspnea, tachycardia).
• Suggest morning dosage to prevent insomnia.
• Monitor pulse rate and blood pressure.
• In children, sleeping pulse and basal morning temperature are guides to treatment.

---

thyrotropin
Thyrotron♦♦, Thytropar♦

INDICATIONS & DOSAGE
Diagnosis of thyroid cancer remnant with ^{131}I *after surgery*—10 international units I.M. or S.C. for 3 to 7 days.
Differential diagnosis of primary and secondary hypothyroidism—10 units I.M. or S.C. for 1 to 3 days.
In PBI or ^{131}I *uptake determinations for differential diagnosis of subclinical hypothyroidism or low thyroid reserve*—10 units I.M. or S.C.
Therapy of thyroid carcinoma (local or metastatic) with ^{131}I—10 units I.M. or S.C. for 3 to 8 days.
To determine thyroid status of patient receiving thyroid—10 units I.M. or S.C. for 1 to 3 days.

SIDE EFFECTS
CNS: headache.
CV: *tachycardia,* atrial fibrillation, *angina pectoris, congestive failure,* hypotension.
GI: nausea, vomiting.
Other: thyroid hyperplasia (large doses), fever, menstrual irregularities, allergic reactions (postinjection flare, urticaria, *anaphylaxis*).

INTERACTIONS
None significant.

NURSING CONSIDERATIONS
• Contraindicated in coronary thrombosis, untreated Addison's disease.

Italicized side effects are common or life-threatening.

Use cautiously in angina pectoris, cardiac failure, hypopituitarism, adrenocortical suppression.

• Purified thyrotropic hormone (TSH) is isolated from bovine anterior pituitary. It stimulates the formation and secretion of thyroid hormone and increases thyroidal uptake of iodine: May cause thyroid hyperplasia.

• Diagnostic use: to identify subclinical hypothyroidism or low thyroid reserve, to evaluate need for thyroid therapy, to distinguish between primary and secondary hypothyroidism, and to detect thyroid remnants and metastases of thyroid carcinoma.

• Therapeutic use: management of certain types of thyroid carcinoma and resulting metastases, and in conjunction with radioactive ^{131}I to enhance uptake of ^{131}I by the thyroid.

• 3-day dosage schedule may be used in long-standing pituitary myxedema or with prolonged use of thyroid medication.

54

Thyroid hormone antagonists

iodine
radioactive iodine (sodium
    iodide) ^{131}I
methimazole
propylthiouracil

---

iodine
Potassium Iodide Solution, U.S.P.;
Sodium Iodide, U.S.P.; Strong Iodine
Solution, U.S.P. (Lugol's Solution),
containing 5% iodine and 10% potas-
sium iodide

INDICATIONS & DOSAGE
Preparation for thyroidectomy—
Adults and children: Strong Iodine
Solution, U.S.P., 0.1 to 0.3 ml t.i.d.,
or Potassium Iodide Solution, U.S.P.,
5 drops in water t.i.d. after meals for
2 to 3 weeks before surgery.
Thyroid crisis—
Adults and children: Strong Iodine
Solution, U.S.P., 1 ml in water P.O.
t.i.d. after meals in refractory cases;
Sodium Iodide, U.S.P., 250 to 500 mg
(or up to 2 g) daily, slow I.V. infusion
with antithyroid drugs and propranolol.

SIDE EFFECTS
EENT: acute rhinitis, inflammation
of salivary glands, periorbital edema,
conjunctivitis, hyperemia.
GI: burning, irritation, *nausea,* vom-
iting, *metallic taste.*
Skin: acneiform rash, mucous mem-
brane ulceration.
Other: fever, frontal headache; with
I.V. use (sodium iodide): acute io-

dism, *colloidoclastic shock,* pulmonary edema.

INTERACTIONS
Lithium carbonate: hypothyroidism
may occur. Use with caution.

NURSING CONSIDERATIONS
• Contraindicated in tuberculosis, iodide hypersensitivity, hyperkalemia,
after meals that contain excessive
starch; in laryngeal edema, swelling
of salivary glands.
• Generally use I.V. route only if
patient is vomiting or cannot receive
anything by mouth. Some prefer I.V.
route to prevent GI side effects, especially during critical time at beginning
of treatment.
• Dilute oral doses in milk to prevent
gastric irritation, to hydrate the patient, and to mask the very salty taste.
• Tell patient to ask doctor about using iodized salt and eating shellfish
during treatment.
• Warn patient that sudden withdrawal may precipitate thyroid storm.
• Store in light-resistant container.
• Give iodides through straw to avoid
tooth discoloration.
• Usually given with other antithyroid drugs.

---

radioactive iodine (sodium iodide) ^{131}I

INDICATIONS & DOSAGE
Hyperthyroidism—
Adults: usual dose is 4 to 10 millicu-

ries P.O. Dose based on estimated weight of thyroid gland and thyroid uptake. Treatment may be repeated after 6 weeks, according to serum thyroxine levels.
Thyroid cancer—
Adults: 50 to 150 millicuries P.O. Dose based on estimated malignant thyroid tissue and metastatic tissue as determined by total body scan. Dose may be repeated according to clinical status.

SIDE EFFECTS
EENT: radiation thyroiditis.
Endocrine: hypothyroidism, exacerbation of hyperthyroidism symptoms.

INTERACTIONS
Lithium carbonate: hypothyroidism may occur. Use with caution.

NURSING CONSIDERATIONS
• Contraindicated in pregnancy and lactation unless used to treat thyroid cancer.
• Stop all antithyroid medications, thyroid preparations, and iodine-containing preparations 1 week before 131I dose. If medications are not stopped, patient may receive thyroid-stimulating hormone for 3 days prior to 131I. When treating women of child-bearing age, give dose during menstruation or within 7 days after menstruation.
• Treatment for hyperthyroidism may be administered as outpatient.
• Patient must be hospitalized for thyroid cancer treatment.
• After therapy for hyperthyroidism, patient should not resume antithyroid drugs, but should continue propranolol or other drugs used to treat symptoms of hyperthyroidism until onset of full 131I effect (usually 6 weeks).
• Monitor thyroid function with serum thyroxine levels.
• After dose for hyperthyroidism, patient's urine and saliva are slightly

radioactive for 24 hours. Tell patient to avoid coughing or expectorating.
• After dose for thyroid cancer, patient's urine and saliva remain radioactive for 3 days. Isolate patient and observe following precautions: pregnant personnel should not take care of patient; use disposable eating utensils and linens; stress good bathroom habits (urine may be flushed down toilet). Limit contact with patient to 30 minutes per shift per person the first day. May increase time to 1 hour second day and longer on third day.

---

methimazole
Tapazole

INDICATIONS & DOSAGE
Hyperthyroidism—
Adults: 5 mg P.O. t.i.d. if mild; 10 to 15 mg P.O. t.i.d. if moderately severe; and 20 mg P.O. t.i.d. if severe. Continue until patient euthyroid, then start maintenance dose of 5 mg daily to t.i.d. Maximum dose 150 mg daily.
Children: 0.4 mg/Kg/day divided q 8 hours. Continue until patient euthyroid, then start maintenance dose of 0.2 mg/Kg/day divided q 8 hours.
Preparation for thyroidectomy—
Adults and children: same doses as for hyperthyroidism until patient is euthyroid; then iodine is added for 10 days before surgery.
Thyrotoxic crisis—
Adults and children: same doses as for hyperthyroidism, with concomitant iodine therapy and propranolol.

SIDE EFFECTS
Blood: *agranulocytosis,* leukopenia, granulopenia, thrombocytopenia (appear to be dose-related).
CNS: headache, drowsiness, vertigo.
GI: diarrhea, nausea, vomiting (may be dose-related).
Skin: rash, urticaria, skin discoloration.

Other: arthralgia, myalgia, salivary gland enlargement, loss of taste, drug fever, jaundice, lymphadenopathy.

INTERACTIONS
None significant.

NURSING CONSIDERATIONS
• Use cautiously in pregnancy. Pregnant women may require less drug as pregnancy progresses. Monitor thyroid function studies closely. Thyroid may be added to regimen. Drugs may be stopped during last few weeks of pregnancy.
• Watch for signs of hypothyroidism (mental depression, cold intolerance, hard, nonpitting edema). Dose may need to be adjusted.
• Monitor CBC periodically to detect impending leukopenia, thrombocytopenia, and agranulocytosis.
• Warn patient to report immediately fever, sore throat, or mouth sores (possible signs of developing agranulocytosis). Agranulocytosis can develop too rapidly to be detected by periodic blood cell counts. Tell him also to report immediately skin eruptions (sign of hypersensitivity).
• Drug should be stopped if severe rash or enlarged cervical lymph nodes develop.
• Tell patient to ask doctor about using iodized salt and eating shellfish during treatment.
• Warn patient against over-the-counter cough medicines; many contain iodine.
• Give with meals to reduce GI side effects.
• Store in light-resistant container.

---

propylthiouracil (PTU)
Propyl-Thyracil♦ ◆

INDICATIONS & DOSAGE
Hyperthyroidism—
Adults: 100 mg P.O. t.i.d.; up to

300 mg q 8 hours has been used in severe cases. Continue until patient euthyroid, then start maintenance dose of 100 mg daily to t.i.d.
Children over 10 years: 100 mg P.O. t.i.d. Continue until patient euthyroid, then start maintenance dose of 25 mg t.i.d. to 100 mg b.i.d.
Children 6 to 10 years: 50 to 150 mg P.O. divided doses q 8 hours.
Preparation for thyroidectomy—
Adults and children: same doses as for hyperthyroidism, with iodine added 10 days before surgery.
Thyrotoxic crisis—
Adults and children: same doses as for hyperthyroidism, with concomitant iodine therapy and propranolol.

SIDE EFFECTS
Blood: *agranulocytosis,* leukopenia, thrombocytopenia (appear to be dose-related).
CNS: headache, drowsiness, vertigo.
EENT: visual disturbances.
GI: diarrhea, *nausea, vomiting* (may be dose-related).
Skin: rash, urticaria, skin discoloration, pruritus.
Other: arthralgia, myalgia, salivary gland enlargement, loss of taste, drug fever, lymphadenopathy, jaundice.

INTERACTIONS
None significant.

NURSING CONSIDERATIONS
• Use cautiously in pregnancy. Pregnant women may require less drug as pregnancy progresses. Monitor thyroid function studies closely. Thyroid may be added to regimen. Drugs may be stopped during last few weeks of pregnancy.
• Watch for signs of hypothyroidism (mental depression, cold intolerance, hard, nonpitting edema). Dose may need to be adjusted.
• Monitor CBC periodically to detect impending leukopenia, thrombocytopenia, and agranulocytosis.

Italicized side effects are common or life-threatening.

• Warn patient to report immediately fever, sore throat, or mouth sores (possible signs of developing agranulocytosis). Agranulocytosis can develop too rapidly to be detected by periodic blood cell counts. Tell him also to report immediately skin eruptions (sign of hypersensitivity).

• Drug should be stopped if severe rash or enlarged cervical lymph nodes develop.

• Tell patient to ask doctor about using iodized salt and eating shellfish during treatment.

• Warn patient against over-the-counter cough medicines; many contain iodine.

• Give with meals to reduce GI side effects.

• Store in light-resistant container.

55

Pituitary hormones

corticotropin (ACTH)
cosyntropin
desmopressin
lypressin
somatropin (human growth
   hormone)
vasopressin
vasopressin tannate

corticotropin (ACTH)
Acthar♦, Acton "X"♦♦, Cortigel-80,
Cortrophin Gel, Cortrophin Zinc,
Duracton♦♦, H.P. Acthar Gel

INDICATIONS & DOSAGE
*Diagnostic test of adrenocortical
function—*
Adults: up to 80 units I.M. or S.C. in
divided doses; or a single dose of repository form; or 10 to 25 units
(aqueous form) in 500 ml dextrose 5%
in water I.V. over 8 hours, between
blood samplings.

   Individual dosages generally vary
with adrenal glands' sensitivity to
stimulation as well as with specific
disease. Infants and younger children
require larger doses per kilogram than
do older children and adults.
For therapeutic use—
Adults: 40 units S.C. or I.M. in 4 divided doses (aqueous); 40 units q 12
to 24 hours (gel or repository form).

SIDE EFFECTS
CNS: *convulsions, dizziness,* papilledema, headache, *euphoria, insomnia,* mood swings, personality
changes, depression, psychosis.

CV: hypertension, congestive heart
failure.
EENT: cataracts, glaucoma.
GI: *peptic ulcer with perforation and
hemorrhage,* pancreatitis, abdominal
distention, ulcerative esophagitis,
nausea, vomiting.
GU: menstrual irregularities.
Metabolic: *sodium and fluid retention,* calcium and potassium loss,
hypokalemic alkalosis, negative nitrogen balance.
Skin: *impaired wound healing,* thin
fragile skin, petechiae, ecchymoses,
facial erythema, increased sweating,
acne, hyperpigmentation, allergic
skin reactions, hirsutism.
Other: muscle weakness, steroid my-
opathy, loss of muscle mass, osteoporosis, vertebral compression fractures, cushingoid state, suppression of
growth in children, *activation of latent
diabetes mellitus,* progressive increase
in antibodies, and loss of ACTH stim-
ulatory effect.

INTERACTIONS
None significant.

NURSING CONSIDERATIONS
• Contraindicated in scleroderma,
osteoporosis, systemic fungal infections, ocular herpes simplex, recent
surgery, peptic ulcer, congestive heart
failure, hypertension, sensitivity to
pork and pork products, concomitant
smallpox vaccination, adrenocortical
hyperfunction or primary insufficiency, or Cushing's syndrome. Use
with caution in pregnant women or
nursing mothers and in women of

childbearing age; patients being immunized; latent tuberculosis or tuberculin reactivity; hypothyroidism; cirrhosis; infection (use anti-infective therapy during and after ACTH treatment); acute gouty arthritis (limit ACTH treatment to a few days, and use conventional therapy during and for several days after ACTH treatment); emotional instability or psychotic tendencies; diabetes; abscess; pyogenic infections; renal insufficiency; myasthenia gravis.

• ACTH treatment should be preceded by verification of adrenal responsiveness and test for hypersensitivity and allergic reactions.
• ACTH should be adjunctive; not sole therapy.
• Unusual stress may require additional use of rapidly acting corticosteroids. Reduce ACTH dosage gradually when reduction is possible to minimize induced adrenocortical insufficiency. Reinstitute therapy if stressful situation occurs shortly after stopping drug.
• Watch neonates of ACTH-treated mothers for signs of hypoadrenalism. Carefully check growth and development of children on long-term ACTH therapy.
• Counteract edema by low-sodium, high-potassium intake; nitrogen loss by high-protein diet; and psychotic changes by reducing ACTH dosage or administering sedatives.
• ACTH may mask signs of chronic disease and decrease host resistance and ability to localize infection.
• Note and record weight changes, fluid exchange, and resting blood pressures until minimal effective dose is achieved.
• Refrigerate reconstituted solution and use within 24 hours.

cosyntropin
Cortrosyn♦, Synacthen Depot♦♦

INDICATIONS & DOSAGE
Diagnostic test of adrenocortical function—
Adults and children: 0.25 to 1 mg I.M. or I.V. (unless label prohibits I.V. administration) between blood samplings.
Children younger than 2 years: 0.125 mg I.M. or I.V.

SIDE EFFECTS
Skin: pruritus.
Other: flushing.

INTERACTIONS
None significant.

NURSING CONSIDERATIONS
• Use cautiously in hypersensitivity to natural corticotropin.
• Drug is synthetic duplication of the biologically active part of the ACTH molecule. It is less likely to produce sensitivity than natural ACTH from animal sources.

desmopressin
DDAVP

INDICATIONS & DOSAGE
Nonnephrogenic diabetes insipidus, temporary polyuria and polydipsia associated with pituitary trauma—
Adults: 0.1 to 0.4 ml intranasally daily in 1 to 3 doses. Adjust morning and evening doses separately for adequate diurnal rhythm of water turnover.
Children 3 months to 12 years: 0.05 to 0.3 ml intranasally daily in 1 or 2 doses.

SIDE EFFECTS
CNS: headache.

CV: slight rise in blood pressure at high dosage.
EENT: nasal congestion, rhinitis.
GI: nausea.
GU: vulval pain.
Other: flushing.

INTERACTIONS
None significant.

NURSING CONSIDERATIONS
• Use with caution in patients with coronary artery insufficiency or hypertensive cardiovascular disease.
• Adjust fluid intake to reduce risk of water intoxication and sodium depletion, especially in very young or old patients.
• Titrate dosage to allow patient sufficient sleep.
• Give intranasally only.
• Overdose may cause oxytocic or vasopressor activity. Withhold drug until effects subside. Furosemide may be used if fluid retention is excessive.
• Not effective in nephrogenic diabetes insipidus.
• Drug of choice for central (neurogenic) diabetes insipidus.

lypressin
Diapid

INDICATIONS & DOSAGE
Nonnephrogenic diabetes insipidus—
Adults and children: 1 or 2 sprays (approximately 2 USP posterior pituitary pressor units per spray) in either or both nostrils q.i.d. and an additional dose at bedtime, if needed, to prevent nocturia. If usual dosage is inadequate, increase frequency rather than number of sprays.

SIDE EFFECTS
CNS: headache, dizziness.
EENT: nasal congestion or ulceration, irritation, pruritus of nasal passages, rhinorrhea, conjunctivitis.

GI: heartburn due to drip of excess spray into pharynx, abdominal cramps, more frequent bowel movements.
GU: possible transient fluid retention due to overdose.
Skin: hypersensitivity reaction.

INTERACTIONS
None significant.

NURSING CONSIDERATIONS
• Use with caution in patients with coronary artery disease.
• Particularly useful if diabetes insipidus is unresponsive to other therapy, or if antidiuretic hormones of animal origin cause adverse reactions.
• Nasal congestion, allergic rhinitis, or upper respiratory infections may diminish drug absorption and require larger dose or adjunctive therapy.
• Inadvertent inhalation of spray may cause tightness in chest, coughing, and transient dyspnea.
• Test patients sensitive to antidiuretic hormone for sensitivity to lypressin.
• To administer a uniform, well-diffused spray, hold bottle upright while patient in vertical position holds head upright.

somatropin (human growth hormone)
Asellacrin, Crescormon

INDICATIONS & DOSAGE
Growth failure due to pituitary growth hormone deficiency—
Children: 2 IU (1 ml) I.M. 3 times weekly, with a minimum of 48 hours between injections. Double dose if growth doesn't exceed 1 inch in 6 months, or recheck diagnosis. Discontinue when epiphyses close, patient achieves satisfactory adult height, or patient fails to respond.

Italicized side effects are common or life-threatening.

SIDE EFFECTS
GU: excess calcium in urine.
Metabolic: hyperglycemia.

INTERACTIONS
None significant.

NURSING CONSIDERATIONS
• Contraindicated in closed epiphyses or intracranial lesions. Use with caution in diabetics or in patients with family history of diabetes. Regular urine testing for glycosuria should be done.
• S.C. administration not recommended.
• Should be used only by doctors experienced in treating patients with pituitary growth hormonal deficiency.
• Concurrent thyroid hormone or androgen therapy may accelerate epiphyseal closure and limit duration of somatropin treatment.
• Monitor bone age progression annually.
• Store powder at or below room temperature.
• Reconstitute with 5 ml of bacteriostatic water per 10-I U vial. Refrigerate unused portion; discard after 1 month. Rotate injection sites.

---

vasopressin
Pitressin Synthetic♦
vasopressin tannate
Pitressin Tannate

INDICATIONS & DOSAGE
Nonnephrogenic, nonpsychogenic diabetes insipidus—
Adults: 5 to 10 units I.M. or S.C. b.i.d. to q.i.d., p.r.n.; or intranasally (spray or cotton balls) in individualized doses, based on response. For chronic therapy, inject 2.5 to 5 units Pitressin Tannate in oil suspension I.M. every 2 to 3 days.
Children: 2.5 to 10 units I.M. or S.C. b.i.d. to q.i.d., p.r.n.; or intra-

nasally (spray or cotton balls) in individualized doses. For chronic therapy, inject 1.25 to 2.5 units Pitressin Tannate in oil suspension I.M. every 2 to 3 days.
Postop abdominal distention—
Adults: 5 units I.M. initially, then q 3 to 4 hours, increasing dose to 10 units, if needed. Reduce dose for children proportionately.
To expel gas before abdominal X-ray—
Adults: inject 10 units S.C. at 2 hours, then again at 30 minutes before X-ray. Enema before first dose may also help to eliminate gas.
Upper GI tract hemorrhage (intra-arterial)—
Adults: 0.2 to 0.4 units/minute. Do not use Tannate in oil suspension.

SIDE EFFECTS
CNS: tremor, dizziness, headache.
CV: *angina in patients with vascular disease,* vasoconstriction. Large doses may cause hypertension, electrocardiographic changes.
GI: abdominal cramps, nausea, vomiting, diarrhea, intestinal hyperactivity.
GU: uterine cramps, anuria.
Skin: circumoral pallor.
Other: water intoxication (drowsiness, listlessness, headache, confusion, weight gain), hypersensitivity reactions (urticaria, angioneurotic edema, bronchoconstriction, fever, rash, wheezing, dyspnea, *anaphylaxis*), sweating.

INTERACTIONS
Lithium, demeclocycline: reduced antidiuretic activity. Use together cautiously.
Chlorpropamide: increased antidiuretic response. Use together cautiously.

NURSING CONSIDERATIONS
• Contraindicated in chronic nephritis with nitrogen retention. Use cautiously in children, the elderly,

pregnant women, and patients with epilepsy, migraine, asthma, cardiovascular disease, or fluid overload.
• Never inject during first stage of labor; may cause ruptured uterus.
• Monitor specific gravity of urine.
• Shake tannate in oil thoroughly or warm in hands to make suspension uniform before withdrawing I.M. injection dose. Use absolutely dry syringe to avoid dilution.
• Give with 1 to 2 glasses of water to reduce side effects and to improve therapeutic response.
• To prevent convulsions, coma, and death, observe patient closely for early signs of water intoxication.

• Overhydration more likely with long-acting tannate oil suspension than with aqueous vasopressin solution.
• Use minimum effective dose to reduce side effects.
• May be used for transient polyuria due to antidiuretic hormone deficiency related to neurosurgery or head injury.
• Synthetic desmopressin is sometimes preferred because of longer duration and less frequent side effects.

56

Parathyroid and parathyroid-like agents

calcitonin (Salmon)
calcitriol
dihydrotachysterol (AT-10)
etidronate disodium
parathyroid hormone

---

calcitonin (Salmon)
Calcimar♦

INDICATIONS & DOSAGE
Paget's disease of bone (osteitis deformans)—
Adults: initially, 100 MRC units daily, S.C. or I.M. Maintenance: 50 to 100 units daily or every other day.
Hypercalcemia—
Adults: 100 to 400 MRC units I.M. once or twice daily.

SIDE EFFECTS
CNS: headaches.
GI: transient nausea with or without vomiting, diarrhea.
GU: transient diuresis.
Metabolic: hyperglycemia
Local: inflammation at injection site, skin rashes.
Other: *facial flushing;* hypocalcemia; swelling, tingling, and tenderness of hands; unusual taste sensation; *anaphylaxis.*

INTERACTIONS
None significant.

NURSING CONSIDERATIONS
• Not recommended for nursing mothers, or women who are or may become pregnant.

• Periodic serum alkaline phosphatase and 24-hour urinary hydroxyproline levels should be determined to evaluate drug effect.
• Skin test is usually done before beginning therapy.
• Systemic allergic reactions possible since hormone is protein. Keep epinephrine handy when administering.
• Facial flushing and warmth occur in 20% to 30% of all patients within minutes of injection; usually last about 1 hour. Reassure patient.
• Monitor calcium levels closely. Watch for signs of hypercalcemic relapse: bone pain, renal calculi, polyuria, anorexia, nausea, vomiting, thirst, constipation, lethargy, bradycardia, muscle hypotonicity, pathologic fracture, psychosis, and coma.
• Periodic examinations of urine sediment advisable.
• Actually derived from the thyroid gland, not the parathyroid.
• Refrigerate solution.

---

calcitriol (1,25-dihydroxycholecalciferol)
Rocaltrol

INDICATIONS & DOSAGE
Management of hypocalcemia in patients undergoing chronic dialysis—
Adults: initially, 0.25 mcg daily. Dosage may be increased by 0.25 mcg/day at 2- to 4-week intervals. Maintenance: 0.25 mcg every other day up to 0.5 to 1.25 mcg daily.

SIDE EFFECTS
Vitamin D intoxication associated with hypercalcemia:
CNS: headache, somnolence.
EENT: conjunctivitis, photophobia, rhinorrhea.
GI: nausea, vomiting, constipation, metallic taste, dry mouth.
GU: polyuria.
Other: weakness, bone and muscle pain.

INTERACTIONS
None significant.

NURSING CONSIDERATIONS
• Contraindicated in hypercalcemia or vitamin D toxicity. Withhold all preparations containing vitamin D in patients taking calcitriol. Not recommended in nursing mothers. Use cautiously in patients on digitalis; hypercalcemia may precipitate cardiac arrhythmias.
• Monitor serum calcium; serum calcium times serum phosphate should not exceed 70. During titration, determine serum levels twice weekly. If hypercalcemia occurs, discontinue, but resume after serum calcium returns to normal. Patient should receive adequate daily intake of calcium, 1,000 mg RDA.
• Protect from heat and light.
• Instruct patient to adhere to diet and calcium supplementation and to avoid unapproved nonprescription drugs.
• Most potent form of vitamin D available.

---

dihydrotachysterol (AT-10)
Hytakerol♦

INDICATIONS & DOSAGE
Familial hypophosphatemia—
Adults and children: 0.5 to 2 mg P.O. daily. Maintenance: 0.3 to 1.5 mg daily.

Hypocalcemia associated with hypoparathyroidism and pseudohypoparathyroidism—
Adults: initially, 0.8 to 2.4 mg P.O. daily for several days. Maintenance: 0.2 to 2 mg daily, as required for normal serum calcium levels. Average dose 0.6 mg daily.
Children: initially, 1 to 5 mg for several days. Maintenance: 0.5 to 1.5 mg daily, as required for normal serum calcium levels.
Renal osteodystrophy in chronic uremia—
Adults: 0.1 to 0.6 mg P.O. daily.

SIDE EFFECTS
Vitamin D intoxication associated with hypercalcemia:
CNS: headache, somnolence.
EENT: conjunctivitis, photophobia, rhinorrhea.
GI: nausea, vomiting, constipation, metallic taste, dry mouth.
GU: polyuria.
Other: weakness, bone and muscle pain.

INTERACTIONS
None significant.

NURSING CONSIDERATIONS
• Contraindicated in hypercalcemia, hypocalcemia associated with renal insufficiency and hyperphosphatemia, renal stones, hypersensitivity to vitamin D, and in nursing mothers.
• Monitor serum and urinary calcium. Watch for signs of hypercalcemia.
• Adequate dietary calcium intake is necessary; usually supplemented with 10 to 15 g oral calcium lactate or gluconate daily.
• Report hypercalcemia reactions to doctor.
• 1 mg equal to 120,000 units ergocalciferol (vitamin D_2).
• Store in tightly closed, light-resistant containers. Don't refrigerate.

Italicized side effects are common or life-threatening.

etidronate disodium
Didronel

INDICATIONS & DOSAGE
Symptomatic Paget's disease—
Adults: 5 mg/Kg/day P.O. as a single dose 2 hours before a meal with water or juice. Patient should not eat for 2 hours after dose. May give up to 10 mg/Kg/day in severe cases. Maximum dose 20 mg/Kg/day.
Heterotrophic ossification in spinal cord injuries—
Adults: 20 mg/Kg/day for 2 weeks, then 10 mg/Kg/day for 10 weeks. Total treatment period 12 weeks.

SIDE EFFECTS
GI: (seen most frequently at 20 mg/Kg/day) diarrhea, increased frequency of bowel movements, nausea.
Other: increased or recurrent bone pain at Pagetic sites, pain at previously asymptomatic sites, increased risk of fracture, elevated serum phosphate.

INTERACTIONS
None significant.

NURSING CONSIDERATIONS
• Use cautiously in enterocolitis, impaired renal function.
• Therapy should not last more than 6 months. After 3 months, resume if needed. Don't give longer than 3 months at doses above 10 mg/Kg/day.
• Don't give drug with food, milk, or antacids; may reduce absorption.
• Monitor renal function before and during therapy.
• Monitor drug effect by serum alkaline phosphatase and urinary hydroxyproline excretion (both lowered if therapy effective).
• Tell patient that improvement may not occur for up to 3 months but may continue for months after drug is stopped. Stress importance of good nutrition, especially high in calcium and vitamin D.

parathyroid hormone
Para-thor-mone, Paroidin

INDICATIONS & DOSAGE
Acute hypoparathyroidism with tetany—
Adults: 20 to 40 units S.C., I.M., or I.V. q 12 hours.
Infants: (with transient congenital idiopathic true hypoparathyroidism) 25 to 50 units I.M. q 12 hours for 1 to 3 days.

SIDE EFFECTS
Allergic: *anaphylactic reactions* (parathyroid hormone is a foreign protein).
Other: hypercalcemia (muscle weakness, bone and flank pain), lethargy, headache, anorexia, nausea, vomiting, diarrhea, abdominal cramps, vertigo, tinnitus, ataxia.

INTERACTIONS
None significant.

NURSING CONSIDERATIONS
• Contraindicated in hypercalcemia, hypercalciuria, tetany unrelated to parathyroid failure, and I.V. administration when serum calcium levels are above normal. Use cautiously in sarcoidosis, renal or cardiac disease, and in digitalized patients.
• Rarely used because calcium salts often effective alone.
• S.C. injections may produce moderate inflammatory reaction.
• Therapy lasts only a few days; patients may soon become refractory to treatment.
• If given I.V., skin-test for sensitivity. If positive, desensitize patient.
• Keep epinephrine injection handy when giving parathyroid hormone.

• Monitor serum calcium and serum phosphate levels, intake and output.
• Know and watch for signs of hypoparathyroidism and calcium deficiency. Test for Chvostek's and Trousseau's signs. Watch for drug-induced hypercalcemia.

• Use seizure precautions in patients with calcium deficiency: padded rails, soft light, no irritating noises until normal calcium level restored.
• Do not dilute with saline solution as a precipitate will form.
• Store ampuls at 2° to 8° C. (36° to 46° F.); do not freeze.

57

Diuretics

acetazolamide
acetazolamide sodium
bendroflumethiazide
benzthiazide
chlorothiazide
chlorthalidone
cyclothiazide
dichlorphenamide
ethacrynate sodium
ethacrynic acid
ethoxzolamide
furosemide
hydrochlorothiazide
hydroflumethiazide
mannitol
mercaptomerin sodium
methazolamide
methyclothiazide
metolazone
polythiazide
quinethazone
spironolactone
triamterene
trichlormethiazide
urea

acetazolamide
Acetazolam♦♦, Diamox♦, Diamox
Sequels♦, Hydrazol
acetazolamide sodium
Diamox Parenteral♦

INDICATIONS & DOSAGE
Narrow-angle glaucoma—
Adults: 250 mg q 4 hours; or 250 mg
b.i.d. P.O., I.M., or I.V. for short-
term therapy.
Edema, in congestive heart failure—

Adults: 250 to 375 mg P.O., I.M., or
I.V. daily in a.m.
Children: 5 mg/Kg daily in a.m.
Epilepsy—
Children: 8 to 30 mg/Kg daily P.O.,
I.M., or I.V. in divided doses.
Open-angle glaucoma—
Adults: 250 mg daily to 1 g P.O.,
I.M., or I.V. divided q.i.d.

SIDE EFFECTS
Blood: *aplastic anemia,* hemolytic
anemia, leukopenia.
CNS: drowsiness, paresthesias.
EENT: transient myopia.
GI: nausea, vomiting, anorexia.
GU: crystalluria, renal calculi.
Metabolic: *hyperchloremic acidosis,*
hypokalemia, asymptomatic hyperuri-
cemia
Skin: rash.

INTERACTIONS
None significant.

NURSING CONSIDERATIONS
• Contraindicated in long-term therapy for chronic noncongestive narrow-angle glaucoma; also in depressed sodium or potassium blood
serum levels, renal or hepatic disease
or dysfunction, adrenal gland failure,
and hyperchloremic acidosis. Use
cautiously in respiratory acidosis, emphysema, chronic lung disease, or
patients receiving other diuretics.
• Monitor intake/output and electrolytes, especially serum potassium.
When used in diuretic therapy, consult with doctor and dietitian to provide high-potassium diet.

• Weigh patient daily. Rapid weight loss may cause hypotension.

• Diuretic effect decreased when acidosis occurs but can be reestablished by withdrawing drug for several days and then restarting, or by utilizing intermittent administration schedules.

• Reconstitute 500 mg vial with at least 5 ml sterile water for injection. Use within 24 hours of reconstitution.

• I.M. injection painful because of alkalinity of solution. Direct I.V. administration preferred (100 to 500 mg/minute).

• Elderly patients are especially susceptible to excessive diuresis.

• May cause false positive urine protein tests by alkalinizing the urine.

• A carbonic anhydrase inhibitor. Its acidotic effects limit usefulness for daily treatment of edema.

---

bendroflumethiazide
Naturetin◆

INDICATIONS & DOSAGE
Edema, hypertension—
Adults: 5 to 20 mg P.O. daily or b.i.d. in divided doses.
Children: initially, 0.1 to 0.4 mg/Kg daily in 1 or 2 doses.
Maintenance: 0.05 to 0.1 mg/Kg daily in 1 or 2 doses.

SIDE EFFECTS
Blood: *aplastic anemia, agranulocytosis,* leukopenia, thrombocytopenia.
CV: *volume depletion and dehydration,* orthostatic hypotension.
GI: anorexia, nausea, pancreatitis.
Hepatic: hepatic encephalopathy.
Metabolic: *hypokalemia, asymptomatic hyperuricemia, hyperglycemia and impairment of glucose tolerance,* fluid and electrolyte imbalances including dilutional hyponatremia and hypochloremia, metabolic alkalosis, hypercalcemia, gout.

Skin: dermatitis, photosensitivity, rash.
Other: hypersensitivity reactions such as pneumonitis and vasculitis.

INTERACTIONS
Cholestyramine, colestipol: intestinal absorption of thiazides decreased. Keep doses as separate as possible.
Diazoxide: increased antihypertensive, hyperglycemic, hyperuricemic effects. Use together cautiously.

NURSING CONSIDERATIONS
• Contraindicated in anuria; hypersensitivity to other thiazides or other sulfonamide-derived drugs. Use cautiously in severe renal disease, impaired hepatic function.

• Monitor intake/output, weight, and serum electrolytes regularly. Monitor serum creatinine and BUN levels regularly. Not effective if these levels are more than twice normal.

• Monitor serum potassium levels; consult with doctor and dietitian to provide high-potassium diet. Watch for signs of hypokalemia (e.g., muscle weakness, cramps). May use with potassium-sparing diuretic to prevent potassium loss.

• Monitor blood sugar. Check insulin requirements in diabetics. May treat severe hyperglycemia with oral antidiabetic agents.

• Monitor blood uric acid levels, especially in patients with a history of gout.

• Give in a.m. to prevent nocturia.

• Elderly patients are especially susceptible to excessive diuresis.

• In hypertension, therapeutic response may be delayed several days.

• A thiazide diuretic.

---

benzthiazide
Aquapres, Aqua-Scrip, Aquasec, Aquatag, Diretic, Exna♦, Hydrex, Lemazide, Marazide, Proaqua, Ridema, S-Aqua, Urazide

INDICATIONS & DOSAGE
Edema—
Adults: 50 to 200 mg P.O. daily or in divided doses.
Children: 1 to 4 mg/Kg daily in 3 divided doses.
Hypertension—
Adults: 50 mg P.O. daily b.i.d., t.i.d., or q.i.d., adjusted to patient's response.

SIDE EFFECTS
Blood: *aplastic anemia, agranulocytosis,* leukopenia, thrombocytopenia.
CV: *volume depletion and dehydration,* orthostatic hypotension.
GI: anorexia, nausea, pancreatitis.
Hepatic: hepatic encephalopathy.
Metabolic: *hypokalemia, asymptomatic hyperuricemia, hyperglycemia and impairment of glucose tolerance,* fluid and electrolyte imbalances including dilutional hyponatremia and hypochloremia, metabolic alkalosis, hypercalcemia, gout.
Skin: dermatitis, photosensitivity, rash.
Other: hypersensitivity reactions such as pneumonitis and vasculitis.

INTERACTIONS
Cholestyramine, colestipol: intestinal absorption of thiazides decreased. Keep doses as separate as possible.
Diazoxide: increased antihypertensive, hyperglycemic, hyperuricemic effects. Use together cautiously.

NURSING CONSIDERATIONS
• Contraindicated in anuria; hypersensitivity to other thiazides or other sulfonamide-derived drugs. Use cautiously in severe renal disease, impaired hepatic function.
• Monitor intake/output, weight, and serum electrolytes regularly. Monitor serum potassium levels; consult with doctor and dietitian to provide high-potassium diet. Watch for signs of hypokalemia (e.g., muscle weakness, cramps). May use with potassium-sparing diuretic to prevent potassium loss.
• Monitor serum creatinine and BUN levels regularly. Not effective if these levels are more than twice normal.
• Monitor blood sugar. Check insulin requirements in diabetics. May treat severe hyperglycemia with oral antidiabetic agents.
• Monitor blood uric acid levels, especially in patients with a history of gout.
• Give in a.m. to prevent nocturia.
• Elderly patients are especially susceptible to excessive diuresis.
• In hypertension, therapeutic response may be delayed several days.
• A thiazide diuretic.

chlorothiazide
Diuril♦, Ro-Chlorozide, SK-Chlorothiazide

INDICATIONS & DOSAGE
Diuresis—
Children over 6 months: 20 mg/Kg P.O. or I.V. daily in divided doses.
Children under 6 months: may require 30 mg/Kg P.O. or I.V. daily in 2 divided doses.
Edema, hypertension—
Adults: 500 mg to 2 g P.O. or I.V. daily or in 2 divided doses.

SIDE EFFECTS
Blood: *aplastic anemia, agranulocytosis,* leukopenia, thrombocytopenia.
CV: *volume depletion and dehydration,* orthostatic hypotension.
GI: anorexia, nausea, pancreatitis.

Hepatic: hepatic encephalopathy.
Metabolic: *hypokalemia, asymptomatic hyperuricemia, hyperglycemia and impairment of glucose tolerance,* fluid and electrolyte imbalances including dilutional hyponatremia and hypochloremia, metabolic alkalosis, hypercalcemia, gout.
Skin: dermatitis, photosensitivity, rash.
Other: hypersensitivity reactions such as pneumonitis and vasculitis.

INTERACTIONS
Cholestyramine, colestipol: intestinal absorption of thiazides decreased. Keep doses as separate as possible.
Diazoxide: increased antihypertensive, hyperglycemic, hyperuricemic effects. Use together cautiously.

NURSING CONSIDERATIONS
• Contraindicated in anuria; hypersensitivity to other thiazides or other sulfonamide-derived drugs; impaired hepatic function; progressive hepatic disease. Use cautiously in severe renal disease.
• Monitor intake/output, weight, and serum electrolytes regularly.
• Monitor potassium levels; consult with doctor and dietitian to provide high-potassium diet. Watch for signs of hypokalemia (e.g., muscle weakness, cramps). May use with potassium-sparing diuretic to prevent potassium loss.
• Monitor blood sugar. Check insulin requirements in diabetics. May treat severe hyperglycemia with oral antidiabetic agents.
• Monitor serum creatinine and BUN levels regularly. Not effective if these levels are more than twice normal.
• Monitor blood uric acid levels, especially in patients with a history of gout.
• Watch for decreased calcium excretion, progressive renal impairment.
• Only injectable thiazide. For I.V. use only—not I.M. or S.C. Reconsti-

tute with 18 ml of sterile water for injection/500 mg vial. May store reconstituted solutions at room temperature up to 24 hours. Compatible with intravenous dextrose or sodium chloride solutions.
• Avoid I.V. infiltration; can be very painful.
• Give in a.m. to prevent nocturia.
• In hypertension, therapeutic response may be delayed several days.
• Elderly patients are especially susceptible to excessive diuresis.
• A thiazide diuretic.
• The only thiazide available in liquid form.

chlorthalidone
Hygroton♦, Novothalidone♦♦, Uridon♦♦

INDICATIONS & DOSAGE
Edema, hypertension—
Adults: 25 to 100 mg P.O. daily, or 100 mg 3 times weekly or on alternate days. Occasionally, up to 200 mg daily may be needed.
Children: 2 mg/Kg P.O. 3 times weekly.

SIDE EFFECTS
Blood: *aplastic anemia, agranulocytosis,* leukopenia, thrombocytopenia.
CV: *volume depletion and dehydration,* orthostatic hypotension.
GI: anorexia, nausea, pancreatitis.
Hepatic: hepatic encephalopathy.
Metabolic: *hypokalemia, asymptomatic hyperuricemia, hyperglycemia and impairment of glucose tolerance,* fluid and electrolyte imbalances including dilutional hyponatremia and hypochloremia, metabolic alkalosis, hypercalcemia, gout.
Skin: dermatitis, photosensitivity, rash.
Other: hypersensitivity reactions such as pneumonitis and vasculitis.

Italicized side effects are common or life-threatening.

INTERACTIONS

Cholestyramine, colestipol: intestinal absorption of thiazides decreased. Keep doses as separate as possible. *Diazoxide:* increased antihypertensive, hyperglycemic, hyperuricemic effects. Use together cautiously.

NURSING CONSIDERATIONS

• Contraindicated in anuria; hypersensitivity to thiazides or other sulfonamide-derived drugs. Use cautiously in severe renal disease, progressive hepatic disease, impaired hepatic function.
• Monitor intake/output, weight, and serum electrolytes regularly.
• Monitor serum potassium levels; consult with doctor and dietitian to provide high-potassium diet. Watch for signs of hypokalemia (e.g., muscle weakness, cramps). May use with potassium-sparing diuretic to prevent potassium loss.
• Monitor serum creatinine and BUN levels regularly. Not effective if these levels are more than twice normal.
• Monitor blood uric acid levels, especially in patients with a history of gout.
• Monitor blood sugar. Check insulin requirements in diabetics. May treat severe hyperglycemia with oral antidiabetic agents.
• In hypertension, therapeutic response may be delayed several days.
• Give in a.m. to prevent nocturia.
• Elderly patients are especially susceptible to excessive diuresis.
• A thiazide-like diuretic.

---

cyclothiazide
Anhydron

INDICATIONS & DOSAGE

Edema—
Adults: 1 to 2 mg P.O. daily. May be used on alternate days as maintenance dose.

Children: 0.02 to 0.04 mg/Kg P.O. daily.
Hypertension—
Adults: 2 mg P.O. daily; up to 2 mg b.i.d. or t.i.d.

SIDE EFFECTS

Blood: *aplastic anemia, agranulocytosis,* leukopenia, thrombocytopenia.
CV: *volume depletion and dehydration,* orthostatic hypotension.
GI: anorexia, nausea, pancreatitis.
Hepatic: hepatic encephalopathy.
Metabolic: *hypokalemia, asymptomatic hyperuricemia, hyperglycemia and impairment of glucose tolerance,* fluid and electrolyte imbalances including dilutional hyponatremia and hypochloremia, metabolic alkalosis, hypercalcemia, gout.
Skin: dermatitis, photosensitivity, rash.
Other: hypersensitivity reactions such as pneumonitis and vasculitis.

INTERACTIONS

Cholestyramine, colestipol: intestinal absorption of thiazides decreased. Keep doses as separate as possible. *Diazoxide:* increased antihypertensive, hyperglycemic, hyperuricemic effects. Use together cautiously.

NURSING CONSIDERATIONS

• Contraindicated in anuria; hypersensitivity to other thiazides or other sulfonamide-derived drugs. Use cautiously in severe renal disease, impaired hepatic function, progressive hepatic disease.
• Monitor intake/output, weight, and serum electrolytes regularly.
• Monitor serum potassium levels; consult with doctor and dietitian to provide high-potassium diet. Watch for signs of hypokalemia (e.g., muscle weakness, cramps). May use with potassium-sparing diuretic to prevent potassium loss.
• Monitor blood sugar. Check insulin requirements in diabetics. May treat

severe hyperglycemia with oral anti-diabetic agents.
• Monitor serum creatinine and BUN levels regularly. Not effective if these levels are more than twice normal.
• Monitor blood uric acid levels, especially in patients with a history of gout.
• In hypertension, therapeutic response may be delayed several days.
• Give in a.m. to prevent nocturia.
• Elderly patients are especially susceptible to excessive diuresis.
• A thiazide diuretic.

dichlorphenamide
Daranide♦, Oratrol

INDICATIONS & DOSAGE
Adjunct in glaucoma—
Adults: initially, 100 to 200 mg P.O., followed by 100 mg q 12 hours until desired response obtained. Maintenance: 25 to 50 mg P.O. daily b.i.d. or t.i.d. Give miotics concomitantly.

SIDE EFFECTS
Blood: *aplastic anemia,* hemolytic anemia, leukopenia.
CNS: drowsiness, paresthesias.
EENT: transient myopia.
GI: nausea, vomiting, anorexia.
GU: crystalluria, renal calculi.
Metabolic: *hyperchloremic acidosis,* hypokalemia, asymptomatic hyperuricemia.
Skin: rash.

INTERACTIONS
None significant.

NURSING CONSIDERATIONS
• Contraindicated in hepatic insufficiency, renal failure, adrenocortical insufficiency, hyperchloremic acidosis, depressed sodium or potassium levels, severe pulmonary obstruction with inability to increase alveolar ventilation, Addison's disease. Long-

term use contraindicated in severe, absolute, or chronic noncongestive narrow-angle glaucoma. Use cautiously in respiratory acidosis, monitoring blood pH and blood gases.
• Monitor electrolytes, especially serum potassium in initial treatment. Usually no problem in long-term glaucoma therapy unless risk for hypokalemia from other causes; potassium supplements may be necessary.
• May cause false positive results in urine protein tests.
• A carbonic anhydrase inhibitor.

ethacrynate sodium
Sodium Edecrin
ethacrynic acid
Edecrin♦

INDICATIONS & DOSAGE
Acute pulmonary edema—
Adults: 50 to 100 mg of ethacrynate sodium I.V. slowly over several minutes.
Edema—
Adults: 50 to 200 mg P.O. daily. Refractory cases may require up to 200 mg b.i.d.
Children: initial dose 25 mg P.O., cautiously, increased in 25 mg increments daily until desired effect is obtained.

SIDE EFFECTS
Blood: *agranulocytosis,* thrombocytopenia.
CV: *volume depletion and dehydration, orthostatic hypotension.*
EENT: transient deafness with too rapid I.V. injection.
GI: abdominal discomfort and pain.
Metabolic: *hypokalemia, hypochloremic alkalosis, asymptomatic hyperuricemia, fluid and electrolyte imbalances including dilutional hyponatremia and hypochloremia, hypocalcemia, hypomagnesemia,* hypergly-

cemia and impairment of glucose tolerance.
Skin: dermatitis.

INTERACTIONS
Aminoglycoside antibiotics: potentiated ototoxic side effects of both ethacrynic acid and aminoglycosides. Use together cautiously.

NURSING CONSIDERATIONS
• Contraindicated in anuria and infants. Use cautiously in electrolyte abnormalities. If electrolyte imbalance, azotemia, or oliguria develops, may require discontinuing drug.
• Monitor intake/output, weight, and serum electrolytes regularly.
• Monitor serum potassium levels; consult with doctor and dietitian to provide high-potassium diet. Watch for signs of hypokalemia (e.g., muscle weakness, cramps).
• I.V. injection painful; may cause thrombophlebitis. Don't give S.C. or I.M. Give slowly through tubing of running infusion over several minutes.
• Salt and potassium chloride supplement may be needed during therapy.
• Reconstitute vacuum vial with 50 ml of 5% dextrose injection or NaCl injection. Discard unused solution after 24 hours. Don't use cloudy or opalescent solutions.
• Elderly patients are especially susceptible to excessive diuresis.
• Give P.O. doses in a.m. to prevent nocturia.
• Monitor blood uric acid levels, especially in patients with history of gout.
• A loop diuretic, especially strong.

ethoxzolamide
Cardrase, Ethamide

INDICATIONS & DOSAGE
Edema (from congestive heart failure)—
Adults: 62.5 to 125 mg P.O. daily in a.m. for 3 consecutive days each week or every other day. Refractory cases may require 250 mg/day.
Glaucoma—
Adults: 62.5 to 250 mg P.O. b.i.d., t.i.d., or q.i.d. Give miotics concomitantly.

SIDE EFFECTS
Blood: *aplastic anemia,* hemolytic anemia, leukopenia.
CNS: drowsiness, paresthesias.
EENT: transient myopia.
GI: nausea, vomiting, anorexia.
GU: crystalluria, renal calculi.
Metabolic: *hyperchloremic acidosis,* hypokalemia, asymptomatic hyperuricemia.
Skin: rash.

INTERACTIONS
None significant.

NURSING CONSIDERATIONS
• Contraindicated in hyperchloremic acidosis, renal failure, hepatic insufficiency, adrenal failure, depressed sodium or potassium blood levels, and long-term therapy for chronic noncongestive narrow-angle glaucoma. Use with caution in advanced pulmonary disease, respiratory acidosis, and concomitantly with other diuretics.
• Monitor electrolytes, especially serum potassium; consult with doctor and dietitian to provide high-potassium diet. Monitor intake/output and weight.
• May cause false positive results in urine protein tests.
• Watch for dehydration, especially in elderly patients.

• A carbonic anhydrase inhibitor. When used on a daily basis for edema, its acidotic effects limit its usefulness.

furosemide
Lasix♦, Novosemide♦♦, Uritol♦♦

INDICATIONS & DOSAGE
Acute pulmonary edema—
Adults: 40 mg I.V. injected slowly; then 40 mg I.V. in 1 to 1½ hours if needed.
Edema—
Adults: 20 to 80 mg P.O. daily in a.m., second dose can be given in 6 to 8 hours; carefully titrated up to 600 mg daily if needed; or 20 to 40 mg I.M. or I.V. Increase by 20 mg q 2 hours until desired response is achieved. I.V. dose should be given slowly over 1 to 2 minutes.
Infants and children: 2 mg/Kg daily; dose increased by 1 to 2 mg/Kg in 6 to 8 hours if needed; carefully titrated up to 6 mg/Kg daily if needed.
Hypertensive crisis, acute renal failure—
Adults: 100 to 200 mg I.V. over 1 to 2 minutes.
Chronic renal failure—
Adults: initially, 80 mg P.O. daily. Increase by 80 to 120 mg daily until desired response is achieved.

SIDE EFFECTS
Blood: *agranulocytosis*, thrombocytopenia.
CV: *volume depletion and dehydration*, orthostatic hypotension.
EENT: transient deafness with too rapid I.V. injection.
GI: abdominal discomfort and pain.
Metabolic: *hypokalemia, hypochloremic alkalosis, asymptomatic hyperuricemia, fluid and electrolyte imbalances including dilutional hyponatremia and hypochloremia, hypocalce-*mia, hypomagnesemia, *hyperglycemia and impairment of glucose tolerance.*
Skin: dermatitis.

INTERACTIONS
Aminoglycoside antibiotics: potentiated ototoxicity. Use together cautiously.
Chloral hydrate: sweating, flushing with I.V. furosemide. Observe patient.
Clofibrate: enhanced furosemide effects. Use cautiously.
Indomethacin: inhibited diuretic response. Use cautiously.

NURSING CONSIDERATIONS
• Use cautiously in cardiogenic shock complicated by pulmonary edema, anuria, hepatic coma, or electrolyte imbalances.
• Potent loop diuretic; can lead to profound water and electrolyte depletion. Monitor blood pressure and pulse during rapid diuresis.
• Sulfonamide-sensitive patients may have allergic reaction to furosemide.
• If oliguria or azotemia increases or develops, may require stopping drug.
• Monitor serum electrolytes, BUN, and CO_2 frequently.
• Monitor serum potassium levels. Watch for signs of hypokalemia (e.g., muscle weakness, cramps). Consult with doctor and dietitian to provide high-potassium diet.
• Monitor blood sugar levels in diabetics. May treat severe hyperglycemia with oral antidiabetic agents.
• Monitor blood uric acid levels, especially in patients with a history of gout.
• Give I.V. doses over 1 to 2 minutes. For doses over 100 mg, give at 10 mg/minute to prevent tinnitus associated with rapid infusion of large doses. In decreased renal function, give I.V. doses at rate of 10 mg/minute or less.
• Don't use parenteral route in in-

fants and children unless oral dosage form is not practical.
- I.M. injection causes transient pain; moderate by using "Z" track to limit leakage into S.C. tissues.
- Give P.O. and I.M. preparations in a.m. to prevent nocturia. Give second doses in early afternoon.
- Elderly patients are especially susceptible to excessive diuresis, with potential for circulatory collapse and thromboembolic complications.
- Store tablets in light-resistant container to prevent discoloration (doesn't affect potency). Don't use discolored (yellow) injectable preparation.
- Promotes calcium excretion. I.V. furosemide often used to treat hypercalcemia.

hydrochlorothiazide
Chlorzide, Diuchlor-H♦♦, Diu-Scrip, Esidrix♦, Hydrid♦♦, HydroAquil♦♦, Hydro Diuril♦, Hydromal, Hydro-Z-25, Hydro-Z-50, Hydrozide♦♦, Hyperetic, Kenazide, Lexor, Neo-Codema♦♦, Novohydrazide♦♦, Oretic, Ro-Hydrazide, Thiuretic, Urozide♦♦, Zide

INDICATIONS & DOSAGE
Edema—
Adults: initially, 25 to 100 mg P.O. daily or intermittently for maintenance to minimize electrolyte imbalance.
Children over 6 months: 2.2 mg/Kg P.O. daily divided b.i.d.
Children under 6 months: up to 3.3 mg/Kg P.O. daily divided b.i.d.
Hypertension—
Adults: 25 to 100 mg P.O. daily or divided dosage. Daily dosage increased or decreased according to blood pressure.

SIDE EFFECTS
Blood: *aplastic anemia, agranulocytosis,* leukopenia, thrombocytopenia.
CV: *volume depletion and dehydration,* orthostatic hypotension.
GI: anorexia, nausea, pancreatitis.
Hepatic: hepatic encephalopathy.
Metabolic: *hypokalemia, asymptomatic hyperuricemia, hyperglycemia and impairment of glucose tolerance,* fluid and electrolyte imbalances including dilutional hyponatremia and hypochloremia, metabolic alkalosis, hypercalcemia, gout.
Skin: dermatitis, photosensitivity, rash.
Other: hypersensitivity reactions such as pneumonitis and vasculitis.

INTERACTIONS
Cholestyramine, colestipol: intestinal absorption of thiazides decreased. Keep doses as separate as possible. *Diazoxide:* increased antihypertensive, hyperglycemic, hyperuricemic effects. Use together cautiously.

NURSING CONSIDERATIONS
- Contraindicated in anuria; hypersensitivity to other thiazides or other sulfonamide derivatives. Use cautiously in severe renal disease, impaired hepatic function, progressive hepatic disease.
- Monitor intake/output, weight, and serum electrolytes regularly.
- Monitor serum potassium levels; consult with doctor and dietitian to provide high-potassium diet. Watch for hypokalemia (e.g., muscle weakness, cramps). May use with potassium-sparing diuretic to prevent potassium loss.
- Monitor serum creatinine and BUN levels regularly. Not effective if these levels are more than twice normal.
- Monitor blood uric acid levels, especially in patients with a history of gout.
- Check insulin requirements in dia-

betics. May treat severe hypergly-
cemia with oral antidiabetic agents.
• In hypertension, therapeutic re-
sponse may be delayed several days.
• Give in a.m. to prevent nocturia.
• Elderly patients are especially sus-
ceptible to excessive diuresis.
• A thiazide diuretic.

---

hydroflumethiazide
Diucardin♦, Saluron

INDICATIONS & DOSAGE
Edema—
Adults: 25 mg to 200 mg P.O. daily in
divided doses. Maintenance doses
may be on intermittent or alternate-
day schedule.
Children: 1 mg/Kg P.O. daily.
Hypertension—
Adults: 50 to 100 mg P.O. daily or
b.i.d.

SIDE EFFECTS
Blood: *aplastic anemia, agranulocytosis,* leukopenia, thrombocytopenia.
CV: *volume depletion and dehydration,* orthostatic hypotension.
GI: anorexia, nausea, pancreatitis.
Hepatic: hepatic encephalopathy.
Metabolic: *hypokalemia, asymptomatic hyperuricemia, hyperglycemia
and impairment of glucose tolerance,*
fluid and electrolyte imbalances including dilutional hyponatremia and
hypochloremia, metabolic alkalosis,
hypercalcemia, gout.
Skin: dermatitis, photosensitivity,
rash.
Other: hypersensitivity reactions
such as pneumonitis and vasculitis.

INTERACTIONS
Cholestyramine, colestipol: intestinal
absorption of thiazides decreased.
Keep doses as separate as possible.
Diazoxide: increased antihypertensive, hyperglycemic, hyperuricemic
effects. Use together cautiously.

NURSING CONSIDERATIONS
• Contraindicated in anuria; hypersensitivity to other thiazides or other
sulfonamide-derived drugs. Use cautiously in severe renal disease, impaired hepatic function, progressive
hepatic disease.
• Monitor intake/output, weight, and
serum electrolytes regularly.
• Monitor serum potassium levels;
consult with doctor and dietitian to
provide high-potassium diet. Watch
for hypokalemia (e.g., muscle weakness, cramps). May use with potassium-sparing diuretic to prevent
potassium loss.
• Monitor serum creatinine and BUN
levels regularly. Not effective if these
levels are more than twice normal.
• Monitor blood uric acid levels, especially in patients with history of
gout.
• Check insulin requirements in diabetics. May treat severe hyperglycemia with oral antidiabetic agents.
• Give in a.m. to prevent nocturia.
• In hypertension, therapeutic response may be delayed several days.
• Elderly patients are especially susceptible to excessive diuresis.
• A long-acting thiazide diuretic.

---

mannitol
Osmitrol♦

INDICATIONS & DOSAGE
Adults, and children over 12:
*Test dose for marked oliguria or sus-
pected inadequate renal function—*
200 mg/Kg or 12.5 g as a 15% or 20%
solution I.V. over 3 to 5 minutes. Response adequate if 30 to 50 ml urine/
hour is excreted over 2 to 3 hours.
Treatment of oliguria— 50 to 100 g
I.V. as a 15% to 20% solution over
90 minutes to several hours.
*Prevention of oliguria or acute renal
failure—* 50 to 100 g I.V. of a concentrated (5% to 25%) solution. Exact

---

Italicized side effects are common or life-threatening.

concentration is determined by fluid requirements.

Edema—100 g as a 10% to 20% solution over 2- to 6-hour period.

To reduce intraocular pressure or intracranial pressure—1.5 to 2 g/Kg as a 15% to 25% solution I.V. over 30 to 60 minutes.

To promote diuresis in drug intoxication—5% to 10% solution continuously up to 200 g I.V., while maintaining 100 to 500 ml urinary output/hour and a positive fluid balance.

SIDE EFFECTS
CNS: rebound increase in intracranial pressure 8 to 12 hours after diuresis, headache, confusion.
CV: *transient expansion of plasma volume during infusion causing circulatory overload and pulmonary edema,* tachycardia, angina-like chest pain.
EENT: blurred vision, rhinitis.
GI: thirst, nausea, vomiting.
GU: urinary retention.
Metabolic: *fluid and electrolyte imbalances, water intoxication, cellular dehydration.*

INTERACTIONS
None significant.

NURSING CONSIDERATIONS
• Contraindicated in anuria, severe pulmonary congestion, frank pulmonary edema, severe congestive heart disease, severe dehydration, metabolic edema, progressive renal disease or dysfunction, progressive heart failure during administration, active intracranial bleeding except during craniotomy.
• Monitor vital signs (including CVP) at least hourly; intake/output hourly (report increasing oliguria); weight daily; renal function; fluid balance; serum and urine Na+ and K+ levels.
• Solution often crystallizes, espe-

cially at low temperatures. To redissolve, warm bottle in hot water bath, shake vigorously. Cool to body temperature before giving. Concentrations greater than 15% have greater tendency to crystallize. Do not use solution with undissolved crystals.
• Infusions should always be given I.V. via an in-line filter.
• Avoid infiltration; observe for inflammation, edema, potential necrosis.
• For maximum pressure reduction before surgery, give 1 to 1½ hours preop.
• Can be used to measure glomerular filtration rate.
• Give frequent mouth care or fluids as permitted to relieve thirst.
• An osmotic diuretic.

---

mercaptomerin sodium
Thiomerin Sodium♦

INDICATIONS & DOSAGE
Edema—
Adults—125 to 250 mg I.M. or S.C. daily. Maintenance with 1 to 2 times weekly dose.
Children: 125 mg/m² I.M.

SIDE EFFECTS
Blood: *agranulocytosis,* leukopenia.
CNS: dizziness, confusion, headache.
CV: volume depletion and dehydration, orthostatic hypotension.
Metabolic: *fluid and electrolyte imbalances including dilutional hyponatremia and hypochloremia, metabolic alkalosis,* asymptomatic hyperuricemia.
Local: pain on injection.
Other: signs of mercury toxicity (albuminuria, hematuria, renal casts, stomatitis, metallic taste, colitis).

INTERACTIONS
None significant.

NURSING CONSIDERATIONS
• Contraindicated in renal insufficiency, acute or subacute nephritis. Use cautiously in impaired hepatic function.
• Rarely used; agents available with less severe side effects.
• Mercurial diuretic. Test for mercury hypersensitivity with 0.5 ml 24 hours before initiating therapy. Watch for signs of mercurialism.
• Monitor urine for albumin, blood cells, and casts. Regularly monitor weight and serum electrolyte levels, especially potassium. Consult with doctor and dietitian to provide high-potassium diet.
• Give in the morning for diuresis within 1 to 2 hours.
• Rotate site of injections, massage gently; avoid edematous or adipose tissue, areas of poor circulation. Do not use I.V.
• Good oral hygiene important to limit or prevent stomatitis.
• Elderly patients are more susceptible to excessive dehydration with potential for circulatory collapse or thromboembolic phenomena.

---

methazolamide
Neptazane

INDICATIONS & DOSAGE
Glaucoma (open-angle, or preop in obstructive or narrow-angle)—
Adults: 50 to 100 mg b.i.d. or t.i.d.

SIDE EFFECTS
Blood: *aplastic anemia,* hemolytic anemia, leukopenia.
CNS: drowsiness, paresthesias.
EENT: transient myopia.
GI: nausea, vomiting, anorexia.
GU: crystalluria, renal calculi.
Metabolic: *hyperchloremic acidosis,* hypokalemia, asymptomatic hyperuricemia
Skin: rash.

INTERACTIONS
None significant.

NURSING CONSIDERATIONS
• Contraindicated in severe or absolute glaucoma; for long-term use in chronic noncongestive narrow-angle glaucoma; in patients with depressed sodium or potassium serum levels, renal or hepatic disease or dysfunction, adrenal gland dysfunction, and hyperchloremic acidosis. Use cautiously in respiratory acidosis, emphysema, chronic lung disease.
• Monitor intake/output, weight, and serum electrolytes frequently.
• May cause false positive urine protein tests by alkalinizing urine.
• A carbonic anhydrase inhibitor.
• Elderly patients are especially susceptible to excessive diuresis.
• Diuretic effect decreases in acidosis.

---

methyclothiazide
Aquatensen, Diuretic♦♦, Enduron

INDICATIONS & DOSAGE
Edema, hypertension—
Adults: 2.5 to 10 mg P.O daily.

SIDE EFFECTS
Blood: *aplastic anemia, agranulocytosis,* leukopenia, thrombocytopenia.
CV: *volume depletion and dehydration,* orthostatic hypotension.
GI: anorexia, nausea, pancreatitis.
Hepatic: hepatic encephalopathy.
Metabolic: *hypokalemia, asymptomatic hyperuricemia, hyperglycemia and impairment of glucose tolerance,* fluid and electrolyte imbalances including dilutional hyponatremia and hypochloremia, metabolic alkalosis, hypercalcemia, gout.
Skin: dermatitis, photosensitivity, rash.
Other: hypersensitivity reactions such as pneumonitis and vasculitis.

Italicized side effects are common or life-threatening.

INTERACTIONS
Cholestyramine, colestipol: intestinal absorption of thiazides decreased. Keep doses as separate as possible.
Diazoxide: increased antihypertensive, hyperglycemic, hyperuricemic effects. Use together cautiously.

NURSING CONSIDERATIONS
• Contraindicated in renal decompensation; anuria; hypersensitivity to other thiazides or other sulfonamide-derived drugs. Use cautiously in potassium depletion, renal disease or dysfunction, impaired hepatic function, progressive hepatic disease.
• Monitor intake/output, weight, and serum electrolytes regularly.
• Monitor serum potassium levels; consult with doctor and dietitian to provide high-potassium diet. Watch for hypokalemia (e.g., muscle weakness, cramps). May use with potassium-sparing diuretic to prevent potassium loss.
• Check insulin requirements in diabetics. May treat severe hyperglycemia with oral antidiabetic agents.
• Monitor serum creatinine and BUN levels regularly. Not effective if these levels are more than twice normal.
• Monitor blood uric acid levels, especially in patients with a history of gout.
• In hypertension, therapeutic response may be delayed several days.
• Give in a.m. to prevent nocturia.
• Elderly patients are especially susceptible to excessive diuresis.
• A thiazide diuretic.

---

metolazone
Diulo, Zaroxolyn♦

INDICATIONS & DOSAGE
Edema (heart failure)—
Adults: 5 to 10 mg P.O. daily.
Edema (renal disease)—
Adults: 5 to 20 mg P.O. daily.

Hypertension—
Adults: 2.5 to 5 mg P.O. daily. Maintenance dose determined by patient's blood pressure.

SIDE EFFECTS
Blood: *aplastic anemia, agranulocytosis,* leukopenia, thrombocytopenia.
CV: *volume depletion and dehydration,* orthostatic hypotension.
GI: anorexia, nausea, pancreatitis.
Hepatic: hepatic encephalopathy.
Metabolic: *hypokalemia, asymptomatic hyperuricemia, hyperglycemia and impairment of glucose tolerance,* fluid and electrolyte imbalances including dilutional hyponatremia and hypochloremia, metabolic alkalosis, hypercalcemia, gout.
Skin: dermatitis, photosensitivity, rash.
Other: hypersensitivity reactions such as pneumonitis and vasculitis.

INTERACTIONS
Cholestyramine, colestipol: intestinal absorption of thiazides decreased. Keep doses as separate as possible.
Diazoxide: increased antihypertensive, hyperglycemic, hyperuricemic effects. Use together cautiously.

NURSING CONSIDERATIONS
• Contraindicated in anuria; hepatic coma or pre-coma; hypersensitivity to thiazides or other sulfonamide-derived drugs. Use cautiously in hyperuricemia or gout and severely impaired renal function.
• Monitor intake/output, weight, and serum electrolytes regularly.
• Monitor serum potassium levels; consult with doctor and dietitian to provide high-potassium diet. Watch for hypokalemia (e.g., muscle weakness, cramps). May use with potassium-sparing diuretic to prevent potassium loss.
• Check insulin requirements in diabetics. May treat severe hyperglycemia with oral antidiabetic agents.

- Monitor blood uric acid levels, especially in patients with a history of gout.
- In hypertension, therapeutic response may be delayed several days.
- Give in a.m. to prevent nocturia.
- Elderly patients are especially susceptible to excessive diuresis.
- A thiazide-related diuretic. However, unlike thiazide diuretics, metolazone is effective in patients with decreased renal function.
- Used as an adjunct in furosemide-resistant edema.

---

polythiazide
Renese♦

INDICATIONS & DOSAGE
Hypertension—
Adults: 2 to 4 mg P.O. daily.
Edema (heart failure, renal failure)—
Adults: 1 to 4 mg P.O. daily.

SIDE EFFECTS
Blood: *aplastic anemia, agranulocytosis,* leukopenia, thrombocytopenia.
CV: *volume depletion and dehydration,* orthostatic hypotension.
GI: anorexia, nausea, pancreatitis.
Hepatic: hepatic encephalopathy.
Metabolic: *hypokalemia, asymptomatic hyperuricemia, hyperglycemia and impairment of glucose tolerance,* fluid and electrolyte imbalances including dilutional hyponatremia and hypochloremia, metabolic alkalosis, hypercalcemia, gout.
Skin: dermatitis, photosensitivity, rash.
Other: hypersensitivity reactions such as pneumonitis and vasculitis.

INTERACTIONS
Cholestyramine, colestipol: intestinal absorption of thiazides decreased. Keep doses as separate as possible.
Diazoxide: increased antihyperten-

sive, hyperglycemic, hyperuricemic effects. Use together cautiously.

NURSING CONSIDERATIONS
- Contraindicated in anuria; hypersensitivity to other thiazides or other sulfonamide-derived drugs. Use cautiously in severe renal disease, impaired hepatic function, allergies.
- Monitor intake/output, weight, and serum electrolytes regularly.
- Monitor serum potassium levels; consult with doctor and dietitian to provide high-potassium diet. Watch for hypokalemia (e.g., muscle weakness, cramps). May use with potassium-sparing diuretic to prevent potassium loss.
- Monitor serum creatinine and BUN levels regularly. Not effective if these levels are more than twice normal.
- Monitor blood uric acid levels, especially in patients with a history of gout.
- Check insulin requirements in diabetics. May treat severe hyperglycemia with oral antidiabetic agents.
- In hypertension, therapeutic response may be delayed several days.
- Give in a.m. to prevent nocturia.
- Elderly patients are especially susceptible to excessive diuresis.
- A long-acting thiazide diuretic.

---

quinethazone
Aquamox♦♦, Hydromox

INDICATIONS & DOSAGE
Edema—
Adults: 50 to 100 mg P.O. daily or 50 mg P.O. b.i.d. Occasionally, up to 150 to 200 mg P.O. daily may be needed.

SIDE EFFECTS
Blood: *aplastic anemia, agranulocytosis,* leukopenia, thrombocytopenia.
CV: *volume depletion and dehydration,* orthostatic hypotension.

Italicized side effects are common or life-threatening.

GI: anorexia, nausea, pancreatitis.
Hepatic: *hepatic encephalopathy.*
Metabolic: *hypokalemia, asymptomatic hyperuricemia, hyperglycemia and impairment of glucose tolerance,* fluid and electrolyte imbalances including dilutional hyponatremia and hypochloremia, metabolic alkalosis, hypercalcemia, gout.
Skin: dermatitis, photosensitivity, rash.
Other: hypersensitivity reactions such as pneumonitis and vasculitis.

INTERACTIONS
Cholestyramine, colestipol: intestinal absorption of thiazides decreased. Keep doses as separate as possible.
Diazoxide: increased antihypertensive, hyperglycemic, hyperuricemic effects. Use together cautiously.

NURSING CONSIDERATIONS
• Contraindicated in anuria; hypersensitivity to quinethazones, thiazides, or other sulfonamide-derived drugs. Use cautiously in severe renal disease, impaired hepatic function, allergies.
• Monitor intake/output, weight, and serum electrolytes regularly.
• Monitor serum potassium levels; consult with doctor and dietitian to provide high-potassium diet. Watch for hypokalemia (e.g., muscle weakness, cramps). May use with potassium-sparing diuretic to prevent potassium loss.
• Monitor serum creatinine and BUN levels regularly. Not effective if these levels are more than twice normal.
• Check insulin requirements in diabetics. May treat severe hyperglycemia with oral antidiabetic agents.
• Monitor blood uric acid levels, especially in patients with a history of gout.
• In hypertension, therapeutic response may be delayed several days.
• Give in a.m. to prevent nocturia.

• Elderly patients are especially susceptible to excessive diuresis.
• A long-acting sulfonamide similar to thiazide diuretics.

spironolactone
Aldactone♦, Altex

INDICATIONS & DOSAGE
Edema—
Adults: 25 to 200 mg P.O. daily in divided doses.
Children: initially, 3.3 mg/Kg P.O. daily in divided doses.
Hypertension—
Adults: 50 to 100 mg P.O. daily in divided doses.
Treatment of diuretic-induced hypokalemia—
Adults: 25 to 100 mg P.O. daily when oral potassium supplements are considered inappropriate.
Detection of primary hyperaldosteronism—
Adults: 400 mg P.O. daily for 4 days (short test) or for 3 to 4 weeks (long test). If hypokalemia and hypertension are corrected, a presumptive diagnosis of primary hyperaldosteronism is made.

SIDE EFFECTS
CNS: headache.
GI: anorexia, nausea, diarrhea.
Metabolic: *hyperkalemia,* dehydration, hyponatremia, transient rise in BUN, acidosis.
Skin: urticaria.
Other: gynecomastia in males, breast soreness and menstrual disturbances in females.

INTERACTIONS
Aspirin: possible blocked spironolactone effect. Watch for diminished spironolactone response.

NURSING CONSIDERATIONS
• Contraindicated in anuria, acute or

progressive renal insufficiency, hyperkalemia. Use cautiously in fluid or electrolyte imbalances, impaired renal function, hepatic disease, pregnancy, lactation. If essential, nursing mother should stop breastfeeding infant.
• Monitor serum potassium levels, electrolytes, intake/output, weight, and blood pressure regularly.
• Potassium-sparing diuretic; useful as an adjunct to other diuretic therapy. Less potent diuretic than thiazide and loop types. Diuretic effect delayed 2 to 3 days when used alone.
• Maximum antihypertensive response may be delayed up to 2 weeks.
• Warn patient to avoid excessive ingestion of potassium-rich foods.
• Elderly patients are more susceptible to excess diuresis.
• Protect drug from light.
• Breast cancer reported in some patients taking spironolactone, but cause-and-effect relationship not confirmed. Warn against taking drug indiscriminately.
• Give with meals to enhance absorption.
• Concomitant potassium supplement can lead to serious hyperkalemia.

triamterene
Dyrenium♦

INDICATIONS & DOSAGE
Diuresis—
Adults: initially, 100 mg P.O. b.i.d. after meals. Total daily dosage should not exceed 300 mg.

SIDE EFFECTS
Blood: megaloblastic anemia related to low folic acid levels.
CNS: dizziness.
CV: hypotension.
EENT: sore throat.
GI: dry mouth, nausea, vomiting.
Metabolic: *hyperkalemia,* dehydra-

tion, hyponatremia, transient rise in BUN, acidosis.
Skin: photosensitivity, rash.
Other: *anaphylaxis,* muscle cramps.

INTERACTIONS
None significant.

NURSING CONSIDERATIONS
• Contraindicated in anuria, severe or progressive renal disease or dysfunction, severe hepatic disease, hyperkalemia. Use cautiously in impaired hepatic function, diabetes mellitus, pregnancy, or lactation.
• Watch for blood dyscrasias.
• Monitor BUN and serum potassium, electrolytes.
• A potassium-sparing diuretic, useful as an adjunct to other diuretic therapy. Less potent than thiazides and loop diuretics. Full diuretic effect delayed 2 to 3 days.
• Warn patients to avoid excessive ingestion of potassium-rich foods.
• Give medication after meals to prevent nausea.
• Should be withdrawn gradually to prevent excessive rebound potassium excretion.
• Concomitant potassium supplement can lead to serious hyperkalemia.

trichlormethiazide
Diurese, Metahydrin, Naqua, Rochlomethiazide, Trichlorex

INDICATIONS & DOSAGE
Edema—
Adults: 1 to 4 mg P.O. daily or in 2 divided dosages.
Hypertension—
Adults: 2 to 4 mg P.O. daily.

SIDE EFFECTS
Blood: *aplastic anemia, agranulocytosis,* leukopenia, thrombocytopenia.
CV: *volume depletion and dehydration,* orthostatic hypotension.

GI: anorexia, nausea, pancreatitis.
Hepatic: hepatic encephalopathy.
Metabolic: *hypokalemia, asymptomatic hyperuricemia, hyperglycemia and impairment of glucose tolerance,* fluid and electrolyte imbalances including dilutional hyponatremia and hypochloremia, metabolic alkalosis, hypercalcemia, gout.
Skin: dermatitis, photosensitivity, rash.
Other: hypersensitivity reactions such as pneumonitis and vasculitis.

INTERACTIONS

Cholestyramine, colestipol: intestinal absorption of thiazides decreased. Keep doses as separate as possible.
Diazoxide: increased antihypertensive, hyperglycemic, hyperuricemic effects. Use together cautiously.

NURSING CONSIDERATIONS

• Contraindicated in anuria; hypersensitivity to other thiazides or other sulfonamide-derived drugs. Use cautiously in severe renal disease, impaired hepatic function.
• Monitor intake/output, weight, and electrolytes regularly.
• Monitor serum potassium levels; consult with doctor and dietitian to provide high-potassium diet. Watch for hypokalemia (e.g., muscle weakness, cramps). May use with potassium-sparing diuretic to prevent potassium loss.
• Monitor serum creatinine and BUN levels regularly. Not effective if these levels are more than twice normal.
• Check insulin requirements in diabetics. May treat severe hyperglycemia with oral antidiabetic agents. Monitor blood sugar.
• Monitor blood uric acid levels, especially in patients with a history of gout.
• In hypertension, therapeutic response may be delayed several days.
• Give in a.m. to prevent nocturia.

• Elderly patients are especially susceptible to excessive diuresis.
• A long-acting thiazide diuretic.

---

urea (carbamide)
Ureaphil

INDICATIONS & DOSAGE

Intracranial or intraocular pressure—
Adults: 1 to 1.5 g/Kg as a 30% solution by slow I.V. infusion over 1 to 2.5 hours.
Children over 2 years: 0.5 to 1.5 g/Kg slow I.V. infusion.
Children under 2 years: as little as 0.1 g/Kg slow I.V. infusion. Maximum 4 ml/minute.
Maximum adult daily dose 120 g. To prepare 135 ml 30% solution, mix contents of 40 g vial of urea with 105 ml dextrose 5% or 10% in water or 10% invert sugar in water. Each ml of 30% solution provides 300 mg urea.

SIDE EFFECTS

CNS: *headache.*
CV: tachycardia, volume expansion.
GI: *nausea, vomiting.*
Metabolic: sodium and potassium depletion.
Local: irritation or necrotic sloughing may occur with extravasation.

INTERACTIONS

None significant.

NURSING CONSIDERATIONS

• Contraindicated in severely impaired renal function, marked dehydration, frank hepatic failure, active intracranial bleeding. Use cautiously in pregnancy, lactation, cardiac disease, hepatic impairment, or sickle cell damage with CNS involvement.
• Avoid rapid I.V. infusion; may cause hemolysis or increased capillary bleeding. Avoid extravasation;

may cause reactions ranging from mild irritation to necrosis.
• Don't administer through the same infusion as blood.
• Don't infuse into leg veins; may cause phlebitis or thrombosis, especially in the elderly.
• Watch for hyponatremia or hypokalemia (muscle weakness, lethargy); may indicate electrolyte depletion before serum levels are reduced.
• Maintain adequate hydration; monitor fluid and electrolyte balance.
• In renal disease, monitor BUN frequently.

• Indwelling urethral catheter should be used in comatose patients to assure bladder emptying.
• If satisfactory diuresis does not occur in 6 to 12 hours, urea should be discontinued and renal function re-evaluated.
• Use freshly reconstituted urea only for I.V. infusion; solution becomes ammonia upon oxidation when standing.
• Use within minutes of reconstitution.

58

Electrolytes and replacement solutions

calcium salts
calcium chloride
calcium gluceptate
calcium gluconate
calcium lactate
dextrans (low molecular weight)
dextrans (high molecular weight)
hetastarch
magnesium sulfate
potassium acetate
potassium bicarbonate
potassium chloride
potassium gluconate
potassium phosphate
Ringer's injection
Ringer's injection, lactated
sodium salts
sodium chloride

---

calcium salts

calcium chloride

calcium gluceptate

calcium gluconate

calcium lactate

INDICATIONS & DOSAGE
Hypocalcemia, hypocalcemic tetany, hypocalcemia during exchange transfusions, cardiac resuscitation for inotropic effect when epinephrine has failed; magnesium intoxication—
Adults and children: initially 500 mg to 1 g elemental calcium I.V., with further dosage based on serum calcium determinations.

Dosage with calcium chloride (1 g [10 ml] yields 13.5 mEq Ca^{++}):
Magnesium intoxication—
Adults and children: initially 500 mg I.V., with further doses based on calcium and magnesium determination.
Cardiac arrest—0.5 to 1 g I.V., not to exceed 1 ml/minute; or 200 to 800 mg into the ventricular cavity.
Hypocalcemia—500 mg to 1 g I.V. at intervals of 1 to 3 days, determined by serum calcium levels.

Dosage with calcium gluconate (1 g [10 ml] yields 4.5 mEq Ca^{++}):
Hypocalcemia—
Adults: 500 mg to 1 g I.V., repeated q 1 to 3 days p.r.n. as determined by serum calcium levels. Further doses depend on serum calcium determination.
Children: 500 mg/Kg I.V. daily. Rate of infusion should not exceed 0.5 ml/min.

Dosage with calcium gluceptate (1.1 g [5 ml] yields 4.5 mEq Ca^{++}) and calcium salts (18 mg [1 ml] yields 0.898 mEq Ca^{++}):
Hypocalcemia—
Adults: initially 5 to 20 ml I.V., with further doses based on serum calcium determinations. If I.V. injection is impossible, 2 to 5 ml I.M. Average adult oral dose, 1 to 2 g/day P.O. in divided doses, t.i.d. or q.i.d. Average oral dose for children, 45 to 65 mg/Kg P.O. daily, in divided doses, t.i.d. or q.i.d.
During exchange transfusions—
Adults and children: 0.5 ml I.V.

after each 100 ml blood exchanged.

SIDE EFFECTS
CNS: from I.V. use, tingling sensations, sense of oppression or heat waves; with rapid I.V. injection, syncope.
CV: mild fall in blood pressure; with rapid I.V. injection, vasodilation, *bradycardia, cardiac arrhythmias, and cardiac arrest.*
GI: with oral ingestion, irritation, hemorrhage, *constipation;* with I.V. administration, chalky taste; with oral calcium chloride, gastrointestinal hemorrhage, nausea, vomiting, thirst, abdominal pain.
GU: hypercalcemia, polyuria, renal calculi.
Skin: local reaction if calcium salts given I.M.: burning, necrosis, sloughing of tissue, cellulitis, soft-tissue calcification.
Local: with S.C. injection, pain and irritation; *with I.V., venous irritation.*

INTERACTIONS
Digitalis glycosides: increased digitalis toxicity; administer calcium very cautiously (if at all) to digitalized patients.

NURSING CONSIDERATIONS
• Contraindicated in ventricular fibrillation, hypercalcemia, renal calculi. Use cautiously in sarcoidosis, renal or cardiac disease, and digitalized patients. Use calcium chloride cautiously in cor pulmonale, respiratory acidosis, or respiratory failure.
• Monitor EKG when giving calcium I.V. Such injections should not exceed 0.7 to 1.5 mEq/minute. Stop if patient complains of discomfort. Following I.V. injection, patient should remain recumbent for a short while.
• I.M. injection should be given in the gluteal region in adults; lateral thigh in infants. I.M. route used only in emergencies when no I.V. route available.

• Monitor blood calcium levels frequently. Report abnormalities.
• Hypercalcemia may result after large doses in chronic renal failure.
• I.V. route generally recommended in children, but not by scalp vein.
• Solutions should be warmed to body temperature.
• Calcium chloride and calcium gluconate should be given I.V. only.
• Severe necrosis and sloughing of tissues follow extravasation. Calcium gluconate is less irritating to veins and tissues than calcium chloride.
• Give oral calcium products 1 to 1½ hours after meals or with milk.
• Oxalic acid (found in rhubarb and spinach), phytic acid (in bran and whole cereals), and phosphorus (in milk and dairy products) may interfere with absorption of calcium. Monitor calcium levels.
• Crash carts usually contain both gluconate and chloride. Make sure doctor specifies form he prefers.

dextrans
(low molecular weight dextrans)
Dextran 40, Gentran 40, LMVD, Rheomacrodex♦

INDICATIONS & DOSAGE
Plasma volume expansion—Dosage of 10% solution by I.V. infusion depends on amount of fluid loss.
First 500 ml of Dextran 40 may be infused rapidly with central venous pressure monitoring. Infuse remaining dose slowly. Total daily dose not to exceed 2 g/Kg body weight. If therapy continued past 24 hours, do not exceed 1 g/Kg daily. Continue for no longer than 5 days.
Reduction of blood sludging—500 ml of 10% solution by I.V. infusion.

SIDE EFFECTS
Blood: *decreased level of hemoglobin*

Italicized side effects are common or life-threatening.

and hematocrit; with higher doses, increased bleeding time.
GI: nausea, vomiting.
GU: tubular stasis and blocking, increased viscosity of urine.
Skin: hypersensitivity reaction, urticaria.
Other: increased SGPT and SGOT levels, *anaphylaxis.*

INTERACTIONS
None significant.

NURSING CONSIDERATIONS
• Contraindicated in marked hemostatic defects; marked cardiac decompensation or pulmonary edema; renal disease with severe oliguria or anuria; or extreme dehydration. Use cautiously in active hemorrhage; may cause additional blood loss.
• Hazardous when given to patients with heart failure, especially if in saline solution. Use dextrose solution instead.
• Works as plasma expander via colloidal osmotic effect, thereby drawing fluid from interstitial to intravascular space. Provides plasma expansion slightly greater than volume infused. Watch for circulatory overload.
• Monitor urine flow rate during administration. If oliguria or anuria occurs or is not relieved by infusion, stop dextran and give osmotic diuretic.
• Hydration should be assessed before starting therapy; otherwise, use urine or serum osmolarity because urine specific gravity is affected by urine dextran concentration.
• Check hemoglobin and hematocrit; don't allow to fall below 30% by volume.
• Draw blood samples *before* starting infusion.
• Store at constant 25° C. (77° F.). May precipitate in storage, but can be heated to dissolve if necessary.

dextrans
(high molecular weight dextrans)
Dextran 70, Dextran 75♦, Gentran 75, Macrodex♦

INDICATIONS & DOSAGE
Plasma expander—
Adults: usual dose 30 g (500 ml of 6% solution) I.V. In emergency situations, may be administered at rate of 1.2 to 2.4 g (20 to 40 ml) per minute. In normovolemic or nearly normovolemic patients, rate of infusion should not exceed 240 mg (4 ml per minute). Total dose during first 24 hours not to exceed 1.2 g/Kg; actual dose depends on amount of fluid loss and resultant hemoconcentration, and must be determined for each patient.

SIDE EFFECTS
Blood: *decreased level of hemoglobin and hematocrit;* with doses of 15 ml/Kg body weight, prolonged bleeding time and significant suppression of platelet function.
GI: nausea, vomiting.
GU: increases specific gravity and viscosity of urine, tubular stasis and blocking.
Skin: hypersensitivity reaction, urticaria.
Other: fever, arthralgia, increased SGPT and SGOT levels, nasal congestion, *anaphylaxis.*

INTERACTIONS
None significant.

NURSING CONSIDERATIONS
• Contraindicated in marked hemostatic defects; marked cardiac decompensation or pulmonary edema; renal disease with severe oliguria or anuria; and extreme dehydration. Use cautiously in active hemorrhage; may cause additional blood loss.
• Hazardous when given to patients with heart failure, especially if in sa-

line solution. Use dextrose solution instead.
• Works as plasma expander via colloidal osmotic effect, thereby drawing fluid from interstitial to intravascular space. Provides plasma expansion slightly greater than volume infused. Watch for circulatory overload.
• Monitor urine flow rate during administration. If oliguria or anuria occurs or is not relieved by infusion, stop dextran and give osmotic diuretic.
• Hydration should be assessed before starting therapy; otherwise, use urine or serum osmolarity because urine specific gravity is affected by the urine dextran concentration.
• Check hemoglobin and hematocrit; don't allow to fall below 30% by volume.
• Draw blood samples *before* starting infusion.
• May precipitate in storage, but can be heated to dissolve if necessary.
• Dextran 70 and Dextran 75 can be used interchangeably. Differ significantly from Dextran 40—do not interchange.

---

hetastarch
Hespan, Volex

INDICATIONS & DOSAGE
Plasma expander—
Adults: 500 to 1,000 ml I.V. dependent on amount of blood lost and resultant hemoconcentration. Total dosage usually not to exceed 1,500 ml/day. Up to 20 ml/Kg/hour may be used in hemorrhagic shock.

SIDE EFFECTS
CNS: headaches.
CV: peripheral edema of lower extremities.
EENT: periorbital edema.
GI: nausea, vomiting.
Skin: urticaria.
Other: wheezing, mild fever.

INTERACTIONS
None significant.

NURSING CONSIDERATIONS
• Contraindicated in severe bleeding disorders or with severe congestive heart failure and renal failure with oliguria and anuria.
• To avoid circulatory overload, monitor patients with impaired renal function carefully.
• Discontinue if allergic or sensitivity reactions occur. If necessary, administer an antihistamine.
• Hetastarch is *not* a substitute for blood or plasma.
• Available in 500 ml I.V. infusion bottles.

---

magnesium sulfate

INDICATIONS & DOSAGE
Hypomagnesemia—
Adults: 1 g, or 8.12 mEq, of 50% solution (2 ml) I.M. q 6 hours for 4 doses, depending on serum magnesium level.
*Severe hypomagnesemia (serum magnesium 0.8 mEq/liter or less, with symptoms)—*6 g, or 50 mEq, of 50% solution I.V. in 1 liter of solution over 4 hours. Subsequent doses depend on serum magnesium levels.
Magnesium supplementation in hyperalimentation—
Adults: 8 to 24 mEq/day added to hyperalimentation solution.
Children over 6 years: 2 to 10 mEq/day added to hyperalimentation solution.
Each 2 ml of 50% solution contains 1 g, or 8.12 mEq, magnesium sulfate.

SIDE EFFECTS
CNS: toxicity: weak or absent deep-tendon reflexes, flaccid paralysis; hypothermia, drowsiness, respiratory depression or paralysis; hypocalcemia

---

Italicized side effects are common or life-threatening.

(perioral paresthesias, twitching carpopedal spasm, tetany, and seizures).
CV: slow, weak pulse; hypocalcemia (cardiac arrhythmias); hypotension.
Skin: flushing, sweating.

INTERACTIONS
None significant.

NURSING CONSIDERATIONS
• Contraindicated in impaired renal function, myocardial damage, heart block, and in actively progressing labor. Use parenteral magnesium with extreme caution in patients receiving digitalis preparations. Treating magnesium toxicity with calcium in such patients could cause serious alterations in cardiac conduction; heart block may result.
• Maximum infusion rate 150 mg/min. Rapid drip causes feeling of heat.
• Keep I.V. calcium available to reverse magnesium intoxication.
• Monitor vital signs every 15 minutes when giving I.V. for severe hypomagnesemia. Watch for respiratory depression and signs of heart block. Respirations should be about 16 per minute before dose is given.
• Monitor intake/output. Output should be 100 ml or more during 4-hour period before dose.
• Test knee jerk and patellar reflexes before each additional dose. If absent, give no more magnesium until reflexes return; otherwise, patient may develop temporary respiratory failure and need cardiopulmonary resuscitation or I.V. administration of calcium.
• Check magnesium levels after repeated doses.
• After giving to toxemic mothers within 24 hours before delivery, watch newborn for signs of magnesium toxicity, including neuromuscular and respiratory depression.

potassium acetate

INDICATIONS & DOSAGE
Potassium replacement—I.V. should be used for life-threatening hypokalemia or when oral replacement not feasible. Give no more than 20 mEq/hour in concentration of 40 mEq/liter or less. Total 24-hour dose should not exceed 150 mEq (3 mEq/Kg in children). Potassium replacement should be done with EKG monitoring and frequent serum K^+ determinations.
Prevention of hypokalemia—
Adults and children: 20 mEq P.O. daily, in divided doses b.i.d., t.i.d., or q.i.d.
Potassium depletion—
Adults and children: usual dose 40 to 100 mEq P.O. daily, in divided doses b.i.d., t.i.d., or q.i.d.

SIDE EFFECTS
Signs of hyperkalemia—
CNS: paresthesias of the extremities, listlessness, mental confusion, weakness or heaviness of legs, flaccid paralysis.
CV: *peripheral vascular collapse with fall in blood pressure, cardiac arrhythmias,* heart block, possible cardiac arrest, EKG changes (prolonged P-R intervals, wide QRS, S-T segment depression, tall tented T waves).
GI: nausea, vomiting, abdominal pain, diarrhea, bowel ulceration.
GU: oliguria.
Skin: cold skin, gray pallor.

INTERACTIONS
None significant.

NURSING CONSIDERATIONS
• Contraindicated in severe renal impairment with oliguria, anuria, azotemia, and untreated Addison's disease; acute dehydration, hyperkalemia, hyperkalemic form of familial periodic paralysis, and conditions as-

sociated with extensive tissue breakdown. Use cautiously in cardiac disease, patients receiving potassium-
sparing diuretics, and those with renal
impairment.
• Monitor EKG for signs of hypokalemia or hyperkalemia; serum potassium level, renal function, BUN, and
serum creatinine; intake/output.
Never give potassium postop until
urine flow is established.
• Give slowly as diluted solution; potentially fatal hyperkalemia may result from too rapid infusion.
• Observe for pain and redness at injection site. Large-bore needle reduces local irritation.
• Parenteral potassium given by infusion only; never I.V. push or I.M.
• Watch for signs of GI ulceration:
obstruction, hemorrhage, pain, distention, severe vomiting, bleeding.
• Reconstitute potassium acetate
powder with liquids; give after meals.

---

potassium bicarbonate
K-Lyte, K-Lyte DS

INDICATIONS & DOSAGE
Hypokalemia—
25 mEq or 50 mEq tablet dissolved in
water 1 to 4 times a day.

SIDE EFFECTS
CNS: paresthesias of the extremities,
listlessness, mental confusion, weakness or heaviness of legs, flaccid
paralysis.
CV: *cardiac arrhythmias,* EKG
changes (prolonged P-R interval, wide
QRS, S-T segment depression, tall
tented T waves).
GI: *nausea, vomiting, abdominal
pain,* diarrhea, ulcerations, hemorrhage, obstruction, perforation.

INTERACTIONS
None significant.

NURSING CONSIDERATIONS
• Contraindicated in severe renal impairment with oliguria, anuria, azotemia, and untreated Addison's disease; also in acute dehydration, hyperkalemia, hyperkalemic familial
periodic paralysis, and conditions associated with extensive tissue breakdown. Use with caution in cardiac disease and patients receiving potassium-sparing diuretics.
• Monitor serum potassium level,
BUN, serum creatinine, and intake/
output.
• Never switch potassium products
without a doctor's order.
• Dissolve potassium bicarbonate
tablets in 6 to 8 ounces of cold water.
• Take with meals and sip slowly over
a 5- to 10-minute period.
• Potassium bicarbonate cannot be
given instead of potassium chloride.
• Potassium bicarbonate does not
correct hypochloremic alkalosis.
• Available in lime or orange flavor.
Check for patient flavor preference.

---

potassium chloride
K-Lor, K-Lyte/Cl, K-10♦, Kaochlor
S-F 10%, Kaochlor 10%, Kaon,
Kaon-Cl, Kaon-Cl 20%, Kato Pow-
der, KayCiel♦, Klor-10%, Kloride,
Klorvess, Klotrix, K Tab, Pfiklor,
SK-Potassium Chloride, Slow K♦

INDICATIONS & DOSAGE
Hypokalemia—
40 to 100 mEq P.O. divided into 3 to
4 doses daily for treatment; 20 mEq
for prevention. Further dose based on
serum potassium determinations.
I.V. route when oral replacement not
feasible or when hypokalemia life-
threatening. Usual dose 20 mEq/hour
in concentration of 40 mEq/liter or
less. Total daily dose not to exceed
150 mEq (3 mEq/Kg in children). Potassium replacement should be done

---

Italicized side effects are common or life-threatening.

only with EKG monitoring and frequent serum K+ determinations.

SIDE EFFECTS
Signs of hyperkalemia:
CNS: paresthesias of the extremities, listlessness, mental confusion, weakness or heaviness of legs, flaccid paralysis.
CV: *peripheral vascular collapse with fall in blood pressure, cardiac arrhythmias, heart block, possible cardiac arrest,* EKG changes (prolonged P-R interval, wide QRS, S-T segment depression, tall tented T waves).
GI: *nausea, vomiting, abdominal pain,* diarrhea, GI ulcerations (possible stenosis, hemorrhage, obstruction, perforation).
GU: oliguria.
Skin: cold skin, gray pallor.

INTERACTIONS
None significant.

NURSING CONSIDERATIONS
• Contraindicated in severe renal impairment with oliguria, anuria, azotemia, and untreated Addison's disease; also in acute dehydration, hyperkalemia, hyperkalemic form of familial periodic paralysis, conditions associated with extensive tissue breakdown. Use with caution in cardiac disease, patients receiving potassium-sparing diuretics.
• Potassium should not be given during immediate postoperative period until urine flow is established.
• Parenteral potassium given by infusion only; never I.V. push or I.M.
• Give slowly as dilute solution; potentially fatal hyperkalemia may result from too rapid infusion.
• Give oral potassium supplements with extreme caution because its many forms deliver varying amounts of potassium. Never switch products without a doctor's order. Tell the doctor if patient tolerates one product better than another.

• Sugar-free liquid available (Kaochlor S-F 10%).
• Have patient sip liquid potassium slowly to minimize GI irritation.
• Give with or after meals with full glass of water or fruit juice to lessen GI distress.
• Make sure powders are completely dissolved before giving.
• Enteric-coated tablets not recommended due to potential GI bleeding and small bowel ulcerations.
• Tablets in wax matrix sometimes lodge in esophagus and cause ulceration in cardiac patients who have esophageal compression due to enlarged left atrium. In such patients and in those with esophageal stasis or obstruction, use liquid form.
• Often used orally with diuretics that cause potassium excretion. Potassium chloride most useful since diuretics waste chloride ion. Hypokalemic alkalosis treated best with potassium chloride.

---

potassium gluconate
Kalinate Elixir, Kaon Liquid, Kaon Tablets♦, Potassium Rougier♦♦

INDICATIONS & DOSAGE
Hypokalemia—40 to 100 mEq P.O. divided into 3 to 4 doses daily for treatment; 20 mEq/day for prevention. Further dose based on serum potassium determinations.

SIDE EFFECTS
CNS: paresthesias of the extremities, listlessness, mental confusion, weakness or heaviness of legs, flaccid paralysis.
CV: cardiac arrhythmias, EKG changes (prolonged P-R interval, wide QRS, S-T segment depression, tall tented T waves).
GI: *nausea, vomiting, abdominal pain,* diarrhea, GI ulcerations with oral products (especially enteric

coated tablets); ulcerations may be accompanied by stenosis, hemorrhage obstruction, perforation.

INTERACTIONS
None significant.

NURSING CONSIDERATIONS
• Contraindicated in severe renal impairment with oliguria, anuria, azotemia, and untreated Addison's disease; also in acute dehydration, hyperkalemia, hyperkalemic form of familial periodic paralysis, and conditions associated with extensive tissue breakdown. Use with caution in cardiac disease; patients receiving potassium-sparing diuretics.
• Monitor serum potassium level, BUN, serum creatinine, and intake/output.
• Give oral potassium supplements with extreme caution because its many forms deliver varying amounts of potassium. Never switch products without doctor's order. If one product is tolerated better than another, tell doctor so brand and dosage can be changed.
• Have patient sip liquid potassium slowly to minimize GI irritation.
• Give with or after meals with full glass of water or fruit juice to lessen GI distress.
• Potassium gluconate does not correct hypokalemic hypochloremic alkalosis.
• Enteric-coated tablets not recommended due to potential for GI bleeding and small-bowel ulcerations.

---

potassium phosphate

INDICATIONS & DOSAGE
Hypokalemia—I.V. should be used when oral replacement not feasible or when hypokalemia life-threatening. Dosage up to 20 mEq/hour in concentration of 60 mEq/liter or less. Total daily dose not to exceed 150 mEq. Should be done only with EKG monitoring and frequent serum K⁺ determinations.
Average P.O. dose: 40 to 100 mEq.
Hypophosphatemia—3 mM/ml is administered I.V. after diluting in a larger volume of fluid. Dosage is adjusted according to individual needs of patient.

SIDE EFFECTS
Signs of hyperkalemia—
CNS: paresthesias of the extremities, listlessness, mental confusion, weakness or heaviness of legs, flaccid paralysis; hypocalcemia—perioral paresthesias, twitching, carpopedal spasm, tetany, and seizures.
CV: *peripheral vascular collapse with fall in blood pressure, cardiac arrhythmias, heart block, possible cardiac arrest,* EKG changes (prolonged P-R interval, wide QRS, S-T segment depression, tall tented T waves).
GI: nausea, vomiting, abdominal pain, diarrhea.
GU: oliguria.
Skin: cold skin, gray pallor.
Other: soft tissue calcification.

INTERACTIONS
None significant.

NURSING CONSIDERATIONS
• Contraindicated in severe renal impairment with oliguria, anuria, azotemia, and untreated Addison's disease; also acute dehydration, hyperkalemia, hyperkalemic form of familial periodic paralysis, extensive tissue damage, hypocalcemia. Use with caution in cardiac disease, patients receiving potassium-sparing diuretics.
• Never give potassium postop until urine flow is established.
• Monitor EKG for indications of tissue potassium levels; plasma potassium and calcium levels as well as BUN and creatinine for renal func-

---

Italicized side effects are common or life-threatening.

tion; inorganic phosphorus levels; intake/output.
- Give slowly as dilute solution; potentially fatal hyperkalemia may result from too rapid an infusion.
- Parenteral potassium given by infusion only; never I.V. push or I.M.
- Reconstitute powder in juice. Give after meals.

Ringer's injection

INDICATIONS & DOSAGE
Fluid and electrolyte replacement—
Adults and children: dose highly individualized, but generally 1.5 to 3 liters (2% to 6% body weight) infused I.V. over 18 to 24 hours.

SIDE EFFECTS
CV: fluid overload.

INTERACTIONS
None significant.

NURSING CONSIDERATIONS
- Contraindicated in renal failure, except as emergency volume expander. Use cautiously in CHF, circulatory insufficiency, kidney dysfunction, hypoproteinemia, or pulmonary edema.
- Ringer's injection contains sodium, 147 mEq/liter; potassium, 4 mEq/liter; calcium, 4.5 mEq liter; and chloride, 155.5 mEq/liter. This electrolyte content is insufficient for treating severe electrolyte deficiencies.
- May be given with dextrose injection.

Ringer's injection, lactated
(Hartmann's solution)

INDICATIONS & DOSAGE
Fluid and electrolyte replacement—
Adults and children: dose highly

individualized, but generally 1.5 to 3 liters (2% to 6% body weight) infused I.V. over 18 to 24 hours.

SIDE EFFECTS
CV: fluid overload.

INTERACTIONS
None significant.

NURSING CONSIDERATIONS
- Contraindicated in renal failure, except as emergency volume expander. Use cautiously in CHF, circulatory insufficiency, kidney dysfunction, hypoproteinemia, and pulmonary edema.
- Ringer's injection, lactated, contains sodium, 130 mEq/liter; potassium, 4 mEq/liter; calcium, 2.7 mEq/liter; chloride, 109.7 mEq/liter; and lactate, 27 mEq/liter.
- Approximates more closely the electrolyte concentration in blood plasma than Ringer's injection.
- May be given with dextrose injection.

sodium salts

sodium chloride

INDICATIONS & DOSAGE
Highly individualized fluid and electrolyte replacement in hyponatremia due to electrolyte loss or in severe salt depletion—
400 ml of 3% or 5% solutions only with frequent electrolyte determination and only if given slow I.V.;
with 0.45% solution: 3% to 8% of body weight, according to deficiencies, over 18 to 24 hours;
with 0.9% solution: 2% to 6% of body weight, according to deficiencies, over 18 to 24 hours.
Management of "heat cramp" due to excessive perspiration—

Adults: 1 g P.O. with every glass of water.

SIDE EFFECTS
CV: aggravation of congestive heart failure; edema and pulmonary edema if too much given or given too rapidly.
Metabolic: aggravation of existing acidosis with excessive infusion.
Other: hypernatremia with excessive infusion; serious electrolyte disturbance, loss of potassium.

INTERACTIONS
None significant.

NURSING CONSIDERATIONS
• Use with caution in congestive heart failure, circulatory insufficiency, kidney dysfunction, hypoproteinemia.
• Infuse 3% and 5% solutions very slowly and with caution to avoid pulmonary edema. Use only for critical situations. Observe patient constantly.
• Concentrates available for addition to parenteral nutrient solutions. Don't confuse these small volumes of parenterals with sodium chloride injection isotonic 0.9%. *Read label carefully*.

59

Potassium-removing resin

sodium polystyrene sulfonate

sodium polystyrene sulfonate
Kayexalate ♦

INDICATIONS & DOSAGE
Hyperkalemia—
Adults: 15 g daily to q.i.d. in water or sorbitol (3 to 4 ml/g of resin).
Children: 1 g of resin for each mEq of potassium to be removed.
Oral administration preferred since drug should remain in intestine for at least 6 hours; otherwise consider nasogastric administration.
Nasogastric administration: mix dose with appropriate medium: aqueous suspension or diet appropriate for renal failure; instill in plastic tube.
Rectal administration:
Adults: 30 to 50 g/100 ml of sorbitol q 6 hours as warm emulsion deep into sigmoid colon (20 cm). In persistent vomiting or paralytic ileus, high-retention enema of sodium polystyrene sulfonate (30 g) suspended in 200 ml of 10% methylcellulose, 10% dextrose, or 25% sorbitol.

SIDE EFFECTS
GI: *constipation,* fecal impaction (in elderly), anorexia, gastric irritation, nausea, vomiting, *diarrhea (with sorbitol emulsions).*
Other: *hypokalemia,* hypocalcemia, hypomagnesemia, sodium retention.

INTERACTIONS
Antacids and laxatives (nonabsorbable cation-donating type, including magnesium hydroxide): systemic alkalosis, reduced potassium exchange capability. Don't use together.

NURSING CONSIDERATIONS
• Use with caution in elderly patients and those on digitalis therapy, with severe congestive heart failure, severe hypertension, and marked edema.
• Treatment may result in potassium deficiency. Monitor serum potassium at least once daily. Usually stopped when potassium level is reduced to 4 or 5 mEq/liter. Watch for other signs of hypokalemia: irritability, confusion, cardiac arrhythmias, EKG changes, severe muscle weakness and sometimes paralysis, and digitalis toxicity in digitalized patients.
• Monitor for symptoms of other electrolyte deficiencies (magnesium, calcium) since drug is nonselective. Monitor serum calcium determination in patients receiving sodium polystyrene therapy for more than 3 days. Supplementary calcium may be needed.
• Watch for sodium overload. About ⅓ of resin's sodium is retained.
• Use only fresh suspensions. Stir just before use. Discard unused portions after 24 hours.
• Do not heat resin. This will impair effectiveness of drug.
• Chill oral suspension for greater palatability.
• If sorbitol is given, it may be mixed with resin suspension.
• Consider solid form. Resin cookie

recipe is available; perhaps pharmacist or dietitian can supply.
• Watch for constipation in oral or nasogastric administration. Use sorbitol (10 to 20 ml of 70% syrup every 2 hours as needed) to produce 1 or 2 watery stools daily.
• Mix polystyrene-resin only with water and sorbitol for oral or rectal use. Do not use other vehicles (i.e., mineral oil) for rectal administration to prevent impactions. Ion exchange requires aqueous medium. Sorbitol content prevents impaction.
• Prevent fecal impaction in elderly by administering resin rectally. Give cleansing enema before rectal administration. Explain necessity of retaining enema to patient. Retention for 6 to 10 hours is ideal, but 30 to 60 minutes is acceptable.

• Prepare rectal dose at room temperature. Stir emulsion gently during administration.
• Use French 28 rubber tube for rectal dose; insert 20 cm into sigmoid colon. Tape tube in place. Alternatively consider a 30 ml Foley catheter with balloon inflated distal to anal sphincter to aid in retention. Use gravity flow. Drain returns constantly through Y-tube connection. When giving rectally, place patient in knee-chest position or with hips on pillow for a while if back-leakage occurs.
• After rectal administration, flush with 50 to 100 ml of nonsodium fluid.
• If hyperkalemia is severe, more drastic modalities should be added; for example, dextrose 50% with regular insulin I.V. push. Do not depend solely on polystyrene-resin to lower serum potassium levels in severe hyperkalemia.

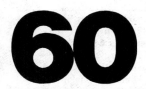

Hematinics

ferrocholinate
ferrous fumarate
ferrous gluconate
ferrous sulfate
iron dextran

---

ferrocholinate
Chel-Iron, Firon, Kelex

INDICATIONS & DOSAGE
Iron deficiency—
Adults: 333 mg tablet P.O. t.i.d.
Children: 6 mg/Kg P.O. daily in divided doses t.i.d.
Prevention of iron deficiency—
Children: 1 mg/Kg P.O. daily as single dose or divided.

SIDE EFFECTS
GI: *nausea,* vomiting, *constipation, black stools.*
Other: stained tooth enamel.

INTERACTIONS
Antacids, cholestyramine resin, pancreatic extracts, vitamin E: decreased iron absorption. Separate doses if possible.
Chloramphenicol: watch for delayed response to iron therapy.
Vitamin C: may increase iron absorption. Beneficial drug interaction.

NURSING CONSIDERATIONS
• Contraindicated in hemosiderosis, hemochromatosis, and hemolytic anemia. Usually contraindicated in peptic ulcer or ulcerative colitis. Use cautiously on long-term basis.

• GI upset related to dose. Between-meal dosing preferable, but can be given with some foods although absorption may be decreased. Enteric-coated products reduce GI upset but also reduce amount of iron absorbed.
• Iron is toxic; parents should be aware of iron poisoning in children.
• Dilute liquid preparations in juice or water, but not in milk or antacids.
• Check for constipation; record color and amount of stool. Teach dietary measures for preventing constipation.
• Tell patient to have frequent blood tests.
• To avoid staining teeth, give liquid iron preparations with glass straw.

---

ferrous fumarate
Eldofe, F&B Caps, Farbegen, Feco-T, Feostat, Feroton♦♦, Ferranol, Ferro-fume♦♦, Fersamal♦♦, Fumasorb, Fumerin, Hematon♦♦, Hemocyte, Ircon, Laud-Iron, Maniron, Novofumar♦♦, Palafer♦♦, Palmiron, Span-FF, Toleron

INDICATIONS & DOSAGE
Iron deficiency states—
Adults: 200 mg P.O. daily t.i.d. or q.i.d.

SIDE EFFECTS
GI: *nausea,* vomiting, *constipation, black stools.*
Other: stained tooth enamel.

INTERACTIONS
Antacids, cholestyramine resin, pancreatic extracts, vitamin E: decreased iron absorption. Separate doses if possible.
Chloramphenicol: watch for delayed response to iron therapy.
Vitamin C: may increase iron absorption. Beneficial drug interaction.

NURSING CONSIDERATIONS
• Contraindicated in peptic ulcer, regional enteritis, ulcerative colitis, hemosiderosis, and hemochromatosis. Use cautiously on long-term basis and in anemic patients.
• GI upset related to dose. Between-meal dosing preferable, but can be given with some foods although absorption may be decreased. Enteric-coated products reduce GI upset but also reduce amount of iron absorbed.
• Iron is toxic; parents should be aware of iron poisoning in children.
• Dilute liquid preparations in juice or water, but not in milk or antacids.
• Check for constipation; record color and amount of stool. Teach dietary measures for preventing constipation.
• Tell patient to have frequent blood tests.
• Combination products, Simron, Ferro-Sequels, Ferocyl, Fer-Regules, contain stool softeners to help prevent constipation. Fermalox contains antacids to help relieve GI upset, if present; don't use this product unless absolutely necessary because of decreased iron absorption.

---

ferrous gluconate
Entron, Fergon♦, Ferralet, Ferrous-G, Fertinic♦♦, Novoferrogluc♦♦

INDICATIONS & DOSAGE
Iron deficiency—
Adults: 200 to 600 mg P.O., t.i.d.

Children 6 to 12 years: 300 to 900 mg P.O. daily.
Children under 6 years: 100 to 300 mg P.O. daily.
1 tablet contains 320 mg ferrous gluconate (37 mg elemental iron).
5 ml of elixir contains 300 mg ferrous gluconate (35 mg elemental iron).

SIDE EFFECTS
GI: *nausea,* vomiting, *constipation, black stools.*
Other: elixir may stain teeth.

INTERACTIONS
Antacids, cholestyramine resin, pancreatic extracts, vitamin E: decreased iron absorption. Separate doses if possible.
Chloramphenicol: watch for delayed response to iron therapy.
Vitamin C: may increase iron absorption. Beneficial drug interaction.

NURSING CONSIDERATIONS
• Contraindicated in peptic ulcer, regional enteritis, ulcerative colitis, hemosiderosis, and hemochromatosis. Use cautiously on long-term basis and in patients with anemia.
• GI upset related to dose. Between-meal dosing preferable but can be given with some foods although absorption may be decreased. Enteric-coated products reduce GI upset but also reduce amount of iron absorbed.
• Iron is toxic; parents should be aware of iron poisoning in children.
• Dilute liquid preparations in juice or water, but not in milk or antacids.
• Check for constipation; record color and amount of stool. Teach dietary measures for preventing constipation.
• Tell patient to have frequent blood tests.

Italicized side effects are common or life-threatening.

ferrous sulfate
Arne Modified Caps, Feosol, Fer-In-Sol♦, Fero-Grad♦♦, Fero-Gradumet, Ferolix, Ferospace, Ferralyn, Fesofor♦♦, Irospan, Mol-Iron, Novo-ferrosulfa♦♦, Slow-Fe♦♦, Telefon

INDICATIONS & DOSAGE
Iron deficiency—
Adults: 750 mg to 1.5 g P.O. daily divided t.i.d.; or 225 to 525 mg P.O. sustained-release preparations once daily or q 12 hours.
Children 6 to 12 years: 600 mg P.O. daily in divided doses.
Prophylaxis for iron-deficiency anemia—
Pregnant women: 300 to 600 mg P.O. daily in divided doses.
Premature or undernourished infants: 3 to 6 mg/Kg P.O. daily in divided doses.

SIDE EFFECTS
GI: *nausea,* vomiting, *constipation, black stools.*
Other: elixir may stain teeth.

INTERACTIONS
Antacids, cholestyramine resin, pancreatic extracts, vitamin E: decreased iron absorption. Separate doses if possible.
Chloramphenicol: watch for delayed response to iron therapy.
Vitamin C: may increase iron absorption. Beneficial drug interaction.

NURSING CONSIDERATIONS
• Contraindicated in peptic ulcer, ulcerative colitis, regional enteritis, hemosiderosis and hemochromatosis. Use cautiously on long-term basis and in patients with anemia.
• GI upset related to dose. Between-meal dosing preferable, but can be given with some foods although absorption may be decreased. Enteric-coated products reduce GI upset but also reduce amount of iron absorbed.
• Iron is toxic; parents should be aware of iron poisoning in children.
• Dilute liquid preparations in juice or water, but not in milk or antacids.
• Check for constipation; record color and amount of stool. Teach dietary measures for preventing constipation.
• Tell patient to have frequent blood tests.

iron dextran
Hematran, Hydextran, Imferon♦, K-FeRON

INDICATIONS & DOSAGE
Iron deficiency anemia—
Adults: I.M. or I.V. injections of iron are advisable only for patients for whom oral administration is impossible or ineffective. Test dose (0.5 ml) required before administration.
I.M. (by Z-track): inject 0.5 ml test dose. If no reactions, next daily dose should ordinarily not exceed 0.5 ml (25 mg) for infants under 5 Kg; 1 ml (50 mg) for children under 9 Kg; 2 ml (100 mg) for patients under 50 Kg; 5 ml (250 mg) for patients over 50 Kg.
I.V. push: inject 0.5 ml test dose. If no reactions, within 2 to 3 days the dosage may be raised to 2 ml per day I.V., 1 ml/minute undiluted and infused slowly until total dose is achieved. No single dose should exceed 100 mg of iron.
I.V. infusion: dosages expressed in terms of elemental iron. A dosage guide based on body weight and the severity of the anemia. Dilute in 250 to 1,000 ml of normal saline solution; dextrose increases local vein irritation. Infuse test dose of 25 mg slowly over 5 minutes. If no reaction occurs in 5 minutes, infusion may be started. Infuse total dose slowly over approxi-

mately 6 to 12 hours. 1 ml iron dextran = 50 mg elemental iron.

SIDE EFFECTS
CNS: headache, transitory paresthesias, arthralgia, myalgia, dizziness, malaise, syncope.
CV: *hypotensive reaction, peripheral vascular flushing with overly rapid I.V. administration, tachycardia.*
GI: nausea, vomiting, metallic taste, transient loss of taste perception.
Local: *soreness and inflammation at injection site (I.M.); brown skin discoloration at injection site (I.M.); local phlebitis at injection site (I.V.).*
Other: *anaphylaxis.*

INTERACTIONS
None significant.

NURSING CONSIDERATIONS
• Contraindicated in all anemias other than iron deficiency anemia. Use with extreme caution in impaired hepatic function and rheumatoid arthritis.
• Watch vital signs for drug reaction. Reactions are varied and severe, ranging from pain, inflammation, and myalgia to hypotension, shock, and death.

• Inject deeply into upper outer quadrant of buttock—never into arm or other exposed area—with a 2- to 3-inch, 19- or 20-gauge needle. Use Z-track technique to avoid leakage into subcutaneous tissue and tattooing of skin.
• Hemoglobin concentration, hematocrit, and reticulocyte count should be determined periodically.
• Use I.V. in these situations: insufficient muscle mass for deep intramuscular injection; impaired absorption from muscle due to stasis or edema; possibility of uncontrolled intramuscular bleeding from trauma (as may occur in hemophilia); and when massive and prolonged parenteral therapy is indicated (as may be necessary in cases of chronic substantial blood loss).
• Patient should rest 15 to 30 minutes after I.V. administration.
• Check hospital policy before administering I.V. In some hospitals, only doctor may administer iron I.V.
• Not removed by hemodialysis.

Italicized side effects are common or life-threatening.

61

Anticoagulants and heparin antagonist

anisindione
dicumarol
heparin sodium
phenindione
phenprocoumon
protamine sulfate
warfarin potassium
warfarin sodium

---

anisindione
Miradon

INDICATIONS & DOSAGE
Treatment of pulmonary emboli; prevention and treatment of deep-vein thrombosis, myocardial infarction, rheumatic heart disease with heart valve damage, atrial arrhythmias—
Adults: 300 mg P.O. first day, 200 mg P.O. second day, 100 mg P.O. third day. Maintenance dose: 25 to 250 mg daily based on prothrombin times.

SIDE EFFECTS
Blood: *hemorrhage with excessive dosage, agranulocytosis,* leukopenia, leukocytosis, eosinophilia.
CNS: headache.
CV: myocarditis, tachycardia.
EENT: conjunctivitis, blurred vision, paralysis of ocular accommodation.
GI: diarrhea, sore mouth and throat.
GU: *nephropathy with renal tubular necrosis,* albuminuria.
Hepatic: jaundice.
Skin: *rash, severe exfoliative dermatitis.*
Other: *fever.*

INTERACTIONS
Allopurinol, clofibrate, dextrothyroxine, thyroid drugs, heparin, anabolic steroids, disulfiram, aminosalicylic acid, glucagon, inhalation anesthetics, sulfonamides: increased prothrombin time. Monitor patient carefully. Consider anticoagulant dose reduction.
Ethacrynic acid, indomethacin, mefenamic acid, oxyphenbutazone, phenylbutazone, salicylates: increased prothrombin time; ulcerogenic effects. Don't use together.
Antipyrine, carbamazepine, antacids, griseofulvin, haloperidol, paraldehyde, rifampin: decreased prothrombin time. Monitor patient carefully.
Phenytoin, glutethimide, chloral hydrate, triclofos sodium, alcohol, diuretics: increased or decreased prothrombin time. Avoid use if possible, or monitor patient carefully.
Barbiturates: inhibition of hypoprothrombinemic effect of anticoagulants. If barbiturates are withdrawn, reduce anticoagulant dose; inhibition may last for weeks after anticoagulant is withdrawn, but fatal hemorrhage can occur when inhibiting effect disappears.
Cholestyramine: decreased response when administered too close together. Administer 6 hours after oral anticoagulants.

NURSING CONSIDERATIONS
• Contraindicated in hemophilia, thrombocytopenic purpura, leukemia with pronounced bleeding tendency, open wounds or ulcers, impaired he-

patic or renal function, severe hypertension, acute nephritis, subacute bacterial endocarditis. Use cautiously in pregnancy, lactation, during menses, during use of any drainage tube in any orifice, and in any patient in whom slight bleeding is dangerous. Use with extreme caution (if at all) in psychiatric patients, debilitated patients, or cachectic patients.
- Use caution when adding or stopping any drug for patient receiving anticoagulants. May change the clotting status and result in hemorrhage.
- Fever and skin rash signal severe complications.
- Give drug at same time daily. Stress importance of complying with recommended dosage and keeping follow-up appointments. Patient should carry a card that identifies him as a potential bleeder.
- Regularly inspect patient for bleeding gums, bruises on arms or legs, petechiae, nosebleeds, melena, tarry stools, hematuria, hematemesis. Tell patient and family to watch for these signs and notify doctor immediately.
- Warn patient to avoid over-the-counter products containing aspirin, other salicylates, or any drugs that may interact with anisindione.
- Because onset of action is delayed, heparin sodium is often given during first few days of treatment. When heparin is being given simultaneously, don't draw blood for prothrombin times within 5 hours of I.V. heparin administration.
- Schedule doses according to prothrombin time (PT). Doctors usually try to maintain PT at 1.5 to 2 times normal. Numerical PT values depend on procedure and reagents used in individual laboratory.
- Tell patient to notify doctor if menses is heavier than usual. May require adjusting dose.
- Tell patient to use electric razor when shaving to avoid scratching

skin, and to brush teeth with a soft toothbrush.
- Warn patient that urine may turn red-orange.
- Duration of action 1.5 to 5 days.
- Light to moderate alcohol intake does not significantly affect prothrombin times.

---

dicumarol
Dufalone♦ ♦

INDICATIONS & DOSAGE
Treatment of pulmonary emboli; prevention and treatment of deep-vein thrombosis, myocardial infarction, rheumatic heart disease with heart valve damage, atrial arrhythmias—
Adults: 200 to 300 mg P.O. on first day, 25 to 200 mg P.O. daily thereafter, based on prothrombin times.

SIDE EFFECTS
Blood: *hemorrhage with excessive dosage,* leukopenia, *agranulocytosis.*
GI: anorexia, nausea, vomiting, cramps, *diarrhea,* mouth ulcers.
GU: hematuria.
Skin: dermatitis, urticaria, *rash.*
Other: alopecia, *fever.*

INTERACTIONS
Allopurinol, clofibrate, dextrothyroxine, thyroid drugs, heparin, anabolic steroids, disulfiram, aminosalicylic acid, glucagon, inhalation anesthetics, sulfonamides: increased prothrombin time. Monitor patient carefully. Consider anticoagulant dose reduction.
Ethacrynic acid, indomethacin, mefenamic acid, oxyphenbutazone, phenylbutazone, salicylates: increased prothrombin time; ulcerogenic effects. Don't use together.
Antipyrine, carbamazepine, antacids, griseofulvin, haloperidol, paraldehyde, rifampin: decreased prothrombin time. Monitor patient carefully.

Italicized side effects are common or life-threatening.

Phenytoin, glutethimide, chloral hydrate, triclofos sodium: increased or decreased prothrombin time. Avoid use if possible, or monitor patient carefully.

Barbiturates: inhibition of hypoprothrombinemic effect of anticoagulants. If barbiturates are withdrawn, reduce anticoagulant dose; inhibition may last weeks after anticoagulant withdrawn, but fatal hemorrhage can occur when inhibiting effect disappears.

Cholestyramine: decreased response when administered too close together. Administer 6 hours after oral anticoagulants.

NURSING CONSIDERATIONS
• Contraindicated in hemophilia, thrombocytopenic purpura, leukemia with pronounced bleeding tendency, open wounds or ulcers, impaired hepatic or renal function, severe hypertension, acute nephritis, subacute bacterial endocarditis. Use cautiously in pregnancy, lactation, during menses, during use of any drainage tube, and in any patient in whom slight bleeding is dangerous. Use with extreme caution (if at all) in psychiatric patients, debilitated patients, or cachectic patients.
• Use caution when adding or stopping any drug for patient receiving anticoagulants. May change the clotting status and result in hemorrhage.
• Fever and skin rash signal severe complications.
• Give drug at same time daily. Stress importance of complying with recommended dosage and keeping follow-up appointments. Patient should carry a card that identifies him as a potential bleeder.
• Regularly inspect patient for bleeding gums, bruises on arms or legs, petechiae, nosebleeds, melena, tarry stools, hematuria, hematemesis. Tell patient and family to watch for these signs and notify doctor immediately.

• Warn patient to avoid over-the-counter products containing aspirin, other salicylates, or drugs that may interact with dicumarol.
• Because onset of action is delayed, heparin sodium is often given during first few days of treatment. When heparin is being given simultaneously, don't draw blood for prothrombin times within 5 hours of I.V. heparin administration.
• Dose given depends on prothrombin times (PT). Doctors usually try to maintain PT at 1.5 to 2 times normal. PT values depend on procedure and reagents used in individual laboratory.
• Tell patient to notify doctor if menses is heavier than usual. May require adjusting dose.
• Tell patient to use electric razor when shaving to avoid scratching skin and to brush teeth with a soft toothbrush.
• May turn urine red-orange.
• Duration of action 2 to 6 days.
• Light to moderate alcohol intake does not significantly affect prothrombin times.

---

heparin sodium
Hepalean♦♦, Heprinar, Lipo-Hepin, Liquaemin Sodium, Panheprin

INDICATIONS & DOSAGE
Treatment of deep vein thrombosis, myocardial infarction—
Adults: initially, 5,000 to 7,500 units I.V. push, then adjust dose according to PTT results and give dose I.V. q 4 hours (usually 4,000 to 5,000 units); or 5,000 to 7,500 units I.V. bolus, then 1,000 units/hour by I.V. infusion pump. Wait 8 hours following bolus dose, and adjust hourly rate according to PTT.
Treatment of pulmonary embolism—
Adults: initially, 7,500 to 10,000 units I.V. push, then adjust

dose according to PTT results and give dose I.V. q 4 hours (usually 4,000 to 5,000 units); or 7,500 to 10,000 units I.V. bolus, then 1,000 units/ hour by I.V. infusion pump. Wait 8 hours following bolus dose, and adjust hourly rate according to PTT.

Prophylaxis of embolism—
Adults: 5,000 units S.C. q 12 hours.
Open heart surgery—
Adults: (total body perfusion) 150 to 300 units/Kg continuous I.V infusion.
Treatment of pulmonary emboli; prevention and treatment of deep-vein thrombosis—
Children: initially, 50 units/Kg I.V. drip. Maintenance dose 100 units/Kg I.V. drip q 4 hours. Constant infusion: 20,000 units/m² daily. Dosages adjusted according to PTT.
Heparin dosing is highly individualized, depending upon disease state, age, renal and hepatic status.

SIDE EFFECTS
Blood: *hemorrhage with excessive dosage, overly prolonged clotting time, thrombocytopenia.*
Local: irritation, mild pain.
Other: hypersensitivity reactions include chills, fever, pruritus, rhinitis, burning of feet, conjunctivitis, lacrimation, arthralgia, urticaria.

INTERACTIONS
Salicylates: increased anticoagulant effect. Don't use together.
Anticoagulants, oral: additive anticoagulation. Monitor prothrombin time and partial thromboplastin time.

NURSING CONSIDERATIONS
• Conditionally contraindicated in active bleeding; blood dyscrasias; or bleeding tendencies such as hemophilia, thrombocytopenia, or hepatic disease with hypoprothrombinemia; suspected intracranial hemorrhage; suppurative thrombophlebitis; inaccessible ulcerative lesions (especially of GI tract); open ulcerative wounds; extensive denudation of skin; ascorbic acid deficiency and other conditions causing increased capillary permeability; during or after brain, eye, or spinal cord surgery; during continuous tube drainage of stomach or small intestine; in subacute bacterial endocarditis; shock; advanced kidney disease; threatened abortion; severe hypertension. While the use of heparin is clearly hazardous in these conditions, a decision to use it depends on the comparative risk in failure to treat the coexisting thromboembolic disorder.
• Use cautiously during menses; in mild hepatic or renal disease; alcoholism; in patients in occupations with the risk of physical injury; immediately postpartum; in past history of allergies, asthma, or GI ulcers.
• Monitor platelet counts regularly. Thrombocytopenia caused by heparin may be associated with arterial thrombosis.
• Measure partial thromboplastin time (PTT) carefully and regularly. Anticoagulation present when PTT values are 1½ to 2 times control values.
• Drug requirements are higher in early phases of thrombogenic diseases and febrile states; lower when patient becomes stabilized.
• Regularly inspect patient for bleeding gums, bruises on arms or legs, petechiae, nosebleeds, melena, tarry stools, hematuria, hematemesis. Tell patient and family to watch for these signs and notify doctor immediately.
• Tell patient to avoid over-the-counter medications containing aspirin, other salicylates, or drugs that may interact with heparin.
• Heparin comes in various concentrations. Check order and vial carefully.
• Low-dose injections given sequentially between iliac crest in lower abdomen deep into S.C. fat. Inject drug

slowly S.C. into fat pad. Leave needle in place for 10 seconds; withdraw needle. Alternate site every 12 hours—right for a.m., left for p.m.
• Don't massage after S.C. injection. Watch for signs of bleeding at injection site. Rotate sites and keep accurate record.
• Check constant I.V. infusions regularly, even when pumps are in good working order, to prevent over- or underdosage.
• I.M. administration not recommended.
• I.V. administration preferred because of long-term effect and irregular absorption when given S.C. Whenever possible, administer I.V. heparin in infusion pump to provide maximum safety.
• Concentrated heparin solutions (greater than 100 units/ml) can irritate blood vessels.
• Place sign above patient's bed to inform I.V. team or lab personnel to apply pressure dressings after taking blood.
• Avoid excessive I.M. injections to avoid or minimize hematomas. If possible, don't give I.M. injections at all.
• Elderly patients should usually start at lower doses.
• When I.V. intermittent therapy is utilized, always draw blood ½ hour before next scheduled dose to avoid falsely elevated PTTs.
• PTTs can be drawn any time after 8 hours of initiation of continuous I.V. heparin therapy. Never draw blood for PTTs from the I.V. tubing of the heparin infusion, or from vein of infusion. Falsely elevated PTT will result. Always draw blood from opposite arm.
• Give on time; try not to skip a dose. If I.V. is out, get it restarted as soon as possible, and reschedule dose immediately.
• Never piggyback other drugs into an infusion line while heparin infusion is running. Many antibiotics and other drugs inactivate heparin. Never mix any drug with heparin in syringe when bolus therapy is used.

---

phenindione
Danilone♦♦, Eridione, Hedulin

INDICATIONS & DOSAGE
Treatment of pulmonary emboli; prevention and treatment of deep-vein thrombosis, myocardial infarction, rheumatic heart disease with heart valve damage, atrial arrhythmias—
Adults: 300 mg P.O. first day; 200 mg P.O. second day. Maintenance dose: 50 to 150 mg daily, based on prothrombin times.

SIDE EFFECTS
Blood: *hemorrhage with excessive dosage, agranulocytosis,* leukopenia, leukocytosis, eosinophilia.
CNS: headache.
CV: myocarditis, tachycardia.
EENT: conjunctivitis, blurred vision, paralysis of ocular accommodation.
GI: diarrhea, sore mouth and throat.
GU: *nephropathy with renal tubular necrosis,* albuminuria.
Hepatic: jaundice.
Skin: *rash, severe exfoliative dermatitis.*
Other: *fever.*

INTERACTIONS
Allopurinol, clofibrate, dextrothyroxine, thyroid drugs, heparin, anabolic steroids, disulfiram, aminosalicylic acid, glucagon, inhalation anesthetics, sulfonamides: increased prothrombin time. Monitor patient carefully. Consider anticoagulant dose reduction.
Ethacrynic acid, indomethacin, mefenamic acid, oxyphenbutazone, phenylbutazone, salicylates: increased prothrombin time; ulcerogenic effects. Don't use together.

Antipyrine, carbamazepine, antacids, griseofulvin, haloperidol, paraldehyde, rifampin: decreased prothrombin time. Monitor patient carefully.
Phenytoin, glutethimide, chloral hydrate, triclofos sodium, alcohol, diuretics: increased or decreased prothrombin time. Avoid use if possible, or monitor patient carefully.
Barbiturates: inhibition of hypoprothrombinemic effect of anticoagulants. If barbiturates are withdrawn, reduce anticoagulant dose; inhibition may last weeks after anticoagulant withdrawn, but fatal hemorrhage can occur when inhibiting effect disappears.
Cholestyramine: decreased response when administered too close together. Administer 6 hours after oral anticoagulants.

NURSING CONSIDERATIONS
• Contraindicated in hemophilia, thrombocytopenic purpura, leukemia with pronounced bleeding tendency, open wounds or ulcers, impaired hepatic or renal function, severe hypertension, acute nephritis, and subacute bacterial endocarditis. Use cautiously in pregnancy, lactation, during menses, during use of any drainage tube in any orifice, and in any patient in whom slight bleeding is dangerous. Use with extreme caution (if at all) in psychiatric patients, debilitated patients, or cachectic patients.
• Use caution when adding or stopping any drug. May cause alteration in clotting status and result in hemorrhage.
• Fever and skin rash signal severe complications.
• Give drug at same time daily. Stress importance of complying with recommended dosage and keeping follow-up appointments. Patient should carry a card that identifies him as a potential bleeder.
• Regularly inspect patient for bleeding gums, bruises on arms or legs, pe-

techiae, nosebleeds, melena, tarry stools, hematuria, hematemesis. Tell patient and family to watch for these signs and notify doctor immediately.
• Warn patient to avoid over-the-counter products containing aspirin, salicylates, or other drugs that may interact with phenindione.
• Because onset of action is delayed, heparin sodium is often given during first few days of treatment. When heparin is being given simultaneously, don't draw blood for prothrombin times within 5 hours of I.V. heparin administration.
• Dose given depends on prothrombin times (PT). Doctors usually try to maintain PT at 1.5 to 2 times normal. Numerical PT values depend on procedure and reagents used in individual laboratory.
• Tell patient to notify doctor if menses is heavier than usual. May require adjusting dose.
• Tell patient to use electric razor when shaving to avoid scratching skin and to brush teeth with a soft toothbrush.
• Warn patient that urine may turn red-orange.
• Duration of action is 2 to 4 days.
• Light to moderate alcohol intake does not significantly affect prothrombin times.

---

phenprocoumon
Liquamar, Marcumar♦♦

INDICATIONS & DOSAGE
Treatment of pulmonary emboli; prevention and treatment of deep-vein thrombosis, myocardial infarction, rheumatic heart disease with heart valve damage, atrial arrhythmias—
Adults: initially, 24 mg P.O. Maintenance dose: 0.75 to 6 mg daily, based on prothrombin time.

SIDE EFFECTS

Blood: *hemorrhage with excessive dosage, agranulocytosis,* leukopenia.
GI: paralytic ileus and intestinal obstruction (both resulting from hemorrhage), nausea, vomiting, cramps, diarrhea, mouth ulcers.
GU: nephropathy, hematuria.
Skin: *rash,* necrosis.
Other: alopecia, *fever.*

INTERACTIONS

Allopurinol, clofibrate, dextrothyroxine, thyroid drugs, heparin, anabolic steroids, disulfiram, aminosalicylic acid, glucagon, inhalation anesthetics, sulfinpyrazone, sulindac, sulfonamides: increased prothrombin time. Monitor patient carefully. Consider anticoagulant dose reduction.
Ethacrynic acid, indomethacin, mefenamic acid, oxyphenbutazone, phenylbutazone, salicylates: increased prothrombin time; ulcerogenic effects. Don't use together.
Antipyrine, carbamazepine, antacids, griseofulvin, haloperidol, paraldehyde, rifampin: decreased prothrombin time. Monitor patient carefully.
Phenytoin, glutethimide, chloral hydrate, triclofos sodium: increased or decreased prothrombin time. Avoid use if possible, or monitor patient carefully.
Barbiturates: inhibition of hypoprothrombinemic effect of anticoagulants. If barbiturates are withdrawn, reduce anticoagulant dose; inhibition may last for weeks after anticoagulant is withdrawn, but fatal hemorrhage can occur when inhibiting effect disappears.
Cholestyramine: decreased response when administered too close together. Administer 6 hours after oral anticoagulants.

NURSING CONSIDERATIONS

• Contraindicated in hemophilia, thrombocytopenic purpura, leukemia with pronounced bleeding tendency, open wounds or ulcers, impaired hepatic or renal function, severe hypertension, acute nephritis, and subacute bacterial endocarditis. Use cautiously in pregnancy, lactation, during menses, during use of any drainage tube in any orifice, and in any patient in whom slight bleeding is dangerous. Use with extreme caution (if at all) in psychiatric, debilitated, or cachectic patients.
• Use caution when adding or stopping any drug for patient receiving anticoagulants. May change the clotting status and result in hemorrhage.
• Fever and skin rash signal severe complications.
• Give drug at same time daily. Stress importance of complying with recommended dosage and keeping follow-up appointments. Patient should carry a card that identifies him as a potential bleeder.
• Regularly inspect patient for bleeding gums, bruises on arms or legs, petechiae, nosebleeds, melena, tarry stools, hematuria, hematemesis. Tell patient and family to watch for these signs and notify doctor immediately.
• Warn patient to avoid over-the-counter products containing aspirin, other salicylates, or drugs that may interact with phenprocoumon.
• Because onset of action is delayed, heparin sodium is often given during first few days of treatment. When heparin is being given simultaneously, don't draw blood for protrombin times within 5 hours of I.V. heparin administration.
• Dose given depends on prothombin times (PT). Doctors usually try to maintain PT at 1.5 to 2 times normal. Numerical PT values depend on procedure and reagents used in individual laboratory.
• Tell patient to notify doctor if menses is heavier than usual. May require adjusting dose.
• Tell patient to use electric razor when shaving to avoid scratching skin

512   NURSING81 DRUG HANDBOOK

and to brush teeth with a soft tooth-brush.
- Warn patient that urine may turn orange-red.
- A coumarin derivative.
- Duration of action is 4 to 7 days.
- Light to moderate alcohol intake does not significantly affect pro-thrombin times.

protamine sulfate

INDICATIONS & DOSAGE
Heparin overdose—
Adults: dosage based on venous blood coagulation studies, generally 1 mg for each 78 to 95 units of heparin. Give diluted to 1% (10 mg/ml) slow I.V. injection over 1 to 3 minutes. Maximum 50 mg/10 minutes.

SIDE EFFECTS
CV: fall in blood pressure, brady-cardia.
Other: transitory flushing, feeling of warmth, dyspnea.

INTERACTIONS
None significant.

NURSING CONSIDERATIONS
- Use cautiously in allergy to fish or after cardiac surgery.
- Doctor gives this drug. Should be given slowly to reduce side effects. Have equipment available to treat shock.
- Monitor patient continually. Check vital signs frequently.
- Watch for spontaneous bleeding, especially in dialysis patients and patients after cardiac surgery (heparin "rebound").
- Protamine sulfate may act as anticoagulant in very high doses.
- 1 mg of protamine neutralizes 78 to 95 units of heparin.
- Heparin antagonist.

warfarin potassium
Athrombin-K♦
warfarin sodium
Coumadin♦♦, Panwarfin, Warfilone Sodium♦♦, Warnerin Sodium♦♦

INDICATIONS & DOSAGE
Treatment of pulmonary emboli; prevention and treatment of deep-vein thrombosis, myocardial infarction, rheumatic heart disease with heart valve damage, atrial arrhythmias—
Adults: 10 to 15 mg P.O. for 3 days, then dosage based on daily prothrombin times. Usual maintenance dose 2 to 10 mg P.O. daily. Alternate regimen: initially, 40 to 60 mg P.O. daily; then 2 to 10 mg daily based on PT determinations.
Warfarin sodium also available for I.V. use (50 mg per vial). Reconstitute with sterile water for injection. I.V. form rarely used and may be in periodic short supply.

SIDE EFFECTS
Blood: *hemorrhage with excessive dosage,* leukopenia.
GI: paralytic ileus, intestinal obstruction (both resulting from hemorrhage), diarrhea, vomiting, cramps, nausea.
GU: excessive uterine bleeding.
Skin: dermatitis, urticaria, *rash,* necrosis.
Other: *fever,* alopecia.

INTERACTIONS
Allopurinol, clofibrate, dextrothyroxine, thyroid drugs, heparin, anabolic steroids, cimetidine, disulfiram, aminosalicylic acid, glucagon, inhalation anesthetics, sulfinpyrazone, sulindac, sulfonamides: increased prothrombin time. Monitor patient carefully. Consider anticoagulant dose reduction.
Ethacrynic acid, indomethacin, mefenamic acid, oxyphenbutazone, phenylbutazone, salicylates: increased pro-

thrombin time; ulcerogenic effects.
Don't use together.
Griseofulvin, haloperidol, paraldehyde, rifampin: decreased prothrombin time. Monitor patient carefully.
Glutethimide, chloral hydrate, triclofos sodium: increased or decreased prothrombin time. Avoid use if possible, or monitor patient carefully.
Barbiturates: inhibition of hypoprothrombinemic effect of anticoagulants. If barbiturates are withdrawn, reduce anticoagulant dose; inhibition may last weeks after anticoagulant withdrawn, but fatal hemorrhage can occur when inhibiting effect disappears.
Cholestyramine: decreased response when administered too close together. Administer 6 hours after oral anticoagulants.

NURSING CONSIDERATIONS
• Contraindicated in bleeding or hemorrhagic tendencies resulting from open wounds, visceral cancer, GI ulcers, severe hepatic or renal disease, severe uncontrolled hypertension, subacute bacterial endocarditis, vitamin K deficiency; after recent operations in eye, brain, or spinal cord. Use cautiously in diverticulitis, colitis, mild or moderate hypertension, mild or moderate hepatic or renal disease, lactation, in presence of drainage tubes in any orifice, with regional or lumbar block anesthesia, or any condition increasing risk of hemorrhage.
• Observe nursing infants of mothers on drug for unexpected bleeding.
• PT determinations essential for proper control. High incidence of bleeding when PT exceeds 2.5 times control values. Doctors usually try to maintain PT at 1.5 to 2 times normal.
• May divide large doses to reduce GI distress.
• Give at same time daily. Stress importance of complying with recom-

mended dosage and keeping follow-up appointments. Patient should carry a card that identifies him as a potential bleeder.
• Elderly patients and patients in renal or hepatic failure are especially sensitive to warfarin effect.
• Half-life of warfarin is 36 to 44 hours.
• Warfarin effect can be neutralized by vitamin K injections.
• Regularly inspect patient for bleeding gums, bruises on arms or legs, petechiae, nosebleeds, melena, tarry stools, hematuria, hematemesis. Tell patient and family to watch for these signs and notify doctor immediately.
• Warn patient to avoid over-the-counter products containing aspirin, other salicylates, or drugs that may interact with warfarin potassium or warfarin sodium.
• Because onset of action is delayed, heparin sodium is often given during first few days of treatment. When heparin is being given simultaneously, don't draw blood for prothrombin times within 5 hours of I.V. heparin administration.
• Fever and skin rash signal severe complications.
• Tell patient to notify doctor if menses is heavier than usual. May require adjusting dose.
• Tell patient to use electric razor when shaving to avoid scratching skin and to brush teeth with a soft toothbrush.
• Best oral anticoagulant when patient must receive antacids or phenytoin.
• Light to moderate alcohol intake does not significantly affect prothrombin times.
• Possibly effective in treatment of transient cerebral ischemic attacks.

62

Hemostatics

absorbable gelatin sponge
aminocaproic acid
antihemophilic factor (AHF)
carbazochrome salicylate
Factor IX complex
microfibrillar collagen hemostat
negatol
oxidized cellulose
thrombin

---

absorbable gelatin sponge
Gelfoam

INDICATIONS & DOSAGE
Adults:
Decubitus ulcers—place aseptically
deep into ulcer. Don't disturb or re-
move; may add extra p.r.n.
*To provide hemostasis in surgery (ad-
junct)*— apply saturated with isotonic
NaCl injection or thrombin solution.
Hold in place for 10 to 15 seconds.
When bleeding is controlled, allow
material to remain in place.

SIDE EFFECTS
None reported.

INTERACTIONS
None significant.

NURSING CONSIDERATIONS
• Contraindicated in frank infection,
as sole hemostatic agent in abnormal
bleeding, or in postpartum bleeding
or hemorrhage.
• Avoid overpacking when placed
into body cavities or closed tissue
spaces.

• Systemically absorbed; no need to
remove.

---

aminocaproic acid
Amicar♦

INDICATIONS & DOSAGE
*Excessive bleeding resulting from
hyperfibrinolysis*—
Adults: initially, 5 g P.O. or slow I.V.
infusion, followed by 1 to 1.25 g
hourly until bleeding is controlled.
Maximum dose 30 g daily.

SIDE EFFECTS
Blood: generalized thrombosis.
CNS: dizziness, headache.
CV: hypotension.
EENT: tinnitus, nasal stuffiness, con-
junctival suffusion.
GI: nausea, cramps, diarrhea.
Skin: rash.
Other: malaise.

INTERACTIONS
Oral contraceptives: increased proba-
bility of hypercoagulability. Use together cautiously.

NURSING CONSIDERATIONS
• Contraindicated in active intravascular clotting. Use cautiously in
thrombophlebitis and cardiac, hepatic, or renal disease.
• Monitor coagulation studies, heart
rhythm, and blood pressure. Notify
doctor of any change immediately.
• Also used as antidote for streptoki-

nase or urokinase toxicity; beneficial in the treatment of thrombocytopenia.
• Dilute solution with sterile water for injection, normal saline injection, 5% dextrose in water, or Ringer's injection.

---

antihemophilic factor (AHF)
Antihemophilic Globulin (AHG), Factorate, Hemofil, Humafac Koate, Profilate

INDICATIONS & DOSAGE
Hemophilia A (Factor VIII deficiency)—
Adults and children: 10 to 20 units/Kg I.V. push or infusion q 8 to 24 hours. Maintenance doses may be less. Infusion rate usually 10 to 20 ml reconstituted solution per 3 minutes. Dosage varies with individual needs.

SIDE EFFECTS
CNS: headache, paresthesias, clouding or loss of consciousness.
CV: tachycardia, hypotension, possible intravascular hemolysis in patients with blood type A, B, or AB.
EENT: disturbed vision.
GI: nausea, vomiting.
Skin: erythema, urticaria.
Other: *chills, fever, backache, flushing,* constriction in chest; hypersensitivity.

INTERACTIONS
None significant.

NURSING CONSIDERATIONS
• Use cautiously in neonates, infants, and patients with hepatic disease because of susceptibility to hepatitis, which may be transmitted in antihemophilic factor.
• Have blood typed and crossmatched to treat possible hemorrhage.
• Monitor vital signs regularly. Take pulse rate before I.V. administration.

If pulse rate increases significantly, flow rate should be reduced or administration stopped.
• Monitor patient for allergic reactions.
• For I.V. use only. Use plastic syringe; drug may interact with glass syringe, causing binding of ground-glass surface.
• Refrigerate concentrate until ready to use, but not after reconstituted. Before reconstituting, concentrate and diluent bottles should be warmed to room temperature. Reconstituted solution unstable; use within 3 hours. Store away from heat. Don't shake or mix with other I.V. solutions.
• Monitor coagulation studies before and during therapy.

---

carbazochrome salicylate
Adrenosem Salicylate

INDICATIONS & DOSAGE
Surgery with excessive capillary bleeding or oozing—
Adults, and children over 12 years: 10 mg I.M. preoperatively on night before surgery and with on-call medication, and 5 mg P.O. or I.M. postop q 2 to 4 hours.
Children under 12 years: 5 mg I.M. preoperatively on night before surgery and with on-call medication, and 2.5 mg P.O. or I.M. postop q 2 to 4 hours.

SIDE EFFECTS
Local: pain at I.M. injection site.

INTERACTIONS
None significant.

NURSING CONSIDERATIONS
• Contraindicated in hypersensitivity to salicylates.
• Obtain patient history concerning allergies, especially to salicylates.

• Has no effect on blood-clotting time, prothrombin, vitamin K levels.

Factor IX complex
Konyne, Proplex

INDICATIONS & DOSAGE
Factor IX deficiency (hemophilia B or Christmas disease), anticoagulant overdosage—
Adults and children: units required equal 0.6 x body weight in Kg x percentage of desired increase of Factor IX level, by slow I.V. infusion or I.V. push. Dosage is highly individualized, depending on degree of deficiency, level of Factor IX desired, weight of patient, and severity of bleeding.

SIDE EFFECTS
CNS: headache.
CV: possible intravascular hemolysis in patients with blood types A, B, AB.
Other: *transient fever, chills, flushing, tingling,* hypersensitivity.

INTERACTIONS
None significant.

NURSING CONSIDERATIONS
• Contraindicated in hepatic disease, intravascular coagulation, or fibrinolysis. Use cautiously in neonates and infants because of susceptibility to hepatitis, which may be transmitted with Factor IX complex.
• Have blood typed and crossmatched to treat possible hemorrhage. If given to patients with blood types A, B, AB, intravascular hemolysis may occur.
• Monitor patient for allergic reactions and vital signs regularly.
• Avoid rapid infusion. If tingling sensation develops during I.V. infusion, decrease flow rate.
• Reconstitute with 20 ml sterile water for injection for each vial of lyophilized drug. Keep refrigerated until

ready to use; warm to room temperature before reconstituting. Use within 3 hours of reconstitution. Unstable in solution. Don't shake, refrigerate, or mix reconstituted solution with other I.V. solutions. Store away from heat.

microfibrillar collagen hemostat
Avitene

INDICATIONS & DOSAGE
To provide hemostasis in surgery (adjunct)—
Adults and children: amount depends on severity of bleeding. Compress area with dry sponges. Apply drug directly to bleeding site for 1 to 5 minutes. Gently remove excess. Reapply if needed.

SIDE EFFECTS
Blood: hematoma.
Local: exacerbation of wound dehiscence, abscess formation, foreign body reaction, adhesion formation.
Other: advanced infection in contaminated wounds, mediastinitis, hypersensitivity.

INTERACTIONS
None significant.

NURSING CONSIDERATIONS
• Contraindicated in closure of skin incisions.
• Not for injection.
• Don't spill on nonbleeding surfaces.
• Don't dilute. Always apply dry.
• Adheres to wet gloves, instruments, or tissue surfaces. Handle and apply with smooth, dry forceps. Apply directly to source of bleeding.

Italicized side effects are common or life-threatening.

negatol
Negatan

INDICATIONS & DOSAGE
Cervical bleeding—
Women: apply 1-inch gauze dipped in 1:10 dilution of drug; insert in cervical canal. If tolerated, may increase to full-strength solution. Remove pack after 24 hours; give 2-quart douche of dilute negatol or vinegar.
Oral ulcers—
Adults and children: apply to dried lesion with applicator, leave for 1 minute, then neutralize with large amounts of water.

SIDE EFFECTS
Local: *burning sensation.*
Skin: erythema, superficial desquamation when applied to skin.

INTERACTIONS
None significant.

NURSING CONSIDERATIONS
• Grayish vaginal membrane after vaginal use.
• When used in vagina, patient should wear a perineal pad to prevent soiling of clothing.
• When used for oral ulcers, may apply topical anesthetic first to prevent burning sensation.
• Always clean and dry area to be treated.
• Astringent, styptic, and protein denaturant; highly acidic.

oxidized cellulose
Oxycel♦, Surgicel

INDICATIONS & DOSAGE
To provide hemostasis in surgery (adjunct)—
Adults and children: apply with sterile technique, p.r.n. Remove after hemostasis, if possible, with dry sterile forceps. Leave in place if necessary.

SIDE EFFECTS
CNS: headache when used as packing for epistaxis, or after rhinologic procedures or application to surface wounds.
EENT: sneezing, epistaxis or stinging, burning when used as packing for rhinologic procedures; nasal membrane necrosis or septal perforation.
Local: encapsulation of fluid, foreign body reaction, burning or stinging after application to surface wounds.
Other: possible prolongation of drainage in cholecystectomies.

INTERACTIONS
None significant.

NURSING CONSIDERATIONS
• Contraindicated in controlling hemorrhage from large arteries; in non-hemorrhagic, serous, oozing surfaces; in implantation in bone defects.
• Don't pack or wad unless it will be removed after hemostasis. Don't apply too tightly when used as wrap sheet in vascular surgery. Apply loosely against bleeding surface.
• Always remove after hemostasis when used in laminectomies or near optic nerve chain.
• Don't autoclave this product.
• Use only amount needed to produce hemostasis. Remove excess before surgical closure.
• Use minimal amounts in urologic procedures.
• In large wounds, don't overlap skin edges.
• Remove with sterile technique from open wounds after hemostasis.
• Don't moisten. Hemostatic effect is greater when applied dry.
• Should not be used for permanent packing in fractures because it may result in cyst formation.

thrombin
Fibrindex

INDICATIONS & DOSAGE
Bleeding from parenchymatous tissue, cancellous bone, dental sockets, nasal and laryngeal surgery, and in plastic surgery and skin-grafting procedures—
Adults: apply 100 units per ml of sterile isotonic NaCl solution or sterile distilled water to area where clotting needed (or may apply dry powder in bone surgery); in major bleeding, apply 1,000 to 2,000 units/ml sterile isotonic NaCl solution. Sponge blood from area before application, but avoid sponging area after application.
GI hemorrhage—
Adults: give 2 oz of milk, followed by 2 oz of milk containing 10,000 to 20,000 units thrombin. Repeat t.i.d. for 4 to 5 days or until bleeding is controlled.

SIDE EFFECTS
Systemic: hypersensitivity and fever.

INTERACTIONS
None significant.

NURSING CONSIDERATIONS
• Contraindicated in hypersensitivity to thrombin or bovine products.
• Obtain patient history of past reactions to thrombin or bovine products.
• Monitor patient for allergic reactions and vital signs regularly.
• Have blood typed and crossmatched to treat possible hemorrhage.
• Don't inject topical thrombin or allow it to enter large blood vessels. I.V. injection may cause death because of severe intravascular clotting.
• May be used with absorbable gelatin sponge but not with oxidized cellulose. Check sponge labeling before use.
• Neutralize stomach acids before oral use in GI hemorrhage.
• Keep refrigerated, preferably frozen, until ready to use. Unstable in solution. Use within 24 hours of reconstitution; discard after 48 hours. Store away from heat.
• Broken down by diluted acid, alkali, and salts of heavy metals.

63

Blood derivatives

normal serum albumin
plasma protein fraction

normal serum albumin 5%
Albuconn 5%, Albuminar 5%, Albumisol 5%, Albuspan 5%, Albutein 5%, Buminate 5%, Plasbumin 5%
normal serum albumin 25%
Albuconn 25%, Albuminar 25%, Albumisol 25%, Buminate 25%, Plasbumin 25%

INDICATIONS & DOSAGE
Shock—
Adults: initially, 500 ml (5% solution) by I.V. infusion, repeat q 30 minutes, p.r.n. Dose varies with patient's condition and response.
Children: 25% to 50% adult dose in nonemergency.
Hypoproteinemia—
Adults: 1,000 to 1,500 ml 5% solution by I.V. infusion daily, maximum rate 5 to 10 ml/minute; or 25 to 100 g 25% solution by I.V. infusion daily, maximum rate 3 ml/minute. Dose varies with patient condition and response.
*Burns—*dosage varies according to extent of burn and patient's condition. Generally maintain plasma albumin at 2 to 3 g/100 ml.
Hyperbilirubinemia—
Infants: 1 g albumin (4 ml 25%)/Kg before transfusion.

SIDE EFFECTS
CV: *vascular overload after rapid infusion,* hypotension, altered pulse rate.
GI: increased salivation, nausea, vomiting.
Skin: urticaria.
Other: chills, fever, altered respiration.

INTERACTIONS
None significant.

NURSING CONSIDERATIONS
• Contraindicated in severe anemia, heart failure. Use cautiously in low cardiac reserve, absence of albumin deficiency, restricted salt intake.
• Do not give more than 250 g in 48 hours.
• Watch for hemorrhage or shock if used after surgery or injury.
• Monitor vital signs carefully.
• Watch for signs of hypervolemia (heart failure or pulmonary edema).
• Patient should be properly hydrated before infusion of solution.
• Avoid rapid I.V. infusion.
• Dilute with sterile water for injection, 0.9% NaCl, or 5% dextrose injection. Use solution promptly; contains no preservatives. Discard unused solution.
• Don't use cloudy solutions or those containing sediment. Solution should be clear amber color.
• Freezing may cause bottle to break. Follow storage instructions on bottle.
• One volume of 25% albumin is equivalent to 5 volumes of 5% albumin in producing hemodilution and relative anemia.

• This product is very expensive, and random supply shortages occur often.

---

plasma protein fraction
Plasmanate, Plasmatein, Protenate

INDICATIONS & DOSAGE
Shock—
Adults: varies with patient's condition and response, but usual dose is 250 to 500 ml (12.5 to 25 g protein), usually not faster than 10 ml/minute.
Children: 22 to 33 ml/Kg I.V. infused at rate of 5 to 10 ml/minute.
Hypoproteinemia—
Adults: 1,000 to 1,500 ml I.V. daily. Maximum infusion rate 8 ml/minute.

SIDE EFFECTS
CNS: headache.
CV: variable effects on blood pressure after rapid infusion or intra-arterial administration; *vascular overload after rapid infusion.*
GI: nausea, vomiting, hypersalivation.
Skin: erythema, urticaria.
Other: flushing, chills, fever, back pain, dyspnea.

INTERACTIONS
None significant.

NURSING CONSIDERATIONS
• Contraindicated in severe anemia, heart failure, patients undergoing cardiac bypass. Use cautiously in hepatic or renal failure, low cardiac reserve, restricted salt intake.
• Monitor blood pressure. Infusion should be slowed or stopped if sudden hypotension occurs.
• Vital signs should return to normal gradually; monitor hourly.
• Watch for signs of vascular overload (heart failure or pulmonary edema).
• Monitor intake and output. Watch for decreased urinary output.
• Check expiration date on container before using. Discard solutions in containers that have been opened for more than 4 hours. Solution contains no preservatives.
• Don't use solutions that are cloudy, contain sediment, or have been frozen.
• If patient is dehydrated, give additional fluids either P.O. or I.V.
• Do not give more than 250 g (5,000 ml 5%) in 48 hours.
• Contains 130 to 160 mEq sodium/liter.

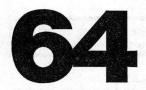

Thrombolytic enzymes

streptokinase
urokinase

streptokinase
Kabikinase, Streptase

INDICATIONS & DOSAGE
Arteriovenous cannula occlusion—
Adults: 250,000 IU in 2 ml I.V. solution by I.V. pump infusion into each occluded limb of the cannula over 25 to 35 minutes. Clamp off cannula for 2 hours. Then aspirate contents of cannula; flush with saline and reconnect.
Venous thrombosis, pulmonary embolism, and arterial thrombosis and embolism—
Adults: loading dose: 250,000 IU I.V. infusion over 30 minutes. Sustaining dose: 100,000 IU/hour I.V. infusion for 72 hours for deep venous thrombosis and 100,000 IU/hour over 24 to 72 hours by I.V. infusion pump for pulmonary embolism.

SIDE EFFECTS
Blood: *bleeding, decreased hematocrit.*
EENT: periorbital swelling.
Local: *phlebitis at injection site.*
Skin: urticaria.
Other: *hypersensitivity to drug, anaphylaxis,* musculoskeletal pain, minor breathing difficulty, bronchospasms, angioneurotic edema.

INTERACTIONS
Anticoagulants: concurrent use of anticoagulants with streptokinase is not recommended. Reversing the effects of oral anticoagulants must be considered before beginning therapy, and heparin must be stopped and its effect allowed to diminish.
Aspirin, indomethacin, phenylbutazone, drugs affecting platelet activity: increased risk of bleeding. Do not use together.

NURSING CONSIDERATIONS
• Contraindicated in ulcerative wounds, active internal bleeding, and cerebrovascular accident; recent trauma with possible internal injuries; visceral or intracranial malignancy; ulcerative colitis; diverticulitis; severe hypertension; acute or chronic hepatic or renal insufficiency; uncontrolled hypocoagulable state; chronic lung disease with cavitation; subacute bacterial endocarditis or rheumatic valvular disease; recent cerebral embolism, thrombosis, or hemorrhage. Also contraindicated within 10 days after intra-arterial diagnostic procedure or any surgery, including liver or kidney biopsy, lumbar puncture, thoracentesis, paracentesis, or extensive or multiple cutdowns.
• Use cautiously when treating arterial emboli that originate from left side of heart because of danger of cerebral infarction.
• I.M. injections contraindicated during streptokinase therapy.
• Before initiating therapy, draw blood to determine PTT and PT. Rate of I.V. infusion depends on thrombin time and streptokinase resistance.

• If the patient has had a recent streptococcal infection or recent treatment
with streptokinase, a higher loading
dose may be necessary.
• Preparation of I.V. solution: reconstitute each vial with 5 ml sodium
chloride for injection. Further dilute
to 45 ml. Don't shake; roll gently to
mix. Use within 24 hours. Store at
room temperature.
• Monitor patient for excessive
bleeding; if evident, stop therapy.
Pretreatment with heparin or drugs
affecting platelets causes high risk of
bleeding.
• Have crossmatched and typed
packed red cells and whole blood
available to treat possible hemorrhage.
• Keep aminocaproic acid (Amicar)
available to treat bleeding. Corticosteroids are used to treat allergic
reactions.
• Before using streptokinase to clear
an occluded arteriovenous cannula,
try flushing with heparinized saline
solution.
• Bruising more likely during therapy; avoid unnecessary handling.
• Keep puncture sites to a minimum;
use pressure dressing on puncture
sites for at least 15 minutes.
• Monitor vital signs frequently.
• Watch for signs of hypersensitivity.
Notify doctor immediately.
• Heparin by continuous infusion is
usually started within an hour after
stopping streptokinase. Use infusion
pump to administer heparin.
• Should be used only by doctors
with wide experience in thrombotic
disease management where clinical
and laboratory monitoring can be performed.
• Store at room temperature. When
reconstituted, store in refrigerator.

urokinase
Abbokinase, Breokinase, Win-Kinase

INDICATIONS & DOSAGE
*Lysis of acute massive pulmonary
emboli and lysis of pulmonary emboli
accompanied by unstable hemo-
dynamics—*
Adults: for I.V. infusion only by constant infusion pump that will deliver a
total volume of 195 ml.
Priming dose: 4,400 IU/Kg/hour of
urokinase-normal saline admixture
given over 10 minutes.
Follow with 4,400 IU/Kg/hour for 12
to 24 hours. Total volume should not
exceed 200 ml.
Follow therapy with continuous I.V.
infusion of heparin, then oral anticoagulants.

SIDE EFFECTS
Blood: *bleeding, decreased
hematocrit.*
Local: *phlebitis at injection site.*
Other: hypersensitivity (not as frequent as streptokinase), musculoskeletal pain, bronchospasm, *anaphylaxis.*

INTERACTIONS
Anticoagulants: concurrent use of
anticoagulants with urokinase is not
recommended. Reversing the effects
of oral anticoagulants must be considered before beginning therapy, and
heparin must be stopped and its effect
allowed to diminish.
*Aspirin, indomethacin, phenylbuta-
zone, other drugs affecting platelet activity:* increased risk of bleeding. Do
not use together.

NURSING CONSIDERATIONS
• Contraindicated in ulcerative
wounds, active internal bleeding, and
cerebrovascular accident; recent
trauma with possible internal injuries;
visceral or intracranial malignancy;

Italicized side effects are common or life-threatening.

pregnancy and first 10 days postpartum; ulcerative colitis; diverticulitis; severe hypertension; acute or chronic hepatic or renal insufficiency; uncontrolled hypocoagulation; chronic lung disease with cavitation; subacute bacterial endocarditis or rheumatic valvular disease; and recent cerebral embolism, thrombosis, or hemorrhage. Also contraindicated within 10 days after intra-arterial diagnostic procedure or any surgery, including liver or kidney biopsy, lumbar puncture, thoracentesis, paracentesis, or extensive or multiple cutdowns.
• I.M. injections are contraindicated during urokinase therapy.
• Preparation of I.V. solution: add 5.2 ml sterile water for injection to vial. Dilute further with 0.9% saline solution before infusion. Don't use bacteriostatic water for injection to reconstitute; it contains preservatives.
• Monitor patient for bleeding. Pretreatment with drugs affecting platelets puts patient at high risk of bleeding.

• Have crossmatched and typed red cells and whole blood available to treat possible hemorrhage.
• Keep aminocaproic acid (Amicar) available to treat bleeding. Corticosteroids are used to treat allergic reactions.
• Watch for signs of hypersensitivity. Notify doctor immediately.
• Monitor vital signs.
• Keep puncture sites to a minimum; use pressure dressing on puncture sites for at least 15 minutes.
• Heparin by continuous infusion usually started within an hour after urokinase has been stopped. Use infusion pump to administer heparin.
• Bruising during therapy more likely; avoid unnecessary handling of patient.
• Should be used only by doctors with wide experience in thrombotic disease management where clinical and laboratory monitoring can be performed.

65

Alkylating agents

busulfan
carmustine (BCNU)
chlorambucil
cisplatin (cis-platinum)
cyclophosphamide
dacarbazine (DTIC)
lomustine (CCNU)
mechlorethamine hydrochloride
    (nitrogen mustard)
melphalan
pipobroman
thiotepa
uracil mustard

busulfan
Myleran◆

INDICATIONS & DOSAGE
Chronic myelocytic (granulocytic) leukemia—
Adults: 4 to 6 mg P.O. daily up to 8 mg P.O. daily until WBC falls to 10,000/mm³; stop drug until WBC rises to 50,000/mm³, then resume treatment as before; or 4 to 8 mg P.O. daily until WBC falls to 10,000 to 20,000/mm³, then reduce daily dose as needed to maintain WBC at this level (usually 2 mg daily).
Children: 0.06 to 0.12 mg/Kg or 2.3 to 4.6 mg/m²/day P.O.; adjust dose to maintain WBC at 20,000/mm³, but never less than 10,000/mm³.

SIDE EFFECTS
Blood: WBC begins to fall after about 10 days and continues for 2 weeks after stopping drug; *thrombocytopenia,* pancytopenia, anemia.

GI: nausea, vomiting, diarrhea, cheilosis, glossitis.
GU: amenorrhea, testicular atrophy, impotence.
Metabolic: Addison-like wasting syndrome. Profound hyperuricemia due to increased cell lysis.
Skin: transient hyperpigmentation, anhidrosis.
Other: gynecomastia; alopecia; *irreversible pulmonary fibrosis, commonly termed "busulfan lung."*

INTERACTIONS
None significant.

NURSING CONSIDERATIONS
• Use cautiously in patients recently given other myelosuppressive drugs or radiation treatment, and in those with depressed neutrophil or platelet count.
• Watch for signs of infection (fever, sore throat).
• Warn patient that side effects may be delayed for 4 to 6 months.
• Persistent cough, progressive dyspnea with alveolar exudate may result from drug toxicity, not pneumonia.
• Monitor uric acid and CBC.
• Patient response usually begins within 1 to 2 weeks (increased appetite, sense of well-being, decreased total leukocyte, reduction in size of spleen).
• Can cause false positive cytology in all body secretions.
• Anticoagulants should be used cautiously. Watch closely for signs of bleeding.

- Avoid all I.M. injections when platelets are low.

carmustine (BCNU)
BiCNU♦

INDICATIONS & DOSAGE
Brain, colon, and stomach cancer; Hodgkin's disease; non-Hodgkin's; lymphomas; melanomas; multiple myeloma; and hepatoma—
Adults: 100 mg/m² I.V. by slow infusion daily for 2 days; repeat q 6 weeks if platelets are above 100,000/mm³ and WBC is above 4,000/mm³. Dose is reduced 50% when WBC less than 2,000/mm³ and platelets less than 25,000/mm³. Alternate therapy: 200 mg/m² I.V. slow infusion as a single dose, repeated q 6 to 8 weeks; or 40 mg/m² I.V. slow infusion for 5 consecutive days, repeated q 6 weeks.

SIDE EFFECTS
Blood: *cumulative bone marrow depression, delayed 4 to 6 weeks, lasts 1 to 2 weeks; leukopenia; thrombocytopenia.*
GI: *nausea, which lasts 2 to 6 hours after giving (can be severe); vomiting.*
Hepatic: hepatotoxicity.
Metabolic: hyperuricemia may occur in lymphoma patients when rapid cell lysis occurs.
Local: *intense pain at infusion site.*

INTERACTIONS
None significant.

NURSING CONSIDERATIONS
- To reduce pain on infusion, dilute further or slow infusion rate.
- Warn patient to watch for signs of infection and bone marrow toxicity (fever, sore throat, anemia, fatigue, easy bruising, nose or gum bleeds, melena). Take temperature daily.
- Monitor uric acid, CBC.

- To reduce nausea, give antiemetic before administering.
- Don't mix with other drugs during administration.
- To reconstitute, dissolve 100 mg carmustine in 3 ml absolute alcohol. Dilute solution with 27 ml sterile water for injection. Resultant solution contains 3.3 mg carmustine/ml in 10% alcohol. Dilute in normal saline solution or dextrose 5% in water for I.V. infusion. Give at least 250 ml over 1 to 2 hours.
- May store reconstituted solution in refrigerator for 24 hours.
- If powder liquefies or appears oily, it is sign of decomposition. Discard.
- Can cause false positive cytology in all body secretions.
- To prevent hyperuricemia with resulting uric acid nephropathy, allopurinol may be used with adequate hydration and alkalinization of urine. Screen urine for stones.
- Avoid contact with skin, as carmustine will cause a brown stain. If drug comes into contact with skin, wash off thoroughly.
- Anticoagulants should be used cautiously. Watch closely for signs of bleeding.
- Avoid all I.M. injections when platelets are low.

chlorambucil
Leukeran♦

INDICATIONS & DOSAGE
Chronic lymphocytic leukemia, lymphosarcoma, giant follicular lymphoma, Hodgkin's disease, ovarian carcinoma, mycosis fungoides—
Adults: 0.1 to 0.2 mg/Kg P.O. daily for 3 to 6 weeks, then adjust for maintenance (usually 2 mg daily).
Children: 0.1 to 0.2 mg/Kg/day or 4.5 mg/m²/day P.O. as single dose or in divided doses.

SIDE EFFECTS

Blood: leukopenia, delayed up to
3 weeks, lasts up to 10 days after last
dose; thrombocytopenia; anemia;
myelosuppression (usually moderate,
gradual, and rapidly reversible).
Metabolic: hyperuricemia.
Skin: *exfoliative dermatitis.*
Other: allergic febrile reactions.

INTERACTIONS

None significant.

NURSING CONSIDERATIONS

• Myelosuppression reversible up to
cumulative dose of 6.5 mg/Kg.
• Monitor uric acid, CBC.
• To prevent hyperuricemia with resulting uric acid nephropathy, allopurinol may be used with adequate hydration and alkalinization of urine.
Screen urine for stones.
• Can cause false positive cytology in
all body secretions.
• Avoid I.M. injections when platelets are low.
• Anticoagulants should be used cautiously. Watch closely for signs of
bleeding.

---

cisplatin (cis-platinum)
Platinol

INDICATIONS & DOSAGE

*Adjunctive therapy in metastatic
testicular cancer—*
Adults: 20 mg/m² I.V. daily for
5 days. Repeat every 3 weeks for
3 cycles or longer.
*Adjunctive therapy in metastatic ovar-
ian cancer—*100 mg/m² I.V. Repeat
every 4 weeks; or 50 mg/m² I.V. every
3 weeks with concurrent doxorubicin
HCl therapy. Give as I.V. infusion in 2
liters normal saline with 37.5 g mannitol over 6 to 8 hours.
Note: Prehydration and mannitol diuresis may reduce renal toxicity and
ototoxicity significantly.

SIDE EFFECTS

Blood: *reversible myelosuppression in
25% to 30% of patients, leukopenia,
thrombocytopenia,* anemia; nadirs in
circulating platelets and leukocytes
on days 18 to 23, with recovery by
day 39.
CNS: peripheral neuritis, loss of
taste, seizures.
EENT: *tinnitus, hearing loss.*
GI: *nausea, vomiting, beginning 1 to
4 hours after dose and lasting
24 hours; diarrhea.*
GU: *renal toxicity becomes more prolonged and severe with repeated
courses of therapy.*
Other: anaphylactoid reaction.

INTERACTIONS

None significant.

NURSING CONSIDERATIONS

• Use cautiously in preexisting renal
impairment, myelosuppression, and
hearing impairment.
• Hydrate patient with normal saline
before giving drug. Maintain urine
output of 100 ml/hour for 4 consecutive hours before therapy and for
24 hours after therapy.
• Don't use aluminum needles for reconstitution or administration of cisplatin; a black precipitate may form.
• Mannitol may be given as 12.5 g
I.V. bolus before starting cisplatin infusion. Follow by infusion of mannitol
at rate up to 10 g/hour p.r.n. to maintain urine output during and 6 to
24 hours after cisplatin infusion.
• Do not repeat dose unless platelets
are over 100,000/mm³, WBC is over
4,000/mm³, creatinine is under 1.5
mg%, or BUN is under 25 mg%.
• Monitor CBC, platelets, and renal
function studies before initial and
subsequent doses.
• Tell patient to report tinnitus immediately to prevent permanent hearing
loss. Do audiometry before and during treatment.
• Nausea and vomiting may be severe

Italicized side effects are common or life-threatening.

and protracted (up to 24 hours). Continue I.V. hydration until patient can tolerate adequate oral intake.
• Reconstitute with sterile water for injection. Stable for 24 hours in normal saline at room temperature. Don't refrigerate.
• Given with bleomycin and vinblastine for testicular cancer and with doxorubicin HCl for ovarian cancer.
• Renal toxicity becomes more severe with repeated doses. Renal function must return to normal before next dose can be given.
• Avoid all I.M. injections when platelets are low.

cyclophosphamide
Cytoxan♦, Procytox♦ ♦

INDICATIONS & DOSAGE

Breast, colon, head, neck, lung, ovarian, and prostatic cancer; Hodgkin's disease; chronic lymphocytic leukemia; chronic myelocytic leukemia; acute lymphoblastic leukemia; neuroblastoma; retinoblastoma; non-Hodgkin's lymphomas; multiple myeloma; mycosis fungoides; sarcomas—
Adults: 40 to 50 mg/Kg P.O. or I.V. in single dose or in 2 to 5 daily doses, then adjust for maintenance; or 2 to 4 mg/Kg P.O. daily for 10 days, then adjust for maintenance. Maintenance dose 1.5 to 3 mg/Kg/day P.O.; or 10 to 15 mg/Kg q 7 to 10 days I.V.; or 3 to 5 mg/Kg twice weekly I.V.
Children: 2 to 8 mg/Kg/day or 60 to 250 mg/m²/day P.O. or I.V. for 6 days (dose depends on susceptibility of neoplasm); divide oral dosages; give I.V. dosages once weekly. Maintenance dose 2 to 5 mg/Kg or 50 to 150 mg/m² twice weekly P.O.

SIDE EFFECTS

Blood: *leukopenia,* nadir between days 8 to 15, recovery in 17 to 28 days; thrombocytopenia; anemia.

CV: *cardiotoxicity* (with very high doses and in combination with doxorubicin).
GI: anorexia; *nausea and vomiting begin within 6 hours, last 4 hours;* stomatitis; mucositis.
GU: gonadal suppression (may be irreversible), *hemorrhagic cystitis,* bladder fibrosis, sterility, nephrotoxicity.
Metabolic: hyperuricemia; syndrome of inappropriate ADH secretion (with high doses).
Other: *alopecia in 50% of patients, especially with high doses;* secondary malignancies, *pulmonary fibrosis (high doses).*

INTERACTIONS

Corticosteroids, chloramphenicol: reduced activity of cyclophosphamide. Use cautiously.
Allopurinol: may produce excessive cyclophosphamide effect. Monitor for enhanced toxicity.

NURSING CONSIDERATIONS

• Use cautiously in severe leukopenia, thrombocytopenia, malignant cell infiltration of bone marrow, recent radiation therapy or chemotherapy, hepatic or renal disease.
• Advise male and female patients to practice contraception while taking this drug and for 4 months after; drug is potentially teratogenic.
• Monitor uric acid, CBC, renal and hepatic functions.
• To reduce nausea, give antiemetic before administering.
• Push fluid (3 liters daily) to prevent hemorrhagic cystitis. Don't give drug at bedtime, since voiding is too infrequent to avoid cystitis. If hemorrhagic cystitis occurs, drug is stopped. Cystitis can occur months after therapy has been stopped.
• Reconstituted solution is stable 6 days refrigerated or 24 hours at room temperature.

- Can cause false positive cytology in all body secretions.
- Avoid all I.M. injections when platelets are low.
- Can be given by direct I.V. push into a running I.V. line or by infusion in normal saline solution or dextrose 5% in water.
- To prevent hyperuricemia with resulting uric acid nephropathy, keep patient well hydrated; alkalinize the urine.
- Warn patient that alopecia is likely to occur.
- Anticoagulants should be used cautiously. Watch closely for signs of bleeding.
- Has been used successfully to treat many nonmalignant conditions.

dacarbazine (DTIC)
DTIC-Dome♦

INDICATIONS & DOSAGE
Hodgkin's disease, metastatic malignant melanoma, neuroblastoma, sarcomas—
Adults: 2 to 4.5 mg/Kg or 70 to 160 mg/m² I.V. daily for 10 days, then repeat q 4 weeks as tolerated; or 250 mg/m² I.V. daily for 5 days, repeated at 3-week intervals.

SIDE EFFECTS
Blood: *WBC falls for up to 5 weeks, recovers in 2 weeks; thrombocytopenia.*
GI: *severe nausea and vomiting begin within 1 to 3 hours in 90% of patients, last 1 to 12 hours; anorexia.*
Local: severe pain if I.V. infiltrates or if solution is too concentrated; tissue damage.
Other: *flu-like syndrome* (fever, malaise, myalgia begin 7 days after treatment stopped and may last 7 to 21 days), alopecia.

INTERACTIONS
None significant.

NURSING CONSIDERATIONS
- Use lower dose if renal function or bone marrow is impaired. Stop drug if WBC falls to 3,000/mm³ or platelets drop to 100,000/mm³.
- Take temperature daily.
- Monitor uric acid, CBC.
- Discard refrigerated solution after 72 hours, room temperature solution after 8 hours.
- Can cause false positive cytology in all body secretions.
- Avoid all I.M. injections when platelets are low.
- Give I.V. infusion in 50 to 100 ml dextrose 5% in water over 30 minutes. May dilute further or slow infusion to decrease pain at infusion site. Make sure drug does not infiltrate.
- For Hodgkin's disease, usually given with bleomycin, vinblastine, doxorubicin.
- Anticoagulants should be used cautiously. Watch closely for signs of bleeding.
- Nausea and vomiting usually subside after several doses.

lomustine (CCNU)
CeeNU♦

INDICATIONS & DOSAGE
Brain, colon, lung, and renal cell cancer; Hodgkin's disease; lymphomas; melanomas; multiple myeloma—
Adults and children: 130 mg/m² P.O. as single dose q 6 weeks. Reduce dose according to bone marrow depression. Repeat doses should not be given until WBC is more than 4,000/mm³ and platelet count is more than 100,000/mm³.

SIDE EFFECTS
Blood: *leukopenia, delayed up to 6 weeks, lasts 1 to 2 weeks; thrombo-*

*cytopenia, delayed up to 4 weeks,
lasts 1 to 2 weeks.*
GI: *nausea and vomiting begin within
4 to 5 hours, last 24 hours;* stomatitis.
Other: alopecia.

INTERACTIONS
None significant.

NURSING CONSIDERATIONS
• Give 2 to 4 hours after meals. To
avoid nausea, give antiemetic before
administering.
• May be useful in cancer involving
CNS, since CSF level equals 30% to
50% of plasma level 1 hour after
administration.
• Monitor blood counts weekly.
Don't give more often than every
6 weeks; bone marrow toxicity is
cumulative and delayed.
• Monitor uric acid, CBC.
• Can cause false positive cytology in
all body secretions.
• Avoid all I.M. injection when platelets are low.
• For Hodgkin's disease, usually
given with mechlorethamine.
• Anticoagulants should be used cautiously. Watch closely for signs of
bleeding.

mechlorethamine hydrochloride (nitrogen mustard)
Mustargen♦

INDICATIONS & DOSAGE
*Breast, lung, and ovarian cancer;
Hodgkin's disease; non-Hodgkin's
lymphomas; lymphosarcoma—*
Adults: 0.4 mg/Kg or 10 mg/m² I.V.
as single or divided dose q 3 to
6 weeks. Give through running I.V.
infusion. Dose reduced in prior radiation or chemotherapy to 0.2 to 0.4
mg/Kg. Dose based on ideal or actual
body weight, whichever is less.
Neoplastic effusions—
Adults: 10 to 20 mg intracavitarily.

SIDE EFFECTS
Blood: *nadir of leukopenia, thrombocytopenia, myelosuppression occurs
by days 4 to 10, lasts 10 to 21 days;*
mild anemia begins in 2 to 3 weeks,
may last 7 weeks.
EENT: tinnitus, *metallic taste,* immediately after dose; deafness in high
doses.
GI: *nausea, vomiting, and anorexia*
begin within minutes, last 8 to
24 hours.
Metabolic: hyperuricemia.
Local: *thrombophlebitis, sloughing,
severe irritation if drug extravasates or
touches skin.*
Other: may precipitate herpes zoster,
alopecia.

INTERACTIONS
None significant.

NURSING CONSIDERATIONS
• Use cautiously in severe anemia,
depressed neutrophil or platelet
count, patients recently treated with
radiation or chemotherapy.
• Avoid contact with skin or mucous
membranes. If contact occurs, wash
with copious amounts of water.
• Giving antiemetic before drug not
always effective in reducing nausea.
• Be sure I.V. doesn't infiltrate. If
drug extravasates, apply cold compresses.
• When given intracavitarily, turn patient from side to side every 15 minutes to 1 hour to distribute drug.
• Monitor uric acid, CBC.
• Severe herpes zoster may require
stopping drug.
• Very unstable solution. Prepare immediately before infusion. Use within
15 minutes. Discard unused solution.
• To prevent hyperuricemia with resulting uric acid nephropathy, allopurinol may be given; keep patient well
hydrated; alkalinize the urine.
• Can cause false positive cytology in
all body secretions.

- Avoid all I.M. injections when platelets are low.
- One of the most effective drugs in treatment of Hodgkin's disease.
- Has been used topically in treatment of mycosis fungoides.
- Anticoagulants should be used cautiously. Watch closely for signs of bleeding.

- Avoid all I.M. injections when platelets are low.
- May need dose reduction in renal impairment.
- Drug of choice in multiple myeloma.
- Anticoagulants should be used cautiously. Watch closely for signs of bleeding.

melphalan
Alkeran♦

INDICATIONS & DOSAGE
Multiple myeloma, malignant melanoma, testicular seminoma, reticulum cell sarcoma, osteogenic sarcoma, breast and ovarian cancer—
Adults: 6 mg P.O. daily for 2 to 3 weeks, then stop drug for up to 4 weeks or until WBC and platelets stop dropping and begin to rise again; resume with maintenance dose of 2 to 4 mg daily. Stop drug if WBC below 3,000/mm^3 or platelets below 100,000/mm^3. Alternate therapy: 0.15 mg/Kg/day P.O. for 7 days, wait for WBC and platelets to recover, then resume with 0.05 mg/Kg/day P.O.

SIDE EFFECTS
Blood: *thrombocytopenia, leukopenia, agranulocytosis.*
GI: anorexia, nausea, vomiting.

INTERACTIONS
None significant.

NURSING CONSIDERATIONS
- Not recommended in severe leukopenia, thrombocytopenia, or anemia, chronic lymphocytic leukemia, patients with suppurative inflammation.
- To reduce nausea, give antiemetic before administering.
- Monitor uric acid, CBC.
- Can cause false positive cytology in all body secretions.

pipobroman
Vercyte♦

INDICATIONS & DOSAGE
Polycythemia vera—
Adults, and children over 15 years: 1 mg/Kg P.O. daily for 30 days; may increase to 1.5 to 3 mg/Kg P.O. daily until hematocrit reduced to 50% to 55%, then 0.1 to 0.2 mg/Kg daily maintenance.
Chronic myelocytic leukemia—
Adults, and children over 15 years: 1.5 to 2.5 mg/Kg P.O. daily until WBC drops to 10,000/mm^3, then start maintenance 7 to 175 mg daily. Stop drug if WBC below 3,000/mm^3 or platelets below 150,000/mm^3.

SIDE EFFECTS
Blood: *leukopenia and thrombocytopenia, delayed up to 4 weeks or longer.*
GI: nausea, vomiting, cramping, diarrhea, anorexia.
Skin: rash.

INTERACTIONS
None significant.

NURSING CONSIDERATIONS
- Use cautiously in bone marrow depression.
- Do WBC and platelet count until desired response or toxicity occurs (platelets less than 150,000/mm^3 or WBC less than 3,000/mm^3).
- Monitor CBC.
- Anticoagulants should be used cau-

Italicized side effects are common or life-threatening.

tiously. Watch closely for signs of bleeding.

---

thiotepa
Thiotepa♦

INDICATIONS & DOSAGE
Adults, and children over 12 years:
Breast, lung, and ovarian cancer; Hodgkin's disease; lymphomas—
0.2 mg/Kg I.V. daily for 5 days; then maintenance dose of 0.2 mg/Kg I.V. q 1 to 3 weeks.
Bladder tumor—60 mg in 60 ml water instilled in bladder once weekly for 4 weeks.
Neoplastic effusions—10 to 15 mg intracavitarily, p.r.n. Stop drug or decrease dosage if WBC below 4,000/mm³ or if platelets below 150,000/mm³.

SIDE EFFECTS
Blood: *leukopenia begins within 5 to 30 days; thrombocytopenia; neutropenia.*
GI: nausea, vomiting, anorexia.
GU: amenorrhea, decreased spermatogenesis.
Metabolic: hyperuricemia.
Skin: hives, rash.
Local: intense pain at administration site.
Other: headache, fever, tightness of throat, dizziness.

INTERACTIONS
None significant.

NURSING CONSIDERATIONS
• Use cautiously in bone marrow depression, chronic lymphocytic leukemia, renal or hepatic dysfunction.
• Do WBC, RBC counts weekly for at least 3 weeks after last dose. Warn patient to report even mild infections.
• GU side effects reversible in 6 to 8 months.

• May require use of local anesthetic at injection site if intense pain occurs.
• For bladder instillation: dehydrate patient 8 to 10 hours before therapy. Instill drug into bladder by catheter; ask patient to retain solution for 2 hours. Volume may be reduced to 30 ml if discomfort is too great with 60 ml. Reposition patient every 15 minutes for maximum area contact.
• Toxicity delayed and prolonged because drug binds to tissues and stays in body several hours.
• Monitor uric acid, CBC.
• Refrigerate dry powder; protect from light.
• Use only sterile water for injection to reconstitute. Refrigerated solution stable 5 days.
• To prevent hyperuricemia with resulting uric acid nephropathy, allopurinol may be given; keep patient well hydrated; alkalinize the urine.
• Can cause false positive cytology in all body secretions.
• Avoid all I.M. injections when platelets are low.
• Can be given by all parenteral routes, including direct injection into the tumor.
• Anticoagulants should be used cautiously. Watch closely for signs of bleeding.

---

uracil mustard

INDICATIONS & DOSAGE
Chronic lymphocytic and myelocytic leukemia; Hodgkin's disease; non-Hodgkin's lymphomas of the histiocytic and lymphocytic types; reticulum cell sarcoma; lymphomas; mycosis fungoides; polycythemia vera; cancer of ovaries, cervix, and lungs—
Adults: 1 to 2 mg P.O. daily for 3 months or until desired response or toxicity; maintenance 1 mg daily for 3 out of 4 weeks until optimum response or relapse; or 3 to 5 mg P.O.

---

for 7 days not to exceed total dose
0.5 mg/Kg, then 1 mg daily until response, then 1 mg daily 3 out of
4 weeks.

SIDE EFFECTS
Blood: bone marrow depression, delayed 2 to 4 weeks; *thrombocytopenia; leukopenia;* anemia.
CNS: irritability, nervousness, mental
cloudiness and depression.
GI: *nausea, vomiting, diarrhea,
epigastric distress,* abdominal pain,
anorexia.
Metabolic: hyperuricemia.
Skin: pruritus, dermatitis, hyperpigmentation, alopecia.

INTERACTIONS
None significant.

NURSING CONSIDERATIONS
• Not recommended in severe thrombocytopenia, aplastic anemia or leukopenia, acute leukemias.

• Give at bedtime to reduce nausea.
• Watch for signs of ecchymoses,
easy bruising, petechiae.
• Monitor uric acid. Do regular platelet count. Do CBC 1 to 2 times
weekly for 4 weeks; then 4 weeks after stopping drug.
• Don't give drug within 2 to 3 weeks
after maximum bone marrow depression from past radiation or chemotherapy.
• To prevent hyperuricemia and resulting uric acid nephropathy, allopurinol can be given; keep patient hydrated; alkalinize the urine.
• Can cause false positive cytology in
all body secretions.
• Avoid all I.M. injections when
platelets are low.
• Anticoagulants should be used cautiously. Watch closely for signs of
bleeding.

Italicized side effects are common or life-threatening.

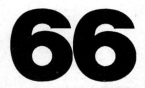

Antimetabolites

azathioprine
cytarabine
floxuridine
fluorouracil
hydroxyurea
mercaptopurine
methotrexate
methotrexate sodium
thioguanine

azathioprine
Imuran ♦

INDICATIONS & DOSAGE
Immunosuppression in renal transplants—
Adults and children: initially, 3 to
5 mg/Kg P.O. daily. Maintain at 1 to
2 mg/Kg/day (dose varies considerably according to patient response).

SIDE EFFECTS
Blood: *leukopenia, bone marrow depression,* anemia, pancytopenia, thrombocytopenia.
GI: nausea, vomiting, anorexia, pancreatitis, ascites, steatorrhea, mouth ulceration, esophagitis.
Hepatic: hepatoxicity, jaundice.
Skin: rash.
Other: *immunosuppression (possibly profound),* arthralgia, muscle wasting, alopecia, pancreatitis.

INTERACTIONS
Allopurinol: impaired inactivation of azathioprine. Decrease azathioprine dose to ¼ or ⅓ normal dose.

NURSING CONSIDERATIONS
• Use cautiously in hepatic or renal dysfunction.
• Watch for clay-colored stools, dark urine, pruritus, yellow skin and sclera, and for increased alkaline phosphatase, bilirubin, SGOT, SGPT.
• In renal homotransplants, start drug 1 to 5 days before surgery.
• Hemoglobin, WBC, platelet count should be done at least once a week; more often at beginning of treatment. Drug should be stopped immediately when WBC is less than 3,000/mm³ to prevent extension to irreversible bone marrow depression.
• This is a potent immunosuppressant. Warn patient to report even mild infections (coryza, fever, sore throat, malaise).
• Patient should avoid conception during and up to 4 months after stopping therapy.
• Warn patient that some thinning of hair is possible.
• Avoid all I.M. injections in patients with severely depressed platelet counts (thrombocytopenia) to prevent bleeding.

cytarabine (ARA-C, cytosine arabinoside)
Cytosar-U ♦

INDICATIONS & DOSAGE
Acute myelocytic and other acute leukemias—
Adults and children: 2 to 3 mg/Kg
(100 mg/m²) I.V. or S.C. b.i.d. for

7 days; 2 to 3 mg/Kg (100 mg/m²) daily for 7 days by 24-hour continuous infusion; or 10 to 30 mg/m² intrathecally, up to 3 times weekly. Maintenance 2 to 3 mg/Kg I.V. or S.C. b.i.d. for 5 days.

SIDE EFFECTS
Blood: WBC nadir occurs 5 to 7 days after drug stopped; *leukopenia, anemia, thrombocytopenia,* reticulocytopenia; platelet nadir occurs day 10; *megaloblastosis.*
GI: *nausea, vomiting,* diarrhea, dysphagia; reddened area at juncture of lips, followed by sore mouth, oral ulcers in 5 to 10 days; high dose given via rapid I.V. may cause projectile vomiting.
Hepatic: hepatotoxicity (usually mild and reversible).
Other: flu-like syndrome.

INTERACTIONS
None significant.

NURSING CONSIDERATIONS
• Use cautiously in inadequate bone marrow reserve. Use cautiously in renal or hepatic disease and after other chemotherapy or radiation.
• Watch for signs of infection (leukoplakia, fever, sore throat).
• Excellent mouth care can help prevent oral side effects.
• Monitor intake/output carefully. Maintain high fluid intake and give allopurinol to avoid urate nephropathy in leukemia induction therapy.
• Check uric acid, CBC with platelets, and hepatic function.
• Use preservative-free normal saline for intrathecal use.
• Optimum schedule is continuous infusion.
• To reduce nausea, give antiemetic before administering.
• Store dry powder in refrigerator; refrigerated, reconstituted solution stable 48 hours. Discard cloudy reconstituted solution.

• Avoid all I.M. injections in patients with severely depressed platelet count (thrombocytopenia) to prevent bleeding.
• Modify or discontinue therapy if polymorphonuclear granulocyte count is 1,000/mm³ or if platelet count is 50,000/mm³.

floxuridine
FUDR

INDICATIONS & DOSAGE
Brain, breast, head, neck, liver, gallbladder, and bile duct cancer—
Adults: 0.1 to 0.6 mg/Kg daily by intra-arterial infusion (use pump for continuous, uniform rate); or 0.4 to 0.6 mg/Kg daily into hepatic artery.

SIDE EFFECTS
Blood: *leukopenia, anemia,* thrombocytopenia.
CNS: cerebellar ataxia, vertigo, nystagmus, convulsions, depression, hemiplegia, hiccups, lethargy.
EENT: blurred vision.
GI: *stomatitis, cramps, nausea, vomiting, diarrhea, bleeding, enteritis.*
Skin: *erythema,* dermatitis, pruritus, rash.

INTERACTIONS
None significant.

NURSING CONSIDERATIONS
• Use cautiously in poor nutritional state, bone marrow depression, or serious infection. Use cautiously following high-dose pelvic irradiation or use of alkylating agent, and in impaired hepatic or renal function.
• Severe skin and GI side effects require stopping drug. Use of antacid eases but probably won't prevent GI distress.
• Excellent mouth care can help prevent oral side effects.

- Monitor intake/output, CBC, and renal and hepatic function.
- Discontinue if WBC falls below 3,500/mm³ or if platelet count below 100,000/mm³.
- Therapeutic effect may be delayed 1 to 6 weeks.
- Reconstitute with sterile water for injection. Dilute further in 5% dextrose in water or normal saline for actual infusion.
- Always use infusion pump.
- Avoid all I.M. injections in patients with thrombocytopenia to prevent bleeding.
- Refrigerated solution stable no more than 2 weeks.
- Observe precautions for catheter line care in arterial perfused area. Check line for bleeding, blockage, displacement, or leakage.

---

fluorouracil (5-fluorouracil)
Adrucil, 5-FU

INDICATIONS & DOSAGE
Colon, rectal, breast, ovarian, cervical, bladder, liver, and pancreatic cancer—
Adults: 12.5 mg/Kg I.V. daily for 3 to 5 days q 4 weeks; or 15 mg/Kg weekly for 6 weeks. (Doses recommended based on lean body weight.) Maximum single recommended dose is 800 mg, although higher single doses (up to 1.5 g) have been used. The injectable form has been given orally but is not recommended.

SIDE EFFECTS
Blood: *leukopenia, thrombocytopenia,* anemia. WBC nadir occurs days 9 to 14 after first dose; platelet nadir occurs days 7 to 14.
GI: *stomatitis, GI ulcer may precede leukopenia, nausea, vomiting in 30% to 50% of patients; diarrhea.*
Skin: *dermatitis,* hyperpigmentation

(especially in Blacks), nail changes, pigmented palmar creases.
Other: *alopecia in 5% to 20% of patients, weakness, malaise.*

INTERACTIONS
None significant.

NURSING CONSIDERATIONS
- Use cautiously following major surgery, in poor nutritional state, serious infections, bone marrow depression. Use cautiously following high-dose pelvic irradiation or use of alkylating agents, in impaired hepatic or renal function, or widespread neoplastic infiltration of bone marrow.
- Watch for stomatitis or diarrhea (signs of toxicity). May use topical oral anesthetic to soothe lesions. Discontinue if diarrhea occurs.
- Give antiemetic before administering to reduce GI side effects.
- Do WBC and platelet counts daily. Drug should be stopped when WBC is less than 3,500/mm³. Watch for ecchymoses, petechiae, easy bruising, and anemia. Drug should be stopped if platelet count is less than 100,000/mm³.
- Skin and ocular side effects reversible when drug is stopped. Patient should use highly protective sun blockers to avoid inflammatory erythematous dermatitis.
- Therapeutic concentrations don't reach cerebrospinal fluid.
- Slowing infusion rate so it takes from 2 to 8 hours lessens toxicity but also lessens efficacy compared with rapid injection.
- Monitor intake/output, CBC, and renal and hepatic functions.
- Do not refrigerate 5-FU.
- Don't use cloudy solution. If crystals form, redissolve by warming.
- Sometimes ordered as 5-FU. The number 5 is part of the drug name and should not be confused with dosage units.
- Sometimes administered via he-

patic arterial infusion in treatment of hepatic metastases.
• Warn patient that alopecia may occur but is reversible.
• To prevent bleeding, avoid all I.M. injections in patients with thrombocytopenia.
• 5-FU toxicity is delayed for 1 to 3 weeks.

---

hydroxyurea
Hydrea

INDICATIONS & DOSAGE
Melanoma; resistant chronic myelocytic leukemia; recurrent, metastatic, or inoperable ovarian cancer—
Adults: 80 mg/Kg P.O. as single dose q 3 days; or 20 to 30 mg/Kg P.O. daily.

SIDE EFFECTS
Blood: *leukopenia,* thrombocytopenia, anemia, *megaloblastosis; bone marrow depression is dose-limiting and dose-related, recovery rapid.*
CNS: drowsiness.
GI: *anorexia, nausea, vomiting, diarrhea,* stomatitis.
GU: increased BUN, serum creatinine.
Metabolic: hyperuricemia.
Skin: rash, pruritus.

INTERACTIONS
None significant.

NURSING CONSIDERATIONS
• Use cautiously following other chemotherapy or radiation therapy.
• Use with caution in renal dysfunction. Discontinue if WBC is less than 2,500/mm³ or if platelet count is less than 100,000/mm³.
• If patient can't swallow capsule, he may empty contents into water and take immediately.
• Monitor intake/output; keep patient hydrated.

• Routinely measure BUN, uric acid, serum creatinine.
• Drug passes blood-brain barrier.
• Auditory and visual hallucinations and blood toxicity increase when decreased renal function exists.
• May exacerbate postirradiation erythema.
• Avoid all I.M. injections when platelets are low.

---

mercaptopurine
Purinethol♦

INDICATIONS & DOSAGE
Acute lymphoblastic leukemia (in children), acute myeloblastic leukemia, chronic myelocytic leukemia—
Adults: 80 to 100 mg/m² P.O. daily as a single dose up to 5 mg/Kg/day.
Children: 70 mg/m² P.O. daily. Usual maintenance for adults and children: 1.5 to 2.5 mg/Kg/day.

SIDE EFFECTS
Blood: *decreased RBC; leukopenia, thrombocytopenia, bone marrow hypoplasia; all may persist several days after drug is stopped.*
GI: *nausea, vomiting, and anorexia in 25% of patients;* painful oral ulcers.
Hepatic: *jaundice, hepatic necrosis.*
Metabolic: hyperuricemia.

INTERACTIONS
Allopurinol: slowed inactivation of mercaptopurine. Decrease mercaptopurine to ¼ or ⅓ normal dose.

NURSING CONSIDERATIONS
• Use cautiously following chemotherapy or radiation therapy, in depressed neutrophil or platelet count, impaired hepatic or renal function.
• Observe for signs of bleeding and infection.
• Hepatic dysfunction reversible when drug is stopped. Watch for jaundice, clay-colored stools, frothy dark

---

Italicized side effects are common or life-threatening.

urine. Drug should be stopped if hepatic tenderness occurs.
- Do weekly blood counts; watch for precipitous fall.
- Monitor intake/output. Push fluids (3 liters daily).
- Sometimes ordered as 6-mercaptopurine or 6-MP. The number 6 is part of drug name and does not signify number of dosage units.
- Improvement may take 2 to 4 weeks or longer.
- GI side effects less common in children.
- Avoid all I.M. injections when platelets are low.

---

methotrexate

methotrexate sodium
Mexate

INDICATIONS & DOSAGE
Trophoblastic tumors (choriocarcinoma, hydatidiform mole)—
Adults: 15 to 30 mg P.O. or I.M. daily for 5 days. Repeat after 1 or more weeks, according to response or toxicity.
Acute lymphoblastic and lymphatic leukemia—
Adults and children: 3.3 mg/m² P.O., I.M., or I.V. daily for 4 to 6 weeks or until remission occurs; then 20 to 30 mg/m² P.O. or I.M. twice weekly.
Meningeal leukemia—
Adults and children: 0.2 to 0.5 mg/Kg intrathecally q 2 to 5 days until cerebrospinal fluid is normal. Use only 20, 50, or 100 mg vials of powder with no preservatives, and dilute to concentration of 1 mg/ml using 0.9% NaCl injection *without* preservatives. Use only new vials of drug and diluent. Use immediately.
Burkitt's lymphoma (Stage I or II)—
Adults: 10 to 25 mg P.O. daily for 4 to 8 days with 1-week rest intervals.

Burkitt's lymphoma (Stage III)—
Adults: up to 1 g/m²/day with cyclophosphamide and prednisolone.
Lymphosarcoma (Stage III)—
Adults: 0.625 to 2.5 mg/Kg daily P.O., I.M., or I.V.
Mycosis fungoides—
Adults: 2.5 to 10 mg P.O. daily or 50 mg I.M. weekly; or 25 mg I.M. twice weekly.
Psoriasis—
Adults: 10 to 25 mg P.O., I.M., or I.V. as single weekly dose. To detect idiosyncratic reactions, 5 to 10 mg test dose recommended 1 week before methotrexate regimen.

SIDE EFFECTS
Blood: WBC and platelet nadir occurs day 7; anemia, *leukopenia, thrombocytopenia* (all dose-related).
CNS: *arachnoiditis within hours of intrathecal use;* subacute neurotoxicity may begin a few weeks later; necrotizing demyelinating leukoencephalopathy a few years later.
GI: *stomatitis* (common); *diarrhea leading to hemorrhagic enteritis and intestinal perforation.*
GU: *tubular necrosis.*
Hepatic: hepatic dysfunction leading to cirrhosis or hepatic fibrosis.
Metabolic: hyperuricemia.
Skin: exposure to sun may aggravate psoriatic lesions, rash, photosensitivity.
Other: alopecia; *pulmonary interstitial infiltrates;* long-term use in children may cause osteoporosis.

INTERACTIONS
Alcohol: increased hepatotoxicity; warn patient not to drink alcoholic beverages.
Probenecid, phenylbutazone, salicylates, sulfonamides: increased methotrexate toxicity; don't use together if possible.

NURSING CONSIDERATIONS
- Use cautiously in impaired hepatic

---

or renal function, bone marrow depression, aplasia, leukopenia, thrombocytopenia, anemia. Use cautiously in infection, peptic ulcer, ulcerative colitis, and in very young, old, or debilitated patients.
• Warn patient to avoid conception during and immediately following therapy because of potential possible abortion or congenital anomalies.
• GI side effects may require stopping drug.
• Rash, redness, or ulcerations in mouth or pulmonary side effects may signal serious complications.
• Monitor uric acid.
• Check thirst and urinary frequency.
• Monitor intake/output daily. Force fluids (2 to 3 liters daily).
• Alkalinize urine by giving NaHCO₃ tablets to prevent precipitation of drug, especially with high doses. Maintain urine pH at more than 6.5. Reduce dose if BUN 20 to 30 mg% or creatinine 1.2 to 2 mg%. Stop drug if BUN more than 30 mg% or creatinine more than 2 mg%.
• Watch SGOT, SGPT, alkaline phosphatase; may signal hepatic dysfunction.
• Watch for bleeding (especially GI) and infection.
• Warn patient to use highly protective sun blocker when exposed to sun.
• Take temperature daily, and watch for cough, dyspnea, cyanosis; corticosteroids may help reduce pulmonary side effects.
• Leucovorin rescue: Leucovorin calcium (folinic acid) is given within 4 hours of administration of methotrexate and is usually continued 24 to 72 hours. Don't confuse with folic acid. This rescue technique is effective against systemic toxicity but does not interfere with the tumor cells' absorption of the methotrexate.

• Avoid all I.M. injections in patients with thrombocytopenia.

---

thioguanine
Lanvis♦ ♦

INDICATIONS & DOSAGE
Acute leukemia, chronic granulocytic leukemia—
Adults and children: initially, 2 mg/Kg/day P.O. (usually calculated to nearest 20 mg); then increased gradually to 3 mg/Kg/day if no toxic effects occur.

SIDE EFFECTS
Blood: *leukopenia,* anemia, *thrombocytopenia* (occurs slowly over 2 to 4 weeks).
GI: nausea, vomiting, stomatitis, diarrhea, anorexia.
Hepatic: hepatotoxicity, jaundice.
Metabolic: hyperuricemia.

INTERACTIONS
None significant.

NURSING CONSIDERATIONS
• Use cautiously in renal or hepatic dysfunction.
• Stop drug if hepatotoxicity or hepatic tenderness occurs. Watch for jaundice; may reverse if drug stopped promptly.
• Do CBC daily during induction, then weekly during maintenance therapy.
• Monitor serum uric acid.
• Sometimes ordered as 6-thioguanine. The number 6 is part of drug name and does not signify dosage units.
• Avoid all I.M. injections when platelets are low.

Italicized side effects are common or life-threatening.

67

Antibiotic-like antineoplastic agents

bleomycin sulfate
dactinomycin (actinomycin D)
daunorubicin hydrochloride
doxorubicin hydrochloride
mithramycin
mitomycin
procarbazine hydrochloride

bleomycin sulfate
Blenoxane ◆

INDICATIONS & DOSAGE
Dosage and indications may vary.
Check patient's protocol with doctor.
*Cervical, esophageal, head, neck, and
testicular cancer—*
Adults: 10 to 20 units/m² I.V., I.M.,
or S.C. 1 or 2 times weekly to total
300 to 400 units.
Hodgkin's disease— 10 to 20 units/m²
I.V., I.M., or S.C. 1 or 2 times
weekly. After 50% response, maintenance 1 unit I.M. or I.V. daily or 5
units I.M. or I.V. weekly.
Lymphomas— first 2 doses should be
5 units or less, and patient should be
monitored for any allergic reaction. If
no reaction, then follow above dosing
schedule.

SIDE EFFECTS
CNS: hyperesthesia of scalp and fingers, headache.
GI: *stomatitis in 22% to 50% of
patients, prolonged anorexia in 13%
of patients, nausea, vomiting,*
diarrhea.
Skin: *erythema, vesiculation, and
hardening and discoloration of pal-*
*mar and plantar skin in 8% of pa-
tients;* desquamation of hands, feet,
and pressure areas; *hyperpigmentation; acne.*
Other: *alopecia,* swelling of interpha-
langeal joints, *pulmonary fibrosis in
10% of patients, pulmonary side effects (fine rales, fever, dyspnea), leukocytosis and non-productive cough,
allergic reaction (fever up to 106° F.
[41.1° C.], with chills up to 5 hours
after injection; anaphylaxis in 1%
to 6% of patients).*

INTERACTIONS
None significant.

NURSING CONSIDERATIONS
• Use cautiously in renal or pulmonary impairment.
• Drug concentrates in keratin of
squamous epithelium. To prevent
linear streaking, don't use adhesive
dressings on skin.
• Allergic reactions may be delayed
for several hours, especially in
lymphoma.
• Monitor chest X-ray and listen to
lungs.
• Pulmonary function tests should be
performed to establish baseline. Drug
should be stopped if pulmonary function test shows a marked decline.
• Pulmonary side effects common in
patients over 70 years and in patients
who receive a total dose of more than
400 mg.
• Warn patient that alopecia may
occur.
• Refrigerated, reconstituted solution
stable 4 weeks; at room temperature,

stable 2 weeks. Solutions prepared in ampules should be discarded if not used immediately.
• Fatal pulmonary fibrosis occurs in 1% of patients, especially when cumulative dose exceeds 400 mg.
• Bleomycin-induced fever is common and may be treated with antipyretics.

dactinomycin (actinomycin D)
Cosmegen♦

INDICATIONS & DOSAGE
Dosage and indications may vary. Check patient's protocol with doctor.
Melanomas, sarcomas, trophoblastic tumors in women, testicular cancer—
Adults: 500 mcg I.V. daily for 5 days; wait 2 to 4 weeks and repeat; or 2 mg I.V. single weekly dose for 3 weeks; wait for bone marrow recovery, then repeat in 3 to 4 weeks.
Wilms' tumor, rhabdomyosarcoma—
Children: 15 mcg/Kg I.V. daily for 5 days. Maximum dose 500 mcg daily. Wait for marrow recovery.

SIDE EFFECTS
Blood: anemia, *leukopenia, thrombocytopenia, pancytopenia.*
GI: *anorexia, nausea, vomiting,* abdominal pain, diarrhea, *stomatitis.*
Skin: *erythema;* desquamation; *hyperpigmentation of skin, especially in previously irradiated areas; acne-like eruptions (reversible).*
Local: phlebitis, severe damage to soft tissue.
Other: reversible alopecia.

INTERACTIONS
None significant.

NURSING CONSIDERATIONS
• Contraindicated in renal, hepatic, or bone marrow impairment; viral infection; or during chicken pox or herpes zoster infection. Use cau-

tiously in metastatic testicular tumors, in combination with chlorambucil and methotrexate therapy. Extreme bone marrow and GI toxicity can occur with this combined therapy.
• Stomatitis, diarrhea, leukopenia, thrombocytopenia may require stopping therapy.
• Give antiemetic before administering to reduce nausea.
• Monitor renal, hepatic functions.
• Monitor CBCs daily and platelet counts every third day.
• Observe for signs of bleeding.
• Warn patient that alopecia may occur but is usually reversible.
• Use only sterile water (without preservatives) as diluent for injection.
• Administer through a running I.V. infusion. Avoid infiltration.

daunorubicin hydrochloride
Cerubidine♦

INDICATIONS & DOSAGE
Dosage and indications may vary. Check patient's protocol with doctor.
Remission induction in acute nonlymphocytic leukemia (myelogenous, monocytic, erythroid) in adults—
As a single agent: 60 mg/m²/day I.V. on days 1, 2, 3 q 3 to 4 weeks.
In combination: 45 mg/m²/day I.V. on days 1, 2, 3, of the first course and on days 1, 2 of subsequent courses with cytosine arabinoside infusions.
Note: Dose should be reduced if hepatic function is impaired.

SIDE EFFECTS
Blood: *bone marrow depression* (lowest blood counts 10 to 14 days after administration).
CV: *cardiomyopathy (dose-related), EKG changes, arrhythmias,* pericarditis, myocarditis.
GI: *nausea, vomiting, stomatitis, esophagitis,* anorexia, diarrhea.
Skin: rash.

Italicized side effects are common or life-threatening.

Local: *severe cellulitis* o *tissue slough if drug ext* ~~...~~*ates.*
Other: *gene~~...~~ alopecia, fever,*
chills

~~...~~IONS

~~...~~*in:* don't mix. May form a precipitate.

NURSING CONSIDERATIONS
• Use cautiously in myelosuppression, impaired cardiac function.
• Stop drug immediately in signs of congestive heart failure or cardiomyopathy. Prevent by limiting cumulative dose to 550 mg/m²; 450 mg/m² when patient has been receiving radiation therapy that encompasses the heart or any other cardiotoxic agent.
• Monitor EKG before treatment, monthly during therapy.
• Note if resting pulse is high: a sign of cardiac side effects.
• *Avoid extravasation;* inject into tubing of freely flowing I.V. *Never* give I.M. or S.C.
• Monitor CBC and hepatic function.
• Warn patient urine may be red for 1 to 2 days.
• Warn patient that alopecia may occur.
• Don't use a scalp tourniquet or apply ice to prevent alopecia. May compromise effectiveness of drug.
• Nausea and vomiting may be very severe and last 24 to 48 hours.
• Refrigerated, reconstituted solution stable for at least 36 hours; 24 hours at room temperature. Optimally, use within 8 hours of preparation.
• Reddish color looks very similar to doxorubicin (Adriamycin). *Do not confuse the two drugs.*

doxorubicin hydrochloride
Adriamycin♦

INDICATIONS & DOSAGE
Dosage and indications may vary. Check patient's protocol with doctor. *Bladder, breast, cervical, head, neck, liver, lung, ovarian, prostatic, stomach, testicular, and thyroid cancer; Hodgkin's disease; acute lymphoblastic and myeloblastic leukemia; Wilms' tumor; neuroblastomas; lymphomas; sarcomas*—
Adults: 60 to 75 mg/m² I.V. as single dose q 3 weeks; or 30 mg/m² I.V. in single daily dose, days 1 to 3 of 4-week cycle. Maximum cumulative dose 550 mg/m².

SIDE EFFECTS
Blood: *leukopenia, especially agranulocytosis, during days 10 to 15, with recovery by day 21; thrombocytopenia.*
CV: *cardiac depression, seen in such EKG changes as sinus tachycardia, T-wave flattening, S-T segment depression, voltage reduction; arrhythmias in 11% of patients; cardiomyopathy (sometimes with pulmonary edema) with mortality of 30% to 75%.*
GI: *nausea, vomiting,* diarrhea, *stomatitis,* esophagitis.
GU: red-colored urine, enhancement of cyclophosphamide-induced bladder injury.
Skin: *hyperpigmentation of skin, especially in previously irradiated areas.*
Local: *severe cellulitis or tissue slough if drug extravasates.*
Other: hyperpigmentation of nails and dermal creases, *complete alopecia within 3 to 4 weeks;* hair may regrow 2 to 5 months after drug is stopped.

INTERACTIONS
None significant.

NURSING CONSIDERATIONS

- Use cautiously in myelosuppression, impaired cardiac function.
- Stop drug or slow rate of infusion if tachycardia develops.
- Stop drug immediately in signs of congestive heart failure or cardiomyopathy. Prevent by limiting cumulative dose to 550 mg/m²; 450 mg/m² when patient is also being treated with cyclophosphamide.
- Monitor EKG before treatment, monthly during therapy.
- Note if resting pulse is high: a signal of cardiac side effects.
- *Avoid extravasation;* inject into tubing of freely flowing I.V. *Never* give I.M. or S.C.
- Monitor CBC and hepatic function.
- Warn patient urine will be red for 1 to 2 days.
- Dose should be reduced in hepatic dysfunction.
- Warn patient that alopecia will occur. A scalp tourniquet or application of ice may decrese alopecia. However, DO NOT use if treating leukemias or other neoplasms where tumor stem cells may be present in scalp.
- Refrigerated, reconstituted solution stable 48 hours; at room temperature, stable 24 hours.
- If cumulative dose exceeds 550 mg/m² body surface area, 30% of patients develop cardiac side effects, which begin 2 weeks to 6 months after stopping drug.
- Decrease dose if serum bilirubin is increased: 50% dose when bilirubin is 1.2 to 3 mg/100 ml; 25% dose when bilirubin is > 3 mg/100 ml.
- Esophagitis very common in patients who have also received radiation therapy.

mithramycin
Mithracin

INDICATIONS & DOSAGE
Dosage and indications may vary. Check patient's protocol with doctor.
Hypercalcemia—
Adults: 25 mcg/Kg I.V. daily for 1 to 4 days.
Testicular cancer—
Adults: 25 to 30 mcg/Kg I.V. daily for up to 8 to 10 days (based on ideal body weight or actual weight, whichever is less).
I.V. infusions should be in 5% dextrose in water or 0.9% normal saline solution (1,000 ml over 4 to 6 hours).

SIDE EFFECTS
Blood: *thrombocytopenia; bleeding syndrome, from epistaxis to generalized hemorrhage; facial flushing.*
GI: *nausea, vomiting,* anorexia, diarrhea, stomatitis.
GU: proteinuria; increased BUN, serum creatinine.
Metabolic: *decreased serum calcium,* potassium, and phosphorus.
Skin: periorbital pallor, usually the day before toxic symptoms occur.
Local: extravasation causes irritation, cellulitis.

INTERACTIONS
None significant.

NURSING CONSIDERATIONS
- Contraindicated in thrombocytopenia; coagulation and bleeding disorders. Use cautiously in renal, hepatic, or bone marrow impairment.
- Slow infusion reduces nausea that develops with I.V. push.
- Monitor LDH, SGOT, SGPT, alkaline phosphatase, BUN, creatinine, potassium, calcium, phosphorus.
- Monitor platelet count and prothrombin time before and during therapy.

Italicized side effects are common or life-threatening.

- Observe for signs of bleeding. Facial flushing early indicator of bleeding.
- Give antiemetic before administering to reduce nausea.
- Avoid extravasation. If I.V. infiltrates, stop immediately; use ice packs. Restart I.V.
- Avoid contact with skin or mucous membranes.
- Therapeutic effect in hypercalcemia may not be seen for 24 to 48 hours; may last 3 to 15 days.
- Precipitous drop in calcium possible. Monitor patient for tetany, carpopedal spasm, Chvostek's sign, muscle cramps; check serum calcium levels.
- Store lyophilized powder in refrigerator. Remains stable after reconstitution for 24 hours; 48 hours in refrigerator.

mitomycin
Mutamycin♦

INDICATIONS & DOSAGE
Dosage and indications may vary. Check patient's protocol with doctor.
Breast, colon, head, neck, lung, pancreatic, and stomach cancer; malignant melanoma—
Adults: 2 mg/m² I.V. daily for 5 days. Stop drug for 2 days, then repeat dose for 5 more days; or 20 mg/m² as a single dose. Repeat cycle 6 to 8 weeks. Stop drug if WBC less than 4,000/mm³ or platelets less than 75,000/mm³.

SIDE EFFECTS
Blood: *thrombocytopenia, leukopenia* (may be delayed up to 8 weeks).
CNS: paresthesias.
GI: nausea, vomiting, anorexia, stomatitis.
Local: desquamation, induration, pruritus, *pain at site of injection.* Extravasation causes cellulitis, ulceration, sloughing.

Other: *alopecia.*

INTERACTIONS
None significant.

NURSING CONSIDERATIONS
- Use cautiously when platelet count is less than 75,000/mm³, WBC is less than 4,000/mm³; in coagulation or bleeding disorders, serious infections, impaired renal function.
- Continue CBC and blood studies at least 7 weeks after therapy is stopped. Observe for signs of bleeding.
- Warn patient that alopecia may occur.
- Reconstituted solution stable 1 week at room temperature, 2 weeks refrigerated.

procarbazine hydrochloride
Matulane, Natulan♦♦

INDICATIONS & DOSAGE
Dosage and indications may vary. Check patient's protocol with doctor.
Hodgkin's disease, lymphomas, brain and lung cancer—
Adults: 100 to 150 mg/m² P.O. for 10 days until WBC falls below 4,000/ mm³ or platelets fall below 100,000/ mm³. After bone marrow recovers, resume maintenance dose 50 to 100 mg P.O. daily.
Children: 50 mg P.O. daily for first week, then 100 mg/m² until response or toxicity occurs. Maintenance dose 50 mg P.O. daily after bone marrow recovery.

SIDE EFFECTS
Blood: bleeding tendency, *leukopenia,* anemia.
CNS: nervousness, depression, insomnia, nightmares, *hallucinations,* confusion.
EENT: retinal hemorrhage, nystagmus, photophobia.
GI: *nausea, vomiting, anorexia,* sto-

matitis, dry mouth, dysphagia, diar-
rhea, constipation.
Skin: dermatitis.
Other: alopecia, pleural effusion.

INTERACTIONS
Alcohol: disulfiram (Antabuse)-like
reaction. Warn patient not to drink
alcohol.

NURSING CONSIDERATIONS
• Use cautiously in inadequate bone
marrow reserve, leukopenia, thrombocytopenia, anemia, impaired hepatic or renal function.
• Observe for signs of bleeding.
• Warn patient that alopecia may
occur.

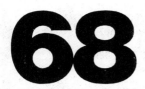

Antineoplastics altering hormone balance

calusterone
dromostanolone propionate
megestrol acetate
mitotane
tamoxifen citrate
testolactone

---

calusterone
Methosarb♦

INDICATIONS & DOSAGE
Postmenopausal breast cancer—
Women: 50 mg P.O. q.i.d. up to
300 mg/day.

SIDE EFFECTS
GI: nausea, vomiting.
GU: clitoral enlargement.
Hepatic: hepatotoxicity, jaundice.
Metabolic: hypercalcemia.
Skin: acne, oily skin.
Other: *virilism (hirsutism, deepened voice, facial hair) in 25% of patients,* increased libido, mild thinning of hair, edema, fever. Brief exacerbation of pain from osseous metastases.

INTERACTIONS
None significant.

NURSING CONSIDERATIONS
• Contraindicated in premenopausal women (unless ovarian function has been terminated) and male breast cancer.
• Monitor hepatic function and serum calcium regularly.
• Monitor for signs of tumor progression.

• Therapy usually lasts for at least 3 months.

---

dromostanolone propionate
Drolban

INDICATIONS & DOSAGE
Advanced, inoperable metastatic breast cancer, 1 to 5 years postmenopausal—
Women: 100 mg deep I.M. 3 times weekly.

SIDE EFFECTS
GU: clitoral enlargement.
Metabolic: hypercalcemia.
Skin: acne.
Other: *virilism (deepened voice, facial hair growth), which may be intense after long-term treatment;* edema, pain at injection site.

INTERACTIONS
None significant.

NURSING CONSIDERATIONS
• Contraindicated by any route other than I.M.; in male breast cancer and premenopausal women. Use cautiously in hepatic disease, cardiac decompensation, nephritis, nephrosis, and prostatic cancer.
• If severe hypercalcemia develops or disease accelerates, drug should be stopped.
• Therapeutic effect may be delayed 8 to 12 weeks. Reassure patient that results are not immediate.

• Do not store in refrigerator; drug precipitates at cold temperatures.

---

megestrol acetate
Megace ♦

INDICATIONS & DOSAGE
Breast cancer—
Women: 40 mg P.O. q.i.d.
Endometrial cancer—
Women: 40 to 320 mg P.O. daily in divided dosages.

SIDE EFFECTS
None reported.

INTERACTIONS
None significant.

NURSING CONSIDERATIONS
• Use cautiously in history of thrombophlebitis.
• Adequate trial is 2 months. Reassure patient that therapeutic response isn't immediate.

---

mitotane
Lysodren ♦

INDICATIONS & DOSAGE
Inoperable adrenal cortical cancer—
Adults: 9 to 10 g P.O. daily, divided t.i.d. to q.i.d. If severe side effects appear, reduce dose until maximum tolerated dose is achieved (varies from 2 to 16 g/day but is usually 8 to 10 g/day).

SIDE EFFECTS
CNS: *depression, somnolence, vertigo;* brain damage and dysfunction in long-term, high-dose therapy.
GI: *severe nausea, vomiting,* diarrhea, anorexia.
Metabolic: adrenal insufficiency.
Skin: dermatitis.

INTERACTIONS
None significant.

NURSING CONSIDERATIONS
• Use cautiously in hepatic disease.
• Drug should be stopped if shock or trauma occurs. Use of corticosteroids may avoid acute adrenocorticoid insufficiency.
• Assess and record behavioral and neurologic signs for baseline data daily throughout therapy.
• Give antiemetic before administering to reduce nausea.
• Dosage may be reduced if GI or skin side effects are severe.
• Obese patients may need higher dosage and may have longer-lasting side effects, since drug distributes mostly to body fat.
• Warn ambulatory patient of CNS side effects; advise him to avoid hazardous tasks requiring mental alertness or physical coordination.
• Monitor effectiveness by reduction in pain, weakness, anorexia.
• Adequate trial is at least 3 months, but therapy can continue if clinical benefits are observed.

---

tamoxifen citrate
Nolvadex ♦

INDICATIONS & DOSAGE
Advanced pre- and postmenopausal breast cancer—
Women: 10 to 20 mg P.O. b.i.d.

SIDE EFFECTS
Blood: transient fall in WBC or platelets.
GI: nausea in 10% of patients, vomiting, anorexia.
GU: vaginal discharge and bleeding.
Skin: rash.
Other: temporary bone or tumor pain, hot flashes in 7% of patients. Brief exacerbation of pain from osseous metastases.

Italicized side effects are common or life-threatening.

INTERACTIONS
None significant.

NURSING CONSIDERATIONS
• Use cautiously in preexisting leukopenia, thrombocytopenia.
• Use analgesic to relieve pain.
• Monitor WBC and platelet counts.
• Acts as an "anti-estrogen." Best results in patients with positive estrogen receptors.
• Side effects are usually minor and are well tolerated.
• Reassure patient that acute exacerbation of bone pain during tamoxifen therapy usually indicates drug will produce good response.

---

testolactone
Teslac♦

INDICATIONS & DOSAGE
Advanced postmenopausal breast cancer—
Women: 100 mg deep I.M. 3 times weekly; or 250 mg P.O. q.i.d.

SIDE EFFECTS
Local: pain, inflammation at injection site.

INTERACTIONS
None significant.

NURSING CONSIDERATIONS
• Contraindicated in male breast cancer and not recommended in premenopausal females.
• Adequate trial is 3 months. Reassure patient that therapeutic response isn't immediate.
• Monitor fluids and electrolytes, especially calcium levels.
• Immobilized patients more prone to hypercalcemia. Exercise may prevent it. Push fluids to aid calcium excretion.
• Shake vial vigorously before drawing up injections. Do not refrigerate.
• Use 1.5-inch needle and inject into upper outer quadrant of gluteal region. Rotate injection sites.
• No advantage over testosterone, except less virilization.
• Higher than recommended doses do not increase incidence of remission.

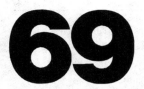

Vinca alkaloids and asparaginase

asparaginase (L-asparaginase)
vinblastine sulfate
vincristine sulfate

**asparaginase
(or L-asparaginase)**
Elspar

INDICATIONS & DOSAGE
Acute lymphocytic leukemia (when used along with other drugs)—
Adults and children: 1,000 international units (IU)/Kg I.V. daily for 10 days, injected over 30 minutes or by slow I.V. push; or 6,000 IU/m² I.M. at intervals specified in protocol.
Sole induction agent—200 IU/Kg I.V. daily for 28 days.

SIDE EFFECTS
Blood: *hypofibrinogenemia* and depression of other clotting factors, thrombocytopenia, *leukopenia,* depression of serum albumin.
GI: *vomiting (may last up to 24 hours),* anorexia, *nausea,* cramps, weight loss.
GU: *azotemia,* renal failure, uric acid nephropathy, glucosuria, polyuria.
Metabolic: elevated SGOT, SGPT, alkaline phosphatase, and bilirubin (direct and indirect); increase or decrease in total lipids; *hyperglycemia; increased blood ammonia.*
Skin: *rash, urticaria.*
Other: *hemorrhagic pancreatitis, hepatotoxicity, anaphylaxis (relatively common).*

INTERACTIONS
None significant.

NURSING CONSIDERATIONS
• Contraindicated in pancreatitis, previous hypersensitivity unless desensitized. Use cautiously in preexisting hepatic dysfunction.
• Should be administered in hospital setting with close supervision.
• Don't use as sole agent to induce remission unless combination therapy is inappropriate. Not recommended for maintenance therapy.
• Risk of hypersensitivity increases with repeated doses. Patient may be desensitized, but this doesn't rule out risk of allergic reactions. Routine administration of 2 unit I.V. test dose may identify high-risk patients.
• Intravenous administration of asparaginase with or immediately before vincristine or prednisone may increase toxicity reactions.
• Give I.V. injection over 30-minute period through a running infusion of sodium chloride injection or 5% dextrose injection.
• For I.M. injection, limit dose at single injection site to 2 ml.
• Due to vomiting, patient may need parenteral fluids for 24 hours or until oral fluids are tolerated.
• Monitor blood count and bone marrow levels. Bone marrow regeneration may take 5 to 6 weeks.
• Obtain frequent serum amylase determinations to check pancreatic status. If elevated, asparaginase should be discontinued.
• Watch for uric acid nephropathy.

Prevent occurrence by increasing fluid intake, alkalinization of urine. Allopurinol may be ordered.
- Watch for signs of bleeding, such as petechiae and melena.
- Monitor blood sugar and test urine for sugar before and during therapy. Watch for signs of hyperglycemia such as glucosuria, polyuria.
- Reconstitute with 2 to 5 ml sterile water for injection or sodium chloride injection.
- Don't shake vial. May cause loss of potency. Don't use cloudy solutions.
- Refrigerate unopened dry powder. Reconstituted solution stable 6 hours at room temperature, 24 hours refrigerated.
- Keep epinephrine, diphenhydramine, and I.V. corticosteroids available for treatment of anaphylaxis.

---

vinblastine sulfate (VLB)
Velban, Velbe♦♦

INDICATIONS & DOSAGE
Breast or testicular cancer, generalized Hodgkin's disease, choriocarcinoma, lymphosarcoma, neuroblastoma, mycosis fungoides, histiocytosis—
Adults and children: 0.1 mg/Kg or 3.7 mg/m² I.V. weekly or q 2 weeks. May be increased to maximum dose (adults) of 0.5 mg/Kg or 18.5 mg/m² I.V. weekly according to response. Dose should not be repeated if WBC less than 4,000/mm³.

SIDE EFFECTS
Blood: *leukopenia* (nadir days 4 to 10 and lasts another 7 to 14 days), *thrombocytopenia.*
CNS: depression, *paresthesias, peripheral neuropathy and neuritis, numbness, loss of deep tendon reflexes, muscle pain and weakness.*
EENT: pharyngitis.
GI: *nausea, vomiting, stomatitis,* ulcer and bleeding, *constipation, ileus, anorexia, weight loss,* abdominal pain.
GU: oligospermia, aspermia, urinary retention.
Skin: dermatitis, vesiculation.
Local: *irritation, phlebitis,* cellulitis, necrosis if I.V. extravasates.
Other: reversible alopecia in 5% to 10% of patients; *pain in tumor site,* low fever.

INTERACTIONS
None significant.

NURSING CONSIDERATIONS
- Contraindicated in severe leukopenia, bacterial infection. Use cautiously in jaundice or hepatic dysfunction.
- Give antiemetic before administering to reduce nausea.
- Drug should be stopped if stomatitis occurs.
- Give laxatives as needed. May use stool softeners prophylactically.
- Don't repeat dose more frequently than every 7 days or severe leukopenia will develop.
- Less neurotoxic than vincristine.
- Should be injected directly into vein or tubing of running I.V. over 1 minute. May also be given in 50 ml dextrose in water or normal saline and infused over 15 minutes. If extravasation occurs, stop infusion. Apply ice packs on and off every 2 hours for 24 hours.
- Warn patient that alopecia may occur but is usually reversible.
- Adequate trial 12 weeks; reassure patient that therapeutic response isn't immediate.
- Reconstitute 10 mg vial with 10 ml of sodium chloride injection or sterile water. This yields 1 mg/ml.
- Refrigerate reconstituted solution. Discard after 30 days.
- Don't confuse vinblastine with vincristine or the investigational agent vindesine.

---

vincristine sulfate
Oncovin♦

INDICATIONS & DOSAGE
Acute lymphoblastic and other leukemias, Hodgkin's disease, lymphosarcoma, reticulum cell sarcoma, neuroblastoma, rhabdomyosarcoma, Wilms' tumor, osteogenic and other sarcomas, lung and breast cancer—
Adults: 1 to 2 mg/m² I.V. weekly.
Children: 1.5 to 2 mg/m² I.V. weekly. Maximum single dose (adults and children) is 2 mg.

SIDE EFFECTS
Blood: rapidly reversible mild anemia and leukopenia.
CNS: *peripheral neuropathy,* sensory loss, *deep tendon reflex loss, paresthesias, wrist and foot drop,* ataxia, cranial nerve palsies (headache, *jaw pain,* hoarseness, vocal cord paralysis, visual disturbances), *muscle weakness and cramps,* depression, agitation, insomnia.
EENT: diplopia, optic and extraocular neuropathy, ptosis.
GI: *constipation, cramps,* ileus that mimics surgical abdomen, *nausea, vomiting,* anorexia, *stomatitis,* weight loss, dysphagia.
GU: urinary retention.
Local: *phlebitis,* cellulitis.
Other: *reversible alopecia (up to 71% of patients).*

INTERACTIONS
None significant.

NURSING CONSIDERATIONS
• Use cautiously in jaundice or hepatic dysfunction, neuromuscular disease, infection, or with other neurotoxic drugs.
• Because of neurotoxicity, don't give drug more than once a week. Children more resistant to neurotoxicity than adults.
• Should be given directly into vein or tubing of running I.V. slowly over 1 minute. May also be given in 50 ml dextrose in water or normal saline and infused over 15 minutes. If drug infiltrates, apply ice packs on and off every 2 hours for 24 hours.
• Check for depression of Achilles tendon reflex, numbness, tingling, foot or wrist drop, difficulty in walking, ataxia, slapping gait. Also check ability to walk on heels. Support patient when walking.
• Monitor bowel function. Give stool softener, laxative, or water before dosing.
• Reconstitute with sodium chloride injection, physiologic saline, or sterile water.
• Refrigerate reconstituted solution. Discard after 14 days.
• Warn patient that alopecia may occur but is usually reversible.
• Be extremely careful about doses. Don't confuse vincristine with vinblastine or the investigational agent vindesine.

Italicized side effects are common or life-threatening.

70

Ophthalmic anti-infectives

bacitracin
benzalkonium chloride
boric acid
chloramphenicol
chlortetracycline hydrochloride
erythromycin
gentamicin sulfate
idoxuridine (IDU)
natamycin
neomycin sulfate
polymyxin B sulfate
silver nitrate 1%
sulfacetamide sodium
tetracycline hydrochloride
trifluridine
vidarabine

---

bacitracin
Baciguent Ophthalmic Ointment♦

INDICATIONS & DOSAGE
Ocular infections—
Adults and children: apply small amount into conjunctival sac several times a day or p.r.n. until favorable response is observed.

SIDE EFFECTS
Eye: slowed corneal wound healing, temporary visual haze.
Other: overgrowth of nonsusceptible organisms.

INTERACTIONS
Heavy metals (silver nitrate): inactivate bacitracin. Don't use together.

NURSING CONSIDERATIONS
• Use cautiously in patients with hereditary predisposition to antibiotic hypersensitivity.
• Warn patient to avoid sharing washcloths, etc. with family members.
• Always wash hands before and after applying ointment.
• Tell patient to watch for signs of sensitivity, such as itching lids or constant burning. Patient who develops such signs should stop drug and notify doctor immediately.
• Show patient how to apply. Stress importance of compliance with recommended therapy.
• Warn patient not to touch tip of tube to any part of eye or surrounding tissue.
• Solution not commercially available but may be prepared by pharmacy. May be stored up to 3 weeks in refrigerator.
• Bactericidal or bacteriostatic, depending on concentration and infection.
• Store in tightly closed, light-resistant container.

---

benzalkonium chloride
Spensomide, Zephiran♦

INDICATIONS & DOSAGE
To increase transcorneal penetration of drugs—
Adults and children: 1:5,000 to 1:2,000 concentration used in some irrigating solutions for its antiseptic as well as its surface-active qualities.
To sterilize ophthalmic solutions: use 1:5,000 concentration.

An ingredient in germicidal cleaning solutions for contact lens.

SIDE EFFECTS
Eye: toxic to abraded cornea and to endothelial cells of cornea if introduced into anterior chamber.

INTERACTIONS
Fluorescein: destroys benzalkonium chloride antibacterial activity. May cause corneal staining. Don't use together.
Sulfonamides (ophthalmic): incompatible. Don't apply at same time.

NURSING CONSIDERATIONS
• Never prepare a straight benzalkonium chloride solution for use in eye.
• Warn patient to avoid sharing washcloths, etc. with family members.
• Don't use concentrations greater than 1:5,000 in the eye; may be irritating.
• Tell patient to watch for signs of sensitivity, such as itching lids or constant burning. If he develops such signs, patient should stop drug and notify doctor immediately.
• Warn patient not to touch applicator to eye or surrounding tissue.
• Always wash hands before and after applying drug.
• Present in most combination topical eye preparations commercially available.

boric acid
Blinx, Collyrium, Neo-Flo

INDICATIONS & DOSAGE
For irrigation following tonometry, gonioscopy, foreign body removal, or use of fluorescein; used to soothe and cleanse the eye; used in conjunction with contact lens—
Adults: irrigate eye with 2% solution or apply 5% or 10% ointment, p.r.n.

SIDE EFFECTS
Note: toxic if absorbed from abraded skin areas, granulating wounds, or ingestion.

INTERACTIONS
Polyvinyl alcohol (Liquifilm): may form insoluble complex. Check with pharmacy on contents in eye drugs and contact lens wetting solutions.

NURSING CONSIDERATIONS
• Contraindicated in eye abrasions.
• Don't apply to abraded cornea or skin.
• Lethal dose is 5 to 6 g in infants and 15 to 20 g in adults.
• Always wash hands before and after instilling solution or ointment.
• Not for use with soft contact lenses.
• Weak bacteriostatic, fungistatic agent.

chloramphenicol
Antibiopto, Chloromycetin Ophthalmic♦, Chloroptic Ophthalmic♦, Chloroptic S.O.P., Econochlor Ophthalmic, Fenicol♦♦, Isopto Fenicol♦♦, Nova-Phenicol♦♦, Ophthoclor Ophthalmic, Pentamycetin♦♦

INDICATIONS & DOSAGE
Surface bacterial infection involving conjunctiva or cornea—
Adults and children: instill 2 drops of solution in eye q 1 hour until condition improves, or instill q.i.d., depending on severity of infection. Apply small amount of ointment to lower conjunctival sac at bedtime as supplement to drops. May use ointment alone by applying a small amount of ointment to lower conjunctival sac q 3 to 6 hours or more frequently, if necessary. Continue until condition improves.

SIDE EFFECTS

Note: systemic adverse reactions have not been reported with short-term topical use.

Blood: *bone marrow hypoplasia with prolonged use*.

Eye: optic atrophy in children, stinging or burning of eye after instillation.

Other: overgrowth of nonsusceptible organisms; hypersensitivity, including itching and burning eye, dermatitis, angioedema.

INTERACTIONS

None significant.

NURSING CONSIDERATIONS

• Not for long-term use. Notify doctor if no improvement in 3 days.

• If patient has more than a superficial infection, systemic therapy should be used also.

• Bacteriostatic.

• One of the safest topical ocular antibiotics, especially for endophthalmitis.

• Warn patient to avoid sharing washcloths, etc. with family members.

• Always wash hands before and after applying ointment or solution.

• Tell patient to watch for signs of sensitivity, such as itching lids or constant burning. Patient who develops such signs should stop drug and notify doctor immediately.

• Show patient how to instill. Stress importance of compliance with recommended therapy.

• Warn patient not to touch tip of applicator to eye or surrounding tissue.

• If chloramphenicol drops are to be given q 1 hour, then tapered, follow order closely to ensure adequate anterior chamber levels.

• Store in tightly closed, light-resistant container.

chlortetracycline hydrochloride
Aureomycin Ophthalmic

INDICATIONS & DOSAGE

Superficial ocular infection—

Adults and children: apply 1% ointment to eye q 2 hours or more, p.r.n.

SIDE EFFECTS

Eye: itching and burning.

Other: overgrowth of nonsusceptible organisms with long-term use, dermatitis.

INTERACTIONS

None significant.

NURSING CONSIDERATIONS

• Contraindicated in tetracycline hypersensitivity.

• *Pseudomonas, Proteus,* and *Staphylococcus* resistant to drug. Used mainly for trachoma in conjunction with oral therapy. Trachoma treatment may continue 2 months or more. Trachoma may cause blindness if untreated or if treated improperly.

• Warn patient to avoid sharing washcloths, etc. with family members.

• Always wash hands before and after applying ointment.

• Tell patient to watch for signs of sensitivity, such as itching lids or constant burning. Patient who develops such signs should stop drug and notify doctor immediately.

• Show patient how to instill. Stress importance of compliance with recommended therapy.

• Warn patient not to touch tip of tube to eye or surrounding tissue.

• Bacteriostatic.

• Store in tightly closed, light-resistant container.

erythromycin
Ilotycin Ophthalmic♦

INDICATIONS & DOSAGE
Acute and chronic conjunctivitis, other eye infections—
Adults and children: apply 0.5% ointment 1 or more times daily, depending upon severity of infection.

SIDE EFFECTS
Eye: slowed corneal wound healing.
Other: overgrowth of nonsusceptible organisms with long-term use; hypersensitivity, including itchy and burning eye, urticaria, dermatitis, angioedema.

INTERACTIONS
None significant.

NURSING CONSIDERATIONS
• Bacteriostatic but may be bactericidal in high concentrations or against highly susceptible organisms.
• Has a limited antibacterial spectrum. Use only when sensitivity studies show it is effective against infecting organisms. Don't use in infections of unknown etiology.
• Warn patient to avoid sharing washcloths, etc. with family members.
• Always wash hands before and after applying ointment.
• Tell patient to watch for signs of sensitivity, such as itching lids or constant burning. Patient who develops such signs should stop drug and notify doctor immediately.
• Show patient how to apply. Stress importance of compliance with recommended therapy.
• Warn patient not to touch tube to eye or surrounding tissue.
• Store at room temperature in tightly closed, light-resistant container.

gentamicin sulfate
Garamycin Ophthalmic♦, Genoptic

INDICATIONS & DOSAGE
External ocular infections (conjunctivitis, keratoconjunctivitis, corneal ulcers, blepharitis, blepharoconjunctivitis, meibomianitis, and dacryocystitis) due to susceptible organisms, especially Pseudomonas aeruginosa, Proteus sp., Klebsiella pneumoniae, Escherichia coli—
Adults and children: instill 1 to 2 drops in eye q 4 hours. In severe infections, may use up to 2 drops q 1 hour. Apply ointment to lower conjunctival sac b.i.d. to t.i.d.

SIDE EFFECTS
Note: systemic absorption from excessive use may cause systemic toxicities.
Eye: burning or stinging with ointment, transient irritation from solution.
Other: hypersensitivity, overgrowth of nonsusceptible organisms with long-term use.

INTERACTIONS
None significant.

NURSING CONSIDERATIONS
• Contraindicated in aminoglycoside hypersensitivity. Use cautiously in impaired renal function.
• Have culture taken before giving drug.
• Stress importance of following recommended therapy. *Pseudomonas* infections can cause complete vision loss within 24 hours if infection is not controlled.
• Warn patient to avoid sharing washcloths, etc. with family members.
• Always wash hands before and after applying ointment or solution.
• Tell patient to watch for signs of sensitivity, such as itching lids or con-

stant burning. Patient who develops such signs should stop drug and notify doctor immediately.
- Show patient how to instill.
- Warn patient not to touch tip of tube or dropper to eye or surrounding tissue.
- Store away from heat.

---

idoxuridine (IDU)
Dendrid, Herplex, Stoxil♦

INDICATIONS & DOSAGE
Herpes simplex keratitis—
Adults and children: instill 1 drop of solution into conjunctival sac q 1 hour during day and q 2 hours at night, or apply ointment to conjunctival sac q 4 hours or 5 times daily, with last dose at bedtime. A response should be seen in 7 days; if not, discontinue and begin alternate therapy. Therapy should not be continued longer than 21 days.

SIDE EFFECTS
Eye: temporary visual haze; irritation, pain, burning, or inflammation of eye; mild edema of eyelid or cornea; photosensitivity; small punctate defects in corneal epithelium; slowed corneal wound healing with ointment.
Other: hypersensitivity.

INTERACTIONS
None significant.

NURSING CONSIDERATIONS
- Contraindicated in deep ulceration.
- Not for long-term use.
- Idoxuridine should not be mixed with other medications.
- Don't use old solution; causes ocular burning and has no antiviral activity.
- Warn patient to avoid sharing washcloths, etc. with family members.
- Always wash hands before and after applying ointment or solution.

- Tell patient to watch for signs of sensitivity, such as itching lids or constant burning. Patient who develops such signs should stop drug and notify doctor immediately.
- Show patient how to apply. Stress importance of compliance with recommended therapy.
- Warn patient not to touch tip of tube or dropper to eye or surrounding tissue.
- Refrigerate idoxuridine 0.1% solution. Store in tightly closed, light-resistant container.

---

natamycin
Natacyn

INDICATIONS & DOSAGE
Treatment of fungal keratitis—
Adults: initial dosage 1 drop instilled in conjunctival sac q 1 to 2 hours. After 3 to 4 days, reduce dosage to 1 drop 6 to 8 times daily.

SIDE EFFECTS
Eye: ocular edema, hyperemia

INTERACTIONS
None significant.

NURSING CONSIDERATIONS
- Only antifungal available as ophthalmic preparation.
- Treatment of choice for fungal keratitis. May also be used to treat fungal blepharitis and conjunctivitis.
- Therapy should be continued for 14 to 21 days, or until active disease subsides.
- Reduce dosage gradually at 4- to 7-day intervals to assure that organism has been eliminated.
- If infection does not improve with 7 to 10 days of therapy, clinical and laboratory reevaluation is recommended.

---

neomycin sulfate
Myciguent Ophthalmic

polymyxin B sulfate
Aerosporin♦

INDICATIONS & DOSAGE
Used alone or in combination with other antibiotics in treating superficial ocular infections involving conjunctiva or cornea—
Adults and children: apply ointment to lower conjunctival sac daily to t.i.d.

SIDE EFFECTS
Other: hypersensitivity reactions (itching and burning eye, erythema, dermatitis, urticaria); after long-term use, overgrowth of nonsusceptible organisms.

INTERACTIONS
None significant.

NURSING CONSIDERATIONS
• Contraindicated in aminoglycoside hypersensitivity.
• Effective against gram-positive and gram-negative organisms.
• Warn patient to avoid sharing washcloths, etc. with family members.
• Always wash hands before and after applying ointment.
• Tell patient to watch for signs of sensitivity, such as itching lids or constant burning. Patient who develops such signs should stop drug and notify doctor immediately.
• Show patient how to apply. Stress importance of compliance with recommended therapy.
• Warn patient not to touch tip of tube to eye or surrounding tissue.
• Bactericidal.

INDICATIONS & DOSAGE
Used alone or in combination with other agents for treating corneal ulcers resulting from Pseudomonas infection or other gram-negative organism infections—
Adults and children: instill 1 to 3 drops of 0.1% to 0.25% (10,000 to 25,000 units per ml) q 1 hour. Increase interval according to patient response; or up to 10,000 units subconjunctivally daily by doctor.

SIDE EFFECTS
Eye: eye irritation, conjunctivitis.
Other: overgrowth of nonsusceptible organisms, hypersensitivity (local burning, itching).

INTERACTIONS
None significant.

NURSING CONSIDERATIONS
• One of the most effective antibiotics against gram-negative organisms, especially *Pseudomonas.*
• Often used in combination with neomycin sulfate.
• Warn patient to avoid sharing washcloths, etc. with family members.
• Always wash hands before and after instilling solution.
• Tell patient to watch for signs of sensitivity, such as itching lids and lashes or constant burning. Patient who develops such signs should stop drug and notify doctor immediately.
• Show patient how to instill. Stress importance of compliance with recommended therapy.
• Warn patient not to touch tip of dropper to eye or surrounding tissue.
• Bactericidal.
• Not commercially available. Polymyxin B sulfate powder must be reconstituted with sterile water for in-

---

Italicized side effects are common or life-threatening.

jection or normal saline solution.
Refrigerated solutions stable for
6 months.

---

silver nitrate 1%

INDICATIONS & DOSAGE
*Prevention of gonorrheal ophthalmia
neonatorum—*
Neonates: cleanse lids thoroughly;
instill 1 drop of 1% solution into each
eye.

SIDE EFFECTS
Eye: periorbital edema, temporary
staining of lids and surrounding tissue, conjunctivitis (with concentrations greater than 1%).

INTERACTIONS
Bacitracin: inactivates silver nitrate.
Don't use together.

NURSING CONSIDERATIONS
• Legally required for neonates in
most states.
• Don't use repeatedly.
• If 2% solution is accidentally used
in eye, prompt irrigation with isotonic
sodium chloride is advised to prevent
eye irritation.
• May delay instillation slightly to
allow neonate to bond with mother.
• Always wash hands before instilling solution.
• Store wax ampules away from light
and heat.
• Bacteriostatic, germicidal, and astringent.
• Don't irrigate eyes after
instillation.

---

sulfacetamide sodium 10%
Bleph-10 Liquifilm Ophthalmic♦,
Cetamide Ophthalmic♦, 10% Sodium
Sulamyd Ophthalmic, Sulf-10
Ophthalmic♦
sulfacetamide sodium 15%
Isopto Cetamide Ophthalmic♦,
Sulfacel-15 Ophthalmic
sulfacetamide sodium 30%
Sodium Sulamyd 30% Ophthalmic♦

INDICATIONS & DOSAGE
*Inclusion conjunctivitis, corneal ul-
cers, trachoma, prophylaxis to ocular
infection—*
Adults and children: instill 1 to
2 drops of 10% solution into lower
conjunctival sac q 2 to 3 hours during
day, less often at night; or instill 1 to
2 drops of 15% solution into lower
conjunctival sac q 1 to 2 hours initially, increasing interval as condition
responds; or instill 1 drop of 30% solution into lower conjunctival sac q 2
hours. Instill ½ to 1 inch of 10% ointment into conjunctival sac q.i.d. and
at bedtime. May use ointment at night
along with drops during the day.

SIDE EFFECTS
Eye: slowed corneal wound healing
(ointment), pain on instilling eye
drop.
Other: hypersensitivity (including
itching or burning), overgrowth of
nonsusceptible organisms.

INTERACTIONS
*Local anesthetics (procaine, tetra-
caine), p-aminobenzoic acid derivatives:* decreased sulfacetamide sodium
action. Wait for ½ to 1 hour after instilling anesthetic or *p*-aminobenzoic
acid derivative before instilling sulfacetamide.

NURSING CONSIDERATIONS
• Contraindicated in sulfonamide
hypersensitivity.

- Often used with systemic tetracycline in treating trachoma and inclusion conjunctivitis.
- Replaced by antibiotics in treating major ocular infections; still used in minor ocular infections.
- Purulent exudate interferes with sulfacetamide action. Remove as much exudate as possible from lids before instilling sulfacetamide.
- Incompatible with silver preparations.
- Warn patient eyedrop is painful.
- Warn patient to avoid sharing washcloths, etc. with family members.
- Always wash hands before and after applying ointment or solution.
- Tell patient to watch for signs of sensitivity, such as itching lids or constant burning. Patient who develops such signs should stop drug and notify doctor immediately.
- Show patient how to instill. Stress importance of compliance with recommended therapy.
- Warn patient not to touch tip of tube or dropper to eye or surrounding tissue.
- Store in tightly closed, light-resistant container away from heat.
- Don't use discolored (dark brown) solution.

tetracycline hydrochloride
Achromycin Ophthalmic ♦

INDICATIONS & DOSAGE
Adults and children:
Superficial ocular infections and inclusion conjunctivitis— instill 1 to 2 drops in eye b.i.d., q.i.d., or more often, depending on severity of infection.
Trachoma—instill 2 drops in each eye b.i.d., t.i.d., or q.i.d. Continue for 1 to 2 months or longer, or use 1% ointment t.i.d. to q.i.d. for 30 days.

SIDE EFFECTS
Eye: itching.
Other: hypersensitivity (eye itching and dermatitis), overgrowth of nonsusceptible organisms with long-term use.

INTERACTIONS
None significant.

NURSING CONSIDERATIONS
- Tell patient or family that trachoma therapy should continue for 1 to 2 months or longer. Trachoma may cause blindness if left untreated or if not treated properly.
- Warn patient to avoid sharing washcloths, etc. with family members.
- Always wash hands before and after applying solution.
- Tell patient to watch for signs of sensitivity, such as itching lids or constant burning. Patient who develops such signs should stop drug and notify doctor immediately.
- Show patient how to instill. Stress importance of compliance with recommended therapy.
- Warn patient not to touch tip of dropper to eye or surrounding tissue.
- Store in tightly closed, light-resistant container.

trifluridine
Viroptic Ophthalmic Solution 1%

INDICATIONS & DOSAGE
Primary keratoconjunctivitis and recurrent epithelial keratitis due to herpes simplex virus, types 1 and 2—
Adults 1 drop of solution q 2 hours while patient is awake, to a maximum of 9 drops daily until re-epithelialization of the corneal ulcer occurs; then 1 drop q 4 hours (minimum 5 drops daily) for an additional 7 days.

Italicized side effects are common or life-threatening.

SIDE EFFECTS
Eye: stinging upon instillation, edema of eyelids.

INTERACTIONS
None significant.

NURSING CONSIDERATIONS
• Should be prescribed only for those patients with clinical diagnosis of herpetic keratitis.
• Consider another form of therapy if improvement doesn't occur after 7 days' treatment or complete re-epithelialization after 14 days' treatment. Trifluridine shouldn't be used more than 21 days continuously due to potential ocular toxicity.
• Reassure patient that mild local irritation of the conjunctiva and cornea that occurs when solution is instilled is usually temporary.
• More effective drug than vidarabine with fewer side effects.

---

vidarabine
Vira-A Ophthalmic◆

INDICATIONS & DOSAGE
Acute keratoconjunctivitis, superficial keratitis, and recurrent epithelial keratitis resulting from herpes simplex types 1 and 2—
Adults and children: instill ½ inch ointment into lower conjunctival sac 5 times daily at 3-hour intervals.

SIDE EFFECTS
Eye: temporary visual burning, itching, mild irritation of eye, lacrimation, foreign body sensation, conjunctival injection, superficial punctate keratitis, eye pain, photosensitivity. **Other:** hypersensitivity.

INTERACTIONS
None significant.

NURSING CONSIDERATIONS
• Not for long-term use.
• A relatively new alternative in treating herpes simplex ocular infections.
• Warn patient not to exceed recommended frequency or duration of dosage.
• Not effective against RNA virus or adenoviral ocular infections, or against bacterial, fungal, or chlamydial infections.
• Warn patient to avoid sharing washcloths, etc. with family members.
• Always wash hands before and after applying ointment.
• Tell patient to watch for signs of sensitivity, such as itching lids or constant burning. Patient who develops such signs should stop drug and notify doctor immediately.
• Show patient how to instill.
• Warn patient not to touch tip of tube to eye or surrounding tissue.
• Available in 3% ointment.
• Store in tightly closed, light-resistant container.

71

Ophthalmic anti-inflammatory agents

dexamethasone
dexamethasone sodium phosphate
fluorometholone
hydrocortisone
hydrocortisone acetate
medrysone
prednisolone acetate
prednisolone sodium phosphate

---

dexamethasone
Maxidex Ophthalmic Suspension♦
dexamethasone sodium phosphate
Decadron Phosphate Ophthalmic♦,
Maxidex Ophthalmic♦, Novadex♦♦,
Opto-Methasone♦♦

INDICATIONS & DOSAGE
Uveitis; iridocyclitis; inflammatory condition of eyelids, conjunctiva, cornea, anterior segment of globe; to prevent corneal scarring in visual axis; corneal injury from chemical or thermal burns, or penetration of foreign bodies; allergic conjunctivitis—
Adults and children: instill 1 to 2 drops into conjunctival sac. In severe disease, drops may be used hourly, tapering to discontinuation as condition improves. In mild conditions, drops may be used up to 4 to 6 times daily. Treatment may extend from a few days to several weeks.

SIDE EFFECTS
Eye: increased intraocular pressure, especially in elderly patients; thinning of cornea, interference with corneal wound healing, increased susceptibility to viral or fungal corneal infection, corneal ulceration; with excessive or long-term use, glaucoma exacerbations, cataracts, visual acuity and visual field defects, optic nerve damage.
Other: systemic effects and adrenal suppression with excessive or long-term use.

INTERACTIONS
None significant.

NURSING CONSIDERATIONS
• Contraindicated in acute superficial herpes simplex (dendritic keratitis), vaccinia, varicella, or other fungal or viral diseases of cornea and conjunctiva; presence of active diabetes; ocular tuberculosis, or any acute, purulent, untreated infection of the eye. Use cautiously in corneal abrasions, since these may be infected (especially with herpes); glaucoma patients (any form), due to possibility of increasing intraocular pressure (miotic medication drug regimen may need to be increased to compensate).
• Viral and fungal infections of the cornea may be exacerbated by the application of steroids.
• Warn patient to call doctor immediately and to stop drug if visual acuity changes or visual field diminishes.
• Not for long-term use.
• May use eye pad with ointment for increased effect.
• Watch for corneal ulceration; may require stopping drug.
• Dexamethasone has greater anti-

inflammatory effect than dexamethasone sodium phosphate.

---

fluorometholone
FML Liquifilm Ophthalmic♦

INDICATIONS & DOSAGE
Inflammatory and allergic conditions of cornea, conjunctiva, sclera, anterior uvea—
Adults and children: instill 1 to 2 drops q 1 hour for first 1 to 2 days, then b.i.d., t.i.d., or q.i.d.

SIDE EFFECTS
Eye: increased intraocular pressure, especially in elderly patients; thinning of cornea, interference with corneal wound healing, corneal ulceration, increased susceptibility to viral or fungal corneal infections; with excessive or long-term use, glaucoma exacerbations, cataracts, decreased visual acuity, diminished visual field; optic nerve damage.
Other: systemic effects and adrenal suppression in excessive or long-term use.

INTERACTIONS
None significant.

NURSING CONSIDERATIONS
• Contraindicated in vaccinia, varicella, acute superficial herpes simplex (dendritic keratitis), or other fungal or viral eye diseases; ocular tuberculosis; or any acute, purulent, untreated eye infection. Use cautiously in corneal abrasions since they are commonly contaminated (e.g., especially with herpes).
• Not for long-term use.
• Less likely to cause increased intraocular pressure with long-term use than other ophthalmic anti-inflammatory drugs (except medrysone).
• Store in tightly covered, light-resistant container.

• Warn patient to call doctor immediately and to stop drug if visual acuity decreases or visual field diminishes.
• Shake well before using.

---

hydrocortisone
Optef
hydrocortisone acetate
Cortamed♦♦, Hydrocortone♦

INDICATIONS & DOSAGE
Uveitis, iridocyclitis, inflammatory condition of eyelids, conjunctiva, cornea, anterior segment of globe; to prevent corneal scarring in visual axis; corneal injury from chemical or thermal burns, or penetration of foreign bodies; allergic conjunctivitis—
Adults and children: instill 1 to 3 drops into conjunctival sac q 1 hour during the day and q 2 hours during the night in acute situations. May be decreased to 1 drop t.i.d. or q.i.d.; or instill ointment t.i.d. to q.i.d. initially. May decrease to daily or b.i.d.

SIDE EFFECTS
Eye: increased intraocular pressure, especially in elderly patients; thinning of cornea, interference with corneal wound healing, increased susceptibility to viral or fungal corneal infection, corneal ulceration; with excessive or long-term use, glaucoma exacerbations, cataracts, visual acuity and visual field defects, optic nerve damage.
Other: systemic effects and adrenal suppression with excessive or long-term use.

INTERACTIONS
None significant.

NURSING CONSIDERATIONS
• Contraindicated in acute superficial herpes simplex (dendritic keratitis), vaccinia, varicella, or other fungal or viral diseases of cornea and conjunc-

---

tiva; presence of active diabetes; ocular tuberculosis; or any acute, purulent, untreated eye infection. Use cautiously in corneal abrasions since they are commonly contaminated (e.g., especially with herpes).
• Viral and fungal infections of the cornea may be exacerbated by the application of steroids.
• Keep in mind possibility of increasing intraocular pressure.
• Warn patient to call doctor immediately and to stop drug if visual acuity changes or visual field diminishes.
• Not for long-term use.
• May use eye pad with ointment for increased effect.
• Watch for corneal ulceration; may require stopping drug.

medrysone
HMS Liquifilm Ophthalmic♦

INDICATIONS & DOSAGE
Allergic conjunctivitis, vernal conjunctivitis, episcleritis, ophthalmic epinephrine sensitivity reaction—
Adults and children: instill 1 drop in conjunctival sac b.i.d. to q.i.d. May use q hour during first 1 to 2 days if needed.

SIDE EFFECTS
Eye: thinning of cornea, interference with corneal wound healing, increased susceptibility to viral or fungal corneal infection, corneal ulceration; with excessive or long-term use, glaucoma exacerbations, cataracts, visual acuity and visual field defects, optic nerve damage.
Other: systemic effects and adrenal suppression with excessive or long-term use.

INTERACTIONS
None significant.

NURSING CONSIDERATIONS
• Contraindicated in vaccinia, varicella, acute superficial herpes simplex (dendritic keratitis), viral diseases of conjunctiva and cornea, ocular tuberculosis, fungal or viral eye diseases, iritis, uveitis, or any acute, purulent, untreated eye infection. Use cautiously in corneal abrasions since they are commonly contaminated (e.g., especially with herpes).
• Shake well before using. Don't freeze.

prednisolone acetate (suspensions)
Econopred Ophthalmic, Econopred Plus Ophthalmic, Pred-Forte♦, Pred Mild Ophthalmic♦, Prednicon♦♦, Predulose Ophthalmic
prednisolone sodium phosphate (solutions)
Hydeltrasol Ophthalmic, Inflamase Forte♦, Inflamase Ophthalmic♦, Metreton Ophthalmic, Nova-Pred Forte♦♦

INDICATIONS & DOSAGE
Inflammation of palpebral and bulbar conjunctiva, cornea, and anterior segment of globe—
Adults and children: instill 2 drops in eye. In severe conditions, may be used hourly, tapering to discontinuation as inflammation subsides. In mild conditions, may be used up to 4 to 6 times daily.

SIDE EFFECTS
Eye: increased intraocular pressure, especially in elderly patients; thinning of cornea, interference with corneal wound healing, increased susceptibility to viral or fungal corneal infection, corneal ulceration; with excessive or long-term use, glaucoma exacerbations, cataracts, visual acuity and visual field defects, optic nerve damage.

Other: systemic effects and adrenal suppression with excessive or long-term use.

INTERACTIONS
None significant.

NURSING CONSIDERATIONS
• Contraindicated in acute untreated purulent ocular infections, acute superficial herpes simplex (dendritic keratitis), vaccinia, varicella, or other viral or fungal eye diseases, ocular tuberculosis. Use cautiously in corneal abrasions since they are commonly contaminated (e.g., especially with herpes).
• Tell patient on long-term therapy to have frequent tonometric exams.
• Shake suspensions before using, and store in tightly covered container.
• Don't stop therapy prematurely.

72

Miotics

acetylcholine chloride
carbachol
demecarium bromide
echothiophate iodide
isoflurophate
physostigmine salicylate
pilocarpine hydrochloride
pilocarpine nitrate

---

acetylcholine chloride
Miochol ♦

INDICATIONS & DOSAGE
Anterior segment surgery—
Adults and children: doctor instills
0.5 to 2 ml of 1% solution gently in
anterior chamber of eye.

SIDE EFFECTS
None reported with 1% concentration.
Iris atrophy possible with higher con-
centrations.

INTERACTIONS
None significant.

NURSING CONSIDERATIONS
• Shake vial gently until clear solu-
tion is obtained.
• Reconstitute immediately before
using.
• Discard any unused solution.
• Complete miosis within seconds.
• Don't gas sterilize vial. Ethylene
oxide may produce formic acid.

---

carbachol (intraocular)
Miostat
carbachol (topical)
Carbacel, Isopto Carbachol ♦

INDICATIONS & DOSAGE
*Ocular surgery (to produce pupillary
miosis)—*
Adults: doctor should gently instill
0.5 ml into the anterior chamber for
production of satisfactory miosis. It
may be instilled before or after secur-
ing sutures.
*Open-angle or narrow-angle
glaucoma—*
Adults: instill 1 drop into eye daily,
b.i.d., t.i.d., or q.i.d. Ointment form
also available with b.i.d. dosage.

SIDE EFFECTS
CNS: headache.
Eye: accommodative spasm, conjunc-
tival vasodilation, eye and brow pain.
GI: abdominal cramps, diarrhea.
Other: sweating, flushing, asthma.

INTERACTIONS
None significant.

NURSING CONSIDERATIONS
• Contraindicated in acute iritis, corneal abrasion. Use cautiously in acute
cardiac failure, bronchial asthma,
peptic ulcer, hyperthyroidism, GI
spasm, urinary tract obstruction,
Parkinson's disease.
• A cholinergic agent.
• Used in glaucoma, especially when

patient is resistant or allergic to pilocarpine HCl or nitrate.
- Warn patient not to exceed recommended dosage.
- For single-dose intraocular use only. Premixed; discard unused portions.
- Warn patient not to touch tip of dropper to eye or surrounding tissue.
- Tell glaucoma patient that long-term use may be necessary. Stress compliance. Tell him to remain under medical supervision for periodic tonometric readings.
- In case of toxicity, atropine should be given parenterally.
- Show patient how to instill.

---

demecarium bromide
Humorsol

INDICATIONS & DOSAGE
Glaucoma, postiridectomy—
Adults: instill 1 drop 0.125% or 0.25% solution in eyes twice weekly up to b.i.d., depending on intraocular pressure.
Accommodative esotropia—
Children: instill 1 drop 0.125% solution in each eye daily for 2 to 3 weeks, taper to 1 drop q 2 days for 3 to 4 weeks, then 1 drop twice weekly. Therapy should be discontinued after 4 months if control of condition still requires q other day therapy or if patient shows no response.

SIDE EFFECTS
CNS: headache.
CV: hypotension, bradycardia.
Eye: iris cysts (reversible with discontinuation), lens opacity, ciliary or accommodative spasm, blurred vision, eye or brow pain, photosensitivity, eyelid twitching, congestive iritis, iridocyclitis, conjunctival and intraocular hyperemia, ocular pain, photophobia, acute attack of congestive glaucoma.

GI: nausea, vomiting, abdominal pain, diarrhea, excessive salivation.
GU: frequent urination.
Skin: contact dermatitis.
Other: flushing, bronchial constriction.

INTERACTIONS
Systemic anticholinesterase for myasthenia gravis: additive effects. Monitor for signs of toxicity.
Echothiophate iodide: decreased duration of miosis if demecarium bromide is given first. Give echothiophate iodide first.
Organophosphate insecticides: additive effects. Warn patient exposed to these insecticides of this danger.
Pilocarpine: interferes with miosis. Do not use together.
Succinylcholine: respiratory or cardiovascular collapse. Don't use together.

NURSING CONSIDERATIONS
- Contraindicated in active uveal inflammation, narrow-angle glaucoma, secondary glaucoma resulting from iridocyclitis, ocular hypertension, vasomotor instability, bronchial asthma, spastic GI conditions, peptic ulcer, severe bradycardia, hypotension, recent myocardial infarction, epilepsy, parkinsonism, history of retinal detachment. Use cautiously in myasthenia gravis patients on systemic anticholinesterase therapy; in patients exposed to organophosphate insecticides.
- Systemic absorption may be minimized by compressing inner canthus of eye for 1 to 2 minutes after instilling drops.
- Dangerous drug capable of producing cumulative systemic side effects. Closely follow prescribed concentration and dosage schedule and monitor patient carefully.
- Atropine sulfate S.C. or I.V. or pralidoxine chloride is antidote of choice.
- Tell patient to stop drug and report

---

immediately if excessive salivation, diaphoresis, urinary incontinence, diarrhea, or muscle weakness occurs.
• Instruct patient to take at bedtime since drug blurs vision.
• Warn patient not to exceed recommended dosage.
• Warn patient not to touch tip of dropper to eye or surrounding tissue.
• Stop drug at least 2 weeks preoperatively.
• If solution contacts skin, wash promptly with large amount of water.
• Wash hands immediately before and after administering.
• Monitor patient for lenticular opacities every 6 months.
• Instruct patient that close and constant medical supervision is vital.
• Treat any extraocular pressure changes with rapid instillation of 1% to 2% epinephrine at 5-minute intervals.
• Antidote for atropine for glaucoma or preglaucoma patients, and used to control preop and postop intraocular pressure tension of glaucoma.
• Store in tightly closed container.
• An extremely potent, long-acting anticholinesterase drug.
• Show patient how to instill.

---

echothiophate iodide
Echodide, Phospholine Iodide♦

INDICATIONS & DOSAGE
Open-angle glaucoma, conditions obstructing aqueous outflow, accommodative esotropia—
Adults and children: instill 1 drop 0.03% to 0.125% solution into conjunctival sac daily. Maximum 1 drop b.i.d. Use lowest possible dosage to continuously control intraocular pressure.

SIDE EFFECTS
CNS: fatigue, muscle weakness, paresthesias, headache.

CV: bradycardia, hypotension.
Eye: ciliary or accommodative spasm, ciliary or conjunctival injection, nonreversible cataract formation (time- and dose-related), reversible iris cysts, pupillary block, blurred or dimmed vision, eye or brow pain, lid-twitching, hyperemia, photosensitivity, lens opacities, lacrimation, retinal detachment.
GI: diarrhea, nausea, vomiting, abdominal pain, intestinal cramps, salivation.
GU: frequent urination.
Other: flushing, sweating, bronchial constriction.

INTERACTIONS
Organophosphate insecticides (parathion, malathion): may have an additive effect that could cause systemic effects. Warn patient exposed to these insecticides of this danger.
Succinylcholine: respiratory and cardiovascular collapse. Don't use together.
Systemic anticholinesterase for myasthenia gravis: effects may be additive. Monitor patient for signs of toxicity.

NURSING CONSIDERATIONS
• Contraindicated in narrow-angle glaucoma, angle-closure glaucoma, epilepsy, vasomotor instability, parkinsonism, iodide hypersensitivity, active uveal inflammation, ocular hypertension with intraocular inflammatory processes, bronchial asthma, spastic GI conditions, urinary tract obstruction, peptic ulcer, severe bradycardia or hypotension, vascular hypertension, myocardial infarction, history of retinal detachment. Use cautiously in patients routinely exposed to organophosphate insecticides. May cause nausea, vomiting, and diarrhea, progressing to muscle weakness and respiratory difficulty. Use cautiously in myasthenia gravis patients on anticholinesterase therapy.
• Toxicity is cumulative. Toxic sys-

Italicized side effects are common or life-threatening.

temic symptoms don't appear for weeks or months after initiating therapy.
- Reconstitute powder carefully to avoid contamination. Use only diluent provided. Discard refrigerated, reconstituted solution after 6 months; solution at room temperature after 1 month.
- Warn patient that transient browache or dimmed or blurred vision is common at first but usually disappears within 5 to 10 days.
- Systemic absorption may be minimized by compressing inner canthus of eye for 1 to 2 minutes after instilling drops.
- Instill at bedtime since drug causes transient blurred vision.
- Tell patient to remain under constant medical supervision. Warn him not to exceed recommended dosage.
- Report salivation, diarrhea, profuse sweating, urinary incontinence, or muscle weakness.
- Stop drug at least 2 weeks preoperatively.
- Atropine sulfate (S.C., I.M., or I.V.) is antidote of choice.
- A potent, long-acting, irreversible anticholinesterase.
- Warn patient not to touch tip of dropper to eye or surrounding tissue.
- Show patient how to instill.

---

isoflurophate
Floropryl

INDICATIONS & DOSAGE
Glaucoma—
Adults and children: instill ¼-inch strip 0.025% ointment in conjunctival sac q 8 to 72 hours.
Esotopia uncomplicated by amblyopia or anisometropia—
Adults and children: ¼-inch of ointment every night for 2 weeks.

SIDE EFFECTS
CNS: headache, muscle weakness.
Eye: moderate conjunctival hyperemia, eye pain, ciliary spasm causing discomfort, iris cysts, cataract formation, retinal detachment, paradoxical increase in intraocular pressure; precipitates attacks of acute congestive glaucoma.
GI: diarrhea, salivation.
Other: sweating, bronchial constriction.

INTERACTIONS
Demecarium, physostigmine: competitive action. Decreased duration of miosis if isoflurophate given second. Give isoflurophate first.
Pilocarpine: interferes with miosis. Use cautiously for ciliary spasm.
Succinylcholine: respiratory or cardiovascular collapse. Don't use together.
Systemic anticholinesterase for myasthenia gravis: additive effects. Monitor patient for signs of toxicity.

NURSING CONSIDERATIONS
- Contraindicated in hypersensitivity to organophosphorous compounds and to peanut oil and polyethylene mineral oil, uveal inflammation, narrow-angle glaucoma, ocular hypertension, bronchial asthma, peptic ulcer, severe bradycardia, hypotension, recent MI, epilepsy, parkinsonism, or history of retinal detachment. Use cautiously in patients exposed to organophosphate insecticides; myasthenia gravis patients on concurrent anticholinesterase drugs.
- Tell glaucoma patient to use at bedtime if possible because of blurred vision and ciliary spasm.
- Don't touch tip of tube to eye, surrounding tissues, or moist surface.
- Warn patient that close, constant medical supervision is vital and not to exceed prescribed dosage.
- Treat paradoxical pressure changes

---

with rapid instillation of 1% to 2% epinephrine at 5-minute intervals.
• Instruct patient to stop therapy at once and notify doctor if he experiences excessive salivation, diarrhea, sweating, muscle weakness.
• Systemic absorption may be minimized by compressing inner canthus of eye for 1 to 2 minutes after instilling drops.
• Unstable and inactivated in the presence of water.
• Store in tightly closed container.
• Rapidly absorbed through skin.
• A potent parasympathomimetic, or anticholinesterase, drug.
• Show patient how to instill.

---

physostigmine salicylate
Eserine Salicylate, Isopto Eserine

INDICATIONS & DOSAGE
Atropine mydriasis, acute angle-closure glaucoma—
Adults and children: instill ¼ inch 0.25% ophthalmic ointment in conjunctival sac, or instill 1 to 2 drops 0.25% to 0.5% solution in conjunctival sac t.i.d. Repeat p.r.n. to obtain miosis.

SIDE EFFECTS
CNS: headache.
Eye: twitching of eyelids, conjunctival irritation, reversible depigmentation of lid skin in Blacks allergic to ointment, eye and brow pain, marked lacrimation, dimmed or blurred vision, follicular cysts.
Skin: allergic dermatitis.

INTERACTIONS
Isoflurophate: decreased miosis if isoflurophate given second. Give isoflurophate first.
Organophosphate insecticides: additive effect. Warn patient exposed to these insecticides of this danger.

Pilocarpine: prolonged miosis. May be used together therapeutically.
Succinylcholine: additive effect. Don't use together.

NURSING CONSIDERATIONS
• Contraindicated in inflammatory diseases of iris or ciliary body, asthma, diabetes mellitus, gangrene, cardiovascular disease, mechanical obstruction of intestinal or urogenital tract, vagotonia, secondary glaucoma. Use cautiously in bradycardia, epilepsy, parkinsonism, and in patients exposed to organophosphate insecticides.
• Glaucoma therapy is long-term. Stress patient compliance. Warn not to exceed dosage.
• Lid-twitching, temporarily blurred vision, and difficulty in seeing in the dark are common side effects.
• Irritating to eye. Watch for signs of conjunctivitis or allergic reactions.
• Don't touch dropper or tip of tube to eye or surrounding tissue.
• Systemic absorption may be minimized by compressing inner canthus of eye for 1 to 2 minutes after instilling drops.
• Discard discolored (rusty or pink-colored) solution or ointment. Aqueous solutions oxidize on exposure to light or air.
• Anticholinesterase.
• Used in ocular myasthenia gravis.
• May be used alternately with atropine as a miotic to break adhesions between the iris and lens.
• Show patient how to instill.

---

pilocarpine hydrochloride

Adsorbocarpine♦, Almocarpine, Is-
opto Carpine♦, Miocarpine♦♦, Nova-
Carpine♦♦, Ocusert Pilo♦, Opto-
Pilo♦♦, Pilocar, Pilocel, Pilomiotin

pilocarpine nitrate

P.V. Carpine Liquifilm♦

INDICATIONS & DOSAGE

*Chronic simple glaucoma, prior to
emergency surgery in acute narrow-
angle glaucoma—*
Adults and children: instill 2 drops
in eye daily b.i.d., t.i.d., q.i.d., or as
directed by doctor.

SIDE EFFECTS

Eye: suborbital headache, *myopia,*
ciliary spasm, *blurred vision,* conjunctival irritation, lacrimation,
changes in visual field, *brow pain.*
GI: nausea, vomiting, abdominal
cramps, diarrhea, salivation.
Other: bronchiolar spasm, pulmonary edema, hypersensitivity.

INTERACTIONS

Carbachol: additive effect. Do not
use together.
Phenylephrine HCl: decreased dilation by phenylephrine HCl. Don't use
together.

NURSING CONSIDERATIONS

• Contraindicated in acute iritis,
acute inflammatory disease of anterior segment of eye, secondary glaucoma. Use cautiously in bronchial
asthma, hypertension.
• Warn patient that vision will be
temporarily blurred.
• Transient browache and myopia are
common at first; usually disappear in
10 to 14 days.
• Warn patient not to exceed recommended dosage.
• Warn patient not to touch dropper
to eye or surrounding tissue.
• Glaucoma therapy is necessarily
prolonged. Stress compliance. Warn
that glaucoma can cause blindness.
• Most widely used drug in initial
treatment of chronic, simple
glaucoma.
• Systemic absorption may be minimized by compressing inner canthus
of eye for 1 to 2 minutes after instilling drops.
• Also used to counteract effects of
mydriatics and cycloplegics after
surgery or ophthalmoscopic examination.
• May be used alternately with atropine to break adhesions between iris
and lens.
• In acute narrow-angle glaucoma
prior to surgery, may be used alone or
with physostigmine or mannitol, urea,
or glycerol.
• Show patient how to instill.

73

Mydriatics

atropine sulfate
cyclopentolate hydrochloride
dipivefrin
epinephrine bitartrate
epinephrine hydrochloride
epinephryl borate
homatropine hydrobromide
hydroxyamphetamine
  hydrobromide
phenylephrine hydrochloride
scopolamine hydrobromide
tropicamide

atropine sulfate
Atropisol, BufOpto Atropine, Isopto
Atropine♦, Opto-Tropinal♦♦

INDICATIONS & DOSAGE
Acute iris inflammation (iritis)—
Adults: 1 to 2 drops of 1% solution or
small amount of ointment 2 to 3 times
daily, b.i.d., or t.i.d.
Children: instill 1 to 2 drops of 0.5%
solution daily, b.i.d., or t.i.d.
Cycloplegic refraction—
Adults: instill 1 to 2 drops of 1% solution 1 hour before refracting.
Children: instill 1 to 2 drops of 0.5%
solution to each eye b.i.d. for 1 to
3 days before eye exam and 1 hour
before refraction, or instill small
amount ointment daily or b.i.d. 2 to
3 days before exam.

SIDE EFFECTS
Eye: increased intraocular pressure,
ocular congestion in long-term use,
conjunctivitis, contact dermatitis,
edema, *blurred vision,* eye dryness,
photophobia.
Systemic: flushing, dry skin and
mouth, fever, tachycardia, abdominal
distention in infants, ataxia, irritability, confusion, somnolence.

INTERACTIONS
None significant.

NURSING CONSIDERATIONS
• Contraindicated in primary glaucoma (shallow anterior chamber or
narrow-angle), increased intraocular
pressure. Use cautiously in infants,
children, elderly or debilitated patients.
• Warn patient vision will be temporarily blurred. Dark glasses ease discomfort of photophobia.
• Not for internal use. Treat drops
and ointment as poison. Keep physostigmine available as antidote for
poisoning.
• Don't touch dropper or tip of tube
to eye or surrounding tissue.
• Watch for signs of glaucoma: increased intraocular pressure, ocular
pain, headache, blurred vision.
• Most potent mydriatic and cycloplegic available; long duration of
action.
• Warn patient not to exceed recommended dosage.
• Systemic absorption may be minimized by compressing inner canthus
of eye for 1 to 2 minutes after instilling drops.
• Show patient how to instill.

cyclopentolate hydrochloride
Cyclogyl♦, Mydplegic♦♦,
Nova-Cyclo ♦♦, Opto-Pentolate♦♦

INDICATIONS & DOSAGE
Diagnostic procedures requiring my-driasis and cycloplegia—
Adults: instill 1 drop 1% solution in
eye, followed by 1 more drop in
5 minutes. Use 2% solution in heavily
pigmented irises.
Children: instill 1 drop of 0.5%, 1%,
or 2% solution in each eye, followed
in 5 minutes with 1 drop 0.5% or 1%
solution, if necessary. Not recommended for children under 6.

SIDE EFFECTS
Eye: burning sensation on instillation,
increased intraocular pressure,
blurred vision, eye dryness, *photo-phobia*, ocular congestion, contact
dermatitis, conjunctivitis.
Systemic: flushing, tachycardia, urinary retention, dry skin, fever, ataxia,
irritability, confusion, somnolence,
convulsions.

INTERACTIONS
None significant.

NURSING CONSIDERATIONS
• Contraindicated in narrow-angle
glaucoma. Use cautiously in elderly
patients.
• Systemic absorption may be minimized by compressing inner canthus
of eye for 1 to 2 minutes after instilling drops.
• Close container after each use to
avoid contamination.
• Potent drug with mydriatic and cycloplegic effect; superior to homatropine hydrobromide and has shorter
duration of action.
• Instruct patient to wear dark
glasses to ease discomfort of photophobia.

• Warn patient drug will burn when
instilled.

dipivefrin
Propine

INDICATIONS & DOSAGE
*To reduce intraocular pressure in
chronic open-angle glaucoma—*
Adults: for initial glaucoma therapy,
1 drop in eye q 12 hours.

SIDE EFFECTS
Eye: burning, stinging.
CV: tachycardia, hypertension.

INTERACTIONS
None significant.

NURSING CONSIDERATIONS
• Contraindicated in narrow-angle
glaucoma.
• Use cautiously in patients with
aphakia.
• Dipivefrin is a prodrug of epinephrine: converted to epinephrine when it
enters the eye.
• May have fewer side effects than
conventional epinephrine therapy.
• Often used concomitantly with
other antiglaucoma drugs.
• Available as a 0.1% solution in
5, 10, and 15 ml dropper bottles.

epinephrine bitartrate
E1, E2, Epitrate♦, Lyophrin,
Murocoll, Mytrate
epinephrine hydrochloride
Epifrin♦, Glaucon♦
epinephryl borate
Epinal♦, Eppy/N♦

INDICATIONS & DOSAGE
Adults and children:
*Intraocular injection—*0.1 to 0.2 ml
of 0.01% or 0.1% epinephrine HCl by
doctor.

Open-angle glaucoma—instill 1 to 2 drops of 1% or 2% bitartrate solution in eye with frequency determined by tonometric readings (once q 2 to 4 days up to q.i.d.), or instill 1 drop 0.5%, 1%, or 2% HCl solution (or 0.25%, 0.5%, or 1% epinephryl borate solution) in eye b.i.d.
During surgery—1 or more drops of 0.1% epinephrine HCl up to 3 times.

SIDE EFFECTS
Eye: corneal or conjunctival pigmentation or corneal edema in long-term use; follicular hypertrophy; chemosis; conjunctivitis; iritis; hyperemic conjunctiva; maculopapular rash; severe stinging, burning, and tearing upon instillation; browache.
Systemic: palpitations, tachycardia.

INTERACTIONS
Cyclopropane or halogenated hydrocarbons: arrhythmias, tachycardia. Use together cautiously, if at all.
Tricyclic antidepressants, antihistamines (diphenhydramine, dexchlorpheniramine): potentiated cardiac effects of epinephrine. Use together cautiously.

NURSING CONSIDERATIONS
• Contraindicated in shallow anterior chamber or narrow-angle glaucoma.
• Use cautiously in diabetes mellitus, hypertension, Parkinson's disease, hyperthyroidism, aphakia (eye without lens), cardiac disease, cerebral arteriosclerosis, elderly patients, or pregnancy.
• May stain soft contact lenses.
• Use with pilocarpine: additive effect in lowering intraocular pressure.
• Monitor blood pressure and other systemic effects.
• Protect from light and heat.
• Don't use darkened solution.
• Also used during surgery to control local bleeding, or injected into the anterior chamber to produce rapid mydriasis during cataract removal.

• Warn patient not to touch dropper to eye or surrounding tissue.

---

homatropine hydrobromide
Homatrocel Ophthalmic, Isopto Homatropine◆

INDICATIONS & DOSAGE
Adults and children:
Cycloplegic refraction—instill 1 to 2 drops 2% or 5% solution in eye; repeat in 5 to 10 minutes.
Uveitis—instill 1 to 2 drops 2% or 5% solution in eye up to every 3 to 4 hours.

SIDE EFFECTS
Eye: eye irritation, *blurred vision, photophobia.*
Systemic: flushing, dry skin and mouth, fever, tachycardia, ataxia, irritability, confusion, somnolence.

INTERACTIONS
None significant.

NURSING CONSIDERATIONS
• Contraindicated in primary glaucoma (shallow anterior chamber or narrow-angle). Use cautiously in infants, elderly or debilitated patients, or in hypertension, cardiac disease, or increased intraocular pressure.
• Warn patient vision will be temporarily blurred after instillation. Dark glasses should be worn to decrease photophobia.
• Long-term frequent use may produce symptoms of atropine SO_4 poisoning, such as dryness of mouth, increase in heart rate.
• Not for internal use. Treat as poison. Keep physostigmine available as antidote for poisoning.
• Systemic absorption may be minimized by compressing inner canthus of eye for 1 to 2 minutes after instilling drops.
• Show patient how to instill.

• Warn patient not to touch dropper tip to eye or surrounding tissue.
• Similar to atropine SO₄ but weaker, with a shorter duration of action.

hydroxyamphetamine hydrobromide
Paredrine

INDICATIONS & DOSAGE
Diagnostic in Horner's syndrome—
Adults, and children over 12: instill 1 to 2 drops 1% solution into conjunctival sac.

SIDE EFFECTS
Eye: increased intraocular pressure, blurred vision, *photophobia.*

INTERACTIONS
None significant.

NURSING CONSIDERATIONS
• Contraindicated in narrow-angle glaucoma. Use cautiously in hypertension, hyperthyroidism, diabetes mellitus, increased intraocular pressure.
• Instruct patient to wear dark glasses to ease discomfort of photophobia.
• Store in tightly closed container. Do not use discolored solution.
• If ingested, toxic symptoms include arrhythmias, headache, nausea, vomiting. Contact doctor immediately.

phenylephrine hydrochloride
Mydfrin, Neo-Synephrine♦

INDICATIONS & DOSAGE
Adults and children:
*Mydriasis (without cycloplegia)—*instill 1 drop 2.5% or 10% solution in eye before exam.
*Posterior synechia (adhesion of iris)—*instill 1 drop 10% solution in eye.

Do not use 10% concentration in infants; use cautiously in elderly.

SIDE EFFECTS
Eye: transient burning or stinging on instillation, blurred vision, reactive hyperemia, allergic conjunctivitis, iris floaters, narrow-angle glaucoma, rebound miosis, allergic conjunctivitis, dermatitis.
CNS: headache, browache.
CV: *hypertension,* tachycardia, palpitations, premature ventricular contractions.
Other: pallor, trembling, sweating.

INTERACTIONS
Guanethidine: increased mydriatic and pressor effects of phenylephrine HCl. Use together cautiously.
Levodopa (systemic): reduced mydriatic effect of phenylephrine HCl. Use together cautiously.
MAO inhibitors: may cause arrhythmias due to increased pressor effect. Use together cautiously.
Tricyclic antidepressants: potentiated cardiac effects of epinephrine. Use together cautiously.

NURSING CONSIDERATIONS
• Contraindicated in narrow-angle glaucoma, soft contact lens use. Use cautiously in marked hypertension, cardiac disorders, and in children of low body weight.
• Should be avoided in patients with idiopathic orthostatic hypotension. May produce high blood pressure response.
• Protect from light and heat.
• Warn patient not to exceed recommended dosage. Systemic effects can result. Monitor blood pressure and pulse.
• Warn patient not to touch dropper tip to eye or surrounding tissue.
• Systemic absorption can be minimized by compressing inner canthus of eye for 1 to 2 minutes after instilling drops.

- Potential for systemic side effects less severe with 2.5% solution.
- Show patient how to instill.

scopolamine hydrobromide
Isopto Hyoscine

INDICATIONS & DOSAGE
Cycloplegic refraction—
Adults: instill 1 to 2 drops 0.5% to 1% solution in eye 1 hour before refraction.
Children: instill 1 drop 0.2% or 0.25% solution or ointment b.i.d. for 2 days before refraction.
Iritis—
Adults: 1 to 2 drops of 0.1% solution daily, b.i.d., or t.i.d.

SIDE EFFECTS
Eye: ocular congestion with prolonged use, conjunctivitis, *blurred vision,* eye dryness, increased intraocular pressure, *photophobia,* contact dermatitis.
Systemic: flushing, fever, dry skin and mouth, tachycardia, hallucinations, ataxia, irritability, confusion, delirium, somnolence.

INTERACTIONS
None significant.

NURSING CONSIDERATIONS
- Contraindicated in primary glaucoma (shallow anterior chamber or narrow-angle). Use cautiously in cardiac disease, increased intraocular pressure, and in patients over age 40.
- Observe patient closely for systemic effects (disorientation, delirium).
- Warn patient vision will be temporarily blurred.
- Instruct patient to wear dark glasses to ease discomfort of photophobia.
- Not for internal use.
- May be used when patient is sensi-

tive to atropine. Faster acting and has shorter duration of action.
- Warn patient not to touch dropper tip to eye or surrounding tissue.
- Systemic absorption may be minimized by compressing inner canthus of eye for 1 to 2 minutes after instilling drops.

tropicamide
Mydriacyl♦

INDICATIONS & DOSAGE
Adults and children:
*Cycloplegic refractions—*instill 1 to 2 drops of 1% solution in each eye; repeat in 5 minutes. Additional drop may be instilled in 20 to 30 minutes.
*Fundus exams—*instill 1 to 2 drops 0.5% solution in each eye 15 to 20 minutes before exam.

SIDE EFFECTS
EENT: *transient stinging on instillation,* increased intraocular pressure (less than with other mydriatic agents because of shorter duration of action), *blurred vision, photophobia,* dry mouth and throat.

INTERACTIONS
None significant.

NURSING CONSIDERATIONS
- Contraindicated in narrow-angle and shallow anterior chamber glaucoma. Use cautiously in elderly.
- Shortest acting cycloplegic, but mydriatic effect greater than cycloplegic effect.
- Causes transient stinging; vision temporarily blurred.
- Instruct patient to wear dark glasses if photosensitivity occurs (lasts about 2 hours).
- Store at room temperature in tightly closed container.

74

Ophthalmic vasoconstrictors

epinephrine hydrochloride
naphazoline hydrochloride
phenylephrine hydrochloride
tetrahydrozoline hydrochloride
zinc sulfate

epinephrine hydrochloride
Adrenalin Chloride 0.1%,
Epinephrine 1:1000 0.1%

INDICATIONS & DOSAGE
Preop to control bleeding and conjunctivitis—
Adults and children: 1 or 2 drops of
0.1% solution or injected by doctor
intracamerally 0.01% to 0.1%. Frequency individualized.

SIDE EFFECTS
Eye: corneal or conjunctival pigmentation or corneal edema in long-term
use; follicular hypertrophy; chemosis;
conjunctivitis; iritis; hyperemic conjunctiva; maculopapular rash; severe
stinging, burning, tearing on instillation; browache; hypersensitivity.
Systemic: palpitations, tachycardia,
extrasystoles.

INTERACTIONS
Pilocarpine: additive effect on decreasing intraocular pressure. Monitor blood pressure and side effects.

NURSING CONSIDERATIONS
• Contraindicated in shallow anterior
eye chamber, narrow-angle glaucoma. Use with caution in cardiac disease, hyperthyroidism, hypertension,
diabetes mellitus, and the elderly.
• May cause staining of soft contact
lenses.
• Keep container tightly sealed, away
from light, and in a cool place.
• Discard solution if it is brown or
contains precipitate.
• If signs of hypersensitivity (edema
of lids, itching, discharge, crusting
eyelids) occur, stop drops and contact
doctor.
• If administering in conjunction
with miotic, instill miotic 2 to
10 minutes before epinephrine.

naphazoline hydrochloride
0.012%, 0.1%, 0.02%
Albalon Liquifilm Ophthalmic♦,
Clear Eyes, Naphcon, Naphcon Forte
Ophthalmic♦, Opto-Zoline♦♦, Vasoclear, Vasocon Regular Ophthalmic♦

INDICATIONS & DOSAGE
*Ocular congestion, irritation,
itching—*
Adults: instill 1 to 2 drops in eye q
3 to 4 hours.

SIDE EFFECTS
Eye: transient stinging, pupillary dilation, increased intraocular pressure,
irritation.

INTERACTIONS
MAO inhibitors: hypertensive crisis if
naphazoline HCl is systemically absorbed. Use together cautiously.

NURSING CONSIDERATIONS

• Contraindicated in narrow-angle glaucoma, hypersensitivity to any ingredients. Use cautiously in hyperthyroidism, heart disease, hypertension, diabetes mellitus, elderly patients.
• Can produce marked sedation and coma if ingested by child.
• Advise patient that photophobia may follow pupil dilation if he is sensitive to drug. Tell patient to report this to the doctor if it occurs.
• Warn patient not to exceed recommended dosage. Rebound congestion and rhinitis may occur with frequent or prolonged use.
• Notify doctor if blurred vision, pain, or lid edema develops.
• Store in tightly closed container.
• Most effective and widely used ocular decongestant.
• Show patient how to instill.

phenylephrine hydrochloride
Isopto Frin, Prefrin, Tear-Efrin

INDICATIONS & DOSAGE
Decongestant, minor eye irritations—
Adults and children: 2 drops of 0.12% or 0.25% in affected eye. May repeat in 3 to 4 hours, p.r.n.

SIDE EFFECTS
CNS: headache.
Eye: transient stinging, iris floaters, narrow-angle glaucoma, blurred vision, reactive hyperemia, browache.

INTERACTIONS
MAO inhibitors: may cause hypertensive crisis. Give cautiously.

NURSING CONSIDERATIONS
• Contraindicated in narrow-angle glaucoma, in patients taking tricyclic antidepressants or MAO inhibitors, and in hypersensitivity to any ingredient.

• May exacerbate hypertension in hypertensive patients.
• Do not use butacaine drops as local anesthetic, since phenylephrine and butacaine are incompatible.
• Do not exceed prescribed dose.
• Monitor blood pressure and pulse; watch for overdosage.
• Do not use if solution is dark brown or contains precipitate.
• Keep container tightly sealed and away from light.

tetrahydrozoline hydrochloride
Clear & Bright, Murine 2, Soothe, Tetrasine, Visine

INDICATIONS & DOSAGE
Ocular congestion, irritation, and allergic conditions—
Adults, and children over 2 years: instill 1 to 2 drops in eye b.i.d. or t.i.d., or as directed by doctor.

SIDE EFFECTS
Eye: transient stinging, pupillary dilation, increased intraocular pressure, irritation, iris floaters in elderly.
Systemic: drowsiness, CNS depression, cardiac irregularities, headache, dizziness, tremors, insomnia.

INTERACTIONS
MAO inhibitors: hypertensive crisis if tetrahydrozoline HCl is systemically absorbed. Use together cautiously.

NURSING CONSIDERATIONS
• Contraindicated in patients receiving MAO inhibitors, hypersensitivity to any ingredients, narrow-angle glaucoma. Use cautiously in hyperthyroidism, heart disease, hypertension, diabetes mellitus, elderly patients.
• Do not exceed recommended dosage. Rebound congestion and rhinitis may occur with frequent or prolonged use.
• Warn patient to stop drug and no-

Italicized side effects are common or life-threatening.

tify doctor if relief is not obtained within 48 hours, or if redness or irritation persists or increases.
• Available without prescription.
• Available in 0.05% concentration; less effective than naphazoline hydrochloride 0.1%.
• Warn patient not to touch dropper tip to eye or surrounding tissue.
• Show patient how to instill.

zinc sulfate
Bufopto Zinc Sulfate, Eye-Sed Ophthalmic, Op-Thal-Zin

INDICATIONS & DOSAGE
Ocular congestion, irritation—

Adults and children: solution 0.2%—instill 1 to 2 drops in eye b.i.d. or t.i.d.

SIDE EFFECTS
Eye: irritation.

INTERACTIONS
None significant.

NURSING CONSIDERATIONS
• Use cautiously in patients with a shallow anterior chamber, predisposition to narrow-angle glaucoma.
• A decongestant astringent.
• Store in tightly closed container.
• Warn patient not to touch dropper tip to eye or surrounding tissue.
• Show patient how to instill drops.

75

Topical ophthalmic anesthetics

cocaine hydrochloride
proparacaine hydrochloride
tetracaine hydrochloride

---

cocaine hydrochloride

INDICATIONS & DOSAGE
*Diagnosis of Horner's syndrome,
topical anesthesia for minor surgery
or exams—*
Adults and children: instill 1 to
2 drops 4% solution in eye just before
procedure or exam.

SIDE EFFECTS
Eye: *blurring,* corneal ulceration or
scarring in excessive or long-term
use. Varying effects on intraocular
pressure.
Systemic: excitation; nervousness;
rapid, shallow respirations; emesis;
chills; fever; tachycardia; hypertension; euphoria; anxiety; delirium;
convulsions; respiratory and circulatory failure.

INTERACTIONS
Epinephrine (topical): increased
epinephrine effect. Use together
cautiously.

NURSING CONSIDERATIONS
• Use cautiously and sparingly in patients with known allergies, cardiac
disease, hyperthyroidism, or open
lesions.
• Patient should be given short-acting barbiturate before administering
to avoid CNS stimulation.

• Solutions not commercially available; must be prepared specially by
pharmacist. Rarely used.
• Monitor heart rate after instillation;
observe for systemic effects.
• Warn patient vision will be blurred
for several hours.
• Warn patient not to rub eye for at
least 20 minutes after instillation.
• Protective eye patch recommended
following procedure.
• Solution should be pink-colored.
Return discolored solution to
pharmacy.
• Doesn't require refrigeration.

---

proparacaine hydrochloride
Alcaine♦, Ophthaine♦, Ophthetic♦

INDICATIONS & DOSAGE
Adults and children:
*Anesthesia for tonometry, gonioscopy,
suture removal from cornea, removal
of corneal foreign bodies—*instill 1 to
2 drops 0.5% solution in eye just
before procedure.
*Anesthesia for cataract extraction,
glaucoma surgery—*instill 1 drop
0.5% solution in eye every 5 to
10 minutes for 5 to 7 doses.

SIDE EFFECTS
Eye: occasional conjunctival redness,
transient pain.
Other: hypersensitivity.

INTERACTIONS
None significant.

NURSING CONSIDERATIONS
- Use cautiously in cardiac diseases and hyperthyroidism.
- *Not* for long-term use; may delay wound healing.
- Warn patient not to rub or touch eye while cornea is anesthetized, since this may cause corneal abrasion and greater discomfort when anesthesia wears off.
- Protective eye patch recommended following procedure.
- Warn patient corneal pain is only relieved temporarily in abrasion.
- Systemic reactions unlikely when used in recommended doses.
- Topical ophthalmic anesthetic of choice in diagnostic and minor surgical procedures.
- Don't use discolored solution.
- Store in tightly closed container.
- Ophthaine brand packaged in bottle that looks similar in size and shape to Hemoccult. When taking bottle from shelf, check label carefully.

---

tetracaine hydrochloride
Anacel, Pontocaine♦

INDICATIONS & DOSAGE
Anesthesia for tonometry, gonioscopy, removal of corneal foreign bodies, suture removal from cornea, other diagnostic and minor surgical procedures—
Adults and children: instill 1 to 2 drops 0.5% solution in eye just before procedure.

SIDE EFFECTS
Eye: transient stinging in eye 30 seconds after initial instillation, epithelial damage in excessive or long-term use.
Other: sensitization in repeated use (allergic skin rash, urticaria).

INTERACTIONS
Sulfonamides: interference with sulfonamide antibacterial activity. Wait ½ hour after anesthesia before instilling sulfonamide.

NURSING CONSIDERATIONS
- Systemic absorption unlikely in recommended doses.
- Avoid repeated use.
- Does not dilate the pupil, paralyze accommodation, or increase intraocular pressure.
- Protective eye patch recommended following procedure.
- Don't use discolored solution. Keep container tightly closed.

76

Artificial tears

artificial tears
eye irrigants

- Instruct patient that product should be used by one person only.

artificial tears
Adsorbotear♦, Bro-Lac, Hypotears, Isopto Alkaline, Isopto Plain, Isopto Tears♦, Lacril♦, Liquifilm Forte, Liquifilm Tears, Lyteers, Methulose, Neotears, Tearisol, Tears Naturale♦, Tears Plus, Ultra Tears, Visculose

eye irrigants
Blinx, Collyrium Eye Lotion♦, Dacriose, EyeStream, I-Lite Eye Drops, Lauro, Lavoptik Medicinal Eye Wash, Murine Eye Drops, Neo-Flow, Sterile Normal Saline (0.9%), Zoptic Eye Lotion

INDICATIONS & DOSAGE
Insufficient tear production—
Adults and children: instill 1 to 2 drops in eye t.i.d., q.i.d., or p.r.n.

INDICATIONS & DOSAGE
Eye irrigation—
Adults and children: flush eye with 1 to 2 drops t.i.d., q.i.d., or p.r.n.

SIDE EFFECTS
Eye: discomfort; burning, pain on instillation; blurred vision; crust formation on eyelids and eyelashes in products with high viscosity, such as Adsorbotear, Isopto Tears, and Tearisol.

SIDE EFFECTS
None reported.

INTERACTIONS
Products containing polyvinyl alcohol: may form gel and gummy deposits on the eye. Keep lids clean.

INTERACTIONS
Borate external irrigation solutions: may form gummy deposits on the lid when used with artificial tear products containing polyvinyl alcohol (Liquifilm Forte, Liquifilm Tears). Keep lids clean.

NURSING CONSIDERATIONS
- Contraindicated in hypersensitivity to active ingredient or preservatives.
- Don't touch tip of container to eye, surrounding tissue, or other surface, to avoid contamination.
- Check date of expiration to make sure solution is potent.
- Store in tightly closed, light-resistant container.
- Should be used by one person only.
- When irrigating, have patient turn his head to side and irrigate from inner to outer canthus. Have tissues handy.

NURSING CONSIDERATIONS
- Contraindicated in hypersensitivity to active product or preservatives.
- Show patient how to instill.
- Warn patient not to touch tip of container to eye, surrounding tissue, or other surface, to avoid contamination of solution.

77

Miscellaneous ophthalmics

alpha-chymotrypsin
fluorescein sodium
glycerin-anhydrous
sodium chloride, hypertonic
timolol maleate

alpha-chymotrypsin
Alpha Chymar, Alpha Chymolean♦♦,
Catarase♦, Zolyse♦, Zonulyn♦♦

INDICATIONS & DOSAGE
Zonulysis in cataract surgery—
Adults over 20 years: 1 to 2 ml instilled into posterior chamber under
the iris, by doctor.

SIDE EFFECTS
Eye: transient increase in intraocular
pressure (dose-related), moderate
uveitis, corneal edema and striation.

INTERACTIONS
Alcohol, surgical detergent: inactivated alpha-chymotrypsin. Rinse off
all alcohol or detergents from surgical
instruments and syringe with saline.

NURSING CONSIDERATIONS
• Contraindicated in high vitreous
pressure with gaping incisional
wound; congenital cataract.
• Solutions very unstable. Use only
freshly reconstituted solution. Don't
use if it is cloudy or has precipitated.
Discard unused portions, including
diluent, except for Zonulyn. Retains
potency 1 week at room temperature,
or for 1 month when refrigerated.

• Remove drug by irrigating with
intraocular balanced salt solution.
• Don't autoclave powder or reconstituted solution; excess heat will inactivate the enzyme.
• Delayed healing of incision has
been reported but not confirmed.

fluorescein sodium
Fluorescite, Fluor-I-Strip, Fluor-I-
Strip-A.T.♦, Ful-Glo Strips♦, Fun-
duscein Injections

INDICATIONS & DOSAGE
*Diagnostic in corneal abrasions and
foreign bodies; fitting hard contact
lenses; lacrimal patency; fundus photography; applanation tonometry—*
Topical: Solution: instill 1 drop of 2%
solution followed by irrigation, or
moisten strip with sterile water.
Touch conjunctiva or fornix with
moistened tip. Flush eye with irrigating solution.
Patient should blink several times
after application.
Indicated in retinal angiography—
Adults: 5 ml of 10% solution
(500 mg) or 3 ml of 25% solution
(750 mg) injected rapidly into antecubital vein, by doctor.
Children: 0.077 ml of 10% solution
(7.7 mg/Kg body weight) or 0.044 ml
of 25% solution (11 mg/Kg body
weight) injected rapidly into antecubital vein, by doctor.

SIDE EFFECTS
Topical use:
Eye: stinging, burning.
Intravenous use:
CNS: headache persisting for 24 to 36 hours.
GI: nausea, vomiting.
GU: bright yellow urine (persists for 24 to 36 hours).
Skin: yellowish skin discoloration (fades in 6 to 12 hours).
Local: extravasation at injection site, thrombophlebitis.
Other: hypersensitivity, including urticaria and *anaphylaxis*.

INTERACTIONS
None significant.

NURSING CONSIDERATIONS
• Use with caution in history of allergy or bronchial asthma.
• Use topical anesthetic before instilling to partially relieve burning and irritation.
• Always use aseptic technique. Easily contaminated by *Pseudomonas*.
• Yellow skin discoloration may persist 6 to 12 hours.
• Warn patient urine will be colored bright yellow after I.V. injection.
• Routine urinalysis will be abnormal within 1 hour of I.V. injection.
• A water-soluble dye.
• Don't freeze; store below 80° F. (26.7° C.).
• Defects will appear green under normal light, or bright yellow under cobalt blue illumination. Foreign bodies are surrounded by a green ring. Similar lesions of the conjunctiva are delineated in orange-yellow.
• Keep an emergency tray with antihistamine, epinephrine, and oxygen always available when giving parenterally.

glycerin-anhydrous
Ophthalgan

INDICATIONS & DOSAGE
Corneal edema prior to ophthalmoscopy or gonioscopy in acute glaucoma and bullous keratitis—
Adults and children: instill 1 to 2 drops glycerin-anhydrous after instilling a local anesthetic.

SIDE EFFECTS
Eye: pain if instilled without topical anesthetic.

INTERACTIONS
None significant.

NURSING CONSIDERATIONS
• Use topical tetracaine HCl or proparacaine HCl before instilling to prevent discomfort.
• Don't touch tip of dropper to eye, surrounding tissues, or tear-film; glycerin will absorb moisture.
• Used to temporarily restore corneal transparency when cornea is too edematous to permit diagnosis.
• Store in tightly closed container.

sodium chloride, hypertonic
Adsorbonac Ophthalmic Solution, Hypersal Ophthalmic Solution, Methylcellulose Ophthalmic Solution, Muro Ointment, Murocoll, Sodium Chloride Ointment 5%

INDICATIONS & DOSAGE
Corneal edema (postop) after cataract extraction or corneal transplantation; also in trauma or bullous keratopathy—
Adults and children: instill 1 to 2 drops q 3 to 4 hours, or apply ointment at bedtime.

SIDE EFFECTS
Eye: slight stinging.
Other: hypersensitivity.

INTERACTIONS
None significant.

NURSING CONSIDERATIONS
- An osmotic agent used to reduce corneal edema when repeated instillation is indicated.
- May use few drops of sterile irrigation solution inside bottle cap to prevent caking on dropper bottle tip.
- Store in tightly closed container.
- Don't touch tip of dropper or tube to eye or surrounding tissue.
- Show patient how to instill.

---

timolol maleate
Timoptic Solution

INDICATIONS & DOSAGE
Chronic open-angle glaucoma, secondary glaucoma, aphakic glaucoma, ocular hypertension—
Adults: initially, instill 1 drop 0.25% solution in each eye b.i.d.; reduce to 1 drop daily for maintenance. If patient doesn't respond, instill 1 drop 0.5% solution in each eye b.i.d. If intraocular pressure is controlled, dosage may be reduced to 1 drop in each eye daily.

SIDE EFFECTS
Eye: minor irritation.
CV: slight reduction in resting heart rate.
Other: apnea in infants, respiratory distress (evidence of beta blockade and systemic absorption).

INTERACTIONS
Propranolol HCl, metoprolol tartrate, other oral beta-adrenergic blocking agents: increased ocular and systemic effect. Use together cautiously.
MAO inhibitors, other adrenergic-augmenting psychotropic drugs: hazardous increased effect. Use together cautiously.

NURSING CONSIDERATIONS
- Use cautiously in bronchial asthma, sinus bradycardia, second- and third-degree heart block, cardiogenic shock, right ventricular failure resulting from pulmonary hypertension, congestive heart failure, severe cardiac disease, infants with congenital glaucoma.
- Warn patient not to touch dropper to eye or surrounding tissue.
- Beta-adrenergic blocking agent in ophthalmic solution.
- Can be safely used in glaucoma patients wearing conventional (PMMA) hard contact lenses.
- Show patient how to instill.

78

Otics

acetic acid
benzocaine
boric acid
carbamide peroxide
chloramphenicol
colistin B sulfate
dexamethasone sodium phosphate
hydrocortisone
hydrocortisone acetate
methylprednisolone disodium
 phosphate
neomycin sulfate
oxytetracycline hydrochloride
polymyxin B sulfate
triethanolamine polypeptide oleate-
 condensate

---

acetic acid
Domeboro Otic♦, VoSol Otic♦

INDICATIONS & DOSAGE
External ear canal infection—
Adults and children: 4 to 6 drops
into ear canal t.i.d. or q.i.d., or insert
saturated wick for first 24 hours, then
continue with instillations.
Prophylaxis of swimmers' ear—
Adults and children: 2 drops in each
ear b.i.d.

SIDE EFFECTS
Ear: irritation or itching.
Skin: urticaria.
Other: overgrowth of nonsusceptible
organisms.

INTERACTIONS
None significant.

NURSING CONSIDERATIONS
• Use cautiously in perforated ear-
drum.
• Has anti-infective, anti-inflamma-
tory, and antipruritic effects.
• *Pseudomonas aeruginosa* particu-
larly sensitive to drug.
• Reculture persistent drainage.

---

benzocaine
Americaine-Otic, Auralgan♦,
Aurasol, Eardro, Myringacaine,
Tympagesic

INDICATIONS & DOSAGE
Cerumen removal—
Adults and children: fill ear canal
t.i.d. for 2 days.
Pain from otitis media—
Adults and children: fill ear canal
with solution and plug with cotton.
May repeat q 1 to 2 hours, p.r.n.

SIDE EFFECTS
Ear: irritation or itching.
Skin: urticaria.
Other: edema.

INTERACTIONS
None significant.

NURSING CONSIDERATIONS
• Contraindicated in perforated
eardrum.
• Local anesthetic effect only.
• Use with antibiotic to treat underlying cause of pain, because use alone
may mask more serious condition.

• Tell patient to call doctor if pain lasts longer than 48 hours.
• Avoid touching ear with dropper. Do not rinse dropper.
• Irrigate ear gently to remove impacted cerumen.
• Keep container tightly closed and away from moisture.

boric acid
Ear-Dry, Swim-Ear, Swim 'n Clear

INDICATIONS & DOSAGE
External ear canal infection—
Adults and children: fill ear canal with solution and plug with cotton. Repeat t.i.d. or q.i.d.

SIDE EFFECTS
Ear: irritation or itching.
Skin: urticaria.
Other: overgrowth of nonsusceptible organisms.

INTERACTIONS
None significant.

NURSING CONSIDERATIONS
• Contraindicated in perforated eardrum or excoriated membranes in ear.
• Watch for signs of superinfection (continual pain, inflammation, fever).
• Weak bacteriostatic germicide; also fungistatic agent.
• If cotton plug used, always moisten with medication.

carbamide peroxide
Benadyne Ear, Debrox♦

INDICATIONS & DOSAGE
Impacted earwax—
Adults and children: 5 to 10 drops into ear canal b.i.d. for 3 to 4 days.

SIDE EFFECTS
None reported.

INTERACTIONS
None significant.

NURSING CONSIDERATIONS
• Contraindicated in perforated eardrum.
• Tell patient to call doctor if redness, pain, or swelling persists.
• Cerumenolytic agent.
• Irrigation of ear may be necessary to aid in removal of cerumen.
• Tip of bottle should not touch ear or ear canal.

chloramphenicol
Chloromycetin Otic♦,
Sopamycetin♦♦

INDICATIONS & DOSAGE
External ear canal infection—
Adults and children: 2 to 3 drops into ear canal t.i.d. or q.i.d.

SIDE EFFECTS
Ear: itching or burning.
Local: pruritus, burning, urticaria, vesicular or maculopapular dermatitis.
Systemic: sore throat, angioedema.
Other: overgrowth of nonsusceptible organisms.

INTERACTIONS
None significant.

NURSING CONSIDERATIONS
• Avoid prolonged use.
• Obtain history of past use and reaction to drug.
• Watch for signs of superinfection (continued pain, inflammation, fever).
• Reculture persistent drainage.
• Watch for signs of sore throat (early sign of toxicity).
• Bacteriostatic agent.

Unmarked trade names available in the United States only.
♦ Also available in Canada   ♦♦ Available in Canada only.

colistin B sulfate
available only in combination with
neomycin and hydrocortisone (Coly-
Mycin-S-Otic◆)

INDICATIONS & DOSAGE
*External ear canal infection and otitis
media—*
Adults and children: 3 to 5 drops
into ear canal t.i.d. or q.i.d.

SIDE EFFECTS
Ear: ototoxicity in patient with a
perforated eardrum and in patient undergoing tympanoplasty; irritation,
itching.
Other: overgrowth of nonsusceptible
organisms.

INTERACTIONS
None significant.

NURSING CONSIDERATIONS
• Watch for signs of superinfection
(continued pain, inflammation,
fever).
• Reculture persistent drainage.
• Observe for signs of hearing loss.
• Bactericidal agent.
• Avoid prolonged use.
• Shake well before using.

dexamethasone sodium phosphate
Decadron◆

INDICATIONS & DOSAGE
Inflammation of external ear canal—
Adults and children: 1 to 2 drops
into ear canal t.i.d. or q.i.d.

SIDE EFFECTS
Systemic: adrenal suppression with
long-term use.
Other: masking or exacerbation of
underlying infection.

INTERACTIONS
None significant.

NURSING CONSIDERATIONS
• Contraindicated in perforated ear-
drum, fungal infections, herpes or
other viral infections.
• Use with antibiotic to treat inflam-
mation caused by infection.
• Use alone in allergic otitis externa.
• Anti-inflammatory agent.

hydrocortisone

hydrocortisone acetate
Cortamed◆◆, Otall

INDICATIONS & DOSAGE
Inflammation of external ear canal—
Adults and children: 3 to 5 drops
into ear canal t.i.d. or q.i.d.
Available in 0.25%, 0.5%, and
1% concentrations.

SIDE EFFECTS
Systemic: adrenal suppression with
long-term use.
Other: may mask or exacerbate underlying infection.

INTERACTIONS
None reported.

NURSING CONSIDERATIONS
• Contraindicated in perforated ear-
drum, fungal infections, herpes or
other viral infections.
• Use with antibiotic to treat inflam-
mation caused by infection.
• Use alone in allergic otitis externa.
• Anti-inflammatory agent.

Italicized side effects are common or life-threatening.

methylprednisolone disodium phosphate
Medrol♦♦

INDICATIONS & DOSAGE
Inflammation of external ear canal—
Adults and children: 2 to 3 drops into ear canal t.i.d. or q.i.d.

SIDE EFFECTS
Systemic: adrenal suppression with long-term use.
Other: may mask or exacerbate underlying infection.

INTERACTIONS
None significant.

NURSING CONSIDERATIONS
• Contraindicated in perforated eardrum, fungal, herpes or other viral infections.
• Use with antibiotic to treat inflammation caused by infection.
• Use alone to treat seborrheic, contact, or noninfected eczematoid dermatitis.
• Anti-inflammatory agent.

neomycin sulfate
Otobiotic

INDICATIONS & DOSAGE
External ear canal infection—
Adults and children: 2 to 5 drops into ear canal t.i.d. or q.i.d.

SIDE EFFECTS
Ear: ototoxicity (in patients undergoing tympanoplasty).
Local: burning, erythema, vesicular dermatitis, urticaria.
Other: overgrowth of nonsusceptible organisms.

INTERACTIONS
None significant.

NURSING CONSIDERATIONS
• Contraindicated in perforated eardrum.
• Obtain history of past use and reaction to neomycin.
• Observe for signs of hearing loss.
• Watch for signs of superinfection (continued pain, inflammation, fever).
• Reculture persistent drainage.
• Bactericidal agent.
• Best used in combination with other antibiotics.

oxytetracycline hydrochloride
available only in combination with polymyxin B sulfate (Terramycin) or polymyxin B sulfate and hydrocortisone (Terra-Cortril♦♦)

INDICATIONS & DOSAGE
External ear canal infection—
Adults and children: instill ½ inch of ointment into external ear canal t.i.d. or q.i.d.

SIDE EFFECTS
Ear: irritation, itching, urticaria.
Other: overgrowth of nonsusceptible organisms.

INTERACTIONS
None significant.

NURSING CONSIDERATIONS
• Obtain history of past reaction to tetracyclines.
• Watch for signs of superinfection (continued pain, inflammation, fever).
• Reculture persistent drainage.
• Bacteriostatic agent.

Unmarked trade names available in the United States only.
♦ Also available in Canada   ♦♦ Available in Canada only.

polymyxin B sulfate
Aerosporin♦

INDICATIONS & DOSAGE
Acute and chronic otitis externa, otitis media if tympanic membrane perforated; otomycosis—
Adults and children: 3 to 4 drops t.i.d. or q.i.d.

SIDE EFFECTS
Ear: irritation, itching, urticaria.
Other: overgrowth of nonsusceptible organisms.

INTERACTIONS
None significant.

NURSING CONSIDERATIONS
• Watch for signs of superinfection (continued pain, inflammation, fever).
• Reculture persistent drainage.
• Bactericidal agent.
• Best used in combination with other antibiotics.
• Keep container tightly closed and away from moisture.

triethanolamine polypeptide oleate-condensate
Cerumenex♦

INDICATIONS & DOSAGE
Impacted earwax—
Adults and children: fill ear canal with solution and insert cotton plug. After 15 to 30 minutes, flush ear with warm water.

SIDE EFFECTS
Ear: erythema, pruritus.
Skin: severe eczema.

INTERACTIONS
None significant.

NURSING CONSIDERATIONS
• Contraindicated in perforated eardrum, otitis media, and allergies. Do patch test by placing 1 drop of drug on inner forearm; cover with small bandage. Read in 24 hours. If any reaction (redness, swelling) occurs, don't use drug.
• Tell patient not to use drops more often than prescribed. Flush ear gently with warm water, using soft rubber bulb ear syringe, within 30 minutes after instillation.
• Cerumenolytic agent.
• Moisten cotton plug with medication before insertion.
• Keep container tightly closed and away from moisture.

Italicized side effects are common or life-threatening.

79

Oral and nasal agents

benzocaine
carbamide peroxide
cocaine hydrochloride
dexamethasone sodium phosphate
ephedrine sulfate
epinephrine hydrochloride
lidocaine hydrochloride
naphazoline hydrochloride
oxymetazoline hydrochloride
phenylephrine hydrochloride
piperocaine hydrochloride
tetrahydrozoline hydrochloride
triamcinolone acetonide
xylometazoline hydrochloride

---

benzocaine
Colrex, Dentition Syrup♦♦, Orabase
with Benzocaine, Oracin, Ora-Jel,
Spec-T Anesthetic, Trocaine,
Tyzomint

INDICATIONS & DOSAGE
*Pain from toothache, cold sore,
canker sore, minor sore throat—*
Adults and children: apply syrup or
jelly to affected area, or suck on
lozenges.

SIDE EFFECTS
Skin: hypersensitivity.
Other: possible tolerance.

INTERACTIONS
None significant.

NURSING CONSIDERATIONS
• Contraindicated in infants under
1 year. Use cautiously in children under 6 years and in severe oral trauma
or sepsis.
• Not intended for use in the presence
of infection.
• Obtain history of past reactions to
local anesthetics.
• Watch for allergic reactions, such
as reddening or swelling. If condition
persists, drug should be stopped and
doctor notified.
• Show patient how to apply.

---

carbamide peroxide
Cank-aid, Clear Drops, Gly-Oxide♦,
Proxigel

INDICATIONS & DOSAGE
*Canker sores, herpetic and other le-
sions, gingivitis, denture irritation,
traumatic or surgical wounds—*
Adults, and children over 3 years:
apply, undiluted, to oral mucosa
q.i.d. or p.r.n., leave for several minutes, then expectorate. Don't rinse out
mouth.

SIDE EFFECTS
None reported.

INTERACTIONS
None significant.

NURSING CONSIDERATIONS
• Use only as adjunct to regular
professional care.
• Don't dilute. Gently massage affected area with medication. Show
patient how to apply. Tell him not to

drink or rinse his mouth for 5 minutes after use.
- Warn patient that drug foams in mouth when mixed with saliva.
- Use after meals and at bedtime for best results.
- If severe or persistent inflammation continues, patient should notify doctor or dentist.
- Provides chemomechanical cleansing, debriding action, and has nonselective microbial activity.
- An oxygenating agent.
- Store in cool place.
- Only one person should use same dropper bottle or tube.

cocaine hydrochloride
Controlled Substance Schedule II

INDICATIONS & DOSAGE
Adults and children:
Acute rhinosinusitis—use 1% solution with nasal pack.
Diagnostic nasal examination— apply 4% solution to nasal mucosa.
Local anesthesia of nose or throat— apply 5% to 10% solution to oral and nasal mucosa.

SIDE EFFECTS
CNS: nervousness, excitation, vasomotor collapse.

INTERACTIONS
None significant.

NURSING CONSIDERATIONS
- Store under lock and key with other controlled drugs.
- Patient should be given a short-acting barbiturate before giving cocaine HCl to prevent excess CNS stimulation or vasomotor collapse.
- Nasal surgery performed with cocaine HCl anesthesia may cause a delayed capillary hemorrhage resulting from capillary dilation. Watch for

postoperative nasal bleeding when effect of cocaine wears off.
- Obtain history of past reactions to local anesthetics.

dexamethasone sodium phosphate
Decadron Phosphate♦, Decadron Phosphate Respihaler, Turbinaire

INDICATIONS & DOSAGE
Allergic or inflammatory conditions, nasal polyps—
Adults: 2 sprays in each nostril b.i.d. or t.i.d. Maximum 12 sprays daily.
Children 6 to 12 years: 1 or 2 sprays in each nostril b.i.d. Maximum 8 sprays daily.
Each spray delivers 0.1 mg dexamethasone sodium phosphate equal to 0.084 mg dexamethasone.

SIDE EFFECTS
EENT: nasal irritation, dryness, rebound nasal congestion.
Other: hypersensitivity, systemic side effects with prolonged use (pituitary-adrenal suppression, sodium retention, congestive heart failure, hypertension, hypokalemia, headaches, convulsions, peptic ulcer, ecchymoses, petechiae, masking of secondary infection).

INTERACTIONS
None significant.

NURSING CONSIDERATIONS
- Contraindicated in cutaneous tuberculosis, fungal and herpetic lesions. Use cautiously in diabetes mellitus, peptic ulcer, tuberculosis, as systemic absorption can activate disease.
- Mothers should not breast-feed, as systemic absorption can occur.
- Control underlying bacterial infection with anti-infectives.

Italicized side effects are common or life-threatening.

- Irritation or sensitivity may require stopping drug.
- Don't break, incinerate, or store in extreme heat; contents under pressure.
- Gradually reduce dose as nasal condition improves.
- Fluid retention can occur as a result of systemic absorption.
- Show patient how to apply. Only one person should use same nasal spray.
- Hypertension and hypokalemia can occur with systemic absorption. Monitor blood pressure, serum potassium frequently.
- Should not be used for prolonged periods.

ephedrine sulfate
Ephedsol-1%, I-Sedrin Plain, Isofedrol, Nasdro

INDICATIONS & DOSAGE
Nasal congestion—
Adults and children: apply 3 to 4 drops 0.5% to 3% solution to nasal mucosa. Use no more frequently than q 4 hours.

SIDE EFFECTS
CNS: nervousness, excitation.
CV: *tachycardia.*
EENT: rebound nasal congestion with long-term or excessive use.
Local: mucosal irritation.

INTERACTIONS
MAO inhibitors: hypertensive crisis if ephedrine is absorbed. Don't use together.

NURSING CONSIDERATIONS
- Use cautiously in hyperthyroidism, coronary artery disease, hypertension, or diabetes mellitus, as systemic absorption can occur.
- Tell patient not to exceed recommended dose. Use only when needed.

- Show patient how to apply. Only one person should use same dropper bottle or nasal spray.

epinephrine hydrochloride
Adrenalin Chloride

INDICATIONS & DOSAGE
Nasal congestion, local superficial bleeding—
Adults and children: apply 0.1% solution to oral or nasal mucosa.

SIDE EFFECTS
CNS: nervousness, excitation.
CV: *tachycardia.*
EENT: rebound nasal congestion, slight sting upon application.

INTERACTIONS
None significant.

NURSING CONSIDERATIONS
- Use cautiously in hyperthyroidism, coronary artery disease, hypertension, or diabetes mellitus, as systemic absorption can occur.
- Tell patient not to exceed recommended dose. Use only when needed.
- Show patient how to apply. Only one person should use same dropper bottle or nasal spray.

lidocaine hydrochloride
Xylocaine♦, Xylocaine Viscous♦

INDICATIONS & DOSAGE
Local anesthesia, pain from dental extractions—
Adults and children: apply 2% to 5% solution, ointment, or 15 ml of Xylocaine Viscous q 3 to 4 hours to oral or nasal mucosa.

SIDE EFFECTS
EENT: interference with pharyngeal stage of swallowing.

Other: hypersensitivity (CNS symptoms are excitatory or depressant; CV symptoms are depressant); systemic absorption when used repeatedly.

INTERACTIONS
None significant.

NURSING CONSIDERATIONS
• Use cautiously in cardiac disease, hyperthyroidism, or severe oral or nasal trauma or sepsis, as systemic absorption can occur.
• Chronic, prolonged use for oropharynx anesthesia can lead to systemic absorption and toxicity.
• Instruct patient how to use. Xylocaine Viscous should be swished around in mouth and can be swallowed. Warn patient to eat or drink cautiously within 60 minutes after oral application, to avoid food aspiration.
• Obtain history of past reactions to local anesthetics.
• Taste can be improved by adding a drop of oil of peppermint.

---

naphazoline hydrochloride
Privine♦

INDICATIONS & DOSAGE
Nasal congestion—
Adults: apply 2 drops or sprays of 0.05% to 0.1% solution to nasal mucosa q 3 to 4 hours.
Children 6 to 12 years: 1 to 2 drops or sprays of 0.05% solution. Repeat q 3 to 6 hours, p.r.n. Use no longer than 3 to 5 days.

SIDE EFFECTS
EENT: rebound nasal congestion with excessive or long-term use, sneezing, stinging, dryness of mucosa.
Other: systemic side effects in children after excessive or long-term use; marked sedation.

INTERACTIONS
None significant.

NURSING CONSIDERATIONS
• Contraindicated in glaucoma. Use cautiously in hyperthyroidism, heart disease, hypertension, or diabetes mellitus, as systemic absorption can occur.
• Warn patient not to exceed recommended dosage.
• Tell patient to notify doctor if nasal congestion persists after 5 days.
• Show patient how to apply. Hold container upright. Only one person should use same dropper bottle or nasal spray.
• Do not shake container.

---

oxymetazoline hydrochloride
Afrin, Duration, Nafrine♦ ♦, St. Joseph's Decongestant for Children

INDICATIONS & DOSAGE
Nasal congestion—
Adults, and children over 6 years: apply 2 to 4 drops or sprays 0.05% solution to nasal mucosa b.i.d.
Children 2 to 5 years: apply 2 to 3 drops 0.025% solution to nasal mucosa b.i.d. Use no longer than 3 to 5 days. Dosage for younger children has not been established.

SIDE EFFECTS
CNS: headache, drowsiness, dizziness, insomnia.
CV: palpitations.
EENT: rebound nasal congestion or irritation with excessive or long-term use, dryness of nose and throat, increased nasal discharge, stinging, sneezing.
Other: systemic side effects in children with excessive or long-term use; possible sedation.

INTERACTIONS
None significant.

Italicized side effects are common or life-threatening.

NURSING CONSIDERATIONS
• Use cautiously in hyperthyroidism, heart disease, hypertension, or diabetes mellitus, as systemic absorption can occur.
• Tell patient not to exceed recommended dose. Use only when needed.
• Show patient how to apply. Have patient bend head forward and sniff spray briskly. Only one person should use same dropper bottle or nasal spray.

phenylephrine hydrochloride
Alconefrin, Coricidin Nasal Mist, Coryzine, Ephrine, Isophrin, Neo-Synephrine♦, Pyracort-D, Rhinall, Sinarest Nasal Spray, Sinophen Intranasal, SuperAnahist Nasal Spray, Synasal, Vacon

INDICATIONS & DOSAGE
Nasal congestion—
Adults: 2 to 3 drops or sprays 0.25% to 1% solution; apply jelly or spray to nasal mucosa.
Children 6 to 12 years: apply 2 to 3 drops or sprays of 0.25% solution.
Children under 6 years: apply 2 to 3 drops or sprays 0.125% solution.
Drops, spray, or jelly can be given q 4 hours, p.r.n.

SIDE EFFECTS
CNS: headache, tremors, dizziness, nervousness.
CV: *palpitations, tachycardia,* premature ventricular contractions, hypertension, pallor.
EENT: transient burning, stinging; dryness of nasal mucosa; rebound nasal congestion may occur with continued use.
GI: nausea.

INTERACTIONS
None significant.

NURSING CONSIDERATIONS
• Contraindicated in narrow-angle glaucoma. Use cautiously in hyperthyroidism, hypertension, diabetes mellitus, or ischemic heart disease, as systemic absorption may occur.
• Tell patient not to exceed recommended dose. Use only when needed.
• Show patient how to apply: keep head erect to minimize swallowing of medication. Only one person should use same dropper bottle or nasal spray.

piperocaine hydrochloride
Metycaine HCl

INDICATIONS & DOSAGE
Anesthetic in dental procedures—
Adults and children: apply 5% to 10% solution as a spray or 1% to 2% solution by infiltration to oral or nasal mucosa.
Local anesthetic in rhinolaryngology exams—
Adults and children: apply 2% solution as a spray to oral or nasal mucosa.

SIDE EFFECTS
EENT: interference with pharyngeal stage of swallowing.
Other: hypersensitivity.

INTERACTIONS
None significant.

NURSING CONSIDERATIONS
• Use cautiously in cardiac disease, hyperthyroidism, severe trauma, or sepsis of oral or nasal mucosa, as systemic absorption can occur.
• Obtain history of past reaction to topical anesthetics.
• Warn patient not to eat or drink for 60 minutes after oral application, to prevent possible food aspiration.

tetrahydrozoline hydrochloride
Tyzine HCl, Tyzine Pediatric

INDICATIONS & DOSAGE
Nasal congestion—
Adults, and children over 6 years:
apply 2 to 4 drops 0.1% solution or
spray to nasal mucosa q 4 to 6 hours,
p.r.n.
Children 2 to 6 years: apply 2 to
3 drops 0.05% solution to nasal
mucosa q 4 to 6 hours, p.r.n.

SIDE EFFECTS
EENT: transient burning, stinging;
sneezing, rebound nasal congestion in
excessive or long-term use.

INTERACTIONS
None significant.

NURSING CONSIDERATIONS
• Contraindicated in glaucoma. Use
cautiously in hyperthyroidism, hypertension, diabetes mellitus.
• Don't use 0.1% solution in children
under 6 years.
• Tell patient not to exceed recommended dose. Use only as needed.
• Show patient how to apply.

triamcinolone acetonide
Kenalog in Orabase

INDICATIONS & DOSAGE
*Stomatitis; erosive lichen planus;
traumatic oral lesions, including sore
denture spots—*
Adults and children: press ¼ inch of
0.1% emollient dental paste onto affected area until thin film develops.
Repeat b.i.d. or t.i.d. Don't rub in or
protection of film will be lost.

SIDE EFFECTS
Systemic: with prolonged use, adrenal insufficiency, altered glucose metabolism, peptic ulcer activation.

INTERACTIONS
None significant.

NURSING CONSIDERATIONS
• Contraindicated in oral herpetic or
viral lesions. Use cautiously in diabetes mellitus, peptic ulcer, or tuberculosis, as systemic absorption can
occur.
• Apply after meals and at bedtime
for best results.

xylometazoline hydrochloride
4-Way Long Acting, Neo-Synephrine
II, Otrivin♦, Sine-Off Nasal Spray,
Sinex-L.A.

INDICATIONS & DOSAGE
Nasal congestion—
Adults, and children over 12 years:
apply 2 to 3 drops or 2 sprays of
0.1% solution to nasal mucosa q 8 to
10 hours.
Children under 12 years: apply 2 to
3 drops or 1 spray of 0.05% solution
to nasal mucosa q 8 to 10 hours.

SIDE EFFECTS
EENT: rebound nasal congestion or
irritation with excessive or long-term
use; transient burning, stinging; dryness or ulceration of nasal mucosa;
sneezing.

INTERACTIONS
None significant.

Italicized side effects are common or life-threatening.

NURSING CONSIDERATIONS
• Contraindicated in narrow-angle glaucoma. Use cautiously in hyperthyroidism, heart disease, hypertension, diabetes mellitus, and advanced arteriosclerosis, as systemic absorption can occur.

• Tell patient not to exceed recommended dose.
• Show patient how to apply. Only one person should use same dropper bottle or nasal spray.

80

Local anti-infectives

amphotericin B
bacitracin
carbol-fuchsin solution
chloramphenicol
chlortetracycline hydrochloride
clotrimazole
erythromycin
gentamicin sulfate
gentian violet (methylrosaniline
  chloride)
haloprogin
iodochlorhydroxyquin
mafenide acetate
miconazole nitrate 2%
neomycin sulfate
nitrofurazone
nystatin
silver sulfadiazine
tetracycline hydrochloride
tolnaftate
undecylenic acid (zinc
  undecylenate)

SIDE EFFECTS
Skin: possible drying, contact sensitivity, erythema, burning, pruritus.

INTERACTIONS
None significant.

NURSING CONSIDERATIONS
• Cream or lotion preferred for folds of groin, armpit, neck creases, etc.
• Cream discolors skin slightly when rubbed in; lotion or ointment doesn't. Lotion may stain nail lesions.
• Watch for and report signs of local irritation.
• Avoid occlusive dressings and ointments.
• Store at room temperature; avoid freezing.
• Well tolerated, even by infants, for long periods.
• A fungistatic agent.

---

amphotericin B
Fungizone Cream, Lotion, Ointment
(3% amphotericin B)

INDICATIONS & DOSAGE
Cutaneous or mucocutaneous candidal infections—
Adults and children: apply liberally b.i.d., t.i.d., or q.i.d. for 1 to 3 weeks; up to several months for interdigital lesions, paronychias, and onychomycosis (where relapses are frequent).

---

bacitracin
Baciguent♦, Bacitin♦♦

INDICATIONS & DOSAGE
Topical infections, impetigo, abrasions, cuts, minor wounds, seborrheic dermatitis, acne, contact dermatitis, psoriasis—
Adults and children: apply thin film b.i.d. or t.i.d. or more often, depending on severity of condition.

SIDE EFFECTS
Skin: rashes and other allergic reactions; itching, burning, swelling of lips or face.

Other: *possible systemic side effects when used over large areas for prolonged periods: potentially nephrotoxic and ototoxic;* tightness in chest, hypotension.

INTERACTIONS
None significant.

NURSING CONSIDERATIONS
• Contraindicated in hypersensitivity to any of the components and for application in the external ear canal if the eardrum is perforated.
• If used on burns that cover more than 20% of body surface, and especially if patient suffers impaired renal function, apply only once daily.
• If no improvement or if condition worsens, stop using and tell doctor.
• Prolonged use may result in overgrowth of nonsusceptible organisms.
• Avoid excess application.
• A bacteriostatic agent.

carbol-fuchsin solution
Carfusin, Castaderm, Castellani's Paint

INDICATIONS & DOSAGE
Tinea, dermatophytosis, skin infections—
Adults and children: apply liberally 1 or 2 times daily.

SIDE EFFECTS
Blood: Possibility of bone marrow hypoplasia with use over long periods or at frequent intervals.
Skin: *contact dermatitis.*

INTERACTIONS
None significant.

NURSING CONSIDERATIONS
• Do not use on large areas or on eroded skin.
• Do not continue use after 1 week if

no improvement shown. Toxicities develop in long-term use.
• Poisonous; warn against swallowing.
• Clean and dry skin thoroughly before applying.
• A fungicidal and bactericidal agent.

chloramphenicol
Chloromycetin♦
(1% chloramphenicol)

INDICATIONS & DOSAGE
Superficial skin infections caused by susceptible bacteria—
Adults and children: after thorough cleansing, apply t.i.d. or q.i.d.

SIDE EFFECTS
Skin: possible contact sensitivity; itching, burning, urticaria, angioneurotic edema in patients hypersensitive to any of the components.

INTERACTIONS
None significant.

NURSING CONSIDERATIONS
• Contraindicated in hypersensitivity to any of the components.
• If no improvement or if condition worsens, stop using and report to doctor.
• Prolonged use may result in overgrowth of nonsusceptible organisms.
• For all but very superficial infections, topical use of this drug should be supplemented by appropriate systemic medication.
• A bacteriostatic agent.

chlortetracycline hydrochloride
Aureomycin 3%♦

INDICATIONS & DOSAGE
Superficial infections of the skin caused by susceptible bacteria—
Adults and children: rub into affected area b.i.d. or t.i.d.

SIDE EFFECTS
Skin: *rashes, dermatitis.*

INTERACTIONS
None significant.

NURSING CONSIDERATIONS
• Contraindicated in hypersensitivity to any of the components.
• Prolonged use may result in overgrowth of nonsusceptible organisms.
• If no improvement or if condition worsens, stop using and report to doctor.
• A bacteriostatic agent.

clotrimazole
Canesten♦♦, Gyne-Lotrimin, Lotrimin (1% clotrimazole)

INDICATIONS & DOSAGE
Superficial fungal infections (tinea pedis, tinea cruris, tinea versicolor, candidiasis, and tinea corporis)—
Adults and children: apply thinly and massage into affected and surrounding area, morning and evening, 1 to 8 weeks.
Candidal vulvovaginitis—
Adults: insert 1 applicatorful or 1 tablet intravaginally daily for 7 to 14 days at bedtime. Alternatively, insert 2 tablets once daily for 3 consecutive days.

SIDE EFFECTS
GU: *with vaginal use: mild vaginal burning, irritation.*

Skin: blistering, *erythema,* edema, pruritus, burning, stinging, peeling, urticaria, skin fissures, general irritation.

INTERACTIONS
None significant.

NURSING CONSIDERATIONS
• Contraindicated in hypersensitivity to any of the components.
• Not for ophthalmic use.
• Watch for and report irritation or sensitivity.
• Improvement usually within a week; if none in 4 weeks, diagnosis should be reviewed.
• Shortened dosage schedule with tablets may be used when compliance is a problem.
• A fungicidal agent.

erythromycin
Erythrocin♦♦, Ilotycin♦

INDICATIONS & DOSAGE
Superficial skin infections caused by susceptible organisms—
Adults and children: clean affected area; apply t.i.d. or q.i.d.

SIDE EFFECTS
Skin: sensitivity reactions.

INTERACTIONS
None significant.

NURSING CONSIDERATIONS
• Prolonged use may result in overgrowth of nonsusceptible organisms.
• If no improvement or if condition worsens, stop using and tell doctor.
• Usually a bacteriostatic agent, but in high concentrations or against highly susceptible organisms, may be bactericidal.

Italicized side effects are common or life-threatening.

gentamicin sulfate
Garamycin♦

INDICATIONS & DOSAGE
Primary and secondary bacterial infections, superficial burns, skin ulcers, infected insect bites and stings, infected lacerations and abrasions, wounds from minor surgery—
Adults, and children over 1 year: rub in small amount gently t.i.d. or q.i.d., with or without gauze dressing.

SIDE EFFECTS
Skin: small percentage of minor skin irritation; possible photosensitivity.

INTERACTIONS
None significant.

NURSING CONSIDERATIONS
• Contraindicated in hypersensitivity to any of the components.
• If no improvement or if condition worsens, stop using and report to doctor.
• Avoid use on large skin lesions or over a wide area because of possible systemic toxic effects.
• Prolonged use may result in overgrowth of nonsusceptible organisms.
• May clear bacterial infections that have not responded to other antibacterial agents.
• Useful for treating patients who are sensitive to neomycin.
• Useful for infected skin cysts, preceded by incision and draining.
• Store in cool place.
• A bactericidal agent.
• Remove crusts before application of gentamicin in impetigo contagiosa.

gentian violet (methylrosaniline chloride)
Bismuth Violet solution (1% and 2%), Crystal Violet

INDICATIONS & DOSAGE
Superficial infections of skin; lesions, except ulcerative lesions of face, particularly Candida albicans—
Adults and children: apply with swab b.i.d. or t.i.d. Keep affected area clean, dry, and exposed to air to prevent spread of infection.

SIDE EFFECTS
Skin: *permanent discoloration if applied to granulation tissue;* ulceration of mucous membranes.

INTERACTIONS
None significant.

NURSING CONSIDERATIONS
• Contraindicated in hypersensitivity to any of the components.
• Do not use on ulcerative lesions of the face.
• Apply carefully to avoid undue staining.
• Fungistatic.

haloprogin
Halotex♦

INDICATIONS & DOSAGE
Superficial fungal infections (tinea pedis, tinea cruris, tinea corporis, tinea manuum, and tinea versicolor)—
Adults and children: apply liberally b.i.d. for 2 to 3 weeks.

SIDE EFFECTS
Skin: burning sensation, irritation, vesicle formation, increased maceration, *pruritus or exacerbation of preexisting lesions.*

INTERACTIONS
None significant.

NURSING CONSIDERATIONS
• Contraindicated in hypersensitivity to any of the components.
• Diagnosis should be reconsidered if no improvement in 4 weeks.
• Fungistatic and fungicidal.

---

iodochlorhydroxyquin
Gentleline, Quinoform, Torofor, Vioform

INDICATIONS & DOSAGE
Inflamed skin conditions, including eczema, athlete's foot, other fungal infections; cutaneous or mucocutaneous mycotic infections caused by Candida species (Monilia)—
Adults and children: apply a thin layer b.i.d., t.i.d., q.i.d., or as directed. Continue for 1 week after clinical cure.

SIDE EFFECTS
Skin: *possible burning, itching, acneiform eruptions.*
Systemic: electrolyte imbalance, adrenal suppression.

INTERACTIONS
Systemic corticosteroids: possible increased absorption. Use together cautiously.

NURSING CONSIDERATIONS
• Contraindicated in tuberculosis, vaccinia, and varicella.
• Note all side effects and precautions of each component in the combination antifungals.
• Presence in urine may cause false positive test for phenylketonuria (PKU) or inaccurate thyroid function tests. Discontinue at least 1 month before thyroid function tests.
• Drug will stain fabric and hair.

---

mafenide acetate
Sulfamylon♦

INDICATIONS & DOSAGE
Adjunctive treatment of second- and third-degree burns—
Adults and children: apply $1/_{16}$ inch daily or b.i.d. to cleansed, debrided wounds.

SIDE EFFECTS
Blood: eosinophilia.
Skin: pain, *burning sensation,* rash, itching, swelling, hives, blisters, erythema.
Other: facial edema.

INTERACTIONS
None significant.

NURSING CONSIDERATIONS
• Use with caution in acute renal failure.
• Closely monitor acid-base balance, especially in the presence of pulmonary and renal dysfunction.
• If acidosis occurs, discontinue use for 24 to 48 hours.
• Check for pain and burning; if they occur, notify doctor. If other allergic reactions occur, treatment may have to be temporarily discontinued.
• Cleanse area before applying.
• Accidental ingestion may cause diarrhea.
• Keep burn areas medicated at all times.
• Bathe patient daily, if possible.

---

miconazole nitrate 2%
Micatin

INDICATIONS & DOSAGE
Tinea pedis, tinea cruris, tinea corporis, cutaneous candidiasis (moniliasis), infections from common dermatophytes—

Adults and children: apply sparingly b.i.d. for 2 to 4 weeks.

SIDE EFFECTS
Skin: isolated reports of irritation, burning, maceration.

INTERACTIONS
None significant.

NURSING CONSIDERATIONS
• For external use only. Keep out of eyes.
• Discontinue if sensitivity or chemical irritation occurs.
• Fungistatic.

---

neomycin sulfate
Herisan Antibiotic◆◆,
Mycifradin◆◆, Myciguent◆,
Neocin◆◆

INDICATIONS & DOSAGE
Topical bacterial infections, burns, wounds, skin grafts, following surgical procedure, lesions, pruritus, trophic ulcerations, edema—
Adults and children: rub in small quantity gently b.i.d., t.i.d., or as directed.

SIDE EFFECTS
Skin: *rashes.*
Other: *possible nephrotoxicity, ototoxicity, and neuromuscular blockade; possible systemic absorption when used on extensive areas of the body.*

INTERACTIONS
None significant.

NURSING CONSIDERATIONS
• Contraindicated in hypersensitivity to any of the components, atopy, vaccinia, varicella, fungal or viral lesions.
• If no improvement or if condition

worsens, stop using and report to doctor.
• If used on more than 20% of the body surface and on patient with impaired renal function, apply only once daily.
• Prolonged use may result in overgrowth of nonsusceptible organisms.
• In those combination products that contain corticosteroids, use of occlusive dressings increases the corticosteroid absorption and the likelihood of systemic effect.
• Particularly absorbed on denuded or abraded areas.
• A bactericidal agent.

---

nitrofurazone
Furacin◆, Furazyme

INDICATIONS & DOSAGE
Adjunctive treatment of second- and third-degree burns (especially when resistance to other antibiotics and sulfonamides occurs); skin grafting—
Adults and children: apply directly to lesion daily or every few days, depending on severity of burn.

SIDE EFFECTS
Skin: *erythema, pruritus,* burning, edema, severe reactions (vesiculation, denudation, ulceration).

INTERACTIONS
None significant.

NURSING CONSIDERATIONS
• Contraindicated in previous hypersensitivity to drug.
• If irritation, sensitization, or infection occurs, discontinue use.
• When using wet dressing, protect skin around wound with zinc oxide.
• Cleanse wound as indicated by doctor at each dressing change.
• Remove adherent dressings by flushing with solution of nitrofura-

---

zone and sterile water or sterile normal saline solution.
- Solution should be stored in tight, light-resistant containers (brown bottles). Avoid exposure of solution at all times to direct light, prolonged heat, and alkaline materials.
- Drug may discolor in light but is still usable because it retains its potency.
- Discard cloudy solutions if warming to 55° to 60° C. (131° to 140° F.) does not restore clarity.

---

nystatin
Candex, Mycostatin♦, Nadostine♦♦, Nilstat

INDICATIONS & DOSAGE
Infant eczema, pruritus ani and vulvae, superficial bacterial infections, localized forms of candidiasis—
Adults and children: apply and rub into area b.i.d. for 2 weeks.

SIDE EFFECTS
Skin: occasional contact dermatitis from preservatives present in some formulations.
Systemic: possible nephrotoxicity or ototoxicity with prolonged or frequent use.

INTERACTIONS
None significant.

NURSING CONSIDERATIONS
- Contraindicated in viral diseases of the skin (vaccinia and varicella), fungal lesions (except candidiasis), and markedly impaired circulation.
- Generally well tolerated by all age groups, including debilitated infants.
- Preparation does not stain skin or mucous membranes.
- Cream recommended for intertriginous areas, powder for very moist areas, ointment for dry areas.
- Fungistatic and fungicidal.

silver sulfadiazine
Flamazine♦♦, Silvadene

INDICATIONS & DOSAGE
Prevention and treatment of wound infection for second- and third-degree burns—
Adults and children: apply $^1/_{16}$ inch thickness of ointment to cleansed and debrided burn wound, then apply daily or b.i.d.

SIDE EFFECTS
Blood: *neutropenia (in 3% to 5%).*
Skin: pain, burning, rashes, itching.
Other: fungal infections.

INTERACTIONS
Topical proteolytic enzymes: inactivity of enzymes when used together. Do not use together.

NURSING CONSIDERATIONS
- Contraindicated for premature and newborn infants during first month of life. (Drug may increase possibility of kernicterus.) Use with caution in hypersensitivity to drug or sulfonamides.
- If hepatic or renal dysfunction occurs, consider discontinuing drug.
- Inspect patient's skin daily, and note any changes. Notify doctor if burning or excessive pain develops.
- Use only on affected areas. Keep medicated at all times.
- For patients with extensive burns, monitor serum sulfa concentrations and renal function, and check urine for sulfa crystals.
- Bathe patient daily, if possible.
- Discard darkened cream.
- Should be discontinued if infection is suspected.

---

tetracycline hydrochloride
Achromycin♦, Topicycline

INDICATIONS & DOSAGE
Superficial skin infections caused by susceptible bacteria—
Adults and children: rub into cleansed affected area b.i.d. or t.i.d.
Acne—
Adults: apply Topicycline generously to affected areas b.i.d. until skin is thoroughly wet.

SIDE EFFECTS
Skin: dermatitis with Achromycin; with Topicycline, temporary stinging or burning on application, slight yellowing of treated skin, especially in patients with light complexions; treated skin areas fluoresce under ultraviolet light; severe dermatitis.

INTERACTIONS
None significant.

NURSING CONSIDERATIONS
• Contraindicated in hypersensitivity to any of the components.
• If no improvement or if condition worsens, stop using and tell doctor.
• Prolonged use may result in overgrowth of nonsusceptible organisms.
• Primarily a bacteriostatic agent.
• Patient may continue normal use of cosmetics.
• Store at room temperature, away from excessive heat.
• Medication to be used by one person only. Tell patient not to share with family members.
• Apply in morning and evening. Warn that drug should be used within 2 months.
• Explain that floating plug in bottle of Topicycline—an inert and harmless result of proper reconstitution of the preparation—shouldn't be removed.
• Serum levels of topical tetracycline HCl are much lower than those for orally administered drug, so systemic effects are unlikely.
• To control flow rate of solution, increase or decrease pressure of the applicator against the skin.

tolnaftate
Aftate, Tinactin♦

INDICATIONS & DOSAGE
Superficial fungus infections of the skin, infections due to common pathogenic fungi, tinea pedis, tinea cruris, tinea corporis, tinea manuum, tinea versicolor—
Adults and children: ¼- to ½-inch ribbon of cream or 1 or 3 drops of lotion to cover area of one hand; same amount of cream or 2 to 3 drops of lotion to cover the toes and interdigital webs of one foot. Apply and massage gently into skin b.i.d. for 2 or 3 weeks, up 6 weeks.

SIDE EFFECTS
None significant.

INTERACTIONS
None significant.

NURSING CONSIDERATIONS
• Discontinue if condition worsens. Check with doctor.
• Odorless, greaseless. Won't stain or discolor skin, hair, nails, or clothing.
• Only a small quantity of cream or lotion is needed; area should not be wet with solution when application is completed.
• Fungistatic and fungicidal.
• Commonly available product used to treat athlete's foot (tinea pedis).

undecylenic acid (zinc undecylenate)
Desenex, Ting, Unde-Jen

INDICATIONS & DOSAGE
Athlete's foot and ringworm of the body exclusive of nails and hairy areas—
Adults and children: clean thoroughly. Apply ointment liberally at night and powder during the day. Use regularly to prevent fungus infections.

SIDE EFFECTS
Skin: possible irritation in hypersensitive person.

INTERACTIONS
None significant.

NURSING CONSIDERATIONS
• Consult doctor before using on person with peripheral neuropathy and peripheral vascular diseases or diabetes.

81

Scabicides and pediculicides

benzyl benzoate lotion
copper oleate solution
  (with tetrahydronaphthalene)
crotamiton
gamma benzene hexachloride
  (or lindane)
sulfa in petrolatum

---

benzyl benzoate lotion
Scabanca♦♦

INDICATIONS & DOSAGE
*Parasitic infestation (scabies,
Phthirus pubis)—*
Adults and children: first, scrub entire body with soap and water. Then
apply the 25% lotion undiluted over
entire body, except the face, while
still damp. Be sure to apply around
nails. Let dry. Apply second coat on
the most involved areas. Bathe after
24 to 48 hours. Adults require 30 ml.
Children require 20 ml.
Pediculosis capitis—
Adults and children: apply to scalp
and leave on overnight; shampoo out
in morning. Repeat next night if
necessary.

SIDE EFFECTS
Skin: *irritation, itching; contact dermatitis with repeated applications.*

INTERACTIONS
None significant.

NURSING CONSIDERATIONS
• Contraindicated when skin is raw or
inflamed. Notify doctor immediately
if skin irritation or hypersensitivity
develops; tell patient to discontinue
drug and to wash it off skin.
• Do not apply to face, eyes, mucous
membranes, or urethral meatus. If accidental contact with eyes does occur,
flush with water and notify doctor.
• Instruct patient to change and sterilize (boil, launder, dry clean, or apply very hot iron) all clothing and bed
linen after drug is washed off.
• Itching may continue for several
weeks; does not indicate that therapy
is ineffective. To prevent acaropho-
bia, reassure patient that itching will
cease.
• Tendency to overuse this drug. Estimate amount needed.
• Topical corticosteroids may be
needed if dermatitis develops from
scratching.
• Question other family members
about possible infestation.
• After application, use a fine comb
on hair to remove nits.

**copper oleate solution
(with tetrahydronaphthalene)**
Cuprex

INDICATIONS & DOSAGE
*Parasitic infestation (pediculoses capi-
tis and pubis)—*
Adults and children: first, scrub entire body with soap and water. Apply
gently and sparingly 3 to 4 tablespoonfuls onto affected areas; after
15 minutes wash off with soap and
water.

SIDE EFFECTS
Skin: *irritation with repeated use, or
if used on raw or inflamed skin.*

INTERACTIONS
None significant.

NURSING CONSIDERATIONS
• Contraindicated when skin is raw or
inflamed, or when there is a severe infection. Notify doctor immediately if
skin irritation or hypersensitivity develops; tell patient to discontinue drug
and to wash it off skin.
• Do not apply more than twice
within 48 hours.
• Do not apply to face, eyes, mucous
membranes, or urethral meatus. If accidental contact with eyes does occur,
flush with water and notify doctor.
• Instruct patient to change and sterilize (boil, launder, dry clean, or apply very hot iron) all clothing and bed
linen after application.
• After application, use a fine comb
on hair to remove nits.
• Question other family members
about possible infestation.
• Tendency for overuse of pediculi-
cides. Estimate amount needed.

---

crotamiton
Eurax♦

INDICATIONS & DOSAGE
Parasitic infestation (scabies)—
Adults and children: scrub entire
body with soap and water. Then, apply a thin layer of cream over entire
body, from chin down, with special
attention to folds, creases, interdigital
spaces, genital areas. Apply second
coat within 24 hours. Wait 48 hours,
then wash off.
General itching—apply locally b.i.d.
or t.i.d.

SIDE EFFECTS
Skin: *irritation with repeated use.*

INTERACTIONS
None significant.

NURSING CONSIDERATIONS
• Contraindicated when skin is raw or
inflamed. Notify doctor immediately
if skin irritation or hypersensitivity
develops; tell patient to discontinue
drug and to wash it off skin.
• Do not apply to face, eyes, mucous
membranes, or urethral meatus. If accidental contact with eyes does occur,
flush with water and notify doctor.
• Instruct patient to change and sterilize (boil, launder, dry clean, or apply very hot iron) all clothing and bed
linen after drug is washed off.
• Topical corticosteroids may be
needed if dermatitis develops from
scratching.
• Tendency to overuse scabicides.
Estimate amount needed.
• Question other family members
about possible infestation.

**gamma benzene hexachloride
(or lindane)**
Gamene, gBh♦♦, Kwell, Kwellada♦♦

INDICATIONS & DOSAGE
*Parasitic infestation (scabies, pedicu-
losis)—*
Adults and children: scrub entire
body with soap and water.
Cream or lotion—apply thin layer
over entire skin surface (with special
attention to folds, creases, interdigital
spaces, genital area) for scabies, or to
hairy areas for pediculosis. After 8 to
12 hours wash off drug. If second application needed for scabies, wait
1 week before repeating. For pediculosis, may be repeated after 7 days but
never more than twice in a week.
Shampoo—apply 30 to 60 ml onto affected area and work into lather for
4 to 5 minutes. Rinse thoroughly and
rub with dry towel.

Italicized side effects are common or life-threatening.

SIDE EFFECTS
Skin: *irritation with repeated use.*

INTERACTIONS
None significant.

NURSING CONSIDERATIONS
• Contraindicated when skin is raw or inflamed. Notify doctor immediately if skin irritation or hypersensitivity develops; tell patient to discontinue drug and to wash it off skin. Use cautiously in infants and small children.
• Do not apply to open areas or acutely inflamed skin, or to face, eyes, mucous membranes, or urethral meatus. If accidental contact with eyes does occur, flush with water and notify doctor.
• Warn parents not to let infants or children suck their fingers after drug application.
• Discourage repeated use, which can lead to skin irritation and possible systemic toxicity.
• Warn patient itching may continue several weeks, especially in scabies.
• Topical corticosteroids may be needed if dermatitis develops from scratching.
• Instruct patient to change and sterilize (boil, launder, dry clean, or apply very hot iron) all clothing and bed linen after drug is washed off.
• After application, use a fine comb on hair to remove nits.
• Gamma benzene hexachloride shampoo can be used to clean comb or brushes; wash them thoroughly afterward. Warn patient not to use gamma benzene hexachloride as routine shampoo.
• Question other family members about possible infestation.
• Tendency for overuse. Estimate amount needed.

sulfa (6%) in petrolatum

INDICATIONS & DOSAGE
Parasitic infestation (scabies)—
Adults and children: after taking a soapy bath, patient should apply drug nightly for 2 to 3 nights consecutively. He should take soapy bath 24 hours after last application.

SIDE EFFECTS
Skin: *may produce dermatitis if applied continuously for several days.*

INTERACTIONS
None significant.

NURSING CONSIDERATIONS
• Instruct patient to change and sterilize (boil, launder, dry clean, or iron with a very hot iron) all clothing and bed linen after drug is washed off.
• Warn patient product has an odor, is messy, and will stain clothing.
• Question other members of family about possible infestation.
• Tendency to overuse scabicides. Estimate amount needed.

82

Topical corticosteroids

amcinonide
betamethasone
betamethasone benzoate
betamethasone dipropionate
betamethasone valerate
desonide
desoximetasone
dexamethasone
dexamethasone sodium phosphate
diflorasone diacetate
flumethasone pivalate
fluocinolone acetonide
fluocinonide
fluorometholone
flurandrenolide
halcinonide
hydrocortisone
hydrocortisone acetate
hydrocortisone valerate
methylprednisolone acetate
prednisolone
triamcinolone acetonide

amcinonide
Cyclocort♦

INDICATIONS & DOSAGE
Inflammation of corticosteroid-responsive dermatoses—
Adults and children: apply a light film to affected areas 2 or 3 times daily. Cream should be rubbed in gently and thoroughly until it disappears.

SIDE EFFECTS
Skin: burning, itching, irritation, dryness, folliculitis, hypopigmentation, striae, acneiform eruptions, perioral dermatitis, hypertrichosis, allergic contact dermatitis. *With occlusive dressings: secondary infection, maceration, atrophy, striae, miliaria.*

INTERACTIONS
None significant.

NURSING CONSIDERATIONS
• Use cautiously in viral diseases of skin, such as varicella, vaccinia, herpes simplex; fungal infections; skin tuberculosis; impaired circulation.
• Avoid application in or near eyes.
• Due to alcohol content of vehicle, gel preparations may cause mild, transient stinging without irritation if used on or near excoriated skin.
• Systemic absorption especially likely with occlusive dressings, prolonged treatment, or extensive body-surface treatment.
• Stop drug and notify doctor if patient develops signs of systemic absorption, skin irritation or ulceration, signs of hypersensitivity, infection. (If antifungals or antibiotics are being used with corticosteroids and infection does not respond immediately, corticosteroids should be stopped until infection is controlled.)
• Before applying, gently wash skin. To prevent damage to skin, rub in medication gently, leaving a thin coat. When treating hairy sites, part hair and apply directly to lesion.
• Occlusive dressing: apply cream heavily, then cover with a thin, pliable, nonflammable plastic film; seal to adjacent normal skin with hypoal-

lergenic tape. Minimize adverse reactions by using occlusive dressing intermittently.
• For patient with eczematous dermatitis who may develop irritation with adhesive material, hold dressing in place with gauze, elastic bandages, or stockings.
• Notify doctor and remove occlusive dressing if body temperature rises.
• Occlusive dressings are generally not used in presence of infections or with weeping or exudative lesions.
• Change dressings as ordered by doctor. Inspect skin for infection, striae, and atrophy. Discontinue drug and notify doctor if these occur.
• Treatment should be continued for a few days after clearing of lesions to prevent recurrence.
• Instruct patient to report signs of drug sensitivity.

---

betamethasone
Celestone♦

INDICATIONS & DOSAGE
Inflammation of corticosteroid-responsive dermatoses—
Adults and children: clean area; apply cream sparingly b.i.d. or t.i.d. Massage gently until it disappears. Apply thick layer with occlusive dressing to manage deep-seated dermatoses, such as neurodermatitis.

SIDE EFFECTS
Skin: burning, itching, irritation, dryness, folliculitis, hypopigmentation, acneiform eruptions, hypertrichosis, allergic contact dermatitis. *With occlusive dressings: secondary infection, maceration, skin atrophy, striae, miliaria.*

INTERACTIONS
None significant.

NURSING CONSIDERATIONS
• Use cautiously in viral diseases of skin, such as vaccinia, varicella, herpes simplex; fungal infections; skin tuberculosis; impaired circulation.
• Avoid application in or near eyes.
• Systemic absorption especially likely with occlusive dressings, prolonged treatment, or extensive body-surface treatment.
• Stop drug and notify doctor if patient develops signs of systemic absorption, skin irritation or ulceration, hypersensitivity, infection. (If antifungals or antibacterials are being used with corticosteroids and infection does not respond immediately, corticosteroids should be stopped until infection is controlled.)
• Before applying, gently wash skin. To prevent damage to skin, rub medication in gently, leaving a thin coat.
• Occlusive dressing: apply cream heavily, then cover with a thin, pliable, nonflammable plastic film; seal to adjacent normal skin with hypoallergenic tape. Minimize adverse reactions by using occlusive dressing intermittently.
• For patient with eczematous dermatitis who may develop irritation with adhesive material, hold dressing in place with gauze, elastic bandages, or stockings.
• Notify doctor and remove occlusive dressing if body temperature rises.
• Occlusive dressings are generally not used in presence of infection or with weeping or exudative lesions.
• Change dressing as ordered by doctor. Inspect skin for infection, striae, and atrophy. Discontinue drug and notify doctor if these occur.
• Treatment should be continued for a few days after clearing of lesions to prevent recurrence.
• Instruct patient to report signs of drug sensitivity.

betamethasone benzoate
Beben◆, Benisone, Uticort

INDICATIONS & DOSAGE
Inflammation of corticosteroid-responsive dermatoses—
Adults and children: clean area; apply cream, lotion, or gel sparingly daily to q.i.d.

SIDE EFFECTS
Skin: burning, itching, irritation, dryness, folliculitis, hypopigmentation, striae, acneiform eruptions, perioral dermatitis, hypertrichosis, allergic contact dermatitis. *With occlusive dressings: secondary infection, maceration, atrophy, striae, miliaria.*

INTERACTIONS
None significant.

NURSING CONSIDERATIONS
• Use cautiously in viral diseases of skin, such as varicella, vaccinia, herpes simplex; fungal infections; skin tuberculosis; impaired circulation.
• Avoid application in or near eyes.
• Due to alcohol content of vehicle, gel preparations may cause mild, transient stinging without irritation if used on or near excoriated skin.
• Systemic absorption especially likely with occlusive dressings, prolonged treatment, or extensive body-surface treatment.
• Stop drug and notify doctor if patient develops signs of systemic absorption, skin irritation or ulceration, signs of hypersensitivity, infection. (If antifungals or antibiotics are being used with corticosteroids and infection does not respond immediately, corticosteroids should be stopped until infection is controlled.)
• Before applying, gently wash skin. To prevent damage to skin, rub in medication gently, leaving a thin coat.

When treating hairy sites, part hair and apply directly to lesion.
• Occlusive dressing: apply cream heavily, then cover with a thin, pliable, nonflammable plastic film; seal to adjacent normal skin with hypoallergenic tape. Minimize adverse reactions by using occlusive dressing intermittently.
• For patient with eczematous dermatitis who may develop irritation with adhesive material, hold dressing in place with gauze, elastic bandages, or stockings.
• Notify doctor and remove occlusive dressing if body temperature rises.
• Occlusive dressings are generally not used in presence of infections or with weeping or exudative lesions.
• Change dressings as ordered by doctor. Inspect skin for infection, striae, and atrophy. Discontinue drug and notify doctor if these occur.
• Treatment should be continued for a few days after clearing of lesions to prevent recurrence.
• Instruct patient to report signs of drug sensitivity.

betamethasone dipropionate
Diprosone◆

INDICATIONS & DOSAGE
Inflammation of corticosteroid-responsive dermatoses—
Adults and children: clean area; apply cream, lotion, or ointment sparingly b.i.d.
Aerosol: Direct spray onto affected area from a distance of 6 inches for only 3 seconds t.i.d.

SIDE EFFECTS
Skin: burning, itching, irritation, dryness, folliculitis, hypopigmentation, perioral dermatitis, allergic contact dermatitis, hypertrichosis, acneiform eruptions. *With occlusive dressings:*

Italicized side effects are common or life-threatening.

maceration of skin, secondary infection, atrophy, striae, miliaria.

INTERACTIONS
None significant.

NURSING CONSIDERATIONS
• Use cautiously in viral diseases of skin, such as varicella, vaccinia, herpes simplex; fungal infections; skin tuberculosis; impaired circulation.
• Avoid application in or near eyes.
• Systemic absorption especially likely with occlusive dressings, prolonged treatment, or extensive body-surface treatment.
• Stop drug and notify doctor if patient develops signs of systemic absorption, skin irritation or ulceration, hypersensitivity, infection. (If antifungals or antibiotics are being used with corticosteroids and infection does not respond immediately, corticosteroids should be stopped until infection is controlled.)
• Before applying, gently wash skin. To prevent damage to skin, rub in medication gently, leaving a thin coat. When treating hairy sites, part hair and apply directly to lesion.
• Aerosol preparation contains alcohol and may produce irritation or burning in open lesions. When using about the face, cover patient's eyes and warn against inhalation of spray. To avoid freezing tissues, do not spray longer than 3 seconds or closer than 6 inches.
• For patient with eczematous dermatitis who may develop irritation with adhesive material, hold dressing in place with gauze, elastic bandages, or stockings.
• Occlusive dressings are generally not used in presence of infection or with weeping or exudative lesions.
• Change dressing as ordered by doctor. Inspect skin for infection, striae, and atrophy. Discontinue drug and notify doctor if these occur.

• Instruct patient to report signs of drug sensitivity.

---

betamethasone valerate
Betnovate♦♦, Betnovate 1/2♦♦, Celestoderm-V♦♦, Celestoderm-V/2♦♦, Valisone

---

INDICATIONS & DOSAGE
Inflammation of corticosteroid-responsive dermatoses—
Adults and children: clean area; apply cream, lotion, ointment, or aerosol sparingly daily to q.i.d.
Aerosol: shake can well. Direct spray onto affected area from a distance of 6 inches. Apply for only 3 seconds t.i.d. to q.i.d.
Betnovate 1/2 and Celestoderm V/2 contain less betamethasone.

SIDE EFFECTS
Skin: burning, itching, irritation, dryness, folliculitis, hypopigmentation, hypertrichosis, acneiform eruptions, perioral dermatitis, allergic contact dermatitis. *With occlusive dressings: maceration of skin, secondary infection, atrophy, striae, miliaria.*

INTERACTIONS
None significant.

NURSING CONSIDERATIONS
• Use cautiously in viral diseases of skin, such as varicella, vaccinia, herpes simplex; fungal infections; skin tuberculosis; impaired circulation.
• Avoid application in or near eyes.
• Systemic absorption especially likely with occlusive dressings, prolonged treatment, or extensive body-surface treatment.
• Stop drug and notify doctor if patient develops signs of systemic absorption, skin irritation or ulceration, hypersensitivity, infection. (If antifungals or antibiotics are being used

with corticosteroids and infection does not respond immediately, corticosteroids should be stopped until infection is controlled.)

• Before applying, gently wash skin. To prevent damage to skin, rub in medication gently, leaving a thin coat. When treating hairy sites, part hair and apply directly to lesions.

• Aerosol preparation contains alcohol and may produce irritation or burning in open lesions. When using about the face, cover patient's eyes and warn against inhalation of the spray. To avoid freezing tissues, do not spray longer than 3 seconds or closer than 6 inches.

• Occlusive dressing: apply cream or ointment heavily, then cover with a thin, pliable, nonflammable plastic film; seal to adjacent normal skin with hypoallergenic tape. Minimize adverse reactions by using occlusive dressing intermittently.

• For patient with eczematous dermatitis who may develop irritation with adhesive material, hold dressing in place with gauze, elastic bandages, or stockings.

• Notify doctor and remove occlusive dressing if body temperature rises.

• Occlusive dressings are generally not used in presence of infection or with weeping or exudative lesions.

• Change dressing as ordered by doctor. Inspect skin for infection, striae, and atrophy. Discontinue drug and notify doctor if these occur.

• Treatment should be continued for a few days after clearing of lesions to prevent recurrence.

• Instruct patient to report signs of drug sensitivity.

desonide
Tridesilon♦

INDICATIONS & DOSAGE
Adjunctive therapy for inflammation in acute and chronic corticosteroid-responsive dermatoses—
Adults and children: clean area; apply cream, lotion, or gel sparingly b.i.d. to t.i.d.

SIDE EFFECTS
Skin: burning, itching, irritation, dryness, folliculitis, hypopigmentation, perioral dermatitis, allergic contact dermatitis, hypertrichosis, acneiform eruptions. *With occlusive dressings: maceration of skin, secondary infection, atrophy, striae, miliaria.*

INTERACTIONS
None significant.

NURSING CONSIDERATIONS
• Use cautiously in viral diseases of skin, such as varicella, vaccinia, herpes simplex; fungal infections; skin tuberculosis; impaired circulation.

• Avoid application in or near eyes.

• Systemic absorption especially likely with occlusive dressings, prolonged treatment, or extensive body-surface treatment.

• Stop drug and notify doctor if patient develops signs of systemic absorption, skin irritation or ulceration, hypersensitivity, infection. (If antifungals or antibiotics are being used with corticosteroids and infection does not respond immediately, corticosteroids should be stopped until infection is controlled.)

• Before applying, gently wash skin. To prevent damage to skin, rub in medication gently, leaving a thin coat. When treating hairy sites, part hair and apply directly to lesion.

• Occlusive dressing: apply cream or

ointment heavily, then cover with a thin, pliable, nonflammable plastic film; seal to adjacent normal skin with hypoallergenic tape. Minimize adverse reactions by using occlusive dressing intermittently.
• For patient with eczematous dermatitis who may develop irritation with adhesive material, hold dressing in place with gauze, elastic bandages, or stockings.
• Notify doctor and remove occlusive dressing if body temperature rises.
• Occlusive dressings are generally not used in presence of infection or with weeping or exudative lesions.
• Change dressing as ordered by doctor. Inspect skin for infection, striae, and atrophy. Discontinue drug and notify doctor if these occur.
• Treatment should be continued for a few days after clearing of lesions to prevent recurrence.
• Instruct patient to report signs of drug sensitivity.

---

desoximetasone
Topicort♦

INDICATIONS & DOSAGE
Inflammation of corticosteroid-responsive dermatoses—
Adults and children: clean area; apply cream sparingly b.i.d.

SIDE EFFECTS
Skin: burning, itching, irritation, dryness, folliculitis, hypopigmentation, hypertrichosis, acneiform eruptions, perioral dermatitis, allergic contact dermatitis. *With occlusive dressings: maceration of skin, secondary infection, atrophy, striae, miliaria.*

INTERACTIONS
None significant.

NURSING CONSIDERATIONS
• Use cautiously in viral diseases of

skin, such as varicella, vaccinia, herpes simplex; fungal infections; skin tuberculosis; impaired circulation.
• Avoid application in or near eyes.
• Systemic absorption especially likely with occlusive dressings, prolonged treatment, or extensive body-surface treatment.
• Stop drug and notify doctor if patient develops signs of systemic absorption, skin irritation or ulceration, hypersensitivity, infection. (If antifungals or antibiotics are being used with corticosteroids and infection does not respond immediately, corticosteroids should be stopped until infection is controlled.)
• Before applying, gently wash skin. To prevent damage to skin, rub in medication gently, leaving a thin coat. When treating hairy sites, part hair and apply directly to lesions.
• Occlusive dressing: apply cream heavily, then cover with a thin, pliable, nonflammable plastic film; seal to adjacent normal skin with hypoallergenic tape. To minimize adverse reactions, use occlusive dressing intermittently.
• For patient with eczematous dermatitis who may develop irritation with adhesive material, hold dressing in place with gauze, elastic bandages, or stockings.
• Notify doctor and remove occlusive dressing if body temperature rises.
• Occlusive dressings are generally not used in presence of infection or with weeping or exudative lesions.
• Change dressing as ordered by doctor. Inspect skin for infection, striae, and atrophy. Discontinue drug and notify doctor if these occur.
• Treatment should be continued for a few days after clearing of lesions to prevent recurrence.
• Instruct patient to report signs of drug sensitivity.

dexamethasone
Aeroseb-Dex, Decaderm, Decaspray,
Hexadrol♦

INDICATIONS & DOSAGE
Inflammation of corticosteroid-respon-sive dermatoses—
Adults and children: clean area; apply cream, gel, or aerosol sparingly b.i.d. to q.i.d.
Aerosol use on scalp: shake can well and apply to dry scalp after shampooing. Hold can upright. Slide applicator tube under hair so that it touches scalp. Spray while moving tube to all affected areas, keeping tube under hair and in contact with scalp throughout spraying, which should take about 2 seconds. Inadequately covered areas may be spot sprayed. Slide applicator tube through hair to touch scalp, press and immediately release spray button. Don't massage medication into scalp or spray forehead or eyes.

SIDE EFFECTS
Skin: burning, itching, irritation, dryness, folliculitis, hypopigmentation, hypertrichosis, acneiform eruptions, perioral dermatitis, allergic contact dermatitis. *With occlusive dressings: maceration of skin, secondary infection, atrophy, striae, miliaria.*

INTERACTIONS
None significant.

NURSING CONSIDERATIONS
• Use cautiously in viral diseases of skin, such as varicella, vaccinia, herpes simplex; fungal infections; skin tuberculosis; impaired circulation.
• Avoid application in or near eyes.
• Systemic absorption especially likely with occlusive dressings, prolonged treatment, or extensive body-surface treatment.

• Stop drug and notify doctor if patient develops signs of systemic absorption, skin irritation or ulceration, signs of hypersensitivity, infection. (If antifungals or antibiotics are being used with corticosteroids and infection does not respond immediately, corticosteroids should be stopped until infection is controlled.)
• Before applying, gently wash skin. To prevent damage to skin, rub in medication gently, leaving a thin coat. When treating hairy sites, part hair and apply directly to lesions.
• Occlusive dressing: apply cream heavily and cover with a thin, pliable, nonflammable plastic film; seal to adjacent normal skin with hypoallergenic tape. To minimize adverse reactions, use occlusive dressing intermittently.
• For patient with eczematous dermatitis who may develop irritation with adhesive material, hold dressing in place with gauze, elastic bandages, or stockings.
• Notify doctor and remove occlusive dressing if body temperature rises.
• Change dressing as ordered by doctor. Inspect skin for infection, striae, and atrophy. Discontinue drug and notify doctor if these occur.
• Occlusive dressings are generally not used in presence of infection or with weeping or exudative lesions.
• Aerosol preparation contains alcohol and may produce irritation or burning in open lesions. When using about the face, cover patient's eyes and warn against inhalation of the spray. To avoid freezing tissues, do not spray longer than 3 seconds or closer than 6 inches.
• Treatments should be continued for a few days after clearing of lesions to prevent recurrence.
• Instruct patient to report signs of drug sensitivity.

Italicized side effects are common or life-threatening.

dexamethasone sodium phosphate
Decadron Phosphate♦

INDICATIONS & DOSAGE
Inflammation of corticosteroid-responsive dermatoses—
Adults and children: clean area; apply cream sparingly b.i.d. to t.i.d.

SIDE EFFECTS
Skin: burning, itching, irritation, dryness, folliculitis, hypopigmentation, hypertrichosis, acneiform eruptions, perioral dermatitis, allergic contact dermatitis. *With occlusive dressings: maceration of skin, secondary infection, atrophy, striae, miliaria.*

INTERACTIONS
None significant.

NURSING CONSIDERATIONS
• Use cautiously in viral diseases of skin, such as varicella, vaccinia, herpes simplex; fungal infections; skin tuberculosis; impaired circulation.
• Avoid application in or near eyes.
• Systemic absorption especially likely with occlusive dressings, prolonged treatment, or extensive body-surface treatment.
• Stop drug and notify doctor if patient develops signs of systemic absorption, skin irritation or ulceration, hypersensitivity, infection. (If antifungals or antibiotics are being used along with corticosteroids and infection does not respond immediately, corticosteroids should be stopped until infection is controlled.)
• Before applying, gently wash skin. To prevent damage to skin, rub in medication gently, leaving a thin coat. When treating hairy sites, part hair and apply directly to lesions.
• Occlusive dressing: apply cream heavily, then cover with a thin, pliable, nonflammable plastic film; seal to adjacent normal skin with hypoallergenic tape. To minimize adverse reactions, use occlusive dressing intermittently. Occlusive dressings are generally not used in presence of infection or with weeping or exudative lesions.
• For patient with eczematous dermatitis who may develop irritation with adhesive material, hold dressing in place with gauze, elastic bandages, or stockings.
• Notify doctor and remove occlusive dressing if body temperature rises.
• Change dressing as ordered by doctor. Inspect skin for infection, striae, and atrophy. Discontinue drug and notify doctor if these occur.
• Treatment should be continued for a few days after clearing of lesions to prevent recurrence.
• Instruct patient to report signs of drug sensitivity.

diflorasone diacetate
Florone, Maxiflor

INDICATIONS & DOSAGE
Inflammation of corticosteroid-responsive dermatoses—
Adults and children: clean area; apply ointment daily to t.i.d.; apply cream b.i.d. to q.i.d. Apply sparingly in a thin film.

SIDE EFFECTS
Skin: burning, itching, irritation, dryness, folliculitis, hypopigmentation, perioral dermatitis, hypertrichosis, acneiform eruptions. *With occlusive dressings: maceration, secondary infection, atrophy, striae, miliaria.*

INTERACTIONS
None significant.

NURSING CONSIDERATIONS
• Use cautiously in viral diseases of

skin, such as varicella, vaccinia, herpes simplex; fungal infections; skin tuberculosis; impaired circulation.

- Avoid application in or near eyes.
- Systemic absorption especially likely with occlusive dressings, prolonged treatment, or extensive body-surface treatment.
- Stop drug and notify doctor if patient develops signs of systemic absorption, skin irritation or ulceration, hypersensitivity, infection. (If antifungals or antibiotics are being used concomitantly, corticosteroids should be stopped until infection is controlled.)
- Before applying, gently wash skin. To prevent damage to skin, rub in medication gently, leaving a thin coat. When treating hairy sites, part hair and apply directly to lesion.
- Occlusive dressing: apply cream or ointment heavily, then cover with a thin, pliable, nonflammable plastic film; seal to adjacent normal skin with hypoallergenic tape. Minimize adverse reactions by using occlusive dressing intermittently. Occlusive dressings are generally not used in presence of infection or with weeping or exudative lesions.
- For patient with eczematous dermatitis who may develop irritation with adhesive material, hold dressing in place with gauze, elastic bandages, or stockings.
- Notify doctor and remove occlusive dressing if body temperature rises.
- Change dressing as ordered by doctor. Inspect skin for infection, striae, and atrophy. Discontinue drug and notify doctor if these occur.
- Instruct patient to report signs of drug sensitivity.
- Diflorasone is often effective with once-daily application.

flumethasone pivalate
Locacorten♦♦, Locorten

INDICATIONS & DOSAGE
Inflammation of corticosteroid-responsive dermatoses—
Adults and children: clean area; apply cream sparingly t.i.d. to q.i.d.

SIDE EFFECTS
Skin: burning, itching, irritation, dryness, folliculitis, hypopigmentation, hypertrichosis, acneiform eruptions, perioral dermatitis, allergic contact dermatitis. *With occlusive dressings: maceration of skin, secondary infection, atrophy, striae, miliaria.*

INTERACTIONS
None significant.

NURSING CONSIDERATIONS
- Use cautiously in viral diseases of skin, such as varicella, vaccinia, and herpes simplex; fungal infections; skin tuberculosis; and impaired circulation.
- Avoid application in or near eyes.
- Systemic absorption especially likely with occlusive dressings, prolonged treatment, or extensive body-surface treatment.
- Stop drug and notify doctor if patient develops signs of systemic absorption, skin irritation or ulceration, hypersensitivity, infection. (If antifungals or antibiotics are being used along with corticosteroids and infection does not respond immediately, corticosteroids should be stopped until infection is controlled.)
- Before applying, gently wash skin. To prevent damage to skin, rub in medication gently, leaving a thin coat. When treating hairy sites, part hair and apply directly to lesion.
- Occlusive dressing: apply cream or ointment heavily, then cover with a thin, pliable, nonflammable plastic

---

Italicized side effects are common or life-threatening.

film; seal to adjacent normal skin with hypoallergenic tape. To minimize adverse reactions, use occlusive dressing intermittently. Occlusive dressings are generally not used in presence of infection or with weeping or exudative lesions.

• For patient with eczematous dermatitis who may develop irritation with adhesive material, hold dressing in place with gauze, elastic bandages, or stockings.

• Notify doctor and remove occlusive dressing if body temperature rises.

• Change dressing as ordered by doctor. Inspect skin for infection, striae, and atrophy. Discontinue drug and notify doctor if these occur.

• Treatment should be continued for a few days after clearing of lesions to prevent recurrence.

• Instruct patient to report signs of drug sensitivity.

---

fluocinolone acetonide
Fluonid, Synalar♦, Synalar-HP♦, Synamol♦, Synemol

INDICATIONS & DOSAGE
Inflammation of corticosteroid-responsive dermatoses—
Adults, and children over 2: clean area; apply cream, ointment, or solution sparingly b.i.d. to q.i.d. Treat multiple or extensive lesions sequentially, applying to only small areas at any one time.

SIDE EFFECTS
Skin: burning, itching, irritation, dryness, folliculitis, hypopigmentation, hypertrichosis, acneiform eruptions, perioral dermatitis, allergic contact dermatitis. *With occlusive dressings: maceration of skin, secondary infection, atrophy, striae, miliaria.*

INTERACTIONS
None significant.

NURSING CONSIDERATIONS
• Use cautiously in viral diseases of skin, such as varicella, vaccinia, herpes simplex; fungal infections; skin tuberculosis; impaired circulation.

• Avoid application in or near eyes.

• Systemic absorption especially likely with occlusive dressings, prolonged treatment, or extensive body-surface treatment.

• Stop drug and notify doctor if patient develops signs of systemic absorption, skin irritation or ulceration, hypersensitivity, infection. (If antifungals or antibiotics are being used with corticosteroids and infection does not respond immediately, corticosteroids should be stopped until infection is controlled.)

• Before applying, gently wash skin. To prevent damage to skin, rub in medication gently, leaving a thin coat. When treating hairy sites, part hair and apply directly to lesion.

• Occlusive dressing: apply gently and sparingly to the lesion until cream disappears. Then reapply, leaving a thin coat. Cover with a thin, pliable, nonflammable plastic film; seal to adjacent normal skin with hypoallergenic tape. To minimize adverse reactions, use occlusive dressing intermittently. Occlusive dressings are generally not used in presence of infection or with weeping or exudative lesions.

• For patient with eczematous dermatitis who may develop irritation with adhesive material, hold dressing in place with gauze, elastic bandages, or stockings.

• Notify doctor and remove occlusive dressing if body temperature rises.

• Change dressing as ordered by doctor. Inspect skin for infection, striae, and atrophy. Discontinue drug and notify doctor if these occur.

• Instruct patient to report signs of drug sensitivity.

• Fluonid solution on dry lesions may increase dryness, scaling, or itching;

on denuded or fissured areas, may produce burning or stinging. If burning or stinging persists and dermatitis has not improved, solution should be discontinued.

---

fluocinonide
Lidemol♦♦, Lidex♦, Lidex-E, Topsyn♦

INDICATIONS & DOSAGE
Inflammation of corticosteroid-responsive dermatoses—
Adults and children: clean area; apply cream, ointment, or gel sparingly t.i.d. to q.i.d.

SIDE EFFECTS
Skin: burning, itching, irritation, dryness, folliculitis, hypopigmentation, hypertrichosis, acneiform eruptions, perioral dermatitis, allergic contact dermatitis. *With occlusive dressings: maceration of skin, secondary infection, atrophy, striae, miliaria.*

INTERACTIONS
None significant.

NURSING CONSIDERATIONS
• Use cautiously in viral diseases of skin, such as varicella, vaccinia, and herpes simplex; untreated purulent bacterial skin infections; fungal infections; skin tuberculosis; impaired circulation.
• Avoid application in or near eyes.
• Systemic absorption especially likely with occlusive dressings, prolonged treatment, or extensive body-surface treatment.
• Stop drug and notify doctor if patient develops signs of systemic absorption, skin irritation or ulceration, hypersensitivity, infection. (If antifungals or antibiotics are being used with corticosteroids and infection does not respond immediately, corticosteroids should be stopped until infection is controlled.)
• Before applying, gently wash skin. To prevent damage to skin, rub in medication gently, leaving a thin coat. When treating hairy sites, part hair and apply directly to lesion.
• Occlusive dressing: apply cream or ointment heavily, then cover with a thin, pliable, nonflammable plastic film; seal to adjacent normal skin with hypoallergenic tape. To minimize adverse reactions, use occlusive dressing intermittently. Occlusive dressings are generally not used in presence of infection or with weeping or exudative lesions.
• For patient with eczematous dermatitis who may develop irritation with adhesive material, hold dressing in place with gauze, elastic bandages, or stockings.
• Notify doctor and remove occlusive dressing if body temperature rises.
• Change dressing as ordered by doctor. Inspect skin for infection, striae, and atrophy. Discontinue drug and notify doctor if these occur.
• Treatment should be continued for a few days after clearing of lesions to prevent recurrence.
• Instruct patient to report signs of drug sensitivity.

---

fluorometholone
Oxylone

INDICATIONS & DOSAGE
Inflammation of corticosteroid-responsive dermatoses—
Adults and children: clean area; apply cream sparingly daily to t.i.d.

SIDE EFFECTS
Skin: burning, itching, irritation, dryness, folliculitis, hypopigmentation, hypertrichosis, acneiform eruptions, perioral dermatitis, allergic contact dermatitis. *With occlusive dressings:*

---

maceration of skin, secondary infection, atrophy, striae, miliaria.

INTERACTIONS
None significant.

NURSING CONSIDERATIONS
• Use cautiously in viral diseases of skin, such as varicella, vaccinia, herpes simplex; fungal infections; skin tuberculosis; impaired circulation.
• Avoid application in or near eyes.
• Systemic absorption especially likely with occlusive dressings, prolonged treatment, or extensive body-surface treatment.
• Stop drug and notify doctor if patient develops signs of systemic absorption, skin irritation or ulceration, hypersensitivity, infection. (If antifungals or antibiotics are being used with corticosteroids and infection does not respond immediately, corticosteroids should be stopped until infection is controlled.)
• Before applying, gently wash skin. To prevent damage to skin, rub in medication gently, leaving a thin coat. When treating hairy sites, part hair and apply directly to lesion.
• Occlusive dressing: apply cream heavily, then cover with a thin, pliable, nonflammable plastic film; seal to adjacent normal skin with hypoallergenic tape. To minimize adverse reactions, use occlusive dressing intermittently. Occlusive dressings are generally not used in presence of infection or with weeping or exudative lesions.
• For patient with eczematous dermatitis who may develop irritation with adhesive material, hold dressing in place with gauze, elastic bandages, or stockings.
• Notify doctor and remove occlusive dressing if body temperature rises.
• Change dressing as ordered by doctor. Inspect skin for infection, striae,

and atrophy. Discontinue drug and notify doctor if these occur.
• Treatment should be continued for a few days after clearing of lesions to prevent recurrence.
• Instruct patient to report signs of drug sensitivity.

---

flurandrenolide
Cordran, Cordran SP, Cordran Tape, Drenison♦♦, Drenison ¼♦♦, Drenison Tape♦♦

INDICATIONS & DOSAGE
Inflammation of corticosteroid-responsive dermatoses—
Adults and children: clean area; apply cream, lotion, or ointment sparingly b.i.d. or t.i.d. Apply tape q 12 to 24 hours. Before applying tape, cleanse skin carefully, removing scales, crust, and dried exudates. Allow skin to dry for 1 hour before applying new tape. Shave or clip hair to allow good contact with skin and comfortable removal. If tape ends loosen prematurely, trim off and replace with fresh tape. Lowest incidence of adverse reactions if tape is replaced q 12 hours, but may be left in place for 24 hours if well tolerated and adheres satisfactorily.
Drenison ¼: for maintenance therapy of widespread or chronic lesions.

SIDE EFFECTS
Skin: burning, itching, irritation, dryness, folliculitis, hypopigmentation, hypertrichosis, acneiform eruptions, allergic contact dermatitis. *With occlusive dressings: maceration of skin, secondary infection, atrophy, striae, miliaria.* With tape: purpura, stripping of epidermis, furunculosis.

INTERACTIONS
None significant.

NURSING CONSIDERATIONS

• Use cautiously in viral diseases of skin, such as varicella, vaccinia, herpes simplex; fungal infections; skin tuberculosis; impaired circulation.
• Tape not advised for exudative lesions or those in intertriginous areas.
• Avoid application in or near eyes.
• Systemic absorption especially likely with occlusive dressings, prolonged treatment, or extensive body-surface treatment.
• Stop drug and notify doctor if patient develops signs of systemic absorption, skin irritation or ulceration, hypersensitivity, infection. (If antifungals or antibiotics are being used with corticosteroids and infection does not respond immediately, corticosteroids should be stopped until infection is controlled.)
• Before applying, gently wash skin. To prevent damage to skin, rub in medication gently, leaving a thin coat. When treating hairy sites, part hair and apply directly to lesion.
• Occlusive dressing: apply cream heavily, then cover with a thin, pliable, nonflammable plastic film; seal to adjacent normal skin with hypoallergenic tape. To minimize adverse reactions, use occlusive dressing intermittently. Occlusive dressings are generally not used in presence of infection or with weeping or exudative lesions.
• For patient with eczematous dermatitis who may develop irritation with adhesive material, hold dressing in place with gauze, elastic bandages, or stockings.
• Notify doctor and remove occlusive dressing if body temperature rises.
• Change dressing as ordered by doctor. Inspect skin for infection, striae, and atrophy. Discontinue drug and notify doctor if these occur.
• Treatment should be continued for a few days after clearing of lesions to prevent recurrence.

• Instruct patient to report signs of drug sensitivity.

---

halcinonide
Halciderm, Halog♦

INDICATIONS & DOSAGE

Inflammation of acute and chronic corticosteroid-responsive dermatoses—
Adults and children: clean area; apply cream, ointment, or solution sparingly b.i.d. to t.i.d.

SIDE EFFECTS

Skin: burning, itching, irritation, dryness, folliculitis, hypopigmentation, hypertrichosis, acneiform eruptions, allergic contact dermatitis. *With occlusive dressings: maceration of skin, secondary infection, atrophy, striae, miliaria.*

INTERACTIONS

None significant.

NURSING CONSIDERATIONS

• Use cautiously in viral diseases of skin, such as varicella, vaccinia, herpes simplex; fungal infections; skin tuberculosis; impaired circulation.
• Avoid application in or near eyes.
• Systemic absorption especially likely with occlusive dressings, prolonged treatment, or extensive body-surface treatment.
• Stop drug and notify doctor if patient develops signs of systemic absorption, skin irritation or ulceration, hypersensitivity, infection. (If antifungals or antibiotics are being used with corticosteroids and infection does not respond immediately, corticosteroids should be stopped until infection is controlled.)
• Before applying, gently wash skin. To prevent damage to skin, rub in medication gently, leaving a thin coat.

Italicized side effects are common or life-threatening.

When treating hairy sites, part hair and apply directly to lesion.

- Occlusive dressing with cream: gently rub small amount into lesion until it disappears. Reapply, leaving a thin coating on lesion, and cover with occlusive dressing. With ointment: apply to lesion and cover with occlusive dressing. Cover with a thin, pliable, nonflammable plastic film; seal to adjacent normal skin with hypoallergenic tape. To minimize adverse reactions, use occlusive dressing intermittently; or with extensive lesions, occlude one part of the body at a time.
- Good results have been obtained by applying occlusive dressings in the evening and removing them in the morning (i.e., 12-hour occlusion). Medication should then be reapplied in the morning, without using the occlusive dressings during the day.
- For patient with eczematous dermatitis who may develop irritation with adhesive material, hold dressing in place with gauze, elastic bandages, or stockings.
- Notify doctor and remove occlusive dressing if body temperature rises.
- Occlusive dressings are generally not used in presence of infection or with weeping or exudative lesions.
- Change dressing as ordered by doctor. Inspect skin for infection, striae, and atrophy. Discontinue drug and notify doctor if these occur.
- Treatment should be continued for a few days after clearing of lesions to prevent recurrence.
- Instruct patient to report signs of drug sensitivity.

hydrocortisone
Acticort, Aeroseb-HC♦, Alphaderm, Carmol-HC, Cetacort, Cortaid, Cort-Dome♦, Corticreme♦♦, Cortinal, Cortril♦, Cotacort, Cremesone, Delacort, Dermacort, Dermolate, Durel-Cort, Ecosone, Eldecort, Emo-Cort♦♦, HC Cream, Heb-Cort, HI-COR-2.5, Hycort, Hycortole, Hydrocortex, Hydro-Cortilean♦♦, Hytone, Ivocort, Manticor♦♦, Maso-Cort, Microcort♦, Nutracort♦, Penetrate, Proctocort, Rectocort♦♦, Relecort, Rhus Tox HC, Rocort, Tarcortin, Ulcort, Unicort

INDICATIONS & DOSAGE
Inflammation of corticosteroid-responsive dermatoses; adjunctive typical management of seborrheic dermatitis of scalp—
Adults and children: clean area; apply cream, lotion, ointment, or aerosol sparingly daily to q.i.d.
Aerosol: shake can well. Direct spray onto affected area from a distance of 6 inches. Apply for only 3 seconds (to avoid freezing tissues). Apply to dry scalp after shampooing; no need to massage or rub medication into scalp after spraying. Apply daily until acute phase is controlled, then reduce dosage to 1 to 3 times a week as needed to maintain control.

SIDE EFFECTS
Skin: burning, itching, irritation, dryness, folliculitis, hypopigmentation, hypertrichosis, acneiform eruptions, allergic contact dermatitis. *With occlusive dressings: maceration of skin, secondary infection, atrophy, striae, miliaria.*

INTERACTIONS
None significant.

NURSING CONSIDERATIONS
- Use cautiously in viral diseases of

---

skin, such as varicella, vaccinia, herpes simplex; fungal infections; skin tuberculosis; impaired circulation.
• Avoid application in or near eyes.
• Systemic absorption especially likely with occlusive dressings, prolonged treatment, or extensive body-surface treatment.
• Stop drug and notify doctor if patient develops signs of systemic absorption, skin irritation or ulceration, hypersensitivity, infection. (If antifungals or antibiotics are being used with corticosteroids and infection does not respond immediately, corticosteroids should be stopped until infection is controlled.)
• Before applying, gently wash skin. To prevent damage to skin, rub in medication gently, leaving a thin coat. When treating hairy sites, part hair and apply directly to lesions.
• Occlusive dressing: apply cream heavily, then cover with a thin, pliable, nonflammable plastic film; seal to adjacent normal skin with hypoallergenic tape. To minimize adverse reactions, use occlusive dressing intermittently. Occlusive dressings are generally not used in presence of infection or with weeping or exudative lesions.
• For patient with eczematous dermatitis who may develop irritation with adhesive material, it may be helpful to hold dressing in place with gauze, elastic bandages, or stockings.
• Notify doctor and remove occlusive dressing if body temperature rises.
• Aerosol preparation contains alcohol and may produce irritation or burning in open lesions. When using about the face, cover patient's eyes and warn against inhalation of the spray. To avoid freezing tissues, do not spray longer than 3 seconds or closer than 6 inches.
• Change dressing as ordered by doctor. Inspect skin for infection, striae,

and atrophy. Discontinue drug and notify doctor if these occur.
• Treatment should be continued for a few days following clearing of lesions to prevent recurrence.
• Instruct patient to report signs of drug sensitivity.
• The 0.5% strength is available without prescription.

---

hydrocortisone acetate
Cortifoam, Cortiprel, Cortef Acetate, Epifoam, Hydrocortisone Acetate, Hydrocortone Acetate, My-Cort Lotion
hydrocortisone valerate
Westcort Cream

INDICATIONS & DOSAGE
Inflammation of corticosteroid-responsive dermatoses—
Adults and children: clean area; apply lotion, cream, ointment, or foam (acetate) sparingly daily to q.i.d. Massage gently (valerate) 2 to 3 times daily p.r.n.

SIDE EFFECTS
Skin: burning, itching, irritation, dryness, folliculitis, hypopigmentation, hypertrichosis, acneiform eruptions, perioral dermatitis, allergic contact dermatitis. *With occlusive dressings: maceration of skin, secondary infection, atrophy, striae, miliaria.*

INTERACTIONS
None significant.

NURSING CONSIDERATIONS
• Use cautiously in viral diseases of skin, such as varicella, vaccinia, herpes simplex; fungal infections; skin tuberculosis; impaired circulation.
• Avoid application in or near eyes.
• Systemic absorption especially likely with occlusive dressings, pro-

---

Italicized side effects are common or life-threatening.

longed treatment, or extensive body-surface treatment.

• Stop drug and notify doctor if patient develops signs of systemic absorption, skin irritation or ulceration, hypersensitivity, infection. (If antifungals or antibiotics are being used with corticosteroids and infection does not respond immediately, corticosteroids should be stopped until infection is controlled.)

• Before applying, gently wash skin. To prevent damage to skin, rub in medication gently, leaving a thin coat. When treating hairy sites, part hair and apply directly to lesion.

• Occlusive dressing: apply cream or ointment heavily, then cover with a thin, pliable, nonflammable plastic film; seal to adjacent normal skin with hypoallergenic tape. To minimize adverse reactions, use occlusive dressings intermittently. Occlusive dressings are generally not used in presence of infection or with weeping or exudative lesions.

• For patient with eczematous dermatitis who may develop irritation with adhesive material, hold dressing in place with gauze, elastic bandages, or stockings.

• Notify doctor and remove occlusive dressing if body temperature rises.

• Lotions and foams are not used with occlusive dressings.

• Change dressing as ordered by doctor. Inspect skin for infection, striae, and atrophy. Discontinue drug and notify doctor if these occur.

• Treatment should be continued for a few days after clearing of lesions to prevent recurrence.

• Instruct patient to report signs of drug sensitivity.

• The 0.5% strength of hydrocortisone acetate is available without prescription.

methylprednisolone acetate
Medrol Acetate♦

INDICATIONS & DOSAGE
Inflammation of corticosteroid-responsive dermatoses—
Adults and children: clean area; apply ointment daily to t.i.d.

SIDE EFFECTS
Skin: burning, itching, irritation, dryness, folliculitis, hypopigmentation, hypertrichosis, acneiform eruptions, allergic contact dermatitis. *With occlusive dressings: maceration of skin, secondary infection, atrophy, striae, miliaria.*

INTERACTIONS
None significant.

NURSING CONSIDERATIONS
• Use cautiously in viral diseases of skin, such as varicella, vaccinia, herpes simplex; fungal infections; skin tuberculosis; impaired circulation.

• Avoid application in or near eyes.

• Systemic absorption especially likely with occlusive dressings, prolonged treatment, or extensive body-surface treatment.

• Stop drug and notify doctor if patient develops signs of systemic absorption, skin irritation or ulceration, hypersensitivity, infection. (If antifungals or antibiotics agents are being used with corticosteroids and infection does not respond immediately, corticosteroids should be stopped until infection is controlled.)

• Before applying, gently wash skin. To prevent damage to skin, rub in medication gently, leaving a thin coat. When treating hairy sites, part hair and apply directly to lesion.

• Occlusive dressing: apply ointment heavily, then cover with a thin, pliable, nonflammable plastic film; seal

to adjacent normal skin with hypoallergenic tape. To minimize adverse effects, use occlusive dressing intermittently. Occlusive dressings are generally not used in presence of infection or with weeping or exudative lesions.
• For patient with eczematous dermatitis who may develop irritation with adhesive material, hold dressing in place with gauze, elastic bandages, or stockings.
• Notify doctor and remove occlusive dressing if body temperature rises.
• Change dressing as ordered by doctor. Inspect skin for infection, striae, and atrophy. Discontinue drug and notify doctor if these occur.
• Treatment should be continued for a few days after clearing of lesions to prevent recurrence.
• Instruct patient to report signs of drug sensitivity.

---

prednisolone
Meti-Derm

INDICATIONS & DOSAGE
Inflammation of corticosteroid-responsive dermatoses—
Adults and children: clean area; apply cream t.i.d. or q.i.d.

SIDE EFFECTS
Skin: burning, itching, irritation, dryness, folliculitis, hypopigmentation, hypertrichosis, acneiform eruptions, perioral dermatitis, allergic contact dermatitis. *With occlusive dressings: maceration of skin, secondary infection, atrophy, striae, miliaria.*

INTERACTIONS
None significant.

NURSING CONSIDERATIONS
• Use cautiously in viral diseases of skin, such as varicella, vaccinia, herpes simplex; fungal infections; skin tuberculosis; impaired circulation.
• Avoid application in or near eyes.
• Systemic absorption especially likely with occlusive dressings, prolonged treatment, or extensive body-surface treatment.
• Stop drug and notify doctor if patient develops signs of systemic absorption, skin irritation or ulceration, hypersensitivity, infection. (If antifungals or antibiotics are being used with corticosteroids and infection does not respond immediately, corticosteroids should be stopped until infection is controlled.)
• Before applying, gently wash skin. To prevent damage to skin, rub in medication gently, leaving a thin coat. When treating hairy sites, part hair and apply directly to lesions.
• Occlusive dressing: apply cream heavily and cover with a thin, pliable, nonflammable plastic film; seal to adjacent normal skin with hypoallergenic tape. To minimize adverse reactions, use occlusive dressing intermittently. Occlusive dressings are generally not used in presence of infection or with weeping or exudative lesions.
• For patient with eczematous dermatitis who may develop irritation with adhesive material, hold dressing in place with gauze, elastic bandages, or stockings.
• Notify doctor and remove occlusive dressing if body temperature rises.
• Change dressing as ordered by doctor. Inspect skin for infection, striae, and atrophy. Discontinue drug and notify doctor if these occur.
• Treatment should be continued for a few days after clearing of lesions to prevent recurrence.
• Instruct patient to report signs of drug sensitivity.

---

triamcinolone acetonide

Aristocort♦, Aristocort A,
Kenalog♦, Triamalone♦♦

INDICATIONS & DOSAGE

Inflammation of corticosteroid-responsive dermatoses—
Adults and children: clean area; apply cream, ointment, lotion, foam, or aerosol sparingly b.i.d. to q.i.d.
Aerosol: shake can well. Direct spray onto affected area from a distance of approximately 6 inches and apply for only 3 seconds.

SIDE EFFECTS

Skin: burning, itching, irritation, dryness, folliculitis, hypopigmentation, hypertrichosis, acneiform eruptions, perioral dermatitis, allergic contact dermatitis. *With occlusive dressings: maceration of skin, secondary infection, atrophy, striae, miliaria.*

INTERACTIONS

None significant.

NURSING CONSIDERATIONS

• Use cautiously in viral diseases of skin, such as varicella, vaccinia, herpes simplex; fungal infections; skin tuberculosis; impaired circulation.
• Avoid application in or near eyes.
• Systemic absorption especially likely with occlusive dressings, prolonged treatment, or extensive body-surface treatment.
• Stop drug and notify doctor if patient develops signs of systemic absorption, skin irritation or ulceration, hypersensitivity, infection. (If anti-fungals or antibiotics are being used with corticosteroids and infection does not respond immediately, corticosteroids should be stopped until infection is controlled.)
• Before applying, gently wash skin. To prevent damage to skin, rub in medication gently, leaving a thin coat. When treating hairy sites, part hair and apply directly to lesion.
• Aerosol preparation contains alcohol and may produce irritation or burning in open lesions. When using about the face, cover patient's eyes and warn against inhalation of the spray. To avoid freezing tissues, do not spray longer than 3 seconds or closer than 6 inches.
• Occlusive dressing: apply cream or ointment heavily, then cover with a thin, pliable, nonflammable plastic film; seal to adjacent normal skin with hypoallergenic tape. To minimize adverse reactions, use occlusive dressing intermittently. Occlusive dressings are generally not used in presence of infection or with weeping or exudative lesions.
• For patient with eczematous dermatitis who may develop irritation with adhesive material, hold dressing in place with gauze, elastic bandages, or stockings.
• Notify doctor and remove occlusive dressing if body temperature rises.
• Change dressing as ordered by doctor. Inspect skin for infection, striae, and atrophy. Discontinue drug and notify doctor if these occur.
• Treatment should be continued for a few days after clearing of lesions to prevent recurrence.
• Instruct patient to report signs of drug sensitivity.

83

Antipruritics and topical anesthetics

benzocaine
camphor
dibucaine hydrochloride
dimethisoquin hydrochloride
diperodon monohydrate
dyclonine hydrochloride
ethyl chloride
lidocaine
lidocaine hydrochloride
menthol
phenol
pramoxine hydrochloride
tars
tetracaine
tetracaine hydrochloride

INTERACTIONS
None significant.

NURSING CONSIDERATIONS
• Contraindicated in hypersensitivity to procaine or other para-aminobenzoic acid (PABA) derivatives (often used in topical sun-blocking agents).
• Avoid contact with eyes.
• If spray preparation used, hold can 6 to 12 inches from affected area and spray liberally. Avoid inhalation.
• If using rectally, cleanse and thoroughly dry rectal area before applying.

---

benzocaine

Aerocaine, Americaine, Anbesol, Ben-Caine B.B., Benzocol, Col-Vi-Nol, Dermoplast, Hurricaine, Morusan, Rhulicream, Rhulihist, Solarcaine, Urolocaine

INDICATIONS & DOSAGE
Local anesthetic for pruritic dermatoses and localized idiopathic pruritus—
Adults and children: apply locally 2 or 3 times a day.
Hemorrhoids or rectal irritation—
Adults and children: apply ointment 2 or 3 times a day.
Suppository: insert well into rectum morning, evening, and after each bowel movement.

SIDE EFFECTS
Blood: methemoglobinemia (infants).
Local: sensitization.

---

camphor

INDICATIONS & DOSAGE
Mild antipruritic and local anesthetic; counterirritant for use in sprains and rheumatic conditions—
Adults and children: apply a 1% to 3% lotion or ointment of camphor, as needed.

SIDE EFFECTS
None reported.

INTERACTIONS
None significant.

NURSING CONSIDERATIONS
• Extremely toxic if taken orally.
• Avoid contact with eyes.
• Do not apply to broken skin or mucous membranes.

dibucaine hydrochloride
D-Caine, Dulzit, Nupercainal
Cream♦, Nupercainal Ointment♦,
Nupercainal Suppositories, Nuporals
(Troches)

INDICATIONS & DOSAGE
*Abrasions, sunburn, hemorrhoids,
and other painful conditions—*
Adults and children: 0.5% to 1%
lotion or ointment applied locally
several times a day.
Suppositories: insert rectally morning, evening, and after every bowel
movement.
Also used as a local anesthetic for
mouth and throat.

SIDE EFFECTS
Local: *hypersensitivity.*

INTERACTIONS
None significant.

NURSING CONSIDERATIONS
• Avoid contact with eyes.
• Before applying cream or ointment
rectally or inserting suppository,
cleanse and thoroughly dry rectal
area.

dimethisoquin hydrochloride
Quotane Cream♦♦, Quotane
Ointment

INDICATIONS & DOSAGE
Surface pain and itching—
Adults and children: 0.5% ointment
or lotion applied topically up to
4 times daily or as directed.

SIDE EFFECTS
Skin: *sensitization and contact dermatitis can develop.*

INTERACTIONS
None significant.

NURSING CONSIDERATIONS
• Don't apply to extensive areas.
• Avoid contact with eyes.
• Avoid prolonged use for patients
with chronic conditions.

diperodon monohydrate
Diothane Ointment♦, Proctodon

INDICATIONS & DOSAGE
*Pain caused by minor burns and cuts
(cream); pain caused by anorectal
disorders (ointment)—*
Adults and children: apply 3 to
4 times a day.

SIDE EFFECTS
Skin: rash, irritation, and other allergic manifestations.

INTERACTIONS
None significant.

NURSING CONSIDERATIONS
• Before applying cream or ointment
rectally, cleanse and thoroughly dry
rectal area.

dyclonine hydrochloride
Dyclone

INDICATIONS & DOSAGE
*To relieve surface pain and itching
caused by minor burns or trauma,
surgical wounds, pruritus ani or vulvae, insect bites, and pruritic dermatoses. Also, to anesthetize mucous
membranes before endoscopic procedures—*
Adults and children: 0.5% solution
or 1% ointment applied 3 or 4 times
daily.
*Urethral dilation or cystourethros-
copy—*
Adults: 10 ml of 0.5% solution may
be instilled into the urethra.

SIDE EFFECTS
Local: *irritation at site of application may occur.*

INTERACTIONS
None significant.

NURSING CONSIDERATIONS
• Avoid prolonged use in patients with chronic conditions.
• May be useful in patients hypersensitive to other local anesthetics because it is a ketone.
• Contraindicated in cystoscopic exams following an IVP. Iodine-containing contrast material will cause precipitate to form with dyclonine.
• Can be combined with diphenhydramine elixir to provide an effective treatment for stomatitis.

---

ethyl chloride
Ethyl Chloride Spray

INDICATIONS & DOSAGE
For irritation—
Adults and children: hold container about 24 inches from skin and spray rhythmically to cover area evenly once or twice. Application may be repeated.
As a local anesthetic in minor operative procedures; relieves pain caused by insect stings and burns, and irritation caused by myofascial and visceral pain syndromes—
Adults and children: dosage varies with different procedures. Use smallest dosage needed to produce desired effect. For local anesthesia, hold container about 12 inches from area to produce a fine spray.
Infants: hold a cotton ball saturated with ethyl chloride to injection site, and make injection when site dries.

SIDE EFFECTS
Skin: sensitization; *frostbite and tis-sue necrosis may occur with prolonged spraying.*
Other: excessive cooling may increase pain and muscle spasms.

INTERACTIONS
None significant.

NURSING CONSIDERATIONS
• Do not apply to broken skin or mucous membrane.
• Protect skin adjacent to treated area with petrolatum to avoid tissue sloughing.
• Avoid use near eyes.
• Avoid inhalation when spraying.
• Highly flammable; do not use in areas where open flames or sparks are possible.

---

lidocaine

lidocaine hydrochloride
Lida-Mantle Cream, Stanacaine, Xylocaine Jelly (2%), Xylocaine Ointment (2.5%)♦, Xylocaine Ointment (5%)♦, Xylocaine Solution (4%)♦, Xylocaine Viscous Solution (2%)

INDICATIONS & DOSAGE
Local anesthesia of skin or mucous membrane—
Adults and children: apply liberally.
In procedures involving the male or female urethra—
Adults: instill about 15 ml (male) or 3 to 5 ml (female) into urethra.
Pain, burning, or itching caused by burns, sunburn, or skin irritation—
Adults and children: apply liberally.

SIDE EFFECTS
Local: *hypersensitivity.*

INTERACTIONS
None significant.

NURSING CONSIDERATIONS
• Use with caution on severely trau-

Italicized side effects are common or life-threatening.

matized mucosa or where sepsis is present or for anesthesia of oropharyngeal mucosa, since gag reflex may be suppressed and aspiration may occur.
• The 4% solution can be sprayed.

menthol

INDICATIONS & DOSAGE
As an antipruritic—
Adults and children: apply 0.25% to 2% lotion or ointment, as needed.

SIDE EFFECTS
None reported.

INTERACTIONS
None significant.

NURSING CONSIDERATIONS
• Relieves itching by substituting a cooling effect.
• Avoid contact with eyes.

phenol

INDICATIONS & DOSAGE
As an antipruritic—
Adults and children: apply 0.5% to 2% preparations locally several times a day.

SIDE EFFECTS
None at recommended strengths.

INTERACTIONS
None significant.

NURSING CONSIDERATIONS
• Avoid accidental contact with normal skin. If contact occurs, remove phenol with alcohol or vegetable oil.
• Tissue necrosis possible with higher concentration or extensive use.
• Avoid contact with eyes.

pramoxine hydrochloride
Proctofoam, Tronothane♦

INDICATIONS & DOSAGE
Pain and itching caused by dermatoses, minor burns, surgical wounds, and insect bites, hemorrhoids—
Adults and children: apply every 3 to 4 hours.

SIDE EFFECTS
Local: stinging or burning, sensitization.

INTERACTIONS
None significant.

NURSING CONSIDERATIONS
• Can be safely used in those allergic to other local anesthetics.
• May be applied with gauze or sprayed directly on skin. Avoid contact with eyes.
• Cleanse and thoroughly dry rectal area before applying ointment or cream, or inserting suppository.

tars

INDICATIONS & DOSAGE
As an antipruritic—
Adults and children: apply preparations 2 to 3 times daily.

SIDE EFFECTS
Skin: irritation, folliculitis, erythema, photosensitivity.

INTERACTIONS
None significant.

NURSING CONSIDERATIONS
• Use caution in applying tar preparations to patients with exacerbation of psoriasis. May precipitate total body exfoliation.
• Never use under occlusive

dressings.
• Avoid excessive exposure to sunlight. May produce photo-sensitization.
• Darkens color of blond hair when applied to scalp.

---

tetracaine

tetracaine hydrochloride
Pontocaine♦

INDICATIONS & DOSAGE
For relief of pain in hemorrhoids, minor burns, ulcers, and poison ivy—
Adults and children: apply 5% oint-ment or 1% cream—no more than 1 oz for adults or ¼ oz for children in 24 hours.

SIDE EFFECTS
Local: *sensitization.*

INTERACTIONS
None significant.

NURSING CONSIDERATIONS
• Contraindicated in hypersensitivity to procaine or other para-aminoben-zoic acid (PABA) derivatives (often used in topical sun-blocking agents).
• Before applying cream or ointment rectally, cleanse and thoroughly dry rectal area.

84

Astringents

acetic acid lotion
aluminum acetate
aluminum sulfate
hamamelis water
tannic acid

acetic acid lotion
(0.1% glacial acetic acid in alcohol)

INDICATIONS & DOSAGE
Superficial fungal or bacterial infection to toughen skin and prevent bedsores—
Adults and children: apply and work into area, p.r.n.

SIDE EFFECTS
Skin: burning and irritation of denuded skin and mucous membrane.

INTERACTIONS
Heavy metals: causes precipitation of the metal acetate.

NURSING CONSIDERATIONS
• Contraindicated under occlusive dressings.
• Never confuse acetic acid solutions with *glacial* acetic acid solutions. Glacial form is a concentrate.
• Keep away from eyes and mucous membranes.
• Always apply to freshly cleansed area, free of other medications.
• Especially good for treating topical infection due to *Pseudomonas aeruginosa.*

aluminum acetate
(modified Burow's solution)
Acid Mantle Creme and Lotion♦, Buro-sol, Burowets, Burow's Emulsion, Burow's Lotion, Burow's Ointment

INDICATIONS & DOSAGE
Mild skin irritation from exposure to soaps, detergents, chemicals, diaper rash, acne, scaly skin, eczema—
Adults and children: apply p.r.n.
Relieve inflammation of poison ivy, insect bites, athlete's foot—
Adults and children: apply as wet dressing, p.r.n.
Ulcerative skin conditions—
Adults and children: apply ointment, p.r.n.

SIDE EFFECTS
Skin: irritation; extension of inflammation possible.

INTERACTIONS
None significant.

NURSING CONSIDERATIONS
• Contraindicated under occlusive dressings.
• Keep away from eyes and mucous membranes.
• Always apply to freshly cleansed area, free of other medications.
• May be used in place of boric acid ointment.
• Powder must be diluted in water to prescribed concentration.
• Discontinue if irritation develops.

• Clear solution may be stored at room temperature for up to 7 days.

---

aluminum sulfate
Bluboro Powder, Domeboro Powder♦ and Tablets♦, Soy-Sitz Powder

INDICATIONS & DOSAGE
Skin inflammation, insect bites, poison ivy, swelling, athlete's foot—
Adults and children: mix powder with 1 pint of water and apply every 15 to 30 minutes for 4 to 8 hours; bandage loosely.

SIDE EFFECTS
Skin: irritation; extension of inflammation possible.

INTERACTIONS
None significant.

NURSING CONSIDERATIONS
• Contraindicated under occlusive dressings; use open wet dressings only.
• When solution is prepared, immediately decant clear portion. Discard precipitate. Use only clear solution, *not* precipitate, for soaks. Never strain or filter solutions. Decanted portion may be stored at room temperature for up to 7 days.
• In general, no more than a third of the body should be treated at any one time, since excessive wet dressings may cause chilling and hypothermia.
• Keep away from eyes and mucous membranes.
• Discontinue if irritation develops.

---

hamamelis water
(witch hazel)
Hazel-Balm, Mediconet (wipes), Tucks (Cream, Ointment, Pads)

INDICATIONS & DOSAGE
Anal discomfort, itching, burning, minor external hemorrhoidal or outer vaginal discomfort, diaper rash—
Adults and children: apply t.i.d. or q.i.d.

SIDE EFFECTS
Skin: hypersensitivity.

INTERACTIONS
None significant.

NURSING CONSIDERATIONS
• Discontinue if irritation or itching does not improve.
• Use pads or wipes after toilet tissue to help prevent pruritus ani, vulvae.
• Cream can be used by nursing mother for nipple care, but wash area clean before nursing baby.
• Some products contain potential allergic sensitizers. Observe for allergic reactions.

---

tannic acid
Amertan Jelly, Dalidyne Lotion, Tanac

INDICATIONS & DOSAGE
Denture irritation; trench mouth; gingivitis; throat irritation; herpes simplex; oral cavity lesions; adjunctive treatment of second- and third-degree thermal, chemical, or electrical burns—
Adults: apply with cotton applicator. As gargle or mouthwash, ½ teaspoon of solution in ½ glass of warm water, p.r.n.
Cold sores, throat irritation, oral cav-

---

*ity lesions, some second- and third-de-
gree burns—*
Children: apply with cotton
applicator.

SIDE EFFECTS
Local: stinging.
Other: large amounts in burn treat-
ment can cause hepatic damage.

INTERACTIONS
Organic salts of heavy metals: will
precipitate tannate salt of heavy
metal. Do not apply.

NURSING CONSIDERATIONS
• Incompatible with organic salts of
heavy metals. Apply only to surfaces
free of other medication.

• Produces a firm eschar on burned
area that helps protect burned tissue
from infection and loss of body fluids,
and comforts patient.
• Apply only after proper debridement of burn.
• Prepare aqueous solutions freshly,
as they are unstable.
• Light and air cause solution to
darken, which reduces potency.
• Avoid extensive application and
prolonged use on denuded tissue to
decrease possibility of systemic toxicity from absorption.
• Slight stinging on application soon
subsides.

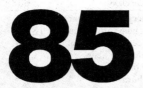

Antiseptics and disinfectants

alcohol, ethyl
alcohol, isopropyl
benzalkonium chloride
boric acid
chlorhexidine gluconate
formaldehyde
glutaraldehyde
hexachlorophene
hydrogen peroxide
iodine
merbromin
nitromersol
oxychlorosene calcium
oxychlorosene sodium
phenylmercuric nitrate
poloxamer iodine
potassium permanganate
povidone-iodine
silver protein, mild
sodium hypochlorite
thiomerosal

alcohol, ethyl
Alcohol, Ethanol

INDICATIONS & DOSAGE
To disinfect skin, instruments, and ampules—disinfect as needed.

SIDE EFFECTS
Skin: dryness.

INTERACTIONS
None significant.

NURSING CONSIDERATIONS
• Effective as fat solvent germicidal; ineffective against spore-forming organisms, tubercle bacilli, viruses.

• Alcohol used as 70% solution known commonly as "rubbing alcohol."
• Don't use on skin before insulin administration. May affect potency of insulin.

alcohol, isopropyl
isopropyl alcohol 99%, isopropyl rubbing alcohol 70%, isopropyl aqueous alcohol 75%

INDICATIONS & DOSAGE
To disinfect skin, instruments, and ampules— disinfect as needed.

SIDE EFFECTS
Skin: dryness.

INTERACTIONS
None significant.

NURSING CONSIDERATIONS
• Isopropyl alcohol is slightly more effective than ethyl alcohol as an antibacterial agent, but it also tends to cause more dryness.
• 75% solution for disinfection and storage of thermometers.
• Not effective against spore-forming organisms, tubercle bacilli, or viruses.
• Combined with formaldehyde, makes effective germicide.

benzalkonium chloride
Benasept, Benzachlor-50♦♦, Benz-All, Drapolex♦♦, Ionax Foam♦♦, Ionax Scrub♦♦, Sabol♦♦, Spensomide, Zalkon, Zalkonium Chloride, Zephiran

INDICATIONS & DOSAGE
Preop disinfection of unbroken skin—apply 1:750 to 1:1,000 tincture or spray.
Disinfection of mucous membranes and denuded skin—apply 1:10,000 to 1:5,000 aqueous solution.
Irrigation of vagina—instill 1:5,000 to 1:2,000.
Irrigation of bladder or urethra—instill 1:20,000 to 1:5,000.
Irrigation of deep infected wounds—instill 1:20,000 to 1:3,000.
Preservation of metallic instruments, ampules, thermometers, and rubber articles—wipe with or soak objects in 1:5,000 to 1:750 solution.
Disinfection of operating room equipment—wipe with 1:5,000 solution.

SIDE EFFECTS
Skin: hypersensitivity.

INTERACTIONS
Soaps: inactivate benzalkonium chloride. Remove soap traces with alcohol.

NURSING CONSIDERATIONS
• Germicidal for some nonspore-forming organisms and fungi. No effect on tubercle bacilli. Limited viricidal use.
• Used as preservative in ophthalmic solutions.
• Before applying to skin, remove all traces of soap with water and apply 70% alcohol.
• Don't store cotton, wool gauze, or sponges in solution. They absorb benzalkonium chloride and reduce the strength of the solution.
• Don't use with occlusive dressings or vaginal packs.
• Store in bottles with screw caps.
• Incompatible with iodine, silver nitrate, fluorescein, nitrates, peroxide, lanolin, potassium permanganate, aluminum, caramel, kaolin, pine oil, zinc sulfate, zinc oxide, and yellow oxide of mercury.
• To prevent rust of metallic instruments stored in benzalkonium chloride, add sodium nitrite to final solution. Change solution weekly.
• Available also as 17% concentrate (Zephiran). Even after dilution, this form of Zephiran should be used only on inanimate objects.

boric acid
Bluboro, boric acid solution 5%, Borofax♦, Ting

INDICATIONS & DOSAGE
Skin conditions (athlete's foot) as a compress, powder, or ointment (2% to 5%)—
Adults and children: apply as directed.

SIDE EFFECTS
Signs of systemic absorption:
CNS: delirium, convulsions, restlessness, headache.
CV: *circulatory collapse,* tachycardia.
GI: irritation, nausea, vomiting, diarrhea.
GU: renal damage.
Other: hypothermia.

INTERACTIONS
None significant.

NURSING CONSIDERATIONS
• Mild antiseptic and astringent.
• Not absorbed through intact skin, but in high concentrations, may be absorbed through abraded skin or granulating wounds.

- Avoid long-term use.
- Ingestion of 5 g (infants) or 20 g (adults) may be fatal.

---

chlorhexidine gluconate
Hibiclens Liquid, Hibitane

INDICATIONS & DOSAGE
Surgical hand scrub, hand wash, skin wound cleanser—use p.r.n.

SIDE EFFECTS
EENT: irritating to eyes. Causes deafness if instilled into middle ear through perforated eardrum.

INTERACTIONS
None significant.

NURSING CONSIDERATIONS
- Bactericidal. Broad spectrum.
- Can be used many times a day without causing irritations or dryness.
- Low potential for producing skin reactions.
- Rinse skin thoroughly after use.
- Keep out of eyes and ears.
- Action is residual. Do not cleanse skin with alcohol after application.

---

formaldehyde
Formalin (37% solution of formaldehyde)

INDICATIONS & DOSAGE
Cold sterilization of equipment—disinfect as needed.
Tissue preservative—cover tissue.

SIDE EFFECTS
EENT: fumes cause eye, nose, and throat irritation.
Skin: irritation.
Other: pungent odor.

INTERACTIONS
None significant.

NURSING CONSIDERATIONS
- 0.5% solution germicidal against all forms of microorganisms, including spores, in 6 to 12 hours; 10% solution used to disinfect inanimate objects.
- Not affected by organic matter.
- Used with alcohol and sodium nitrite to disinfect instruments and articles that can't tolerate heat (cold sterilization).
- Avoid skin or mucous membrane contact with solutions greater than 0.5%.
- Always dilute 37% solution.

---

glutaraldehyde
Cidex ◆

INDICATIONS & DOSAGE
Cold sterilization of surgical instruments—cover instruments with 2% solution.
Fumigate hospital and operating rooms—fog with aerosol.

SIDE EFFECTS
Skin: irritation.

INTERACTIONS
None significant.

NURSING CONSIDERATIONS
- Excellent disinfectant; broad spectrum of activity against gram-positive and gram-negative bacteria (vegetative and spores), viruses, and fungi.
- Use on inanimate objects only.
- Comes with activator that must be mixed before use to yield active acidic glutaraldehyde.
- Not affected by organic matter.
- Whenever possible, use commercially prepared 2% solution rather than diluting the 25% solution.

Italicized side effects are common or life-threatening.

hexachlorophene

Germa-Medica "MG," Hexamead-Ph, pHisoHex♦, pHisoScrub, Sept-Soft, Septisol Soy-Dome Cleanser, WescoHEX

INDICATIONS & DOSAGE

Surgical scrub, bacteriostatic skin cleanser—use as directed in 0.25% to 3% concentrations.

SIDE EFFECTS

Note: systemic absorption can cause neurotoxic effects, including irritability, generalized clonic muscular contractions, decerebrate rigidity, convulsions, optic atrophy. (Systemic absorption has occurred only when used on premature infants, mucous membranes, and broken skin and burns.)
Skin: dermatitis, mild scaling, dryness (especially when combined with excessive scrubbing).

INTERACTIONS

None significant.

NURSING CONSIDERATIONS

• Use with caution in infants (especially premature infants) and burn patients. These patients tend to absorb hexachlorophene through the skin and may develop neurotoxic effects.
• Bacteriostatic agent. Spectrum of activity limited to gram-positive organisms, especially staphylococcus.
• Must be used preop for at least 3 days for maximum effectiveness.
• After cleaning area, rinse thoroughly (especially the scrotum and perineum). Do not apply alcohol or organic solvents to cleansed area.

hydrogen peroxide

3% to 6% solution

INDICATIONS & DOSAGE

Cleansing wound—use 1.5% to 3% solution.
Mouth wash for necrotizing ulcerative gingivitis—gargle with 3% solution.
Cleansing douche—use 2% solution.

SIDE EFFECTS

EENT: excessive use as mouthwash causes "hairy tongue."

INTERACTIONS

None significant.

NURSING CONSIDERATIONS

• Germicidal.
• Don't inject into closed body cavities or abscesses; generated gas can't escape.
• Dilute concentrate with 1 to 4 parts water.
• Useful to remove mucus from inner cannula of tracheostomy tube.
• Store tightly capped in cool dry place. Protect from light and heat.
• Do not shake bottle. This causes decomposition.

iodine

solution (2% iodine and 2.4% sodium and iodide in water)♦, tincture (2% iodine and 2.4% sodium iodide in diluted alcohol), Sepp Antiseptic Applicators (2% mild iodine tincture), strong iodine tincture (7% iodine and 5% potassium iodide in diluted alcohol)

INDICATIONS & DOSAGE

Preop disinfection of skin (small wounds and abraded areas)—apply p.r.n.

SIDE EFFECTS
Skin: irritation, redness, swelling (sign of hypersensitivity).

INTERACTIONS
None significant.

NURSING CONSIDERATIONS
• Microbicidal agent effective against bacteria, fungi, viruses, protozoa, and yeasts.
• If skin reaction develops, remove iodine residue from skin and stop use.
• To prevent skin irritation, do not cover areas treated with iodine.
• Aqueous solution less irritating.
• Sodium thiosulfate renders iodine colorless and is used to remove stains. It is also antidote of choice for accidental ingestion.

merbromin
Mercurochrome (2% aqueous solution)

INDICATIONS & DOSAGE
General antiseptic and first aid prophylactic—
Adults and children: apply p.r.n. as 1% to 2% solution or tincture.

SIDE EFFECTS
Skin: sensitization.

INTERACTIONS
None significant.

NURSING CONSIDERATIONS
• Bacteriostatic.
• Least effective mercurial antiseptic. Its activity is decreased in presence of organic matter.
• Cleanse injury with soap and water before applying. Let dry.
• Stains may be removed with 2% permanganate solution, followed by 5% oxalic acid solution.
• Never heat solution.

• To prepare 1% solution, dilute with equal parts water.

nitromersol
Metaphen

INDICATIONS & DOSAGE
*Disinfection of instruments—*soak in 0.04% solution.
Disinfection of skin— apply 0.2 to 0.5% solution to area p.r.n.
*Irrigation of mucous membranes (eye, urethra)—*instill 0.01 to 0.02% solution as directed.
*Skin antiseptic for abrasions—*apply 0.2% solution to area.

SIDE EFFECTS
Skin: erythematous, papular, or vesicular eruptions indicate hypersensitivity; irritation.

INTERACTIONS
None significant.

NURSING CONSIDERATIONS
• Contraindicated in hypersensitivity to mercury compounds.
• Do not use when aluminum may come in contact with skin.
• Incompatible with permanganates, strong acids, and heavy metal salts.
• Prepare as needed. Solutions tend to precipitate on standing.

oxychlorosene calcium
Clorpactin XCB
oxychlorosene sodium
Clorpactin WCS-90

INDICATIONS & DOSAGE
*Topical antiseptic for local infections, preoperative skin cleanser (sodium salt)—*apply as spray, soak, wet dressing, or irrigation as a 4% solution.
Ophthalmic and urologic irrigant (sodium salt)— 0.1% to 0.2% solution.

Local irrigation during surgery (calcium salt)—use 0.5% solution.

SIDE EFFECTS
Skin: local irritation.

INTERACTIONS
None significant.

NURSING CONSIDERATIONS
• Effective against bacteria, fungi, viruses, yeast, and spores.
• Powder reconstituted in saline.
• Refrigerate dry crystal until reconstitution.

---

phenylmercuric nitrate
Phe-Mer-Nite

INDICATIONS & DOSAGE
Preop disinfection—apply p.r.n. as a 0.1% to 0.2% solution.

SIDE EFFECTS
Skin: rash.

INTERACTIONS
None significant.

NURSING CONSIDERATIONS
• Contraindicated in hypersensitivity to mercury-containing compounds.
• Antiseptic and fungicidal.
• Frequent or prolonged use may cause mercury poisoning.
• Orange stain removed with soap and water.
• Commonly used as a preservative in ophthalmic solutions.

---

poloxamer iodine
Prepodyne, SeptoDyne

INDICATIONS & DOSAGE
Preop skin prep and scrub, wound disinfection—use as directed.

SIDE EFFECTS
None reported.

INTERACTIONS
None significant.

NURSING CONSIDERATIONS
• Contraindicated in hypersensitivity to iodines.
• Prolonged germicidal action.
• Water-soluble solution releases iodine at predetermined rate, causing prolonged action.
• Relatively nonirritating to skin.

---

potassium permanganate

INDICATIONS & DOSAGE
Topical antiseptic—apply 1:10,000 to 1:500 solution.
Vaginal douche—instill 1:5,000 to 1:1,000 solution as directed.

SIDE EFFECTS
Skin: solutions greater than 1:5,000 are irritating to skin.

INTERACTIONS
Iodine: precipitates iodine salt. Do not use together.

NURSING CONSIDERATIONS
• Antiseptic astringent with fungicidal properties.
• Germicidal effects reduced by organic matter.
• Stains caused by potassium permanganate removed with dilute acids (lemon juice, oxalic acid, or dilute hydrochloric acid).
• Never mix with charcoal or give charcoal as antidote. May explode.

povidone-iodine
ACU-dyne, Aerodine, Betadine♦,
BPS, Bridine♦♦, Efodine, Final Step,
Frepp, Frepp/Sepp, Isodine, Mallisol,
Polydine, Proviodine♦♦, Sepp

INDICATIONS & DOSAGE
*Many uses, including preop skin prep
and scrub, germicide for surface
wounds, postop application to incisions, miscellaneous disinfection—*
Adults: apply p.r.n.

SIDE EFFECTS
Skin: local hypersensitivity reactions.

INTERACTIONS
None significant.

NURSING CONSIDERATIONS
• Germicidal activity of iodine without irritation to skin and mucous
membranes.
• Thought to be superior to soap as a
disinfectant; less effective than
aqueous or alcoholic solutions of
iodine.
• Treated areas may be bandaged or
taped.
• Germicidal activity reduced if area
cleansed with alcohol or other organic
solvents after application of povidone-
iodine.
• Prolonged, excessive use may lead
to systemic absorption and toxicity.

silver protein, mild
Argyrol S.S.♦, Silvol, Solargentum

INDICATIONS & DOSAGE
*Topical application for inflammation
of eye, nose, throat—*
Adults and children: apply p.r.n. as
a 5% to 25% solution.

SIDE EFFECTS
Skin: argyria in long-term use.

INTERACTIONS
None significant.

NURSING CONSIDERATIONS
• Store in amber glass bottles; protect
from light.

sodium hypochlorite
5% solution (instruments, swimming
pools), 0.5% aqueous solution for
wounds, Modified Dakins
Solution

INDICATIONS & DOSAGE
*Athlete's foot, wound irrigation, disin-
fection of walls and floors—*apply as
directed.

SIDE EFFECTS
Skin: irritation.

INTERACTIONS
None significant.

NURSING CONSIDERATIONS
• Germicidal and weakly fungicidal.
• Interferes locally with thrombin
formation, delaying blood clotting.
Dissolves necrotic tissue.
• Unstable in solution. Make fresh
solution and use immediately.
• Avoid contact with hair due to its
bleaching properties.

thiomerosal
Aeroaid Thiomerosal, Merthiolate

INDICATIONS & DOSAGE
*Preop disinfection of skin; antiseptic
for open wounds—*apply or instill to
affected area daily, b.i.d., or t.i.d. as
a 0.1% solution or tincture.

SIDE EFFECTS
Skin: erythematous, vesicular, papular eruptions (indicate hypersensitivity); irritation with tincture.

Italicized side effects are common or life-threatening.

INTERACTIONS
None significant.

NURSING CONSIDERATIONS
• Contraindicated in hypersensitivity to mercury-containing compounds.
• Do not use when aluminum may come in contact with skin.
• Incompatible with permanganate, strong acids, salts of heavy metals.

• Cleanse wound thoroughly before applying tincture.
• To prevent skin irritation, allow tincture to dry completely before applying dressing.
• Can be instilled into body cavities.
• Store in amber glass container.

86

Emollients, demulcents, and protectants

aluminum paste
calamine
collodion, U.S.P.
flexible collodion
compound benzoin tincture
dexpanthenol
glycerin
hydrophilic lotion
hydrophilic ointment
hydrophilic petrolatum
hydrous wool fat lotion
hydrous wool fat and castor oil
liquid petrolatum
methyl salicylate
oatmeal
para-aminobenzoic acid
petrolatum
silicone
starch
talc
urea or carbamide
vitamins A and D ointment
zinc gelatin

aluminum paste
(10% aluminum in zinc oxide ointment with liquid petrolatum)

INDICATIONS & DOSAGE
Emollient and protectant: colostomy area or other surgical sites—apply p.r.n.

SIDE EFFECTS
None.

INTERACTIONS
Topical enzymes: aluminum may inactivate preparations used to debride wounds. Don't use together.

NURSING CONSIDERATIONS
• Zinc oxide paste can be used as an alternative.
• Observe for inflammation or infection since protectants are occlusive layers that retain moisture, exclude air, and trap cutaneous bacteria.
• Skin should be cleaned daily or more often as needed.
• Emollients and protectants may be used alone, as vehicles for medications, or with other topical medications. Check with doctor.

calamine
liniment (15% calamine), lotion (8% calamine), ointment (17% calamine), Rhulihist (3% calamine), Rhulispray (1% calamine)

INDICATIONS & DOSAGE
Topical astringent and protectant: itching, poison ivy and poison oak, nonpoisonous insect bites, mild sunburn, minor skin irritations—apply p.r.n.

SIDE EFFECTS
Skin: transient light stinging, irritation, dry skin.

INTERACTIONS
None significant.

NURSING CONSIDERATIONS

- Contraindicated in hypersensitivity to any of the components.
- Watch for sensitivity reactions to calamine. Preparations containing antihistamines can cause sensitivity.
- Always shake well before use.
- Don't use cotton to apply; it will absorb the solute. Use gauze sponge.
- Do not apply to blistered, raw, or oozing areas of the skin.
- Toxic if taken internally.
- Observe for inflammation or infection since protectants are occlusive layers that retain moisture, exclude air, and trap skin bacteria.
- Skin should be cleaned daily or more often as needed.
- Emollients, demulcents, protectants may be used alone, as vehicles for medications, or with other topical medications. Check with doctor.
- Highly flammable; never use near flame.
- May irritate and dry skin.
- Keep container tightly closed so solvent won't evaporate.

---

collodion, U.S.P.
(5% pyroxylin in 1 part alcohol, 3 parts ether)
flexible collodion
(5% pyroxylin in 1 part alcohol, 3 parts ether plus 20% camphor, 30% castor oil)

INDICATIONS & DOSAGE
Protectant; vehicle for other medicinal agents; and sealant for small wounds— apply to dry skin, p.r.n., or use flexible collodion when a flexible noncontracting film is desired.

SIDE EFFECTS
None.

INTERACTIONS
None significant.

NURSING CONSIDERATIONS

- Observe for inflammation or infection since protectants are occlusive layers that retain moisture, exclude air, and trap cutaneous bacteria.
- Skin should be cleaned daily or more often as needed.
- Protectants may be used alone, as vehicles for medications, or with other topical medications. Check with doctor.
- Camphor in flexible collodion is weakly antiseptic and antipruritic; may irritate and dry skin.
- Highly flammable; never use near flame.
- Keep container tightly closed so solvent won't evaporate.
- Toxic if taken internally.
- Avoid excessive inhalation of vapors.

---

compound benzoin tincture
(10% benzoin in alcohol mixed with glycerin and water)
Benzoin Spray

INDICATIONS & DOSAGE
Demulcent and protectant: cutaneous ulcers, bedsores, cracked nipples, fissures of lips and anus— apply locally once daily or b.i.d.

SIDE EFFECTS
None.

INTERACTIONS
None significant.

NURSING CONSIDERATIONS
- Do not apply to acutely inflamed areas.
- Observe for inflammation or infection since protectants are occlusive layers that retain moisture, exclude air, and trap cutaneous bacteria.
- Skin should be cleaned daily or more often as needed.
- Protectants may be used alone, as

Unmarked trade names available in the United States only.
◆ Also available in Canada　　◆◆ Available in Canada only.

vehicles for medications, or with other topical medications. Check with doctor.
• For demulcent and expectorant action in laryngitis or croup, use in boiling water and have patient inhale vapors.
• Spray is not intended for use as inhalant.
• Can be mixed with magnesium-aluminum hydroxide and applied on bedsores.

dexpanthenol
Panthoderm Cream♦ (dexpanthenol 2% in a water-miscible cream base), Panthoderm Lotion (dexpanthenol 2%, menthol 0.1%, and camphor 0.1%)

INDICATIONS & DOSAGE
Epithelial-bed stimulator in emollient base: itching, wounds, insect bites, poison ivy, poison oak, diaper rash, chafing, mild eczema, decubitus ulcers, dry lesions—apply topically, p.r.n.

SIDE EFFECTS
None.

INTERACTIONS
None significant.

NURSING CONSIDERATIONS
• Contraindicated in wounds of hemophilia patients.
• Before each new application *always* thoroughly cleanse affected area, removing all traces of previously applied medication. Observe for inflammation or infection.
• Dry lesions respond better than oozing lesions.
• May heal skin lesions in mild eczema and dermatoses.

glycerin
Corn Huskers Lotion (tragacanth 1 g, glycerin 30 ml, propylene glycol 10 ml)

INDICATIONS & DOSAGE
Emollient and lubricant: rectal tubes and catheters; dry skin, hands—apply p.r.n.

SIDE EFFECTS
None.

INTERACTIONS
None significant.

NURSING CONSIDERATIONS
• Applied undiluted to inflamed, dehydrated skin. Paradoxically, excessive use may dry the skin.
• Diluted with rose water, glycerin is useful for irritated or dry lips.

hydrophilic lotion
(white petrolatum 4.2 g, stearyl alcohol 4.2 g, methylparaben 0.004 g, propylparaben 0.002 g, sodium lauryl sulfate 0.167 g, propylene glycol 2 ml, perfume q.s., purified water)

INDICATIONS & DOSAGE
Protectant and emollient: dry skin, irritation—apply p.r.n.

SIDE EFFECTS
None.

INTERACTIONS
None significant.

NURSING CONSIDERATIONS
• Observe for inflammation or infection since protectants are occlusive layers that retain moisture, exclude air, and trap skin bacteria.
• Skin should be cleaned daily or more often as needed.

Italicized side effects are common or life-threatening.

• Emollients and protectants may be used alone, as vehicles for medications, or with other topical medications. Check with doctor.

hydrophilic ointment

Cetaphil, Heb Cream Base, Multibase, Neobase, Unibase, Vanibase (methylparaben 0.025 g, propylparaben 0.015 g, stearyl alcohol 25 g, white petrolatum 25 g, propylene glycol 12 g, sodium lauryl sulfate 1 g, purified water)

INDICATIONS & DOSAGE

Protectant and emollient: dry skin, oozing lesions—apply p.r.n.

SIDE EFFECTS

None.

INTERACTIONS

None significant.

NURSING CONSIDERATIONS

• Easily removed with water.
• Use when little penetration of medicinal agent is desired.
• Observe for inflammation or infection since protectants are occlusive layers that retain moisture, exclude air, and trap skin bacteria.
• Skin should be cleaned daily or more often as needed.
• Emollients and protectants may be used alone, as vehicles for medications, or with other topical medications. Check with doctor.

hydrophilic petrolatum

Aquaphor, Hydrosort, Plastibase Hydrophilic, Polysort (cholesterol 3 g, stearyl alcohol 3 g, white wax 8 g, white petrolatum 86 g)

INDICATIONS & DOSAGE

Protectant and emollient: dry skin,
eczema, or psoriasis—mix with other medicinal ingredients as ordered, and apply p.r.n.

SIDE EFFECTS

None.

INTERACTIONS

None significant.

NURSING CONSIDERATIONS

• Not water-soluble; greasy.
• Observe for inflammation or infection since protectants are occlusive layers that retain moisture, exclude air, and trap skin bacteria.
• Skin should be cleaned daily or more often as needed.
• Emollients and protectants may be used alone, as vehicles for medications, or with other topical medications. Check with doctor.

hydrous wool fat

Lanolin Lotion (stearic acid 2 g, triethanolamine 0.8 ml, light liquid petrolatum 10 ml, propylparaben 0.2 g, rose water)

hydrous wool fat and castor oil

(hydrous wool fat 25 g, castor oil 25 g, ceresin wax 5 g, polysorbate 60 5 g, white petrolatum)

INDICATIONS & DOSAGE

Protectant and emollient—apply hydrous wool fat p.r.n.
Protection against hydrocarbons, solvents, and cutting oils—apply hydrous wool fat and castor oil before exposure.

SIDE EFFECTS

Skin: allergic rash.

INTERACTIONS

None significant.

NURSING CONSIDERATIONS
• Contraindicated in hypersensitivity to lanolin.
• Don't confuse with anhydrous wool fat, which will dry skin if applied alone.
• Observe for inflammation or infection since protectants are occlusive layers that retain moisture, exclude air, and trap skin bacteria.
• Skin should be cleaned daily or more often as needed.
• Emollients and protectants may be used alone, as vehicles for medications, or with other topical medications. Check with doctor.

liquid petrolatum
Liquid Petrolatum, U.S.P., Light Liquid Petrolatum, N.F., Mineral Oil

INDICATIONS & DOSAGE
Protectant and emollient—apply locally, full strength, or diluted.

SIDE EFFECTS
None.

INTERACTIONS
None significant.

NURSING CONSIDERATIONS
• Occasionally used with other drugs.
• Exists in two forms: light mineral oil and heavy mineral oil.
• Heavy mineral oil can be used internally as a laxative. Never use light mineral oil as a laxative. Mineral oil used as nose drops can cause lipid pneumonia.
• Observe for inflammation or infection since protectants are occlusive layers that retain moisture, exclude air, and trap skin bacteria.
• Skin should be cleaned daily or more often as needed.
• Emollients and protectants may be used alone, as vehicles for medica-

tions, or with other topical medications. Check with doctor.

methyl salicylate
Banalg, Baumodyne Gel and Ointment, Betula Oil, Gaultheria Oil, Sweet Birch Oil, Wintergreen Oil

INDICATIONS & DOSAGE
Counterirritant: minor pains of osteoarthritis, rheumatism, sprains, muscle and tendon soreness and tightness, lumbago, sciatica—
Adults: apply with gentle massage several times daily.
Not recommended for children.

SIDE EFFECTS
Skin: rash, irritation, burning, blistering.

INTERACTIONS
None significant.

NURSING CONSIDERATIONS
• Never apply directly, undiluted to skin.
• Warning: as little as 4 ml ingested by children can cause fatal toxicity; in adults as little as 30 ml. Since GI absorption may be delayed, treat such ingestion with emetic lavage, then a saline cathartic. Continue lavage until no odor of methyl salicylate can be detected in the washings.
• Absorbed through skin; prolonged increased application can cause toxicity. Toxic effects include hyperpnea leading to respiratory alkalosis, nausea, vomiting, tinnitus, hyperpyrexia, and convulsions.
• Discontinue if rash or redness occurs. Consult doctor if pain or redness persists more than 10 days.
• Avoid getting near eyes, open wounds, mucous membranes.
• Do not use on sunburned membranes.

Italicized side effects are common or life-threatening.

- Do not wrap or bandage treated area.
- Store in tightly closed container.

oatmeal
Aveeno Colloidal, Aveeno Oilated Bath (with liquid petrolatum and hypoallergenic lanolin)

INDICATIONS & DOSAGE
Emollient and demulcent: local irritation—use as a lotion; 1 level tablespoon to a cup of warm water.
Skin irritation, pruritus, common dermatoses, dry skin—
Adults: 1 packet in tub of warm water.
Children: 1 to 2 rounded tablespoons in 3 to 4 inches of bath water.
Infants: 2 or 3 level teaspoons, depending on size of bath.

SIDE EFFECTS
None.

INTERACTIONS
None significant.

NURSING CONSIDERATIONS
- Not to be ingested. Don't confuse with oatmeal as food.
- Instruct patient to exercise caution to avoid slipping in tub.
- Avoid getting in eyes.

para-aminobenzoic acid
PABA♦, Pabagel♦, Pabanol♦, Pre-Sun♦, PreSun Gel, RV Paba Lipstick, Sunbrella Lotion

INDICATIONS & DOSAGE
Topical protectant: sunburn protection, sun-sensitive skin, slow tanning—
Adults: apply evenly to dry skin; follow directions on various products for number and time of application,
which vary from 2 to 6 hours; reapply after swimming.
Not recommended for children.

SIDE EFFECTS
Local: allergic reaction, irritation, sensitization.
Skin: photocontact dermatitis.

INTERACTIONS
None significant.

NURSING CONSIDERATIONS
- Contraindicated in hypersensitivity to any of the components and for persons with damaged or diseased skin.
- Discontinue if skin rash occurs.
- Encourage slow tanning and short exposure to sun.
- Avoid contact with eyes and lids.
- Avoid contact with open flame.
- May stain clothing.
- Observe for inflammation and infection since protectants produce an occlusive layer that retains perspiration, excludes air, and traps cutaneous bacteria, producing sites for anaerobic infections.

petrolatum
Vaseline

INDICATIONS & DOSAGE
Topical protectant and emollient—use alone or with other drugs, as directed.

SIDE EFFECTS
None.

INTERACTIONS
None significant.

NURSING CONSIDERATIONS
- Stable, does not become rancid.
- Observe for inflammation or infection since protectants are occlusive layers that retain moisture, exclude air, and trap skin bacteria.

Unmarked trade names available in the United States only.
♦ Also available in Canada   ♦ ♦ Available in Canada only.

- Skin should be cleaned daily or more often as needed.
- Emollients and protectants may be used alone, as vehicles for medications, or with other topical medications. Check with doctor.

silicone
Silicone and Zinc Oxide Compound, Silon Spray

INDICATIONS & DOSAGE
Topical protectant: dermatoses, diaper rash, decubitus ulcers—apply b.i.d. or t.i.d. in ointment.
Protection against water and corrosive chemicals—apply before exposure.

SIDE EFFECTS
None.

INTERACTIONS
None significant.

NURSING CONSIDERATIONS
- Protect eyes against spray.
- Very difficult to remove from skin; resistant to water and soap.
- Will not protect against oils or solvents.
- Observe for inflammation or infection since protectants are occlusive layers that retain moisture, exclude air, and trap cutaneous bacteria.
- Skin should be cleaned daily or more often as needed.
- Protectants may be used alone, as vehicles for medications, or with other topical medications. Check with doctor.

starch
Linit

INDICATIONS & DOSAGE
Demulcent: minor skin irritations, pruritus associated with common der-matoses—mix 2 cups of starch with 4 cups of water, add to tub of water, and soak affected area for 30 minutes.

SIDE EFFECTS
None.

INTERACTIONS
None significant.

NURSING CONSIDERATIONS
- Instruct patient to exercise caution to avoid slipping in tub.

talc (magnesium silicate)

INDICATIONS & DOSAGE
Topical lubricant, protectant, drying agent, absorbent dusting powder: irritation such as intertrigo prickly heat—sprinkle on affected areas p.r.n. for soothing and lubrication.

SIDE EFFECTS
None.

INTERACTIONS
None significant.

NURSING CONSIDERATIONS
- Don't use on surgical gloves; causes granulation and adhesions in open wounds.
- Avoid dust entering eyes or inhalation of talc dust.
- Should not be used on open, weeping surfaces; it cakes and crusts.

Italicized side effects are common or life-threatening.

urea or carbamide

Aquacare Dry Skin Cream and Lotion♦, Aquacare/HP Cream and Lotion♦, Aqua Lacten, Artra Ashy Skin Cream, Carmol Ten, Carmol Twenty, Gormel Cream, Nutraplus♦, Rea-Lo, Ultra-Mide, Uremol♦♦, Urtex♦♦

INDICATIONS & DOSAGE

Emollient: hard, dry skin on hands, elbows, or knees—

Adults: apply to affected area b.i.d. or t.i.d., particularly after exposure to sun or wind.

Not recommended for children.

SIDE EFFECTS

Skin: transient stinging when applied to irritated or fissured skin.

INTERACTIONS

None significant.

NURSING CONSIDERATIONS

• Contraindicated in viral skin diseases, or in impaired circulation. Use cautiously on face or broken skin.
• Wet skin before application. If irritation persists, discontinue.
• Avoid contact with eyes.
• Emollients produce an occlusive layer that retains perspiration, excludes air, and traps cutaneous bacteria, producing sites for anaerobic infections. Before each new application, *always* thoroughly cleanse affected area, removing all traces of previously applied medication. Observe for inflammation or infection.

vitamins A and D ointment

A&D Balmex, Caldesene Medicated, Clocream, Comfortine, Desitin, Primaderm

INDICATIONS & DOSAGE

Emollient, demulcent, and epithelial- bed stimulant: superficial burns, sunburn, abrasions, slow-healing lesions, chapped skin, diaper rash, skin care of infants or bedridden patients—apply several times a day.

SIDE EFFECTS

Skin: irritation.

INTERACTIONS

None significant.

NURSING CONSIDERATIONS

• Discontinue if skin condition persists or irritation develops.
• Observe for inflammation or infection since emollients and demulcents are occlusive layers that retain moisture, exclude air, and trap cutaneous bacteria.
• Skin should be cleaned daily or more often as needed.
• Emollients and demulcents may be used alone, as vehicles for medications, or with other topical medications. Check with doctor.

zinc gelatin

Dome-Paste, Unna's Boot

INDICATIONS & DOSAGE

*Protectant: varicosities, lesions of lower legs or arms—*heat in hot bath till liquefied, clean skin, dust with talc, and apply gel with paint brush; make three layers, with gauze between each layer; retain 2 weeks. Dome-Paste, in 3- and 4-inch bandages, can be applied directly to arm or leg.

SIDE EFFECTS

None.

INTERACTIONS

None significant.

NURSING CONSIDERATIONS

• Observe for inflammation and in-

---

fection since protectants produce an occlusive layer that retains perspiration, excludes air, and traps cutaneous bacteria, producing sites for anaerobic infections. Before each new application *always* thoroughly cleanse affected area, removing all traces of

previously applied medication.
• Zinc gelatin boot can be removed by unwinding outer bandage and soaking leg or arm in warm water until dressing floats off. Tell patient not to shower or take tub bath with zinc gelatin boot on leg.

87

Keratolytics and caustics

cantharidin
dichloroacetic acid
podophyllum resin
resorcinol
resorcinol monoacetate
salicylic acid
silver nitrate
sulfur
sulfurated lime solution

cantharidin
Cantharone

INDICATIONS & DOSAGE
Adults and children:

Molluscum contagiosum—coat each lesion. Repeat in a week on new or remaining lesions, this time covering with occlusive tape. Remove tape in 6 to 8 hours.

Palpebral warts—apply, leave lesion uncovered.

Plantar warts—pare away keratin, apply generously to affected area, allow to dry, apply protective padding, cover with nonporous tape for a week, then debride. Repeat 3 times, if necessary, on large lesions.

Removal of ordinary and periungual warts and other benign epithelial growths—apply directly to lesion and cover completely. Allow to dry, then cover with nonporous adhesive tape. Remove tape in 24 hours (or less if extreme pain) and replace with loose bandage. Reapply, if necessary.

SIDE EFFECTS
Skin: annular warts, burning, tingling, extreme tenderness, inflammation.

INTERACTIONS
None significant.

NURSING CONSIDERATIONS
• If dropped on normal skin, remove immediately with acetone, alcohol, or tape remover. Scrub with warm, soapy water, and rinse well, as blistering of skin may result.
• If dropped on mucous membranes or in eyes, flush well with water to remove precipitated collodion, then continue to flush with water for 15 minutes.
• Treat only one or two lesions initially to test patient's sensitivity.
• Stop treatment if severe inflammation develops.
• If application causes burning, tenderness, or tingling, remove tape and soak area in cool water for 10 to 15 minutes; repeat, if necessary.
• If annular warts develop, assure patient that lesions are superficial; retreat or substitute another procedure.
• Does not affect tissue layers below the epidermis and leaves no scar.
• Treatment should be supervised by a doctor.

dichloroacetic acid
Bichloracetic Acid

INDICATIONS & DOSAGE
All types of verrucae; calluses, corns; xanthelasma; ingrown toenails; cysts

and benign erosion of the cervix; sebaceous adenoma; infectious granuloma; tattoo marks; epistaxis; spider nevi; tonsil tabs—
Adults: applied only by doctor at his discretion.

SIDE EFFECTS
Local: irritation, inflammation of normal skin.

INTERACTIONS
None significant.

NURSING CONSIDERATIONS
• Contraindicated for treatment of malignant or premalignant lesions.
• Protect adjacent areas with petrolatum, especially when using 50% solutions.
• Sodium bicarbonate is local antidote.
• Thoroughly dry area before application.
• Warn patient that once solution is applied, treated area will turn from white to red in about 4 hours.
• Peeling of skin usually is noticed in 4 days and is completed in a week.
• If acid comes in contact with normal skin, wipe off with cotton gauze and flush area with water.

podophyllum resin
Podoben

INDICATIONS & DOSAGE
Venereal warts and granuloma inguinale—
Adults: apply podophyllum resin preparation to the lesion, cover with waxed paper, and bandage. Leave covered for 8 to 12 hours, then wash lesion to remove medication. Repeat at weekly intervals.

SIDE EFFECTS
Blood: thrombocytopenia, leukopenia when systemically absorbed.

Local: irritation of normal skin.
Other: peripheral neuropathy when systemically absorbed.

INTERACTIONS
Other keratolytics: may cause extensive damage to the skin. Do not use together.

NURSING CONSIDERATIONS
• Resin is irritating and cytotoxic, and should not be applied to normal skin. Petrolatum can be applied to adjacent areas to protect them during treatment.
• Should be applied only by a doctor because of toxicity.
• Do not use on extensive areas or for prolonged therapy; may be absorbed systemically.

resorcinol

resorcinol monoacetate
Euresol, Resorcin

INDICATIONS & DOSAGE
Acute eczema, urticaria, and other inflammatory skin diseases (1% or 2% concentration in alcohol); acne or seborrhea (5% lotion or 10% soap liniment for scalp); chronic eczema, psoriasis (2% to 10% ointment); acne scarring (45% peeling paste)—
Adults and children: apply as directed.

SIDE EFFECTS
Skin: irritation, moderate erythema or scaling.
Other: darkening of light hair (resorcinol only).

INTERACTIONS
None significant.

NURSING CONSIDERATIONS
• Do not use preparations on or near eyes.

Italicized side effects are common or life-threatening.

• If skin irritation persists, discontinue medication.
• Apply lotion with cotton ball to affected area.
• When applying the peeling paste, closely observe the patient and site of application until paste is removed.

salicylic acid
Calicylic, Keralyt♦, Salactic Liquifilm, Salonil

INDICATIONS & DOSAGE
Superficial fungal infections, acne, psoriasis, seborrheic dermatitis, other scaling dermatoses, hyperkeratosis, calluses, warts—
Adults and children: apply to affected area and place under occlusion at night.

SIDE EFFECTS
Skin: irritation, drying.
Other: salicylism with percutaneous absorption.

INTERACTIONS
None significant.

NURSING CONSIDERATIONS
• Use with caution in diabetics or patients with peripheral vascular disease. The skin inflammation that may result is difficult to treat. Limit use for children under 12 years. (Do not exceed 1 oz in 24 hours.)
• Avoid contact with eyes and mucous membranes.
• If excessive skin drying or irritation occurs, apply a bland cream or lotion.
• Rinse hands after application (unless they are being treated).
• Skin should be hydrated for at least 5 minutes before treatment and washed the morning after treatment.
• Most preparations are occlusive, which increases percutaneous absorption. Therefore, do not use on large surface areas for prolonged periods.

silver nitrate

INDICATIONS & DOSAGE
Cauterization of mucous membranes, fissures, aphthous lesions (5% to 10% solution); cauterization of granulomatous tissues and warts (solid form)—
Adults and children: applied only by doctor at his discretion.

SIDE EFFECTS
Local: *argyria (permanent silver discoloration of skin).*

INTERACTIONS
None significant.

NURSING CONSIDERATIONS
• May cause burns. Avoid accidental contact with skin and eyes. If accidental contact with skin occurs, flush with water for at least 15 minutes; accidental contact with eyes, call doctor at once.
• Not to be ingested; may cause altered respiration, coma, convulsions, paralysis, and even death. If ingested, call doctor at once. Give 1 tablespoon salt in warm water; repeat until emesis is clear. Or have patient drink milk or beaten egg whites mixed in warm water. Keep patient warm and lying down.
• Warn that silver nitrate stains skin and clothing.
• Silver nitrate pencils must be moistened with water before use.

sulfur
Acne-Aid♦, Acnomead, Bensulfoid, EpiClear, Liquimat, Postacne♦, Transact, Xerac

INDICATIONS & DOSAGE
Acne, ringworm, psoriasis, seborrheic dermatitis, chigger infestation, sca-

*bies, favus, staphylococcal
folliculitis—*
Adults and children: apply preparation to affected areas b.i.d., t.i.d., or as directed.

SIDE EFFECTS
Local: excessive drying of skin, blackheads, contact dermatitis.

INTERACTIONS
None significant.

NURSING CONSIDERATIONS
• Prolonged use may cause severe contact dermatitis.
• When initiating therapy, use sparingly for patients with sensitive skin.
• Avoid contact with eyes. If accidental contact occurs, flush with water.
• Wash skin thoroughly before application. Tell patient that tingling sensation may be felt upon application.
• Skin is more reactive to drug in cold, dry climates, so decrease frequency of application. In hot, humid climates, increase frequency of application.

sulfurated lime solution
Vlem-Dome, Vleminckx

INDICATIONS & DOSAGE
Acne vulgaris, seborrhea—
Adults and children: dilute 1 packet in 1 pint hot water and apply as hot dressing for 15 to 20 minutes daily.
Generalized furunculosis—
Adults and children: add 30 to 60 ml solution to bath water.

SIDE EFFECTS
Local: may cause excessive drying of skin.

INTERACTIONS
None significant.

NURSING CONSIDERATIONS
• Discontinue use if excessive drying or skin irritation develops.
• Avoid contact with jewelry, metallic objects, or clothing.
• Avoid getting solution in eyes, nose, or mouth.
• Fumes are irritating and malodorous (rotten eggs). Ventilate adequately.

Italicized side effects are common or life-threatening.

88

Miscellaneous

ammoniated mercury
anthralin
benzoyl peroxide
collagenase
dextranomer
fluorouracil
hydroquinone
methoxsalen
scarlet red
selenium sulfide
streptokinase-streptodornase
sutilains
tretinoin (vitamin A acid, retinoic
  acid)

---

ammoniated mercury
Mercuronate 5% ointment

INDICATIONS & DOSAGE
*Psoriasis, seborrheic dermatitis,
impetigo contagiosa, tinea capitis, and
favus—*
Adults and children: apply to affected area b.i.d. or t.i.d.

SIDE EFFECTS
None reported.

INTERACTIONS
None significant.

NURSING CONSIDERATIONS
• Don't apply to large areas of body
or use for extended periods of time.
Mercury poisoning could result.
• Don't apply to highly inflamed
skin, sunburn, or open wounds.
• Has no odor. Doesn't stain.

---

anthralin
Anthra-Derm♦, Lasan

INDICATIONS & DOSAGE
Psoriasis and chronic dermatitis—
Adults and children: apply thinly
daily or b.i.d. Concentrations range
from 0.1% to 1%; start with lowest
and increase, if necessary.

SIDE EFFECTS
GU: possible renal toxicity.
Skin: erythema on healthy skin.

INTERACTIONS
None significant.

NURSING CONSIDERATIONS
• Contraindicated in renal damage.
Should not be used on acute or inflammatory eruptions.
• Partial excretion in urine may cause
renal irritation, casts, and albuminuria. Check urine weekly.
• Discontinue if allergic reaction,
pustular folliculitis, or renal irritation
occurs.
• Don't get in eyes. May cause conjunctivitis, keratitis, corneal opacity.
• Wash hands thoroughly after using.

benzoyl peroxide

Benoxyl♦, Benzac, Benzagel♦, Clear by Design, Dermodex, Desquam-X♦♦, Dry & Clear, Epi-Clear Antiseptic, Oxy-5,-10, Panoxyl♦, Persadex, Persadox HP, Persa-Gel, Xerac BP

INDICATIONS & DOSAGE

Adjunctive treatment of acne—
Adults and children: apply once daily or b.i.d.

SIDE EFFECTS

Skin: transient stinging on application, feeling of warmth, painful irritation.

INTERACTIONS

Tretinoin: reduced effectiveness of benzoyl peroxide. Do not use together.

NURSING CONSIDERATIONS

• Contraindicated in sensitivity to any of the ingredients.
• Don't use on eyelids, mucous membranes, denuded or highly inflamed skin.
• Dryness, redness, peeling should occur 3 to 4 days after starting treatment. If these common reactions cause considerable discomfort, discontinue temporarily until they subside.
• If painful irritation develops, discontinue use.
• Cleanser (4%) may cause bleaching of hair or colored fabric.

collagenase

Santyl♦

INDICATIONS & DOSAGE

Debridement of dermal ulcers and severely burned areas—
Adults and children: apply ointment (250 units/g) to lesion daily or every other day.

SIDE EFFECTS

Skin: slight erythema of surrounding area, especially if ointment is not confined to lesion.
Other: hypersensitivity reactions.

INTERACTIONS

Detergents, hexachlorophene, antiseptics (especially those containing heavy metal ions such as mercury or silver), iodine, soaks or acidic solutions containing metal ions such as aluminum acetate (Burow's solution): decreased enzymatic activity. Do not use together.

NURSING CONSIDERATIONS

• Use with caution in debilitated patients, since debriding enzymes may increase risk of bacteremia; watch for signs of systemic infection.
• Before application, cleanse lesion with gauze saturated in normal saline, neutral buffer solution, or hydrogen peroxide; use topical antibacterial agent (such as neomycin-bacitracin-polymyxin B) if infection is present. Apply to lesion in powder form before using collagenase. If infection persists, discontinue collagenase until infection is healed. Confine collagenase ointment to area of lesion (Lassar's paste may protect surrounding skin). Apply ointment in thin layers to assure contact with necrotic tissue and complete wound coverage; apply collagenase ointment with tongue depressor on deep wounds; with gauze on shallow wounds. Remove any debris that comes off easily. Remove excess ointment, and cover wound with sterile gauze pad.
• Discontinue when sufficient debridement has occurred.
• Observe wound to monitor progress of therapy. Appearance of granulation may indicate effectiveness. Notify doctor if inflammation or color of

drainage indicates any spread of infection.
• Watch for symptoms of protein sensitization (long-term therapy).
• If enzymatic action must be stopped for any reason, apply Burow's solution.
• Avoid getting ointment in eyes. If this occurs, flush with water at once.
• Protect drug from heat.

dextranomer
Debrisan

INDICATIONS & DOSAGE
To clean secreting wounds, such as venous stasis and decubitus ulcers, infected surgical wounds, and burns—
Adults and children: apply to affected area daily, b.i.d., or more often, p.r.n. Apply to ⅛- or ¼-inch thickness, and cover with sterile gauze pad.

SIDE EFFECTS
Skin: temporary pain.

INTERACTIONS
None significant.

NURSING CONSIDERATIONS
• Before application, cleanse wound with sterile water, saline, or other appropriate solution. Do not dry.
• When saturated, medication turns gray-yellow and should be removed.
• To remove, irrigate with sterile water, saline, or other cleansing solution.

fluorouracil
Efudex♦, Fluoroplex♦

INDICATIONS & DOSAGE
Multiple actinic or solar keratoses; superficial basal cell carcinoma—

Adults and children: apply cream (5%) or solution (2% or 5%) b.i.d.

SIDE EFFECTS
Skin: erythema, pain, burning, scaling, pruritus, hyperpigmentation, dermatitis, soreness, suppuration, swelling.

INTERACTIONS
None significant.

NURSING CONSIDERATIONS
• Wash hands immediately after handling medication.
• Avoid use with occlusive dressings.
• Patient should avoid prolonged exposure to sunlight or ultraviolet light.
• Apply with caution near eyes, nose, and mouth.
• Warn patient that treated area may be unsightly during therapy and for several weeks after therapy is stopped. Complete healing may not occur until 1 or 2 months after treatment is stopped.
• Ingestion and systemic absorption may cause leukopenia, thrombocytopenia, stomatitis, diarrhea, or GI ulceration, bleeding, and hemorrhage.
• Topical application to large ulcerated areas may cause systemic toxicity.
• For basal cell carcinoma, use 5% strength.

hydroquinone
Artra Skin Tone Cream, Derma-Blanch, Eldopaque♦, Eldopaque-Forte♦, Eldoquin♦, Eldoquin Forte♦, Esoterica Medicated Cream, Golden Peacock, HQC Kit, Quinnone

INDICATIONS & DOSAGE
Bleaching of blemished skin, lentigo, chloasma, freckles, old-age spots, and other skin conditions due to melanin—
Adults, and children 12 years and

over: apply 2% to 4% concentration daily or b.i.d.

SIDE EFFECTS
Skin: mild irritation, sensitization, rash.

INTERACTIONS
None significant.

NURSING CONSIDERATIONS
• Contraindicated in patients with prickly heat, sunburn, irritated skin; or as depilatory.
• Don't use near eyes.
• If rash or irritation develops, discontinue therapy.
• Sensitivity can be tested by applying a small amount of low-concentration medication on skin before treatment is started. Allergic reactions should appear within 24 hours.
• Patient should protect treated areas from ultraviolet light.
• Use opaque medication during the day; cream or lotion at night.
• Doesn't cause permanent depigmentation.

---

methoxsalen
Oxsoralen♦

INDICATIONS & DOSAGE
Protect against sunburn, enhance pigmentation, and induce repigmentation in vitiligo—
Adults, and children over 12 years: for small, well-defined lesions, apply topically weekly or less often and expose to ultraviolet light gradually, as directed.

SIDE EFFECTS
CNS: nervousness, insomnia, depression.
GI: discomfort, nausea, diarrhea.
Hepatic: liver toxicity.
Skin: edema, erythema, painful blis-

tering, burning, peeling, *photosensitivity*.

INTERACTIONS
Photosensitizing agents: do not use together.

NURSING CONSIDERATIONS
• Contraindicated in hepatic insufficiency, porphyria, acute lupus erythematosus, hydromorphic, polymorphic light eruptions. Use with caution in familial history of sunlight allergy, GI diseases, chronic infection.
• Regulate therapy carefully. Overdosage or overexposure to light can cause serious burning or blistering.
• Topical treatment should be directly supervised by a doctor.
• When applied topically to face or hands, patient should protect area from light (except during treatment exposure).
• Protect eyes and lips during light exposure treatments.
• Monthly liver function tests should be done on patients with vitiligo (especially at beginning of therapy).
• Significant changes require 6 to 9 months of therapy.

---

scarlet red
Decubitex Ointment
(also contains peruvian balsam, zinc oxide, starch, castor oil, petrolatum, xantham gum, sodium propionate, methylparaben, propylparaben, propylene glycol, and water)

INDICATIONS & DOSAGE
Aid in management of decubitus ulcers—
Adults and children: pour a small amount of 3% hydrogen peroxide or normal saline on the affected area. Cleanse thoroughly and apply ointment. Cover with dry sterile gauze.

SIDE EFFECTS
None reported.

INTERACTIONS
None significant.

NURSING CONSIDERATIONS
• Change dressing twice daily, especially where seeping and secretions are present.
• Ointment should be in contact with newly forming tissue for maximum therapeutic results. Wound should be allowed to "breathe" by being loosely covered.
• Using excess ointment or covering the wound completely will retard wound healing.
• Use ointment until healing is complete.
• In more advanced decubitus ulcers, use normal saline solution rather than hydrogen peroxide.

---

selenium sulfide
Exsel♦, Iosel 250, Selsun♦, Selsun Blue, Sul-Blue

INDICATIONS & DOSAGE
Dandruff, seborrheic scalp dermatitis—
Adults and children: massage 1 to 2 teaspoonfuls into clean, wet scalp. Leave on for 2 to 3 minutes. Rinse thoroughly, and repeat application. Apply twice weekly for 2 weeks, then once a week for 2 weeks, or as often as needed to maintain control.

SIDE EFFECTS
Skin: oily or dry scalp and hair, hair discoloration, hair loss, sensitivity reactions.

INTERACTIONS
None significant.

NURSING CONSIDERATIONS
• Contraindicated in sulfur hypersensitivity.
• Use with caution around areas of acute inflammation or exudation to avoid increased absorption.
• If sensitivity reactions occur, discontinue use.
• Reduce or prevent hair discoloration by thorough rinsing after treatment.
• Avoid contact with eyes.
• Highly toxic if ingested.
• Wash hands carefully after handling.
• Protect from heat.

---

streptokinase-streptodornase
Varidase♦

INDICATIONS & DOSAGE
Adjunctive treatment of suppurative surface tissues, including ulcers, radiation necrosis, infected wounds, burns, surgical incisions, skin grafts, and whenever clotted blood, or fibrinous or purulent accumulations are undesirable—
Adults and children: apply on individual basis, depending on area treated and doctor's instructions.

SIDE EFFECTS
Systemic: fever.

INTERACTIONS
Detergents, anti-infectives (such as benzalkonium chloride, hexachlorophene, iodine): decreased enzymatic activity. Do not use together.

NURSING CONSIDERATIONS
• Contraindicated in areas of active hemorrhage.
• Remove exudates carefully and frequently, especially from closed areas, to avoid pyogenesis.
• Not effective on fibrous tissue, mucoproteins, or collagens.

• Refrigerated solution stable for 2 weeks. Room temperature solution stable for 24 hours.
• Use rubber dams or gauze or nylon dressing to keep medication in constant contact with lesion.
• Prolonged use may result in a high antienzyme titer. Dosage may need to be increased.
• Product comes as solution or jelly. Mix to dilution ordered.
• To make jelly, add 5 ml sterile water for injection or sterile physiological saline to 125,000-unit vial streptokinase-streptodornase; mix with 15 ml jar of carboxymethyl cellulose (CMC) jelly 4.5%. The resulting mixture contains 5,000 IU SK and 1,250 IU SD/ml or g.
• Thoroughly cleanse and irrigate wound area with sterile normal saline or water before treatment to remove antiseptics, detergents, and heavy metal antibacterials, which can decrease enzyme activity.
• Moisten wound area for optimal enzymatic activity. Dress wound if necessary, but remove waste products frequently. Observe wound to monitor progress of therapy. Appearance of granulation tissue may indicate effectiveness. Notify doctor if inflammation or color of drainage indicates spread of infection.
• Avoid getting solution in eyes. If this occurs, flood with water at once.
• Protect drugs from heat.

sutilains
Travase ♦

INDICATIONS & DOSAGE
Debridement of second and third-degree burns, adjunctive debridement of decubitus ulcers, pyogenic wounds, or ulcers resulting from peripheral vascular disease—
Adults and children: apply thinly to area extending ¼ to ½ inch beyond area to be debrided. Cover with loose wet dressing t.i.d. or q.i.d.

SIDE EFFECTS
CNS: local paresthesias.
Skin: mild pain, bleeding, transient dermatitis.

INTERACTIONS
Detergents, anti-infectives (such as benzalkonium chloride, hexachlorophene, iodine, and nitrofurazone), and compounds containing metallic ions (such as silver nitrate and thimerosal): adversely affected enzymatic activity. Do not use together.

NURSING CONSIDERATIONS
• Contraindicated in wounds involving major body cavities or containing exposed nerves or nerve tissue, fungating neoplastic ulcers, wounds in women of childbearing age, persons having limited cardiac or pulmonary reserves.
• Use cautiously near eyes. If accidental contact occurs, flush eyes repeatedly with large amounts of normal saline solution or sterile water.
• Before application, cleanse and irrigate affected area with normal saline or sterile water solution to remove antiseptic or heavy metal antibacterial agents.
• May give mild analgesic to reduce painful reactions, but discontinue if pain is severe; also discontinue if bleeding or dermatitis occurs.
• For best response, keep affected area moist.
• In concomitant use of topical antimicrobial agent, apply sutilains first.
• Store at 2° to 10° C. (35.6° to 50° F.).
• Check expiration date.

tretinoin (vitamin A acid, retinoic acid)
Retin-A

INDICATIONS & DOSAGE
Acne vulgaris (especially grades I, II, and III)—
Adults and children: cleanse affected area and lightly apply solution once daily at bedtime.

SIDE EFFECTS
Skin: *feeling of warmth, slight stinging, local erythema, peeling at site,* chapping and swelling, blistering and crusting, temporary hyperpigmentation or hypopigmentation.

INTERACTIONS
None significant.

NURSING CONSIDERATIONS
• Contraindicated in hypersensitivity to any tretinoin component. Use with caution in eczema.

• If severe local irritation develops, discontinue temporarily and readjust dosage when application is resumed.
• Some redness and scaling are normal reactions.
• Beneficial effects should be seen within 6 weeks of treatment.
• When treatment is stopped, relapses generally occur within 3 to 6 weeks.
• Patient should wash face with a mild soap no more than 2 or 3 times a day. Warn against using strong or medicated cosmetics, soaps, or other skin cleansers.
• Exposure to sunlight or ultraviolet rays should be minimal during treatment. If patient is sunburned, delay therapy until sunburn subsides.
• Avoid contact with eyes, mouth, nose, and mucous membranes.
• Warn patient not to use topical products containing alcohol, astringents, spices, and lime. These may interfere with action of tretinoin.

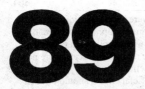

Local anesthetics

bupivacaine hydrochloride
chloroprocaine hydrochloride
dibucaine hydrochloride
etidocaine hydrochloride
lidocaine hydrochloride
mepivacaine hydrochloride
piperocaine hydrochloride
prilocaine hydrochloride
procaine hydrochloride
tetracaine hydrochloride

bupivacaine hydrochloride
Marcaine♦

INDICATIONS & DOSAGE
Available with or without epinephrine. Dosages given are for drug *without* epinephrine.
Epidural:

Sol.	Vol. (ml)	Dose (mg)
0.75%	10 to 20	75 to 150
0.50%	10 to 20	50 to 100
0.25%	10 to 20	25 to 50

Caudal:

Sol.	Vol. (ml)	Dose (mg)
0.50%	15 to 30	75 to 150
0.25%	15 to 30	37.5 to 75

Peripheral nerve block:

Sol.	Vol. (ml)	Dose (mg)
0.50%	5 to 80	25 to 400 (max.)

May repeat dose q 3 hours. Dose and
interval may be increased with epinephrine. Maximum 400 mg daily.

SIDE EFFECTS
Skin: dermatologic reactions.
Other: edema, status asthmaticus, or
anaphylactoid reactions.

Side effects of local anesthetics generally result from high blood levels of
the drug. Examples of these are:
CNS: anxiety, apprehension, nervousness, convulsions followed by
drowsiness, unconsciousness, and *respiratory arrest*.
CV: myocardial depression, *arrhythmias, cardiac arrest*.
EENT: blurred vision.
GI: nausea, vomiting.

INTERACTIONS
*Chloroform, halothane, cyclopro-
pane, trichloroethylene, and related
drugs:* cardiac arrhythmias may occur
when used with bupivacaine *with* epinephrine. Use with extreme caution.
*MAO inhibitors, tricyclic antidepres-
sants:* severe, sustained hypertension
may occur when used with bupivacaine *with* epinephrine. Use
with extreme caution.

NURSING CONSIDERATIONS
• Contraindicated in children under
12 years and for spinal, paracervical
block, or topical anesthesia. Use cautiously in debilitated, elderly, or
acutely ill patients; severe hepatic
disease; drug allergies.
• Use cautiously in cardiovascular
disorders and in body areas with limited blood supply (ears, nose).
• Keep resuscitative equipment and
drugs available.
• Don't use solution with preservatives for caudal or epidural block.
• Onset in 4 to 17 minutes; duration
3 to 7 hours.

• Causes less fetal depression than other local anesthetics.
• Discard partially used vials without preservatives.

chloroprocaine hydrochloride
Nesacaine (for infiltration and regional anesthesia), Nesacaine-CE (for caudal and epidural anesthesia)

INDICATIONS & DOSAGE
Only available without epinephrine.
Infiltration and nerve block:

Sol.	Vol. (ml)	Dose (mg)
1%	3 to 20	30 to 200
2%	2 to 40	20 to 400

Caudal and epidural:

Sol.	Vol. (ml)	Dose (mg)
2% to 3%	15 to 25	300 to 750

May repeat with smaller doses q 40 to 50 minutes. Dose and interval may be increased with epinephrine. Maximum adult dose 800 mg, or 1 g when mixed with epinephrine.

SIDE EFFECTS
Skin: dermatologic reactions.
Other: edema, status asthmaticus, or anaphylactoid reactions.
Side effects of local anesthetics generally result from high blood levels of the drug. Examples of these are:
CNS: anxiety, apprehension, nervousness, convulsions followed by drowsiness, unconsciousness, and *respiratory arrest*.
CV: myocardial depression, *arrhythmias, cardiac arrest*.
EENT: blurred vision.
GI: nausea, vomiting.

INTERACTIONS
None significant.

NURSING CONSIDERATIONS
• Contraindicated in hypersensitivity to procaine, tetracaine, or other *p*-aminobenzoic acid derivatives, and for spinal or topical anesthesia. Epidural and caudal contraindicated in CNS disease. Use cautiously in debilitated, elderly, or acutely ill patients; children; drug allergies; paracervical block; cardiovascular disease.
• Use solutions with epinephrine cautiously in cardiovascular disorders and in body areas with limited blood supply (ears, nose).
• A 3 ml test dose should be injected at least 10 minutes before giving total dose to check for intravascular or subarachnoid injection. Motor paralysis and extensive sensory anesthesia indicate subarachnoid injection.
• Don't use solution with preservatives for caudal or epidural block.
• Don't use discolored solution.
• Keep resuscitative equipment and drugs available.
• Duration 30 to 60 minutes.
• Discard partially used vials without preservatives.

dibucaine hydrochloride
Nupercaine

INDICATIONS & DOSAGE
Only available without epinephrine.
Spinal anesthesia:
Perineum and lower limbs

Sol.	Vol. (ml)	Dose (mg)
0.5%	0.5 to 1	2.5 to 5

Lower abdomen

Sol.	Vol. (ml)	Dose (mg)
0.5%	1 to 1.5	5 to 7.5

Upper abdomen

Sol.	Vol. (ml)	Dose (mg)
0.5%	2	10

Spinal anesthesia:
Lower extremities as high as pelvis

Sol.	Vol. (ml)	Dose (mg)
1:1,500	6	4

Lower abdomen

Sol.	Vol. (ml)	Dose (mg)
1:1,500	10 to 15	6.67 to 10

Upper abdomen

Sol.	Vol. (ml)	Dose (mg)
1:1,500	15 to 18	10 to 12

SIDE EFFECTS

Skin: dermatologic reactions.
Other: edema, status asthmaticus, or anaphylactoid reactions.
Side effects of local anesthetics generally result from high blood levels of the drug. Examples of these are:
CNS: anxiety, apprehension, nervousness, convulsions followed by drowsiness, unconsciousness, and *respiratory arrest.*
CV: myocardial depression, *arrhythmias, cardiac arrest.*
EENT: blurred vision.
GI: nausea, vomiting.

INTERACTIONS

None significant.

NURSING CONSIDERATIONS

• Contraindicated in cerebrospinal disease, septicemia, pernicious anemia with spinal cord symptoms, arthritis, pyogenic skin infection in puncture area. Use cautiously in hysteria, chronic backache, headache of long duration, migraine, shock, hypotension, leaking spinal fluid, cardiac decompensation, pleural effusions, increased abdominal pressure, possibility of hemorrhage.
• Low spinal solution contraindicated in cesarean section or in presence of blood when doing lumbar puncture. Use low spinal solutions cautiously in cardiac or neurologic disease, back problems, uncooperative or hysterical patients.
• Use solutions with epinephrine cautiously in cardiovascular disorders and in body areas with limited blood supply (ears, nose).
• Keep resuscitative equipment and drugs available.
• Don't use for nerve block or infiltration.
• Don't use discolored solution.
• Used primarily for spinal block and as topical anesthetic.

• Onset in 10 to 15 minutes; duration 6 hours.
• Discard partially used vials without preservatives.

---

etidocaine hydrochloride
Duranest

INDICATIONS & DOSAGE

Available with or without epinephrine. Doses cited are for drug *with* epinephrine.
Dose and interval may be decreased without epinephrine.
Infiltration:

Sol.	Vol. (ml)	Dose (mg)
0.5%	1 to 80	5 to 400

Peripheral nerve block:

Sol.	Vol. (ml)	Dose (mg)
0.5%	5 to 80	25 to 400
1%	5 to 40	50 to 400

Central neural block:
Lower limbs, cesarean section, lumbar peridural

Sol.	Vol. (ml)	Dose (mg)
1%	10 to 30	100 to 300
1.5%	10 to 20	150 to 300

Vaginal

Sol.	Vol. (ml)	Dose (mg)
0.5%	10 to 30	50 to 150
1%	5 to 20	50 to 200

Caudal:

Sol.	Vol. (ml)	Dose (mg)
0.5%	10 to 30	50 to 150
1%	10 to 30	100 to 300

SIDE EFFECTS

Skin: dermatologic reactions.
Other: edema, status asthmaticus, or anaphylactoid reactions.
Side effects of local anesthetics generally result from high blood levels of the drug. Examples of these are:
CNS: anxiety, apprehension, nervousness, convulsions followed by drowsiness, unconsciousness, and *respiratory arrest.*
CV: myocardial depression, *arrhythmias, cardiac arrest.*

EENT: blurred vision.
GI: nausea, vomiting.

INTERACTIONS

Chloroform, halothane, cyclopropane, trichloroethylene, and related drugs: cardiac arrhythmias may occur when used with etidocaine *with* epinephrine. Use with extreme caution.
MAO inhibitors, tricyclic antidepressants, phenothiazines: severe, sustained hypertension or hypotension may occur when used with etidocaine solution *with* epinephrine. Use with extreme caution.

NURSING CONSIDERATIONS

• Contraindicated in inflammation or infection in puncture region, children under 14 years, septicemia, severe hypertension, spinal deformities, neurologic disorders, and spinal block. Use cautiously in debilitated, elderly, or acutely ill patients; severe shock; heart block; epidural block in obstetrics; general drug allergies; hepatic and renal disease.
• Use solutions with epinephrine cautiously in cardiovascular disease and in body areas with limited blood supply (nose, ear).
• Don't use solution with preservatives for caudal or epidural block.
• Keep resuscitative equipment and drugs available.
• Onset in 2 to 8 minutes; duration 4½ to 13 hours.

---

lidocaine hydrochloride

Ardecaine, Canocaine, Dilocaine, Dolicaine, L-Caine, Nervocaine, Norocaine, Rocaine, Ultracaine, Xylocaine Hydrochloride♦

INDICATIONS & DOSAGE

Available with or without epinephrine. Doses cited are for drug *without* epinephrine except where indicated.

Caudal *(obstetrics)* **or epidural** *(thoracic):*

Sol.	Vol. (ml)	Dose (mg)
1%	20 to 30	200 to 300

Caudal *(surgery):*

Sol.	Vol. (ml)	Dose (mg)
1.5%	15 to 20	225 to 300

Epidural *(lumbar anesthesia):*

Sol.	Vol. (ml)	Dose (mg)
1.5%	15 to 20	225 to 300
2%	10 to 15	200 to 300

Maximum dose 200 to 300 mg per hour.
For anesthesia other than spinal— maximum single adult dose 4.5 mg/ Kg or 300 mg.
With epinephrine for anesthesia other than spinal— maximum single adult dose 7 mg/Kg or 500 mg. Don't repeat dose more often than q 2 hours.

Spinal surgical anesthesia:

Sol.	Vol. (ml)	Dose (mg)
5% with 7.5% dextrose	1.5 to 2	75 to 100

Dose and interval may be increased with epinephrine.

SIDE EFFECTS

Skin: dermatologic reactions.
Other: edema, status asthmaticus, or anaphylactoid reactions.
Side effects of local anesthetics generally result from high blood levels of the drug. Examples of these are:
CNS: anxiety, apprehension, nervousness, convulsions followed by drowsiness, unconsciousness, and *respiratory arrest.*
CV: myocardial depression, *arrhythmias, cardiac arrest.*
EENT: blurred vision.
GI: nausea, vomiting.

INTERACTIONS

Chloroform, halothane, cyclopropane, trichloroethylene, and related drugs: cardiac arrhythmias may occur when used with lidocaine *with* epinephrine. Use with extreme caution.
MAO inhibitors, tricyclic antidepres-

sants: severe, sustained hypertension may occur when used with lidocaine *with* epinephrine. Use with extreme caution.

NURSING CONSIDERATIONS
• Contraindicated in inflammation or infection in puncture region, septicemia, severe hypertension, spinal deformities, neurologic disorders. Use cautiously in debilitated, elderly, or acutely ill patients; in severe shock; heart block; in obstetrics; general drug allergies; and paracervical block.
• Use solutions with epinephrine cautiously in cardiovascular disorders and in body areas with limited blood supply (nose, ear).
• Keep resuscitative equipment and drugs available.
• A 2- to 5-ml test dose should be injected at least 5 minutes before giving total dose to check for intravascular or subarachnoid injection. Motor paralysis and extensive sensory anesthesia indicate subarachnoid injection.
• Solutions containing preservatives should not be used for spinal, epidural, or caudal block.
• Discard partially used vials without preservatives.

---

mepivacaine hydrochloride
Carbocaine♦, Cavacaine, Isocaine

INDICATIONS & DOSAGE
Available with or without levonordefrin (vasoconstrictor). Doses cited are for drug *without* levonordefrin.
Nerve block:

Sol.	Vol. (ml)	Dose (mg)
1%	5 to 20	50 to 200
2%	5 to 20	100 to 400

Transvaginal block or infiltration *(maximum dose):*

Sol.	Vol. (ml)	Dose (mg)
1%	40	400

Paracervical block *(obstetrics):*

Sol.	Vol. (ml)	Dose (mg)
1%	10	100

Give on each side (200 mg total) per 90-minute period.
Caudal and epidural:

Sol.	Vol. (ml)	Dose (mg)
1%	15 to 30	150 to 300
1.5%	10 to 25	150 to 375
2%	10 to 20	200 to 400

Therapeutic block *(pain management):*

Sol.	Vol. (ml)	Dose (mg)
1%	1 to 5	10 to 50
2%	1 to 5	20 to 100

Adults: maximum single dose 7 mg/Kg up to 550 mg. Don't repeat more often than q 90 minutes. Maximum total dose 1,000 mg daily.
Children: maximum dose 5 to 6 mg/Kg. In children under 3 years or weighing less than 14 Kg, use 0.5% or 1.5% solution only. Dose and interval may be increased with levonordefrin.

SIDE EFFECTS
Skin: dermatologic reactions.
Other: edema, status asthmaticus, or anaphylactoid reactions.
Side effects of local anesthetics generally result from high blood levels of the drug. Examples of these are:
CNS: anxiety, apprehension, nervousness, convulsions followed by drowsiness, unconsciousness, and *respiratory arrest.*
CV: myocardial depression, *arrhythmias, cardiac arrest.*
EENT: blurred vision.
GI: nausea, vomiting.

INTERACTIONS
Chloroform, halothane, cyclopropane, trichloroethylene, and related drugs: cardiac arrhythmias may occur when used with mepivacaine *with* levonordefrin. Use with extreme caution.
MAO inhibitors, tricyclic antidepressants: severe, sustained hypertension may occur when used with mepiva-

caine *with* levonordefrin. Use with extreme caution.

NURSING CONSIDERATIONS
• Contraindicated in sensitivity to methylparaben, in heart block, or for spinal anesthesia. Use cautiously in debilitated, elderly, or acutely ill patients, or for paracervical block.
• Use solutions with levonordefrin cautiously in cardiovascular disease and in body areas with limited blood supply (nose, ear).
• Monitor fetal heart rate when paracervical block used in delivery.
• Keep resuscitative equipment and drugs available.
• Don't use solutions with preservatives for caudal or epidural block.
• Onset in 15 minutes; duration 3 hours.
• Discard partially used vials without preservatives.

---

piperocaine hydrochloride
Metycaine

INDICATIONS & DOSAGE
Caudal block *(obstetrics in women with normal-sized pelvic canals):*

Sol.	Vol. (ml)	Dose (mg)
1.5%	30	450

May give additional 20 ml doses (300 mg) q 30 to 40 minutes, p.r.n.
Infiltration *(maximum dose):*

Sol.	Vol. (ml)	Dose (mg)
0.5%	200	1,000
1%	80	800

For dental infiltration, use a 1% to 2% solution.
For peripheral or sympathetic nerve block, use 0.5% to 2% solution.

SIDE EFFECTS
Skin: dermatologic reactions.
Other: edema, status asthmaticus, or anaphylactoid reactions.
Side effects of local anesthetics gener-

ally result from high blood levels of the drug. Examples of these are:
CNS: anxiety, apprehension, nervousness, convulsions followed by drowsiness, unconsciousness, and *respiratory arrest.*
CV: myocardial depression, *arrhythmias, cardiac arrest.*
EENT: blurred vision.
GI: nausea, vomiting.

INTERACTIONS
None significant.

NURSING CONSIDERATIONS
• Contraindicated in hypersensitivity to procaine, tetracaine, or other *p*-aminobenzoic acid derivatives, CNS diseases, spinal deformity, infection at injection site, extreme obesity, profound anemia, or spinal block, in highly nervous women.
• Don't use solutions with preservatives for caudal block.
• Keep resuscitative equipment and drugs available.
• Effect peaks in 20 to 30 minutes, then decreases over next 10 minutes.
• Dilute 2% solutions to 0.5% or 1% with NaCl injection or Ringer's injection. Don't use sterile water for injection.
• An 8 ml dose of anesthetic solution should be injected a few minutes before giving total dose to check for subarachnoid injection. Motor paralysis and extensive sensory anesthesia indicate subarachnoid injection.
• Discard partially used vials without preservatives.

---

prilocaine hydrochloride
Citanest♦, Propitocaine

INDICATIONS & DOSAGE
Infiltration:

Sol.	Vol. (ml)	Dose (mg)
1% to 2%	20 to 30	200 to 600

Peripheral nerve block (*intercostal or paravertebral*):

Sol.	Vol. (ml)	Dose (mg)
1% to 2%	3 to 5	30 to 100

Peripheral nerve block (*sciatic* [*femoral or brachial plexus*] *or caudal nerve block* [*surgery*])

Sol.	Vol. (ml)	Dose (mg)
2%	20 to 30	400 to 600
3%	15 to 20	450 to 600

Caudal nerve block (*obstetrics*):

Sol.	Vol. (ml)	Dose (mg)
1%	20 to 30	200 to 300

Epidural:

Sol.	Vol. (ml)	Dose (mg)
1%	20 to 30	200 to 300
2%	20 to 30	400 to 600
3%	15 to 20	450 to 600

Maximum single adult dose 8 mg/Kg up to 600 mg. In continuous caudal or epidural anesthesia, don't give maximum dose more often than q 2 hours.

SIDE EFFECTS
Skin: dermatologic reactions.
Other: edema, status asthmaticus, or anaphylactoid reactions.
With 4% solution: swelling and paresthesia of lips and mouth.
At maximum dose: methemoglobinemia.
Side effects of local anesthetics generally result from high blood levels of the drug. Examples of these are:
CNS: anxiety, apprehension, nervousness, convulsions followed by drowsiness, unconsciousness, and *respiratory arrest*.
CV: myocardial depression, *arrhythmias, cardiac arrest*.
EENT: blurred vision.
GI: nausea, vomiting.

INTERACTIONS
None significant.

NURSING CONSIDERATIONS
• Contraindicated in methemoglobinemia, severe shock, heart block, infection at injection site, or for spinal block. Use cautiously in debilitated, elderly, or acutely ill patients; children under 10 years; and in general drug sensitivities.
• Epidural and caudal contraindicated in CNS disease, spinal deformities, septicemia, severe hypertension, and in children.
• Keep resuscitative equipment and drugs available.
• Duration 1 to 3 hours.
• Don't use solutions with preservatives for caudal or epidural block.
• Discard partially used vials without preservatives.
• A 5 ml test dose should be injected at least 5 minutes before giving total dose to check for intravascular or subarachnoid injection. Motor paralysis and extensive sensory anesthesia indicate subarachnoid injection.

---

procaine hydrochloride
Novocain♦, Unicaine

INDICATIONS & DOSAGE
Spinal anesthesia—before using, dilute 10% solution with 0.9% NaCl injection, sterile distilled water, or cerebrospinal fluid.
For hyperbaric technique, use dextrose solution.
Perineum: use 0.5 ml 10% solution and 0.5 ml diluent injected at fourth lumbar interspace.
Perineum and lower extremities: use 1 ml 10% solution and 1 ml diluent injected at third or fourth lumbar interspace.
Up to costal margin: use 2 ml 10% solution and 1 ml diluent injected at second, third, or fourth lumbar interspace.

Epidural block:

Sol.	Vol. (ml)	Dose (mg)
1.5%	25	375

Peripheral nerve block:

Sol.	Vol. (ml)	Dose (mg)
1%	50	250
2%	25	500

Italicized side effects are common or life-threatening.

Infiltration: use 250 to 600 mg 0.25% to 0.5% solution. Maximum initial dose 1 g. Dose and interval may be increased with epinephrine.

SIDE EFFECTS
Skin: dermatologic reactions.
Other: edema, status asthmaticus, or anaphylactoid reactions.
Side effects of local anesthetics generally result from high blood levels of the drug. Examples of these are:
CNS: anxiety, apprehension, nervousness, convulsions followed by drowsiness, unconsciousness, and *respiratory arrest.*
CV: myocardial depression, *arrhythmias, cardiac arrest.*
EENT: blurred vision.
GI: nausea, vomiting.

INTERACTIONS
Echothiophate iodide: reduced hydrolysis of procaine. Use together cautiously.

NURSING CONSIDERATIONS
• Contraindicated in traumatized urethra and in hypersensitivity to chloroprocaine, tetracaine, or other *p*-aminobenzoic acid derivatives. Use cautiously in CNS diseases, infection at puncture site, shock, profound anemia, cachexia, sepsis, hypertension, hypotension, hyperexcitable patients, GI hemorrhage, bowel perforation or strangulation, peritonitis, cardiac decompensation, massive pleural effusions, and increased intra-abdominal pressure.
• Contraindications to obstetric use: pelvic disproportion, placenta previa, abruptio placentae, floating fetal head, intrauterine manipulation.
• Keep resuscitative equipment and drugs available.
• A 1- to 5-ml test dose should be given 5 to 15 minutes before total epidural dose. Motor paralysis and extensive sensory anesthesia indicate subarachnoid injection.

• Use solution without preservatives for epidural block.
• Onset in 2 to 5 minutes; duration 60 minutes.
• Discard partially used vials without preservatives.

---

tetracaine hydrochloride
Pontocaine♦

INDICATIONS & DOSAGE
Low spinal (saddle block) in vaginal delivery: give 2 to 5 mg as hyperbaric solution (in 10% dextrose). Maximum dose 15 mg.
Perineum and lower extremities: give 5 to 10 mg.
Prolonged spinal anesthesia (2 to 3 hours): dilute 1% solution with equal volume of cerebrospinal fluid, or dissolve 5 mg powdered drug in 1 ml cerebrospinal fluid immediately before giving. Give 1 ml/5 seconds.
Up to costal margin: give 15 to 20 mg.

SIDE EFFECTS
Skin: dermatologic reactions.
Other: edema, status asthmaticus, or anaphylactoid reactions.
Side effects of local anesthetics generally result from high blood levels of the drug. Examples of these are:
CNS: anxiety, apprehension, nervousness, convulsions followed by drowsiness, unconsciousness, and *respiratory arrest.*
CV: myocardial depression, *arrhythmias, cardiac arrest.*
EENT: blurred vision.
GI: nausea, vomiting.

INTERACTIONS
None significant.

NURSING CONSIDERATIONS
• Contraindicated in infection at injection site, serious CNS diseases, and in hypersensitivity to procaine, chloroprocaine, tetracaine, or other

---

p-aminobenzoic acid derivatives. Use cautiously in shock, profound anemia, cachexia, hypertension, hypotension, peritonitis, cardiac decompensation, massive pleural effusion, increased intracranial pressure, infection, and in highly nervous patients.
• Saddle block contraindicated in cephalopelvic disproportion, placenta previa, abruptio placentae, intrauterine manipulation, floating fetal head.

• Don't use cloudy, discolored, or crystallized solutions.
• Keep resuscitative equipment and drugs available.
• 10 times as strong as procaine HCl.
• Onset in 15 minutes; duration up to 3 hours.
• When cerebrospinal fluid is added to powdered drug or drug solution during spinal anesthesia, solution may be cloudy.
• Protect from light; store in refrigerator.

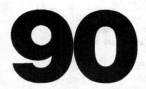

General anesthetics

fentanyl citrate with droperidol
ketamine hydrochloride
methohexital sodium
thiamylal sodium
thiopental sodium

fentanyl citrate with droperidol
Controlled Substance Schedule II
Innovar (Each ml contains [in a 1:50
ratio] fentanyl 0.05 mg as a citrate
and droperidol 2.5 mg.)

INDICATIONS & DOSAGE
Doses vary depending on application
and patient.
Anesthesia—
Adults:
Premedication—0.5 to 2 ml I.M. 45
to 60 minutes before surgery.
Adjunct to general anesthesia—Induction: 1 ml per 20 to 25 lbs body
weight by slow I.V.
Maintenance: not indicated as sole
agent for maintenance of surgical
anesthesia. Used in combination with
other measures. To prevent excessive
accumulation of the relatively long-acting droperidol component, fentanyl alone should be used in increments of 0.025 to 0.05 mg (0.5 to
1 ml) for maintenance of analgesia.
However, during prolonged surgery,
additional 0.5 to 1 ml amounts of
Innovar may be administered with
caution.
Diagnostic procedures—0.5 to 2 ml
I.M. 45 to 60 minutes before procedure. In prolonged procedure, give

0.5 to 1 ml. I.V. with caution and
without a general anesthetic.
Adjunct in regional anesthesia—1 to
2 ml I.M. or slow I.V.
Children:
Premedication—0.25 ml/20 lbs body
weight I.M. 45 to 60 minutes before
surgery.
Adjunct to general anesthesia—0.5 ml
per 20 lbs body weight (total combined dose for induction and maintenance). Following induction with Innovar, fentanyl alone in a dose of ¼ to
⅓ of adult dose should be used to
avoid accumulation of droperidol.
However, during prolonged surgery,
additional amounts of Innovar may be
administered with caution.

SIDE EFFECTS
CNS: emergence delirium and hallucinations, postoperative drowsiness.
CV: vasodilation, *hypotension,* decreased pulmonary arterial pressure,
bradycardia, or tachycardia.
EENT: blurred vision.
GI: *nausea, vomiting.*
Other: *respiratory depression, apnea,*
or *arrest;* drug dependence; muscle rigidity; *laryngospasms;* chills; *shivering;* twitching; diaphoresis.

INTERACTIONS
*CNS depressants (such as barbiturates, tranquilizers, narcotics, and
general anesthetics):* additive or potentiating effect. Dosage should be
reduced.
MAO inhibitors: severe and unpredictable potentiation of Innovar. Do not

use together or within 2 weeks of MAO inhibitor therapy.

NURSING CONSIDERATIONS
• Contraindicated in intolerance to either component. Use with caution in patients with head injuries and increased intracranial pressure, chronic obstructive pulmonary disease, hepatic and renal dysfunction, bradyarrhythmias, elderly or debilitated patients.
• Hypotension is a common side effect. However, if blood pressure drops, also consider hypovolemia as a possible cause. Use appropriate parenteral fluids to help restore blood pressure.
• Vital signs should be monitored requently.
• Be aware that respiratory depression, muscular rigidity of respiratory muscles, and respiratory arrest can occur. Have narcotic antagonist and CPR equipment on hand.
• Maintain airway.
• Postoperative EEG pattern may return to normal slowly.
• Postoperatively, if narcotic analgesics are required, use initially in reduced doses, as low as ¼ to ⅓ those usually recommended.
• When Innovar is given for anesthesia induction, fentanyl (Sublimaze) should be used for maintenance analgesia during the procedure.

---

ketamine hydrochloride
Ketaject, Ketalar♦

INDICATIONS & DOSAGE
Induce anesthesia for procedures, especially short-term diagnostic or surgical, not requiring skeletal muscle relaxation; before giving other general anesthetics or to supplement low-potency agents, such as nitrous oxide—
Adults and children: 1 to 4.5 mg/Kg I.V., administered over 60 seconds; or

6.5 to 13 mg/Kg I.M. To maintain anesthesia, repeat in increments of half to full initial dose.

SIDE EFFECTS
CNS: *tonic and clonic movements resembling convulsions,* respiratory depression.
CV: *increased blood pressure and pulse rate,* hypotension, bradycardia.
EENT: diplopia, nystagmus, slight increase in intraocular pressure, *laryngospasms.*
GI: mild anorexia, nausea, vomiting.
Skin: transient erythema, measleslike rash.
Other: *dream-like states, hallucinations, confusion, excitement,* irrational behavior, psychic abnormalities.

INTERACTIONS
Thyroid hormones: may elevate blood pressure and cause tachycardia. Give cautiously.

NURSING CONSIDERATIONS
• Contraindicated in history of cerebrovascular accident; patients who would be endangered by a significant rise in blood pressure; severe hypertension; severe cardiac decompensation; surgery of the pharynx, larynx, or bronchial tree, unless used with muscle relaxants. Use with caution in chronic alcoholism, alcohol-intoxicated patients, patients with cerebrospinal fluid pressure elevated before anesthesia.
• Discourage giving anything orally at least 6 hours before elective surgery.
• Because of rapid induction, patient should be physically supported during administration.
• Do not inject barbiturates and ketamine HCl from same syringe, as they are chemically incompatible.
• Monitor vital signs before, during, and after anesthesia.
• Check cardiac function in patients

with hypertension or cardiac depression.
• Maintain airway.
• Resuscitation equipment should be available and ready for use.
• Start supportive respiration if respiratory depression occurs. Use mechanical support if possible rather than administering analeptics.
• Keep verbal, tactile, and visual stimulation at a minimum during recovery phase to reduce incidence of emergent reactions.
• A potent hallucinogen. Abused by young adults.

---

methohexital sodium
Controlled Substance Schedule IV
Brevital Sodium, Brietal Sodium♦♦

INDICATIONS & DOSAGE
General anesthetic for short-term procedures (oral surgery, gynecologic and genitourinary examinations); reduction of fractures; before electroconvulsive therapy; for prolonged anesthesia when used with gaseous anesthetics—
Adults and children: 5 to 12 ml 1% solution (50 to 120 mg) I.V. at 1 ml/5 seconds. Dose required for induction may vary from 50 to 120 mg or more; average about 70 mg. Induction dose provides anesthesia for 5 to 7 minutes. Maintenance—intermittent injection: 2 to 4 ml 1% solution (20 to 40 mg) q 4 to 7 minutes; continuous I.V. drip: administer 0.2% solution (1 drop/second).

SIDE EFFECTS
CNS: *muscular twitching,* headache, emergence delirium.
CV: *temporary hypotension, tachycardia,* circulatory depression, *peripheral vascular collapse.*
GI: excessive salivation, *nausea, vomiting.*

Skin: tissue necrosis with extravasation.
Local: pain at injection site, injury to nerves adjacent to injection site.
Other: hiccups, coughing, acute allergic reactions, *laryngospasm, bronchospasm, respiratory depression, apnea, twitching.* Extended use may cause cumulative effect; may be habit-forming.

INTERACTIONS
None significant.

NURSING CONSIDERATIONS
• Contraindicated in severe hepatic dysfunction, hypersensitivity to barbiturates, or porphyria; in shock or impending shock; and in patients for whom general anesthetics would be hazardous. Use with caution in debilitated patients, in patients with asthma, respiratory obstruction, severe hypertension or hypotension, myocardial disease, congestive heart failure, severe anemia, or extreme obesity.
• Maintain pulmonary ventilation.
• Avoid extravascular or intra-arterial injections.
• Monitor vital signs before, during, and after anesthesia.
• Have resuscitative equipment and drugs ready.
• Reduce postoperative nausea by having patient fast before administration.
• Incompatible with silicone; avoid contact with rubber stoppers or parts of syringes that have been treated with silicone.
• Incompatible with lactated Ringer's solution.
• Do not mix with acid solutions such as atropine sulfate.
• Solvents recommended are 5% glucose solution or isotonic (0.9%) sodium chloride instead of distilled water.
• Rate of flow must be individualized for each patient.

• Solutions may be stored and used as long as they remain clear and colorless. Solutions cannot be heated for sterilization.

thiamylal sodium
Controlled Substance Schedule III
Surital♦

INDICATIONS & DOSAGE
General anesthetic for short-term procedures; anesthetic before administering other general anesthetics (dosage individualized to patient's response)—
Adults: 3 to 6 ml 2.5% solution I.V. at 1 ml/5 seconds. Additional intermittent injections of 0.5 to 1 ml. Maximum dose 1 g (40 ml 2.5% solution).
Rectal administration before diagnostic procedures—
Children: 800 mg to 1 g 5% solution/22.5 Kg body weight.
Supplemental anesthetic—
Adults: 0.2% or 0.3% solution continuous I.V. drip. Recovery occurs within 20 to 30 minutes after last injection.

SIDE EFFECTS
CNS: excitement, headache, emergence delirium.
CV: hypotension, *circulatory depression,* thrombophlebitis, *hypoxia.*
GI: nausea, vomiting, excessive salivation.
Skin: rash, urticaria, tissue necrosis with extravasation.
Local: pain at injection site, injury to nerves adjacent to injection site.
Other: hiccups, *laryngospasm, bronchospasm, respiratory depression, apnea.* Extended use can cause cumulative effects; may be habit-forming.

INTERACTIONS
None significant.

NURSING CONSIDERATIONS
• Contraindicated in hepatic dysfunction or disease, traumatic or impending shock, porphyria, hypersensitivity to barbiturates, and in those for whom general anesthetics would be hazardous. Use with caution in respiratory disease or obstruction, obesity, marked disturbance of arterial tension, heart failure, anemia, status asthmaticus, endocrine or renal dysfunction, and in debilitated patients.
• Maintain airway.
• Have resuscitative equipment and drugs ready.
• Monitor vital signs before, during, and after anesthesia.
• Avoid extravascular or intra-arterial injection.
• Incompatible with lactated Ringer's solution or with solutions containing bacteriostatic or buffer agents, which tend to cause precipitation.
• Don't inject air into solution; may cause cloudiness.
• Sterile water is the preferred solvent for injections. For drip maintenance use 5% glucose or isotonic sodium chloride to avoid extreme hypotonicity.
• Solutions of atropine sulfate, *d*-tubocurarine, or succinylcholine may be given concurrently but should not be mixed together.
• Do not heat solutions for sterilization. Solutions should be stored in refrigerator and used within 6 days. If kept at room temperature, use within 24 hours.

thiopental sodium
Controlled Substance Schedule III
Pentothal Sodium♦
(injection and rectal suspension)

INDICATIONS & DOSAGE
*Induce anesthesia before administering other anesthetics—*210 to 280 mg

---

Italicized side effects are common or life-threatening.

(3 to 4 ml/Kg) usually required for average adult (70 Kg).

General anesthetic for short-term procedures—
Adults: 2 to 3 ml 2.5% solution (50 to 75 mg) administered I.V. only at intervals of 20 to 40 seconds, depending on reaction. Dose may be repeated with caution, if necessary.
Convulsive states following anesthesia— 75 to 125 mg (3 to 5 ml of 2.5% solution) immediately following convulsion.
*Psychiatric disorders (narcoanalysis, narcosynthesis)—*100 mg/minute (4 ml/minute 2.5% solution) until confusion occurs and before sleep. Maximum dose 50 ml/minute.
Basal anesthesia by rectal administration—
Adults and children: administer up to 1 g/22.5 Kg (50 lbs) body weight, or 0.5 ml 10% solution/Kg body weight. Maximum 1 to 1.5 g (children weighing 34 Kg or more) and 3 to 4 g (adults weighing 91 Kg or more).
Note: thiopental not recommended by routes other than I.V.

SIDE EFFECTS

CNS: *prolonged somnolence,* retrograde amnesia.
CV: *myocardial depression, arrhythmias.*
Skin: tissue necrosis with extravasation.
Local: pain at injection site.
Other: sneezing, coughing, *shivering, respiratory depression (momentary apnea following each injection is typical), bronchospasm, laryngospasm.* May be habit-forming.

INTERACTIONS
None significant.

NURSING CONSIDERATIONS
• Contraindicated in absence of suitable veins for intravenous administration, hypersensitivity to barbiturates, status asthmaticus, porphyria, respiratory depression or obstruction, decompensated cardiac disease, severe anemia, hepatic cirrhosis, shock, renal dysfunction, intracranial pressure.
• Give test dose (1 to 3 ml 2.5% solution) to assess reaction to drug.
• When used as general anesthetic, give atropine sulfate as premedication to diminish laryngeal reflexes and to prevent spastic abduction of vocal cords.
• Have resuscitative equipment and oxygen ready.
• Avoid extravasation and intra-arterial injection.
• Maintain airway.
• Monitor vital signs before, during, and after anesthesia.
• Solutions of atropine sulfate, *d*-tubocurarine, or succinylcholine may be given concurrently but should not be mixed together.
• Do not heat solutions for sterilization. Solutions should be stored in refrigerator and used within 6 days. If kept at room temperature, use within 24 hours.

91

Vitamins

vitamin A
  oleovitamin A
vitamin B complex
  cyanocobalamin (B_{12})
  cyanocobalamin,
      hydroxocobalamin (B_{12a})
  folic acid (B_9)
  leucovorin calcium
  niacin (B_3)
  niacinamide
  pyridoxine hydrochloride (B_6)
  riboflavin (B_2)
  thiamine hydrochloride (B_1)
vitamin C
  ascorbic acid
vitamin D
  cholecalciferol (D_3)
  ergocalciferol (D_2)
vitamin E
vitamin K analogs
  menadione/menadiol sodium
      diphosphate (K_3)
  phytonadione (K_1)
multivitamins
sodium fluoride
trace elements
  chromium
  copper
  iodine
  manganese
  zinc
  zinc sulfate

oleovitamin A

Acon, Afaxin♦♦, Alphalin,
Aquasol-A♦, Dispatabs, Natola

INDICATIONS & DOSAGE

Severe vitamin A deficiency with xerophthalmia—
Adults, and children over 8 years: 500,000 IU P.O. daily for 3 days, then 50,000 IU P.O. daily for 14 days, then maintenance with 10,000 to 20,000 IU P.O. daily for 2 months, followed by adequate dietary nutrition and RDA vitamin A supplements.

Severe vitamin A deficiency—
Adults, and children over 8 years: 100,000 IU P.O. or I.M. daily for 3 days, then 50,000 IU P.O. or I.M. daily for 14 days, then maintenance with 10,000 to 20,000 IU P.O. daily for 2 months, followed by adequate dietary nutrition and RDA vitamin A supplements.

Children 1 to 8 years: 17,500 to 35,000 IU I.M. daily for 10 days.

Infants under 1 year: 7,500 to 15,000 IU I.M. daily for 10 days.

Maintenance only—
Children 4 to 8 years: 15,000 IU I.M. daily for 2 months, then adequate dietary nutrition and RDA vitamin A supplements.

Children under 4 years: 10,000 IU I.M. daily for 2 months, then adequate dietary nutrition and RDA vitamin A supplements.

SIDE EFFECTS

Side effects are usually seen only with toxicity (hypervitaminosis A).

Blood: hypoplastic anemia, leukopenia.

CNS: irritability, headache, increased intracranial pressure, fatigue, lethargy, malaise.

EENT: miosis, papilledema, exophthalmos.

GI: anorexia, epigastric pain, diarrhea.

GU: hypomenorrhea.

Skin: alopecia; drying, cracking, scaling of skin; pruritus; lip fissures; massive desquamation; increased pigmentation; night sweating.

Other: slow growth, decalcification of bone, fractures, hyperostosis, painful periostitis, premature closure of epiphyses, migratory arthralgia, cortical thickening over the radius and tibia, bulging fontanels, hepatomegaly, jaundice, splenomegaly.

INTERACTIONS

Mineral oil, cholestyramine resin: reduced GI absorption of fat-soluble vitamins. If needed, give mineral oil at bedtime.

NURSING CONSIDERATIONS

• Oral administration contraindicated in presence of malabsorption syndrome; if malabsorption is due to inadequate bile secretion, oral route may be used with concurrent administration of bile salts (dehydrocholic acid). Also contraindicated in hypervitaminosis A. Intravenous administration contraindicated except for special water-miscible forms intended for infusion with large parenteral volumes. Intravenous push of vitamin A of any type is also contraindicated (anaphylaxis or anaphylactoid reactions and death have resulted).

• Caution: evaluate intake from fortified foods, dietary supplements, self-administered drugs, and prescription drug sources.

• In pregnant women, avoid doses exceeding 6,000 IU daily.

• To avoid toxicity, discourage patient self-administration of megavitamin doses without specific indications.

• Watch for side effects if dosage is high.

• Acute toxicity has resulted from single doses of 25,000 IU/Kg of body weight; 350,000 IU in infants and over 2,000,000 IU in adults have also proved acutely toxic.

• Chronic toxicity in infants (3 to 6 months) has resulted from doses of 18,500 IU daily for 1 to 3 months. In adults, chronic toxicity has resulted from doses of 50,000 IU daily for over 18 months; 500,000 IU daily for 2 months; and 1,000,000 IU daily for 3 days.

• Monitor patient closely during vitamin A therapy for skin disorders, since high dosages may induce chronic toxicity.

• Liquid preparations available if nasogastric administration is needed.

• Record eating and bowel habits. Report abnormalities to doctor.

• Adequate vitamin A absorption requires suitable protein intake, bile (give supplemental salts if necessary), concurrent RDA doses of vitamin E, and zinc (multivitamins usually supply zinc, but supplements may be necessary in long-term hyperalimentation).

• Absorption is faster and more complete with water-miscible preparations, intermediate with emulsions, and slowest with oil suspensions.

• In severe hepatic dysfunction, diabetes, and hypothyroidism, use vitamin A rather than carotenes for vitamin therapy because the vitamin itself is more easily absorbed and the diseases adversely affect conversion of carotenes into vitamin A. If carotenes are prescribed, dosage should be doubled.

• Protect from light.

cyanocobalamin (vitamin B₁₂)

Anacobin♦♦, Bedoce, Bedoz♦♦, Berubigen, Betalin-12, Bio-12♦♦, Crystimin, Cyanabin♦♦, Cyanocobalamin, Cyano-Gel, DBH-B₁₂, Dodex, Kaybovite, Neo-Vadrin, Pernavite, Poyamin, Redisol♦, Rhodavite, Rubesol, Rubion♦♦, Rubramin♦, Ruvite, Sigamine, Sytobex, Vibedoz, Vi-Twel

cyanocobalamin, hydroxocobalamin (vitamin B₁₂ₐ)

Alpha Redisol, Alpha-Ruvite, Codroxomin, Droxomin, Neo-Betalin 12, Rubesol-LA, Sytobex-H

INDICATIONS & DOSAGE

Vitamin B₁₂ deficiency due to inadequate diet, subtotal gastrectomy, or any other condition, disorder, or disease except malabsorption related to pernicious anemia or other gastrointestinal disease—
Adults: 25 mcg P.O. daily as dietary supplement, or 30 to 100 mcg S.C. or I.M. daily for 5 to 10 days, depending on severity of deficiency. Maintenance dose: 100 to 200 mcg I.M. once monthly. For subsequent prophylaxis, advise adequate nutrition and daily RDA vitamin B₁₂ supplements.
Children: 1 mcg P.O. daily as dietary supplement, or 1 to 30 mcg S.C. or I.M. daily for 5 to 10 days, depending on severity of deficiency. Maintenance: at least 60 mcg per month I.M. or S.C. For subsequent prophylaxis, advise adequate nutrition and daily RDA vitamin B₁₂ supplements.
Pernicious anemia or B₁₂ malabsorption—
Adults: initially, 100 to 1,000 mcg I.M. daily for 2 weeks, then 100 to 1,000 mcg I.M. once monthly for life. If neurologic complications are present, follow initial therapy with 100 to 1,000 mcg I.M. once every 2 weeks before starting monthly regimen.
Children: 1,000 to 5,000 mcg I.M.

or S.C. given over 2 or more weeks as 100 mcg increments; then 60 mcg I.M. or S.C. monthly for life.
Methylmalonic aciduria—
Neonates: 1,000 mcg I.M. daily for 11 days with a protein-restricted diet.
Diagnostic test for vitamin B₁₂ deficiency without concealing folate deficiency in patients with megaloblastic anemias—
Adults and children: 1 mcg I.M. daily for 10 days with low B₁₂ and folate diet. Reticulocytosis between days 3 to 10 confirms diagnosis of B₁₂ deficiency.
Schilling test flushing dose—
Adults and children: 1,000 mcg I.M. in a single dose.

SIDE EFFECTS

CV: peripheral vascular thrombosis.
GI: transient diarrhea.
Skin: itching, transitory exanthema, urticaria.
Local: pain, burning at S.C. or I.M. injection sites.
Other: *anaphylaxis*, anaphylactoid reactions.

INTERACTIONS

Neomycin, colchicine, para-aminosalicyclic acid and salts, chloramphenicol: malabsorption of vitamin B₁₂. Don't use together.

NURSING CONSIDERATIONS

• Parenteral administration contraindicated in hypersensitivity to vitamin B₁₂ or cobalt. Alternate use of large oral doses of vitamin B₁₂ is controversial and should not be considered routine; combined with intrinsic factor increases risk of hypersensitive reactions and should be avoided. Therapeutic dose contraindicated before proper diagnosis; B₁₂ therapy may mask folate deficiency.
• I.V. administration may cause anaphylactic reactions. Use cautiously and only if other routes are ruled out.
• Use cautiously in anemic patients

with coexisting cardiac, pulmonary, or hypertensive disease; in patients with early Leber's disease; in patients with severe B_{12}-dependent deficiencies, especially those receiving cardiac glycosides (monitor closely the first 2 to 3 days for hypokalemia, fluid overload, pulmonary edema, congestive heart failure, and hypertension); and in patients with gouty conditions (monitor serum uric acid levels for hyperuricemia).
- Don't mix parenteral liquids in same syringe with other medication. Protect from light.
- Repository forms add cost without extra effectiveness and may stimulate antibody formation.
- Infection, tumors, or renal, hepatic, and other debilitating diseases may reduce therapeutic response.
- Deficiencies more common in strict vegetarians and their breastfed infants.
- Stress need for pernicious anemia patients to return for monthly injections. Although total body stores may last 3 to 6 years, anemia will recur if not treated monthly.
- May cause false positive intrinsic factor antibody test.
- Hydroxocobalamin is approved for I.M. use only. Only advantage of hydroxocobalamin over B_{12} is longer duration.
- 50% to 98% of injected dose may appear in urine within 48 hours. Major portion is excreted within first 8 hours.
- Closely observe serum potassium the first 48 hours. Give potassium if necessary.
- Physically incompatible with dextrose solutions, alkaline or strongly acidic solutions, oxidizing and reducing agents, and many other drugs.

folic acid (vitamin B_9)
Folvite♦, Novofolacid♦♦

INDICATIONS & DOSAGE
Megaloblastic or macrocytic anemia secondary to folic acid or other nutritional deficiency, hepatic disease, alcoholism, intestinal obstruction, excessive hemolysis—
Pregnant and lactating women: 0.8 mg P.O., S.C., or I.M. daily.
Adults, and children over 4 years: 1 mg P.O., S.C., or I.M. daily for 4 to 5 days. After anemia secondary to folic acid deficiency is corrected, proper diet and RDA supplements are necessary to prevent recurrence.
Children under 4 years: up to 0.3 mg P.O., S.C., or I.M. daily.
Prevention of megaloblastic anemia of pregnancy and fetal damage—
Women: 1 mg P.O., S.C., or I.M. daily throughout pregnancy.
Nutritional supplement—
Adults: 0.1 mg P.O., S.C., or I.M. daily.
Children: 0.05 mg P.O. daily.
Treatment of tropical sprue—
Adults: 3 to 15 mg P.O. daily.
Test of megaloblastic anemia patients to detect folic acid deficiency without masking pernicious anemia—
Adults and children: 0.1 to 0.2 mg P.O. or I.M. for 10 days while maintaining a diet low in folate and vitamin B_{12}.
(Reticulosis, reversion to normoblastic hematopoesis, and return to normal hemoglobin indicate folic acid deficiency.)

SIDE EFFECTS
Skin: allergic reactions (rash, pruritus, erythema).
Other: *allergic bronchospasms,* general malaise.

INTERACTIONS
Chloramphenicol: antagonism of folic

acid. Monitor for decreased folic acid effect. Use together cautiously.

NURSING CONSIDERATIONS

• Contraindicated in normocytic, refractory, or aplastic anemias; as sole agent in treatment of pernicious anemia (since it may mask neurologic effects); in treatment of methotrexate, pyrimethamine, or trimethoprim overdose; and in undiagnosed anemia (since it may mask pernicious anemia).
• Patients with small bowel resections and intestinal malabsorption may require parenteral administration routes.
• Don't mix with other medications in same syringe for I.M. injections.
• Protect from light.
• May use concurrent folic acid and vitamin B_{12} therapy if supported by diagnosis.
• Proper nutrition is necessary to prevent recurrence of anemia.
• Peak folate activity occurs in the blood in 30 to 60 minutes.
• Hematologic response to folic acid in patients receiving chloramphenicol concurrently with folic acid should be carefully monitored.

---

leucovorin calcium (citrovorum factor or folinic acid)
Calcium Folinate

INDICATIONS & DOSAGE

Overdose of folic acid antagonist—
Adults and children: P.O., I.M., or I.V. dose equivalent to the weight of the antagonist given.
Leucovorin rescue after high methotrexate dose in treatment of malignancy—
Adults and children: dose at doctor's discretion within 6 to 36 hours of last dose of methotrexate.
Toxic effects of methotrexate used to treat severe psoriasis—

Adults and children: 4 to 8 mg I.M. 2 hours after methotrexate dose.
Hematologic toxicity due to pyrimethamine therapy—
Adults and children: 5 mg P.O. or I.M. daily.
Hematologic toxicity due to trimethoprim therapy—
Adults and children: 400 mcg to 5 mg P.O. or I.M. daily.
Megaloblastic anemia due to congenital enzyme deficiency—
Adults and children: 3 to 6 mg I.M. daily, then 1 mg P.O. daily for life.
Folate-deficient megaloblastic anemias—
Adults and children: up to 1 mg of leucovorin I.M. daily. Duration of treatment depends on hematologic response.

SIDE EFFECTS
Skin: allergic reactions (rash, pruritus, erythema).
Other: *allergic bronchospasms.*

INTERACTIONS
None significant.

NURSING CONSIDERATIONS
• Contraindicated in treatment of undiagnosed anemia, since it may mask pernicious anemia. Use cautiously in pernicious anemia; a hemolytic remission may occur while neurologic manifestations remain progressive.
• Do not confuse leucovorin (folinic acid) with folic acid.
• Follow leucovorin rescue schedule and protocol closely to maximize therapeutic response. Generally, leucovorin should not be administered simultaneously with systemic methotrexate.
• Treat overdosage of folic acid antagonists; administer within 1 hour if possible; usually ineffective after 4-hour delay.
• Protect from light, especially reconstituted parenteral preparations.
• Since allergic reactions have been

reported with folic acid, the possibility of allergic reactions to leucovorin should be considered.

niacin (vitamin B₃, nicotinic acid)

niacinamide (nicotinamide)
Diacin, Efacin, Lipo-Nicin, Niac, Nico400, Nicobid, Nicocap, Nicolar, Nico-Span, Ni-Span, Vasotherm, Wampocap

INDICATIONS & DOSAGE
Pellagra—
Adults: 10 to 20 mg P.O., S.C., I.M., or I.V. infusion daily, depending on severity of niacin deficiency. Maximum daily dose recommended, 500 mg; should be divided into 10 doses, 50 mg each.
Children: up to 300 mg P.O. or 100 mg I.V. infusion daily, depending on severity of niacin deficiency.
After symptoms subside, advise adequate nutrition and RDA supplements to avoid recurrence.
Hyperlipoproteinemia types III, IV, and V, and as secondary agent in type II—
Adults: up to 1 g 3 or 4 times a day.
Peripheral vascular disease and circulatory disorders—
Adults: 250 to 800 mg P.O. daily in divided doses.

SIDE EFFECTS
Most side effects are dose-dependent.
CNS: dizziness, transient headache.
CV: *excessive peripheral vasodilation.*
GI: *nausea, vomiting, diarrhea,* possible activation of peptic ulcer, epigastric or substernal pain.
Hepatic: liver dysfunction.
Metabolic: hyperglycemia, hyperuricemia.
Skin: *flushing,* pruritus, dryness.

INTERACTIONS
Antihypertensive drugs of the sympa-
thetic blocking type: may have an additive vasodilating effect and cause postural hypotension. Use together cautiously. Warn patient about postural hypotension.

NURSING CONSIDERATIONS
• Contraindicated in hepatic dysfunction, active peptic ulcer disease, severe hypotension, arterial hemorrhage. Use with caution in patients with gallbladder disease, diabetes mellitus, gout.
• Monitor hepatic function and blood glucose early in therapy.
• Give with meals to minimize GI side effects.
• Timed-release niacin or niacinamide may avoid excessive flushing effects with large doses. Give slow I.V. Explain harmlessness of flushing syndrome to ease patient's mind.
• Stress that medication used to treat hyperlipoproteinemia or to dilate peripheral vessels not "just a vitamin." Explain importance of adhering to therapeutic regimen.

pyridoxine hydrochloride (vitamin B₆)
Bee six, Hexa-Betalin♦, Hexacrest, Hexavibex♦

INDICATIONS & DOSAGE
Dietary vitamin B₆ deficiency—
Adults: 10 to 20 mg P.O., I.M., or I.V. daily for 3 weeks, then 2 to 5 mg daily as a supplement to a proper diet.
Children: 100 mg P.O., I.M., or I.V. to correct deficiency, then an adequate diet with supplementary RDA doses to prevent recurrence.
Seizures related to vitamin B₆ deficiency or dependency—
Adults and children: 100 mg I.M. or I.V. in single dose.
Vitamin B₆-responsive anemias or dependency syndrome (inborn errors of metabolism)—

Adults: up to 600 mg P.O., I.M., or I.V. daily until symptoms subside, then 50 mg daily for life.
Children: 100 mg I.M. or I.V., then 2 to 10 mg I.M. or 10 to 100 mg P.O. daily.
Prevention of B₆ deficiency during isoniazid therapy—
Adults: 25 to 50 mg P.O. daily.
Children: at least 0.5 to 1.5 mg daily.
Infants: at least 0.1 to 0.5 mg daily.
If neurologic symptoms develop in pediatric patients, increase dosage as necessary.
Treatment of B₆ deficiency secondary to isoniazid—
Adults: 100 mg P.O. daily for 3 weeks, then 50 mg daily.
Children: titrate dosages.

SIDE EFFECTS
CNS: drowsiness, paresthesias.

INTERACTIONS
None significant.

NURSING CONSIDERATIONS
• Contraindicated in hypersensitivity to parenteral pyridoxine and in doses larger than 5 mg for patients also receiving levodopa. Caution patient to check dosage, especially in multivitamins.
• Protect from light. Do not use injection solution if it contains a precipitate. Slight darkening is acceptable.
• Excessive protein intake increases daily pyridoxine requirements.
• If sodium bicarbonate is required to control acidosis in isoniazid toxicity, do not mix in same syringe with pyridoxine.
• If prescribed for maintenance therapy to prevent deficiency recurrence, stress importance of compliance and of good nutrition. Explain that pyridoxine in combination therapy with isoniazid has a specific therapeutic purpose and is not "just a vitamin." Emphasize need for adhering to therapeutic regimen.

• Patients taking levodopa alone (not in combination with carbidopa) shouldn't take pyridoxine.

---

riboflavin (vitamin B₂)

INDICATIONS & DOSAGE
Riboflavin deficiency or adjunct to thiamine treatment for polyneuritis or cheilosis secondary to pellagra—
Adults, and children over 12 years: 5 to 50 mg P.O., S.C., I.M., or I.V. daily, depending on severity.
Children under 12 years: 2 to 10 mg P.O., S.C., I.M., or I.V. daily, depending on severity.
For maintenance, increase nutritional intake and supplement with vitamin B complex.

SIDE EFFECTS
GU: high doses make urine yellow.

INTERACTIONS
None significant.

NURSING CONSIDERATIONS
• Protect from light.
• Stress proper nutritional habits to avoid recurrence of deficiency.
• Riboflavin deficiency usually accompanies other B complex deficiencies and may require multivitamin therapy.

---

thiamine hydrochloride (vitamin B₁)
Apatate Drops, Betalin S, Betaxin♦♦, Bewon♦, Megamin♦♦, Thia

INDICATIONS & DOSAGE
Beriberi—
Adults: 10 to 500 mg, depending on severity, I.M. t.i.d. for 2 weeks, followed by dietary correction and multivitamin supplement containing 5 to 10 mg daily thiamine for 1 month.

Children: 10 to 50 mg, depending on severity, I.M. daily for several weeks with adequate dietary intake.
Anemia secondary to thiamine deficiency; polyneuritis secondary to alcoholism, pregnancy, or pellagra—
Adults: 100 mg P.O. daily.
Children: 10 to 50 mg P.O. daily in divided doses.
Wernicke's encephalopathy—
Adults: up to 500 mg to 1 g I.V. for crisis therapy, followed by 100 mg b.i.d. for maintenance.
"Wet beriberi," with myocardial failure—
Adults and children: 100 to 500 mg I.V. emergency treatment.

SIDE EFFECTS
CNS: restlessness.
CV: *hypotension after rapid I.V. injection,* angioneurotic edema, cyanosis.
EENT: tightness of throat (allergic reaction).
GI: nausea, hemorrhage, diarrhea.
Skin: feeling of warmth, pruritus, urticaria, sweating.
Other: *anaphylactic reactions,* weakness, pulmonary edema.

INTERACTIONS
None significant.

NURSING CONSIDERATIONS
• Contraindicated in hypersensitivity to thiamine products. I.V. push contraindicated, except when treating life-threatening myocardial failure in "wet beriberi." Use with caution in I.V. administration of large doses (to avoid anaphylactic reactions); skin-test patients with history of hypersensitivity before therapy.
• Use parenteral administration only when P.O. route is not feasible.
• Clinically significant deficiency can occur in approximately 3 weeks of totally thiamine-free diet. Thiamine deficiency usually requires concurrent treatment for multiple deficiencies.

• Doses larger than 30 mg t.i.d. may not be fully utilized by body. When body tissues saturated with thiamine, it is excreted in urine as pyrimidine.
• If beriberi occurs in a breast-fed infant, both mother and child should be treated with thiamine.
• Unstable in alkaline solutions; should not be used with materials that yield alkaline solutions.

---

ascorbic acid (vitamin C)
Adenex♦♦, Ascorbajen, Ascorbicap, Ascorbineed, Ascoril♦♦, Best-C, Cecon, Cemill, Cenolate, Cetane, Cevalin, Cevi-Bid, Ce-Vi-Sol♦, Cevita, Chew-Cee, C-Ject, C-Long, C-Syrup-500, Liqui-Cee, Megascorb♦♦, Redoxon♦♦, Saro-C, Solucap C, Tega-C, Vitacee, Viterra C

INDICATIONS & DOSAGE
Frank and subclinical manifestations of scurvy—
Adults: 100 mg to 2 g, depending on severity, P.O., S.C., I.M., or I.V. daily, then at least 50 mg daily for maintenance.
Children: 100 to 200 mg, depending on severity, P.O., S.C., I.M., or I.V. daily, then at least 35 mg daily for maintenance.
Infants: 50 to 100 mg P.O., I.M., I.V., or S.C. daily.
Extensive burns, delayed fracture or wound healing, postoperative wound healing, and severe febrile or chronic disease states—
Adults: 200 to 500 mg S.C., I.M., or I.V. daily.
Children: 100 to 200 mg P.O., S.C., I.M., or I.V. daily.
Prevention of vitamin C deficiency in those with poor nutritional habits or increased requirements—
Adults: at least 45 to 50 mg P.O., S.C., I.M., or I.V. daily.
Pregnant or lactating women: at

least 60 mg P.O., S.C., I.M., or I.V. daily.
Children: at least 40 mg P.O., S.C., I.M., or I.V. daily.
Infants: at least 35 mg P.O., S.C., I.M., or I.V. daily.
Potentiation of methenamine in urine acidification—
Adults: 4 to 12 g daily in divided doses.
Preop in gastrectomy patients—
Adults: 1 g daily for 4 to 7 days.

SIDE EFFECTS
CNS: faintness or dizziness with fast I.V. administration.
GI: diarrhea, epigastric burning.
GU: acid urine, oxaluria, renal calculi.
Skin: discomfort at injection site.

INTERACTIONS
None significant.

NURSING CONSIDERATIONS
• Use cautiously in G-6-PD deficiency to avoid possibility of hemolytic anemia.
• Avoid rapid I.V. administration.
• Protect solution from light.
• Discourage self-administration for colds; harmful side effects possible.
• Intravenous form used in some cancer centers investigationally to treat some forms of cancer.

---

vitamin D
(cholecalciferol: vitamin D₃; ergocalciferol: vitamin D₂)

$$\text{vitamin D}$$
$$(\text{cholecalciferol: vitamin } D_3;$$
$$\text{ergocalciferol: vitamin } D_2)$$

Calciferol, Deltalin, Drisdol♦, Radiostol♦♦, Radiostol Forte♦♦

INDICATIONS & DOSAGE
Rickets and other vitamin D deficiency diseases—
Adults: 12,000 IU P.O. or I.M. daily initially, increased as indicated by response up to 500,000 IU daily in most cases and up to 800,000 IU daily for vitamin D-resistant rickets.
Children: 1,500 to 5,000 IU P.O. or I.M. daily for 2 to 4 weeks, repeated after 2 weeks, if necessary. Alternatively, a single dose of 600,000 IU. Monitor serum calcium daily to guide dosage. After correction of deficiency, maintenance includes adequate dietary nutrition and RDA supplements.
Hypoparathyroidism—
Adults and children: 50,000 to 200,000 IU P.O. or I.M. daily, with 4 g calcium supplement.

SIDE EFFECTS
Side effects listed are usually seen in vitamin D toxicity only.
CNS: headache, dizziness, ataxia, weakness, somnolence, decreased libido, overt psychosis, convulsions.
CV: calcifications of soft tissues, including the heart.
EENT: metallic taste, rhinorrhea, conjunctivitis (calcific), photophobia, tinnitus.
GI: anorexia, nausea, constipation, diarrhea.
GU: polyuria, albuminuria, hypercalciuria, nocturia, impaired renal function, renal calculi.
Metabolic hypercalcemia, hyperphosphatemia.
Skin: hyperthermia, pruritus, widespread soft-tissue calcification.
Other: bone and muscle pain, bone demineralization, weight loss.

INTERACTIONS
Mineral oil, cholestyramine resin: inhibited GI absorption of oral vitamin D. Space doses. Use together cautiously.

NURSING CONSIDERATIONS
• Contraindicated in hypercalcemia, hypervitaminosis A, renal osteodystrophy with hyperphosphatemia.
• If I.V. route is necessary, use only water-miscible solutions intended for

---

Italicized side effects are common or life-threatening.

dilution in large-volume parenterals. Use cautiously in cardiac patients, especially if they are receiving glycosides.
• Monitor eating and bowel habits for indications of toxicity.
• Patients with hyperphosphatemia require dietary phosphate restrictions and binding agents to avoid metastatic calcifications and renal calculi.
• Dosage range between therapeutic and toxic effects is narrow. When high therapeutic doses are used, frequent serum and urinary calcium, potassium, and urea determinations should be made.
• Malabsorption due to inadequate bile or hepatic dysfunction may require addition of exogenous bile salts to oral vitamin D.
• Protect solution from light.

vitamin E
Aquasol E♦, D-Alpha-E, Daltose♦♦, E-Ferol, Eprolin, Epsilan-M, Hy-E-Plex, Kell-E, Lethopherol, Maxi-E, Pertropin, Solucap E, Tocopher-Caps, Tokols, Viterra E

INDICATIONS & DOSAGE
Vitamin E deficiency in premature infants and in patients with impaired fat absorption—
Adults: 60 to 75 IU, depending on severity, P.O. or I.M. daily. Maximum 300 IU daily.
Children: 1 mg equivalent per 0.6 g of dietary unsaturated fat P.O. or I.M. daily.

SIDE EFFECTS
None reported.

INTERACTIONS
Mineral oil, cholestyramine resin: inhibited GI absorption of oral vitamin E. Space doses. Use together cautiously.

NURSING CONSIDERATIONS
• Water-miscible forms more completely absorbed in GI tract than other forms.
• Adequate bile is essential for absorption.
• Requirements increase with rise in dietary polyunsaturated acids.
• May protect other vitamins against oxidation.
• Used for a variety of disorders with mixed successes and failures. Dosages not established.
• Megadoses can cause thrombophlebitis.

menadione/menadiol sodium diphosphate (vitamin K₃)
Kappadione, Synkavite♦♦, Synkayvite

INDICATIONS & DOSAGE
Hypoprothrombinemia secondary to vitamin K malabsorption or drug therapy, or when oral administration is desired and bile secretion is inadequate—
Adults: 2 to 10 mg menadione P.O. or 5 to 15 mg menadiol sodium diphosphate P.O. or parenterally, titrated to patient's requirements.

SIDE EFFECTS
CNS: headache, kernicterus.
GI: nausea, vomiting.
Skin: allergic rash, pruritus, urticaria.
Local: pain, hematoma at injection site.

INTERACTIONS
Mineral oil, cholestyramine resin: inhibited GI absorption of oral vitamin K. Space doses. Use together cautiously.

NURSING CONSIDERATIONS
• Contraindicated in treatment of oral anticoagulant overdose; in treatment

for hereditary hypoprothrombinemia (because vitamin K_3 can paradoxically worsen it); in patients with hepatocellular disease, unless it is caused by biliary obstruction; or in treatment of heparin-induced bleeding. Use cautiously during last weeks of pregnancy to avoid toxic reactions in newborns and in G-6-PD deficiency to avoid hemolysis. In severe bleeding, do not delay other measures such as giving fresh frozen plasma or whole blood. Use large doses cautiously in severe hepatic disease.

• Failure to respond to vitamin K_3 may indicate coagulation defects.

• Excessive use of vitamin K_3 may temporarily defeat oral anticoagulant therapy. Higher doses of oral anticoagulant or interim use of heparin may be required.

• Protect parenteral products from light.

• When I.V. route must be used, rate shouldn't exceed 1 mg/minute.

• Effects of I.V. injections more rapid but shorter lived than S.C. or I.M. injections.

• Monitor prothrombin time to determine dosage effectiveness.

• Observe for signs of side effects and report them to doctor.

• Use caution in handling bulk menadione powder. It is irritating to the skin and respiratory tract.

• Leafy vegetables high in vitamin K content. May alter warfarin needs.

---

phytonadione (vitamin K₁)
AquaMephyton♦, Konakion♦, Mephyton♦

INDICATIONS & DOSAGE

Hypoprothrombinemia secondary to vitamin K malabsorption drug therapy or excess vitamin A—
Adults: 2 to 25 mg, depending on severity, P.O. or parenterally, repeated and increased up to 50 mg, if necessary.
Children: 5 to 10 mg P.O. or parenterally.
Infants: 2 mg P.O. or parenterally. I.V. injection rate for children and infants should not exceed 3 mg/m²/minute or a total of 5 mg.
Hypoprothrombinemia secondary to effect of oral anticoagulants—
Adults: 2.5 to 10 mg P.O., S.C., or I.M., based on prothrombin time, repeated, if necessary, 12 to 48 hours after oral dose or 6 to 8 hours after parenteral dose. In emergency, give 10 to 50 mg slow I.V., rate not to exceed 1 mg/minute, repeated q 4 hours, as needed.
Prevention of hemorrhagic disease in neonates—
Neonates: 0.5 to 1 mg S.C. or I.M. immediately after birth, repeated in 6 to 8 hours, if needed, especially if mother received oral anticoagulants or long-term anticonvulsant therapy during pregnancy.
Differentiation between hepatocellular disease or biliary obstruction as source of hypoprothrombinemia—
Adults and children: 10 mg I.M. or S.C.
Prevention of hypoprothrombinemia related to vitamin K deficiency in long-term parenteral nutrition—
Adults: 5 to 10 mg S.C. or I.M. weekly.
Children: 2 to 5 mg S.C. or I.M. weekly.
Prevention of hypoprothrombinemia in infants receiving less than 0.1 mg/liter vitamin K in breast milk or milk substitutes—
Infants: 1 mg S.C. or I.M. monthly.

SIDE EFFECTS
CNS: dizziness, convulsive movement.
CV: *transient hypotension after I.V. administration,* rapid and weak pulse, cardiac irregularities.
GI: nausea, vomiting.

Italicized side effects are common or life-threatening.

Skin: sweating, flushing, erythema.
Local: pain, swelling, and hematoma at injection site.
Other: bronchospasms, dyspnea, cramp-like pain, *anaphylaxis and anaphylactoid reactions, usually after rapid I.V. administration.*

INTERACTIONS
Mineral oil, cholestyramine resin: inhibited GI absorption of oral vitamin K. Use together cautiously.

NURSING CONSIDERATIONS
• Contraindicated in hereditary hypoprothrombinemia; bleeding secondary to heparin therapy or overdose; hepatocellular disease, unless it is caused by biliary obstruction (vitamin K can paradoxically worsen the hypoprothrombinemia). Oral administration contraindicated if bile secretion is inadequate, unless supplemented with bile salts. Use cautiously, if at all, during last weeks of pregnancy to avoid toxic reactions in newborns; in G-6-PD deficiency to avoid hemolysis. Use large doses cautiously in severe hepatic disease.
• Failure to respond to vitamin K may indicate coagulation defects.
• In severe bleeding, don't delay other measures such as fresh frozen plasma or whole blood.
• Protect parenteral products from light. Wrap containers and tubing in foil during infusion.
• Effects of I.V. injections more rapid but shorter lived than S.C. or I.M. injections.
• Monitor prothrombin time to determine dosage effectiveness.
• Observe for signs of side effects and report them to the doctor.
• Phytonadione therapy for hemorrhagic disease in infants causes fewer adverse reactions than do other vitamin K analogs.
• Check brand-name labels for administration route restrictions.
• Administer I.V. by slow infusion.

Mix in normal saline solution, dextrose 5% in water, or dextrose 5% in normal saline.
• Leafy vegetables are high in vitamin K content. May alter warfarin needs.

multivitamins
Available by many brand names. Contain vitamins A, B complex, C, D, and E in varying amounts.

INDICATIONS & DOSAGE
Prevention of vitamin deficiencies in patients with inadequate diets or increased daily requirements; treatment of multiple vitamin deficiencies and prevention of recurrence; additions to parenteral nutrition solutions to meet patient's normal or increased requirements to reduce cost and facilitate patient compliance with therapy involving multiple vitamin deficiencies—
Adults and children: dosage depends on nature and severity of deficiencies and composition of multivitamin preparation.

SIDE EFFECTS
• Multivitamin preparations with ordinary doses of each component are usually nontoxic.
• Megavitamin combinations may promote significant accumulation of fat-soluble vitamins, with resultant toxicity.
• Multivitamins containing therapeutic doses of folic acid may mask pernicious anemia. Unless prescribed otherwise by doctor, patient should avoid folic acid in undiagnosed but suspected pernicious anemia.
• Other side effects depend on specific components and concentrations in each multivitamin preparation.

INTERACTIONS
Refer to each component of the multivitamin combination.

NURSING CONSIDERATIONS
• A single discovered vitamin deficiency usually coexists with others. After initial deficiencies are corrected, stress need for adequate nutrition and multivitamin supplements, if appropriate.
• Tell patient about possible interactions of vitamins in combinations and what precautions to take to avoid problems.
• Stress need to follow doctor's orders regarding daily dosages and follow-up therapy.
• Avoid excessive use of large-volume parenteral solutions of multivitamin supplements containing fat-soluble vitamins to avoid hypervitaminosis. I.V. solutions of water-soluble multivitamins may be used more freely.
• Chewable flavored multivitamins available for children. Prevent use of these drugs as "candy."
• Liquid preparations may contain varying percentages of alcohol. Check label; alert patient to content.
• Warn against overdosing. Encourage patient to eat a well-balanced diet.
• Store vitamins in a cool place in light-resistant containers to limit loss of potency.

---

sodium fluoride
Flo-Tabs, Fluor-A-Day ♦♦, Fluoritabs, Flura-Drops, Karidium♦, Luride Lozi-Tabs, Pediaflor, Pedi-Dent♦, Studafluor

---

INDICATIONS & DOSAGE
Aid in prevention of dental caries—
Oral—
Children 3 years and under: 0.5 mg daily.
Children over 3 years: 1 mg daily.
Topical—
Children 6 to 12 years: 5ml.
Adults, and children over 12 years:

10 ml. Use once daily after thoroughly brushing teeth and rinsing mouth. Rinse around and between teeth for 1 minute, then spit out.

SIDE EFFECTS
CNS: headaches, weakness.
GI: gastric distress.
Skin: hypersensitivity reactions such as atopic dermatitis, eczema, and urticaria.

INTERACTIONS
None significant.

NURSING CONSIDERATIONS
• Contraindicated when fluoride intake from drinking water exceeds 0.7 ppm; sodium-free diets.
• Chronic toxicity (fluorosis) may result from prolonged use of higher than recommended doses.
• Intended for use only where community water supplies are not fluoridated.
• Advise patient to notify dentist if tooth mottling occurs.
• Tablets may be dissolved in mouth, chewed, or swallowed whole.
• Drops may be administered orally undiluted or mixed with fluids or food.
• Topical forms (rinses and gels) should not be swallowed. Most effective when used immediately after brushing teeth.
• Tell patient not to dilute drops or rinses in glass containers but to use plastic instead.
• Used investigationally in the treatment of osteoporosis.

---

trace elements
chromium, copper, iodine (as iodide), manganese, zinc

INDICATIONS & DOSAGE
Prevention of individual trace element

deficiencies in patients receiving long-term hyperalimentation—
Chromium—
Adults: 10 to 15 mcg I.V. daily.
Children: 0.14 to 0.20 mcg/Kg I.V. daily.
Copper—
Adults: 0.5 to 1.5 mg I.V. daily.
Children: 0.05 to 0.2 mg/Kg I.V. daily.
Iodine—
Adults: 1 mcg/Kg I.V. daily.
Manganese—
Adults: 1 to 3 mg I.V. daily.
Zinc—
Adults: 2 to 4 mg I.V. daily.
Children: 0.05 mg/Kg I.V. daily.

SIDE EFFECTS
None reported.

INTERACTIONS
None significant at recommended dosages.

NURSING CONSIDERATIONS
• Check trace element serum levels of patients who have received total parenteral nutrition for 2 months or longer. Give supplement if necessary.
• Normal serum levels are 0.07 to 0.15 mg/ml copper; 0.05 to 0.15 mg/100 ml zinc; 4 to 20 mcg/100 ml manganese.
• Solutions of trace elements are compounded by pharmacy for addition to total parenteral nutrition solutions according to various formulas. One common trace element solution is Shil's solution, which contains copper 1 mg/ml, iodide 0.06 mg/ml, manganese 0.4 mg/ml, and zinc 2 mg/ml.

zinc sulfate
Orazinc

INDICATIONS & DOSAGE
Treatment of zinc deficiency or adjunct to treatment of disorders related to low serum zinc levels, including oral and decubitus leg ulcers, acne, granulomata of the ear, rheumatoid arthritis, idiopathic hypogeusia, anosmia; also, as adjunct to vitamin A therapy when patient fails to respond to vitamin A alone and in acrodermatitis enteropathica—
Adults: 200 to 220 mg P.O. t.i.d. (equivalent to 135 to 150 mg elemental zinc daily, 9 times the adult RDA of 15 mg daily).
Children: dosages not established. RDA is 0.3 mg/Kg daily.

SIDE EFFECTS
GI: distress and irritation, nausea, vomiting with high doses.

INTERACTIONS
None significant.

NURSING CONSIDERATIONS
• Therapeutic benefits result only if patient is zinc-deficient.
• Normal serum levels may not reliably show absence of zinc deficiency.
• Results may not appear for 6 to 8 weeks in zinc-depleted patients.
• If nausea or other GI side effects occur, decreasing dosage to 100 mg b.i.d. may help, since zinc is believed to irritate gastric mucosa.
• Brown bread and dairy products may interfere with zinc absorption.

92

Calorics

amino acid solution
corn oil
dextrose (d-glucose)
essential crystalline amino acid
   solution
fat emulsions
fructose (levulose)
invert sugar
medium-chain triglycerides

amino acid solution
(crystalline amino acid solution)
Aminosyn, Travasol♦, Veinamine

INDICATIONS & DOSAGE
*Total, supportive, or supplemental
and protein-sparing parenteral nutrition when body systems must rest during healing, or when patient can't,
shouldn't, or won't eat at all or eat
enough for adequate nutrition—*
Adults: 1 to 1.5 g/Kg I.V. daily.
Children: 2 to 3 g/Kg I.V. daily. Individualize dosage to metabolic and
clinical response as determined by nitrogen balance and body weight corrected for fluid balance. Add electrolyte and nonprotein caloric solutions
as needed.

SIDE EFFECTS
CNS: mental confusion, unconsciousness, headache, dizziness.
CV: hypervolemia related to congestive heart failure (in susceptible patients), *pulmonary edema,* exacerbation of hypertension (in predisposed
patients).
GI: nausea, vomiting.
GU: glycosuria, osmotic diuresis.
Hepatic: fatty liver.
Metabolic: *rebound hypoglycemia*
(when long-term infusions are
abruptly stopped), *hyperglycemia,*
hypervolemia, metabolic acidosis, alkalosis, hypophosphatemia, *hyperosmolar syndrome, hyperosmolar-
hyperglycemic-nonketotic syndrome,*
hyperammonemia, *electrolyte imbalances,* and dehydration (if hyperosmolar solutions used).
Skin: chills, flushing, feeling of
warmth.
Local: tissue sloughing at infusion
site due to extravasation, *catheter sepsis, thrombophlebitis.*
Other: allergic reactions.

INTERACTIONS
None significant.

NURSING CONSIDERATIONS
• Contraindicated in patients with severe uncorrected electrolyte or acid-
base imbalances, in hyperammonemia, and in decreased circulating
blood volume. Use cautiously in renal
insufficiency or failure, cardiac disease, and hepatic impairment. Long-
term use not advised for infants and
children.
• Monitor serum electrolytes, magnesium, glucose, BUN, renal and hepatic function. Check serum calcium
levels frequently to avoid bone demineralization in children.
• If long-term therapy is needed,
doctor may order trace element and
vitamin supplements. Avoid overuse
of fat-soluble vitamins.

• Refrigerate solution until ready to use.
• Don't mix medications, except electrolytes, with hyperalimentation solution without consulting pharmacist.
• Control infusion rate carefully with infusion pump.
• If infusion rate falls behind, do not attempt to "catch up." Notify doctor.
• Check injection site frequently for irritation, tissue sloughing, necrosis, and phlebitis. Change I.V. sites periodically to prevent irritation; usually given by catheter into subclavian vein.
• Watch closely for signs of fluid overload. Notify doctor promptly.
• Some brands of crystalline amino acid solutions contain large amounts of acetates and lactates; use cautiously in alkalosis or hepatic insufficiency.
• Most side effects are due to mixing amino acids with hypertonic dextrose solutions.

corn oil
Lipomul♦

INDICATIONS & DOSAGE
As energy source—
Adults: 45 ml P.O. b.i.d. to q.i.d. after or between meals, alone or with proteins, milk, or other energy sources.
Children: 30 ml P.O. daily to q.i.d. after or between meals, alone or with proteins, milk, or other energy sources.

SIDE EFFECTS
GI: nausea, vomiting, diarrhea.

INTERACTIONS
Griseofulvin: increased GI absorption of griseofulvin. Space doses.

NURSING CONSIDERATIONS
• Contraindicated in gallbladder calculi or complete GI obstructions. Use cautiously in steatorrhea, partial GI obstruction, enterostomies, hepatic cirrhosis, portacaval shunts.
• To minimize nausea, diarrhea, and vomiting, give more frequent, smaller doses with meals or mixed with milk.

dextrose (d-glucose)

INDICATIONS & DOSAGE
Fluid replacement and caloric supplementation in patient who can't maintain adequate oral intake or is restricted from doing so—
Adults and children: dosage depends on fluid and caloric requirements. Use peripheral I.V. infusion of 2.5%, 5%, or 10% solutions, central I.V. infusion of 20% solution for minimal fluid needs. Use 50% solution to treat insulin-induced hypoglycemia. Solutions from 40% to 70% are used in admixtures, normally with amino acid solutions, for total central I.V. parenteral nutrition.

SIDE EFFECTS
CNS: mental confusion, unconsciousness in hyperosmolar syndrome.
CV: with fluid overload: pulmonary edema, exacerbated hypertension, and congestive heart failure in susceptible patients. *Prolonged or concentrated infusions may cause phlebitis, sclerosis of vein, especially with peripheral route of administration.*
GU: glycosuria, osmotic diuresis.
Metabolic: with rapid infusion of concentrated solution or prolonged infusion: hyperglycemia, hypervolemia, hyperosmolarity. Rapid termination of long-term infusions may cause hypoglycemia from rebound hyperinsulinemia.
Skin: sloughing, if extravasation occurs with concentrated solutions.

INTERACTIONS
None significant.

NURSING CONSIDERATIONS
• Contraindicated in hyperglycemia, diabetic coma, intracranial or intraspinal hemorrhage, delirium tremens. Use cautiously in heart or pulmonary disease, hypertension, renal insufficiency, urinary obstruction, or hypovolemia.
• Control infusion rate carefully. Maximal rate for dextrose infusion is 0.5 g/Kg per hour. Use infusion pump when infusing dextrose with amino acids for total parenteral nutrition.
• Never infuse concentrated solutions rapidly.
• Monitor serum glucose carefully. Prolonged therapy with 5% dextrose can cause depletion of pancreatic insulin production and secretion.
• Never stop abruptly. If necessary, have 10% dextrose available to treat hypoglycemia if rebound hyperinsulinemia occurs.
• Take care to prevent extravasation. Check injection site frequently to prevent irritation, tissue sloughing, necrosis, and phlebitis.
• Watch closely for signs of fluid overload, especially if fluid intake is restricted.
• Monitor intake/output carefully, especially in impaired renal function.
• Check vital signs frequently. Report side effects promptly.
• Don't give dextrose solutions without saline with blood transfusions; may cause clumping of red blood cells.

---

essential crystalline amino acid solution
Nephramine

INDICATIONS & DOSAGE
Management of potentially reversible renal decompensation—

Adults: 0.3 to 0.5 g/Kg I.V., up to 26 g total daily (250 ml with 500 ml 70% dextrose injection), and infuse through central I.V. line at initial rate of 20 to 30 ml/hour, increased in steps of 10 ml/ hour every 24 hours, to a maximum of 60 to 100 ml/hour. Individualize dose and infusion rate to tolerance for glucose, fluid, and nitrogen. Add electrolytes and vitamins as needed.
Children: up to 1 g/Kg daily, individualized to patient's tolerance for glucose, fluid, and nitrogen. Add electrolytes and vitamins as needed.

SIDE EFFECTS
CNS: mental confusion, dizziness, unconsciousness, headache.
CV: hypervolemia related to congestive heart failure (in susceptible patients), *pulmonary edema,* exacerbation of hypertension (in predisposed patients).
GI: nausea, vomiting.
GU: glycosuria, osmotic diuresis.
Metabolic: *rebound hypoglycemia* (when long-term infusions are abruptly stopped), *hyperglycemia,* hypervolemia, metabolic acidosis, alkalosis, hypophosphatemia, hyperosmolar syndrome, *hyperosmolar-hyperglycemic-nonketotic syndrome,* hyperammonemia, *electrolyte imbalances,* and dehydration (if hyperosmolar solutions used).
Skin: chills, flushing, feeling of warmth.
Local: tissue sloughing at infusion site due to extravasation, *catheter sepsis, thrombophlebitis.*
Other: allergic reactions.

INTERACTIONS
None significant.

NURSING CONSIDERATIONS
• Contraindicated in severe uncorrected electrolyte or acid-base imbalances, hyperammonemia, and decreased circulating blood volume.

Italicized side effects are common or life-threatening.

• Monitor serum electrolytes, magnesium, glucose, BUN, renal and hepatic function. Check serum calcium levels frequently to avoid bone demineralization in children.

• In long-term therapy, doctor may order trace element and vitamin supplements. Avoid overuse of fat-soluble vitamins.

• Refrigerate solution until ready to use.

• Don't mix medications, except electrolytes, with hyperalimentation solution without consulting pharmacist.

• Control infusion rate carefully with infusion pump.

• If infusion rate falls behind, do not attempt to "catch up." Notify doctor.

• Check injection site frequently for irritation, tissue sloughing, necrosis, and phlebitis. Change I.V. sites periodically to prevent irritation; usually given by catheter into subclavian vein.

• Watch closely for signs of fluid overload. Notify doctor promptly.

• Essential amino acid solution is used identically to other crystalline amino acid solutions, except that it contains only the essential amino acids. By controlling amino acid content, patients with impaired renal function have decreases in blood urea nitrogen level, minimized deterioration of serum potassium, magnesium, and phosphorus balances. May lead to earlier return of renal function in patients with potentially reversible acute renal failure and may decrease morbidity associated with acute renal failure.

• Most side effects due to mixing essential crystalline amino acid solution with hypertonic dextrose solutions.

fat emulsions
Intralipid♦, Liposyn

INDICATIONS & DOSAGE
Intralipid:
Source of calories adjunctive to total parenteral nutrition—
Adults: 1 ml/minute I.V. for 15 to 30 minutes. If no adverse reactions, increase rate to deliver 500 ml over 4 hours. Infuse only 1,500-ml unit the first day. Total daily dose should not exceed 2.5 g/Kg (25 ml/Kg 10% emulsion).
Children: 0.1 ml/minute for 10 to 15 minutes. If no adverse reactions, increase rate to deliver 10 ml/Kg over 4 hours. Daily dose should not exceed 4 g/Kg (40 ml/Kg 10% emulsion). Equals 60% of daily caloric intake. Protein-carbohydrate hyperalimentation should supply remaining 40%.
Fatty-acid deficiency—
Adults and children: 8% to 10% of total caloric intake I.V.
Liposyn:
Prevention of fatty acid deficiency—
Adults: 500 ml I.V. twice weekly. Infuse initially at a rate of 1 ml/minute for 30 minutes. Rate may be increased but should not exceed 500 ml over 4 to 6 hours.
Children: 5 to 10 ml/Kg I.V. daily. Infuse initially at a rate of 0.1 ml/minute for 30 minutes. Rate may be increased but should not exceed 100 ml per hour.

SIDE EFFECTS
Early reactions:
Blood: hyperlipemia, hypercoagulability, rarely thrombocytopenia in neonates.
CNS: headache, sleepiness, dizziness.
EENT: pressure over eyes.
GI: nausea, vomiting.
Skin: flushing, sweating.
Local: irritation at infusion site.

Other: fever, dyspnea, chest and back pains, cyanosis, allergic reactions, deposition of I.V. fat.
Delayed reactions:
Blood: thrombocytopenia, leukopenia, leukocytosis.
CNS: focal seizures.
CV: shock.
Other: fever, transient increased liver function test, hepatomegaly, splenomegaly.

INTERACTIONS
None significant.

NURSING CONSIDERATIONS
• Contraindicated in hyperlipemia, lipoid nephrosis, and acute pancreatitis accompanied by hyperlipemia. Use cautiously in severe hepatic disease, pulmonary disease, anemia, blood coagulation disorders, or with possible danger of fat embolism.
• Never mix with electrolytes or other nutrient products or dilute manufactured fat emulsions. Infusion may be piggybacked into another I.V. line, but do not place additives in the fat emulsion bottle.
• Do not use an in-line filter when administering this drug.
• Discard fat emulsion if it separates or becomes oily. Keep Intralipid refrigerated until ready to use. Liposyn needs no refrigeration.
• Avoid rapid infusion. Use an infusion pump to regulate rate.
• Check injection site daily. Report signs of inflammation or infection promptly.
• Watch closely for side effects, especially during first half hour of infusion.
• Monitor serum lipids closely when patient is receiving fat emulsion therapy. Lipemia must clear between dosing.
• Check platelet count frequently in neonates receiving fat emulsions I.V.
• Monitor hepatic function carefully in long-term use.

• Intralipid and Liposyn differ mainly by their fatty acid components.

---

fructose (levulose)

INDICATIONS & DOSAGE
Source of carbohydrate calories primarily when fluid replacement is also indicated and as a dextrose substitute for diabetic patients—
Adults and children: dosage depends on caloric needs. I.V. infusion rate should not exceed 1 g/Kg per hour. Single liter 10% solution yields 375 calories.

SIDE EFFECTS
CV: increased pulse rate, precipitation or exacerbation of congestive heart failure in susceptible patients, *pulmonary edema*.
Metabolic: metabolic acidosis, hypervolemia.
Local: extravasation at infusion site may cause sloughing of skin, thrombophlebitis.
Other: increased respiratory rate, enlarged liver.

INTERACTIONS
None significant.

NURSING CONSIDERATIONS
• Contraindicated in hereditary fructose intolerance or in those receiving therapy for hypoglycemia. Use cautiously in heart disease, hypertension, pulmonary disease, hypervolemia, renal insufficiency, or urinary tract obstructions.
• Control infusion rate carefully. Make sure rate does not exceed 1 g/Kg per hour in infants.
• Change injection sites frequently to avoid irritation with prolonged therapy. Take care to avoid extravasation.
• Watch closely for signs of fluid

Italicized side effects are common or life-threatening.

overload, pulmonary edema, or congestive heart failure.
- May be safely used in diabetics.

invert sugar
Travert

INDICATIONS & DOSAGE
Nonelectrolyte fluid replacement and caloric supplementation solution—
Adults and children: dosage depends on patient's age, weight, clinical need. I.V. infusion rate should not exceed 1 g/Kg per hour. Single liter 5% invert sugar yields 375 calories.

SIDE EFFECTS
CNS: mental confusion.
CV: increased pulse rate, precipitation or exacerbation of congestive heart failure in susceptible patients, *pulmonary edema,* hypertension.
GU: glycosuria, osmotic diuresis.
Metabolic: metabolic acidosis, hypervolemia, hyperglycemia, hypoglycemia.
Local: extravasation at infusion site may cause sloughing of skin, thrombophlebitis.
Other: increased respiratory rate.

INTERACTIONS
None significant.

NURSING CONSIDERATIONS
- Contraindicated in hereditary fructose intolerance, hyperglycemia, diabetic coma, intracranial or intraspinal hemorrhage, or delirium tremens. Use cautiously in heart disease, hypertension, pulmonary disease, hypervolemia, renal insufficiency, or urinary tract obstructions.
- Control infusion rate carefully. Make sure rate does not exceed 1 g/Kg per hour in infants.
- Change injection sites frequently to avoid irritation with prolonged therapy. Take care to avoid extravasation.

- Watch closely for signs of fluid overload, pulmonary edema, or congestive heart failure. Monitor blood pressure frequently.
- May be safely used in diabetics.
- Monitor serum glucose closely. Prolonged therapy can cause depletion of pancreatic insulin production and secretion.
- Don't stop abruptly. If necessary, have 10% dextrose available to prevent rebound hyperinsulinemia and subsequent hypoglycemia.
- Monitor intake/output closely, especially if renal function is impaired.
- Check vital signs frequently. Tell doctor promptly if side effects develop.

medium-chain triglycerides
M.C.T. Oil♦

INDICATIONS & DOSAGE
Inadequate digestion or absorption of food fats—
Adults: 15 ml P.O. t.i.d. to q.i.d.

SIDE EFFECTS
CNS: reversible coma and precoma in susceptible patients.
GI: *nausea, vomiting, diarrhea.*

INTERACTIONS
None significant.

NURSING CONSIDERATIONS
- Contraindicated in advanced hepatic disease.
- To minimize GI side effects, give smaller doses more frequently with meals or mixed with fruit juice or salad dressing.
- More easily absorbed than long-chain fats.
- Rapid metabolism provides quick energy.
- May be useful in obesity control and in lowering cholesterol levels.

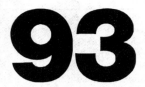

Immune serums

antirabies serum, equine
hepatitis B immune globulin,
    human
immune serum globulin
rabies immune globulin, human
Rh_o (D) immune globulin, human
tetanus immune globulin, human

---

antirabies serum, equine

INDICATIONS & DOSAGE
Rabies exposure—
Adults and children: 40 to 55 units/
Kg at time of first dose of rabies vaccine. Use half dose to infiltrate wound
area. Give remainder I.M. Don't give
vaccine and serum in same syringe or
at same site.

SIDE EFFECTS
Local: pain at injection site.
Systemic: within 6 to 12 days serum
sickness occurs in 15% to 25% of patients. Symptoms are skin eruptions,
arthralgia, pruritus, lymphadenopathy, fever, headache, malaise, abdominal pain, *anaphylaxis.*

INTERACTIONS
None significant.

NURSING CONSIDERATIONS
• In hypersensitivity, use rabies immune globulin, human, instead. If unavailable, desensitize before giving.
Consult doctor or pharmacist.
• Do sensitivity test on all patients
before giving. Dilute serum 1:100 or
1:1,000 with 0.9% sodium chloride

for injection. Inject intradermally on
inner forearm. Inject other arm with
0.1 ml 0.9% sodium chloride for injection intradermally as control. Read
within 20 minutes. Positive reaction:
wheal 10 mm or more and erythematous flare 20 x 20 mm.
• Use only when rabies immune globulin, human, not available.
• Obtain history of animal bite, allergies (especially to horse serum), and
past reaction to immunization.

**hepatitis B immune globulin,
    human**
H-BIG, HyperHep,
Hep-B-Gammagee

INDICATIONS & DOSAGE
Hepatitis B exposure—
Adults and children: 0.06 ml/Kg
I.M. within 7 days after exposure.
Repeat 28 days after exposure.

SIDE EFFECTS
Systemic: *anaphylaxis.*

INTERACTIONS
None significant.

NURSING CONSIDERATIONS
• Buttocks or deltoid areas preferred
injection sites.
• Nurse should receive immunization
if exposed to hepatitis B (e.g., needle-
stick, direct contact).
• Obtain history of allergies and past
reaction to immunization.

immune serum globulin
Gamastan, Gammagee, Gammar,
Gamulin, Immu-G, Immuglobin

INDICATIONS & DOSAGE
Agammaglobulinemia or hypogamma-globulinemia—
Adults: 30 to 50 ml I.M. monthly.
Children: 20 to 40 ml I.M. monthly.
Hepatitis A exposure—
Adults and children: 0.02 to
0.04 ml/Kg I.M. as soon as possible
after exposure. Up to 0.1 ml/Kg may
be given after prolonged or intense
exposure.
Serum hepatitis posttransfusion—
Adults and children: 10 ml I.M.
within 1 week after transfusion and
10 ml I.M. 1 month later.
Measles exposure—
Adults and children: 0.02 ml/Kg
within 6 days of exposure.
Modification of measles—
Adults and children: 0.04 ml/Kg
I.M. within 6 days of exposure.
Measles vaccine complications—
Adults and children: 0.02 to
0.04 ml/Kg I.M.
Poliomyelitis exposure—
Adults and children: 0.3 to
0.4 ml/Kg I.M. within 7 days after
exposure.
Chickenpox exposure—
Adults and children: 0.2 to 1.3 ml/
Kg I.M. as soon as exposed.
*Rubella exposure in first trimester of
pregnancy—*
Women: 0.2 to 0.4 ml/Kg I.M. as
soon as exposed.

SIDE EFFECTS
Skin: urticaria.
Local: pain, erythema, muscle
stiffness.
Systemic: angioedema, headache,
malaise, fever, nephrotic syndrome,
anaphylaxis.

INTERACTIONS
None significant.

NURSING CONSIDERATIONS
• Obtain history of allergies and past
reaction to immunization.
• Have drugs available for anaphylactic reaction.
• Divide dose of more than 10 ml,
and inject into different sites, preferably buttocks.
• Do not give for hepatitis A exposure if 6 weeks or more have elapsed
since exposure or after onset of clinical illness.

rabies immune globulin, human
Hyperab

INDICATIONS & DOSAGE
Rabies exposure—
Adults and children: 20 IU/Kg at
time of first dose of rabies vaccine.
Use half dose to infiltrate wound area.
Give remainder I.M. Don't give vaccine and immune globulin in same
syringe or at same site.

SIDE EFFECTS
Local: pain, redness, induration at
injection site.
Other: slight fever, *anaphylaxis.*

INTERACTIONS
None significant.

NURSING CONSIDERATIONS
• Repeated doses contraindicated
once rabies vaccine started.
• Use only with rabies vaccine and
immediate local treatment of wound.
Give regardless of interval between
exposure and initiation of therapy.
• Obtain history of animal bite, allergies, past reaction to immunization.
• Corticosteroids decrease resistance
to infection and decrease antibody response to vaccine. Stop corticosteroids after possible rabies exposure.

Rh₀ (D) immune globulin, human
Gamulin R, HypRho D,
MICRhoGAM, RhoGam

INDICATIONS & DOSAGE
Rh exposure—
Women postabortion, postmiscarriage, ectopic pregnancy, or postpartum: transfusion unit or blood bank determines fetal packed red blood cell volume entering woman's blood, then gives 1 vial I.M. if fetal packed red blood cell volume was less than 15 ml. More than 1 vial I.M. may be required if there is large fetomaternal hemorrhage. Must be given within 72 hours following delivery or miscarriage.
Transfusion accidents—
Adults and children: consult blood bank or transfusion unit at once. Must be given within 72 hours.
Postabortion or postmiscarriage to prevent Rh antibody formation—
Women: consult transfusion unit or blood bank. Must be given within 3 hours after abortion or miscarriage.

SIDE EFFECTS
Local: discomfort at injection site.
Other: slight fever.

INTERACTIONS
None significant.

NURSING CONSIDERATIONS
• Contraindicated in Rh₀ (D) positive or Dᵘ positive patients and those previously immunized to Rh₀ (D) blood factor.
• Immediately after delivery send infant's cord blood to lab for type and crossmatch. Confirm mother is Rh₀ (D) negative and Dᵘ negative. Infant must be Rh₀ (D) positive or Dᵘ positive.
• Give only to postpartum mother, not infant.

• Obtain history of allergies and past reaction to immunization.
• MICRhoGam recommended for every woman undergoing abortion or miscarriage up to 12 weeks gestation unless she is Rh₀ (D) positive or Dᵘ positive, has Rh antibodies, or the father and/or fetus is Rh negative.
• For I.M. use only.
• Store at 36° to 46° F. (2° to 8° C.). Do not freeze.

tetanus immune globulin, human
Homo-Tet, Hu-Tet, Hyper-Tet, Immu-Tetanus, T-I-Gammagee

INDICATIONS & DOSAGE
Tetanus exposure—
Adults and children: 250 units I.M.
Tetanus treatment—
Adults and children: single doses of 3,000 to 6,000 units have been used, but optimal dosage schedules not established. Do not give at same site as toxoid.

SIDE EFFECTS
Local: pain, stiffness, erythema.
Other: slight fever, allergy, *anaphylaxis.*

INTERACTIONS
None significant.

NURSING CONSIDERATIONS
• Use tetanus immune globulin only if wound is over 24 hours old or patient has had less than 2 previous tetanus toxoid injections.
• Obtain history of injury, past tetanus immunizations, last tetanus toxoid injection, allergies, and past reaction to immunization.
• Thoroughly cleanse and remove all foreign matter from wound.

Italicized side effects are common or life-threatening.

94

Vaccines and toxoids

BCG vaccine
cholera vaccine
diphtheria and tetanus toxoids, adsorbed
diphtheria and tetanus toxoids and pertussis vaccine (DPT)
diphtheria toxoid, adsorbed, pediatric
influenza virus vaccine, trivalent
measles, mumps, and rubella virus vaccine, live
measles (rubeola) and rubella virus vaccine, live attenuated
measles (rubeola) virus vaccine, live attenuated
meningitis vaccines
mumps virus vaccine, live
plague vaccine
pneumococcal vaccine, polyvalent
poliovirus vaccine, live, oral, trivalent
rabies vaccine (duck embryo), dried, killed virus
rabies vaccine, human diploid cell (HDCV)
rubella and mumps virus vaccine, live
rubella virus vaccine, live attenuated (RA 27/3)
smallpox vaccine
staphylococcus toxoid
tetanus toxoid
typhoid vaccine
typhus vaccine
yellow fever vaccine

BCG vaccine

INDICATIONS & DOSAGE
Tuberculosis exposure—
Adults and children: 0.1 ml intradermally.
Newborns: 0.05 ml intradermally.

SIDE EFFECTS
Local: lymphangitis, lymph node and skin abscess, ulceration at site of injection (2 to 3 weeks after injection), lupus reaction.
Other: urticaria of trunk and limbs, *anaphylaxis.*

INTERACTIONS
Isoniazid (INH): inhibited multiplication of BCG. Avoid using together.

NURSING CONSIDERATIONS
- Contraindicated in hypogammaglobulinemia, positive tuberculin reaction, corticosteroid therapy, immunosuppression, fresh smallpox vaccination, and burn patients. Use cautiously in chronic skin disease. Inject in area of healthy skin only.
- Obtain history of allergies and past reaction to immunization.
- Vaccine is of no value in patients with positive tuberculin test.
- Keep epinephrine 1:1,000 available to treat anaphylaxis.
- Recommended injection site is over insertion of deltoid muscle.
- Do not shake vial following reconstitution.

• Expected lesion forms in 7 to 10 days.
• Live vaccine; destroy by autoclaving or formalin solution before disposal.
• Patient should have tuberculin skin test 2 to 3 months after BCG vaccination to determine success of vaccine.

---

cholera vaccine

INDICATIONS & DOSAGE
Primary immunization—
Adults, and children over 10 years: 2 doses of 0.5 ml I.M. or 1 ml S.C., 1 week to 1 month before traveling in cholera area. Booster: 0.5 ml q 6 months as long as protection is needed.
Children 5 to 10 years: 0.3 ml I.M. or S.C.
Children 6 months to 4 years: 0.2 ml I.M. or S.C. Boosters of same dose should be given q 6 months as long as protection needed.

SIDE EFFECTS
Systemic: malaise, fever, flushing, urticaria, tachycardia, hypotension, headache, *anaphylaxis.*
Local: erythema, swelling, pain, induration.

INTERACTIONS
None significant.

NURSING CONSIDERATIONS
• Contraindicated in corticosteroid therapy or in immunosuppression. Defer in acute illness.
• Obtain history of allergies and past reaction to immunization.
• Keep epinephrine 1:1,000 available.
• May be given intradermally, but I.M. and S.C. routes give higher levels of protection.

---

diphtheria and tetanus toxoids, adsorbed

INDICATIONS & DOSAGE
Primary immunization—
Adults, and children 7 years and over: use adult strength; 0.5 ml I.M. 4 to 6 weeks apart for 2 doses and a third dose 1 year later.
Booster: 0.5 ml I.M. q 10 years.
Children under 7 years: use pediatric strength; 0.5 ml I.M. 4 to 8 weeks apart for 2 doses and a third dose 6 to 12 months later.
Booster: 0.5 ml when starting school.

SIDE EFFECTS
Systemic: chills, fever, malaise, *anaphylaxis.*
Local: stinging, edema, erythema, pain, induration.

INTERACTIONS
None significant.

NURSING CONSIDERATIONS
• Contraindicated in immunosuppression, radiation, or corticosteroid therapy. Defer in respiratory illness or polio outbreaks, or acute illness except in emergency. Use single antigen during polio risks. In children under 6 years, use only when diphtheria, tetanus, and pertussis toxoid combination is contraindicated because of pertussis component.
• Verify strength (pediatric or adult) of toxoid used.
• Don't use hot or cold compresses; may increase severity of local reaction.
• Obtain history of allergies and past reaction to immunization.
• Keep epinephrine 1:1,000 available.
• Give in site not previously used for vaccines or toxoids.

Italicized side effects are common or life-threatening.

diphtheria and tetanus toxoids and pertussis vaccine (DPT)
Tri-Immunol, Triogen, Triple Antigen

INDICATIONS & DOSAGE
Primary immunization—
Children 6 weeks to 6 years: 0.5 ml I.M. 2 months apart for 3 doses and a fourth dose 1 year later.
Booster: 0.5 ml I.M. when starting school. Not advised for adults, or children over 6 years.

SIDE EFFECTS
Systemic: slight fever, chills, malaise, *convulsions, encephalopathy, anaphylaxis.*
Local: soreness, redness, expected nodule remaining several weeks.

INTERACTIONS
None significant.

NURSING CONSIDERATIONS
• Contraindicated in corticosteroid therapy or immunosuppression. Defer in acute illness.
• Stop immunization if CNS disorder occurs. Immunization may be continued with diphtheria and tetanus toxoids without pertussis component at doses of 0.05 to 0.1 ml.
• DPT injection may be given at same time as trivalent oral polio vaccine (TOPV).
• Obtain history of allergies and past reaction to immunization.
• Keep epinephrine 1:1,000 available.
• Not to be used for active infection.
• Don't give subcutaneously.
• Shake before using. Refrigerate.

diphtheria toxoid, adsorbed, pediatric

INDICATIONS & DOSAGE
Diphtheria immunization—

Children under 6 years: 0.5 ml I.M. 6 to 8 weeks apart for 2 doses and a third dose 1 year later. Booster: 0.5 ml I.M. at 5- to 10-year intervals. Not advised for adults or children over 6 years; instead, use adult strength of diphtheria toxoid (usually combined with tetanus toxoid).

SIDE EFFECTS
Systemic: fever, malaise, urticaria, tachycardia, flushing, pruritus, hypotension, aches and pains, *anaphylaxis.*
Local: erythema, pain, induration, expected nodule persistent for several weeks.

INTERACTIONS
None significant.

NURSING CONSIDERATIONS
• Contraindicated in immunosuppression, radiation or corticosteroid therapy, children under 12 months with cerebral damage. Defer in acute illness or polio outbreak, except in emergency.
• Don't use hot or cold compresses; may intensify local reaction.
• Obtain history of allergies and past reaction to immunization.
• Keep epinephrine 1:1,000 available to treat anaphylaxis.
• Shake vial well before using. Store in refrigerator.

influenza virus vaccine, trivalent
Fluax♦♦, Fluogen♦,
Fluzone-Connaught
influenza virus, trivalent types A & B

INDICATIONS & DOSAGE
Brazil, Bangkok, and Singapore influenza prophylaxis—
Adults 28 years and over: 0.5 ml whole or split virus I.M. Use adult formula.
Youths 13 to 27 years: 0.5 ml whole

or split virus I.M. Repeat doses in 4 weeks. Those who received the 1979 or 1980 vaccine require only 1 dose.
Children 3 to 12 years: give 0.5 ml split virus I.M. Repeat dose in 4 weeks unless child received 1979 or 1980 vaccine.
Children 6 to 35 months: 0.25 ml split virus I.M. Repeat dose in 4 weeks unless child received 1979 or 1980 vaccine.
Recommendations are for 1981 only. Must check yearly for new recommendations.

SIDE EFFECTS
Systemic: *fever, malaise, myalgia, Guillain-Barré syndrome, anaphylaxis.*
Local: erythema, induration. Side effects occur most often in children and in others not exposed to influenza viruses.

INTERACTIONS
None significant.

NURSING CONSIDERATIONS
• Contraindicated in egg allergy. Defer in acute respiratory or other active infection, or when there is risk of poliomyelitis infection.
• Obtain history of allergies, especially to eggs, and past reaction to immunization.
• Give injections in deltoid or midlateral thigh.
• Keep epinephrine 1:1,000 available.
• Recommended for patients with chronic disease, metabolic disorders, and those over 65 years of age.
• Fever, malaise, and myalgia begin 6 to 12 hours after vaccination and persist 1 to 2 days.
• Allergic reactions, which occur immediately, are extremely rare.
• Paralysis associated with Guillain-Barré syndrome is uncommon, but patient should be made aware of risk as

compared to risk of influenza and its complications.

---

measles, mumps, and rubella virus vaccine, live
M-M-R-II♦

INDICATIONS & DOSAGE
Immunization—
Children over 12 months to puberty: 1 vial (1,000 units) S.C.

SIDE EFFECTS
Systemic: fever, rash, regional lymphadenopathy, urticaria, *anaphylaxis.*
Local: erythema.

INTERACTIONS
Immune serum globulin, whole blood, plasma: antibodies in serum may interfere with immune response. Don't use vaccine within 3 months of transfusion.

NURSING CONSIDERATIONS
• Contraindicated in immunosuppression; cancer; blood dyscrasias; corticosteroid or radiation therapy; gamma globulin disorders; fever; active, untreated tuberculosis. Use cautiously in hypersensitivity to neomycin, chickens, ducks, eggs, or feathers. Defer immunization in acute illness.
• Presence of maternal antibodies may prevent response in children under 12 months.
• Treat fever with antipyretics.
• Store in refrigerator; protect from light. Solution may be used if red, pink, or yellow, but must be clear.
• Use only diluent supplied. Discard 8 hours after reconstituting.
• Obtain history of allergies, especially to ducks, rabbits, antibiotics, and past reaction to immunization.
• Inject in outer aspect of upper arm. Don't give I.V.

Italicized side effects are common or life-threatening.

• Keep epinephrine 1:1,000 available.

measles (rubeola) and rubella virus vaccine, live attenuated
M-R-Vax-II

INDICATIONS & DOSAGE
Immunization—
Children 15 months to puberty:
1 vial (1,000 units) S.C.

SIDE EFFECTS
Systemic: fever, rash, lymphadenopathy, *anaphylaxis.*

INTERACTIONS
Immune serum globulin, whole blood, plasma: antibodies in serum may interfere with immune response. Don't use vaccine within 3 months of transfusion.
Tuberculin skin test: may temporarily decrease response to test. Defer skin testing.

NURSING CONSIDERATIONS
• Contraindicated in immunosuppression; cancer; blood dyscrasias; corticosteroid or radiation therapy; gamma globulin disorders; fever; active, untreated tuberculosis. Use cautiously in hypersensitivity to neomycin, chickens, ducks, eggs, or feathers, and when there is a history of febrile seizures or in cerebral injury. Defer immunization in acute illness.
• Do not give within 1 month of other live virus vaccines, except oral poliovirus vaccine.
• Store in refrigerator and protect from light. Solution may be used if red, pink, or yellow, but must be clear (with no precipitation).
• Use only diluent supplied. Discard 8 hours after reconstituting.
• Inject in outer aspect of upper arm. Don't inject I.V.

measles (rubeola) virus vaccine, live attenuated
Attenuvax ♦ , M-Vac

INDICATIONS & DOSAGE
Immunization—
Adults, and children 15 months or over: 0.5 ml (1,000 units) S.C.

SIDE EFFECTS
Systemic: fever and rash, lymphadenopathy, *anaphylaxis,* febrile convulsions in susceptible children, anorexia, leukopenia.
Local: erythema, swelling, tenderness.

INTERACTIONS
Immune serum globulin, whole blood, plasma: antibodies in serum may interfere with immune response. Don't use vaccine within 3 months of transfusion.
Tuberculin skin test: may temporarily decrease response to test. Defer skin testing.

NURSING CONSIDERATIONS
• Contraindicated in immunosuppression; cancer; blood dyscrasias; corticosteroid or radiation therapy; gamma globulin disorders; active, untreated tuberculosis; fever. Use with caution in hypersensitivity to neomycin, chickens, eggs, or feathers. Defer in acute illness or after administration of blood or plasma.
• Warn patient to avoid pregnancy for 3 months after vaccination.
• Do not give I.V.
• Obtain history of allergies, especially to eggs, and past reaction to immunization.
• Keep epinephrine 1:1,000 available.
• Store in refrigerator and protect from light. Solution may be used if red, pink, or yellow, but must be clear (with no precipitation).
• Use only diluent supplied. Discard 8 hours after reconstituting.

• May be given with oral polio vaccine.

meningitis vaccines
Meningovax-C, Meningovax-A/C, Menomune-A, Menomune-C, Menomune-A/C

INDICATIONS & DOSAGE
Meningococcal meningitis prophylaxis—
Adults, and children over 2 years: 0.5 ml S.C. Use vaccine group C or A, except in highly endemic areas; in these areas use A/C combination.
Children 3 months to 2 years: 0.5 ml S.C. Use vaccine group A.

SIDE EFFECTS
Systemic: headache, malaise, chills, fever, cramps, *anaphylaxis.*
Local: pain, erythema, induration.

INTERACTIONS
None significant.

NURSING CONSIDERATIONS
• Contraindicated in immunosuppression. Defer in acute illness.
• Tell patient to avoid pregnancy for 3 months after vaccination.
• Obtain history of allergies and past reaction to immunization.
• Do not give I.V.
• Keep epinephrine 1:1,000 available.

mumps virus vaccine, live
Mumpsvax ◆

INDICATIONS & DOSAGE
Immunization—
Adults, and children over 12 months: 1 vial (5,000 units) S.C.

SIDE EFFECTS
Systemic: *slight fever,* skin rash, malaise, mild allergic reactions.

INTERACTIONS
Immune serum globulin, whole blood, plasma: antibodies in serum may interfere with immune response. Don't use vaccine within 3 months of transfusion.
Tuberculin skin test: may temporarily decrease response to test. Defer skin testing.

NURSING CONSIDERATIONS
• Contraindicated in immunosuppression; cancer; blood dyscrasias; corticosteroid or radiation therapy; gamma globulin disorders; active, untreated tuberculosis. Use cautiously in hypersensitivity to neomycin, chickens, ducks, eggs, or feathers. Defer in acute illness and for 3 months following transfusions or immune serum globulin.
• Stress importance of avoiding pregnancy for 3 months after immunization. If necessary, provide contraceptive information.
• Treat fever with antipyretics.
• Don't give I.V.
• Store in refrigerator and protect from light. Solution may be used if red, pink, or yellow, but must be clear.
• Use only diluent supplied. Discard 8 hours after reconstituting.
• Obtain history of allergies, especially to antibiotics, and past reaction to immunization.

plague vaccine

INDICATIONS & DOSAGE
Primary immunization and booster—
Adults, and children over 11 years: 1 ml I.M. followed by 0.2 ml in 1 to 3 months, then 0.2 ml 3 to 6 months after second injection.
Booster: 0.1 to 0.2 ml q 6 months while in plague area.
Children under 1 year: $1/_5$ adult primary or booster dose.

Italicized side effects are common or life-threatening.

Children 1 to 4 years: $^2/_5$ adult primary or booster dose.
Children 5 to 10 years: $^3/_5$ adult primary or booster dose.

SIDE EFFECTS
Systemic: malaise, headache, slight fever, lymphadenopathy, *anaphylaxis*.
Local: swelling, induration, erythema.

INTERACTIONS
None significant.

NURSING CONSIDERATIONS
• Contraindicated in immunosuppression. Defer in respiratory infection.
• Deltoid area preferred injection site.
• Obtain history of allergies and past reaction to immunization.
• Keep epinephrine 1:1,000 available.

pneumococcal vaccine, polyvalent
Pneumovax♦, Pnu-Imune

INDICATIONS & DOSAGE
Pneumococcal immunization—
Adults, and children 2 years or over: 0.5 ml I.M. or S.C.
Not recommended for children under 2 years.

SIDE EFFECTS
Systemic: *slight fever, anaphylaxis.*
Local: severe local reaction can occur when revaccination takes place within 3 years.

INTERACTIONS
None significant.

NURSING CONSIDERATIONS
• Check immunization history carefully to avoid revaccination within 3 years.
• Inject in deltoid or midlateral thigh. Don't inject I.V.

• Keep refrigerated. Reconstitution or dilution not necessary.
• Treat fever with mild antipyretics.
• Protects against 14 pneumococcal types, which account for 80% of pneumococcal disease.
• Obtain history of allergies and past reaction to immunization.
• Keep epinephrine 1:1,000 available.

poliovirus vaccine, live, oral, trivalent
Orimune

INDICATIONS & DOSAGE
Poliovirus immunization—
Adults, and children over 6 weeks: 2 drops or 0.5 ml P.O. in 5 ml water or simple syrup, or on sugar cube. Repeat dose in 8 weeks. Give third dose at 18 months. Booster: 2 drops or 0.5 ml P.O.

SIDE EFFECTS
None reported.

INTERACTIONS
Immune serum globulin, whole blood, plasma: antibodies in serum may interfere with immune response. Don't use vaccine within 3 months of transfusion.

NURSING CONSIDERATIONS
• Contraindicated in immunosuppression, cancer, immunoglobulin abnormalities, radiation or corticosteroid therapy. Defer in acute illness, vomiting, or diarrhea.
• Keep frozen until used. Once thawed, if unopened, may store refrigerated up to 30 days. Opened vials may be refrigerated up to 7 days. Thaw before administration.
• Discard if vaccine color changes from red or pink to yellow.
• Obtain history of allergies and past reaction to immunization.
• Not for parenteral use.

rabies vaccine (duck embryo), dried, killed virus

INDICATIONS & DOSAGE
Postexposure immunization for domestic animal bite—
Adults and children: 1 ml S.C. daily for 14 days in the abdomen on alternate sides.
Postexposure immunization for wild animal bite—
Adults and children: 2 ml S.C. daily for 7 days, then 1 ml daily for 7 more days. Supplemental doses may be needed after initial therapy.
Preexposure immunization (for patients constantly exposed to rabies)—
Adults and children: 1 ml S.C. weekly for 3 weeks, then fourth dose 6 months later; or 1 ml S.C. 1 month apart for 2 doses, then third dose 7 months after second. Booster (for patients constantly exposed to rabies): 1 ml q 1 to 2 years.

SIDE EFFECTS
Systemic: peripheral neuritis, dorsolumbar myelitis, acute idiopathic polyneuritis, acute encephalomyelitis, fever, weakness, stiff neck, respiratory distress, *anaphylaxis.*
GI: *nausea, vomiting, diarrhea, abdominal cramps.*
Skin: *urticaria.*
Local: *stinging, pain, erythema, induration,* lymphadenopathy.

INTERACTIONS
None significant.

NURSING CONSIDERATIONS
• Stop corticosteroids during immunization period.
• When postexposure immunization is indicated, pregnancy is not a contraindication.
• Immediate, thorough cleaning of wound is best way to prevent rabies.
• Rabies immune globulin may be given at time of first vaccine dose to provide immediate protection.
• Use 23- or 24-gauge, ½- to ¾-inch needle.
• Obtain history of allergies, especially to eggs, ducks, or proteins, and past reaction to immunization.
• Keep epinephrine 1:1,000 available.

rabies vaccine, human diploid cell (HDCV)

INDICATIONS & DOSAGE
Postexposure antirabies immunization—
Adults and children: 5 1-ml doses of HDCV I.M. (for example, in the deltoid region). Give first dose as soon as possible after exposure; give an additional dose on each of days 3, 7, 14, and 28 after first dose.

SIDE EFFECTS
Systemic: headache, nausea, abdominal pain, muscle aches, dizziness.
Local: *pain, erythema, swelling or itching at injection site.*

INTERACTIONS
None significant.

NURSING CONSIDERATIONS
• Stop corticosteroids during immunization period.
• When postexposure immunization is indicated, pregnancy is not a contraindication.
• Persons with a history of hypersensitivity should be given rabies vaccine with caution. Persons allergic to duck embryo vaccine are less likely to be allergic to HDCV.
• Keep epinephrine 1:1,000 available.
• HDCV is the preferred rabies vaccine because of its presumed greater efficacy and because fewer adverse reactions are known to be associated with it.
• Contact state health department or

Merieux Institute (1-800-327-8387) on vaccine availability.

rubella and mumps virus vaccine, live
Biavax-II

INDICATIONS & DOSAGE
Measles and mumps immunization—
Adults, and children over 12 months: 1 vial (1,000 units) S.C.

SIDE EFFECTS
Systemic: fever, rash, thrombocytopenic purpura, urticaria, arthritis, arthralgia, polyneuritis, *anaphylaxis.*
Local: pain, erythema, induration, lymphadenopathy.

INTERACTIONS
Immune serum globulin, whole blood, plasma: antibodies in serum may interfere with immune response. Don't give vaccine within 3 months of transfusion.
Tuberculin skin test: may temporarily decrease response to test. Defer skin testing.

NURSING CONSIDERATIONS
• Contraindicated in immunosuppression; cancer; blood dyscrasias; corticosteroid or radiation therapy; gamma globulin disorders; active, untreated tuberculosis; fever; pregnancy. Use with caution in hypersensitivity to neomycin, chickens, ducks, eggs, or feathers. Defer in acute illness and after administration of immune serum globulin, blood, or plasma.
• Stress importance of avoiding pregnancy for 3 months after immunization. If necessary, provide contraceptive information.
• Store in refrigerator and protect from light. Solution may be used if red, pink, or yellow, but must be clear.

• Use only diluent supplied. Discard 8 hours after reconstituting.
• Obtain history of allergies, especially to ducks, rabbits, and antibiotics, and past reaction to immunization.
• Inject into outer aspect of upper arm. Don't inject I.V.
• Keep epinephrine 1:1,000 available.

rubella virus vaccine, live attenuated (RA 27/3)
Meruvax-II♦

INDICATIONS & DOSAGE
Measles immunization—
Adults, and children over 12 months: 1 vial (1,000 units) S.C. or I.M.

SIDE EFFECTS
Systemic: fever, rash, thrombocytopenic purpura, urticaria, arthritis, arthralgia, polyneuritis, *anaphylaxis.*
Local: pain, erythema, induration, lymphadenopathy.

INTERACTIONS
Immune serum globulin, whole blood, plasma: antibodies in serum may interfere with immune response. Don't use vaccine within 3 months of transfusion.
Tuberculin skin test: may temporarily decrease response to test. Defer skin testing.

NURSING CONSIDERATIONS
• Contraindicated in immunosuppression; cancer; blood dyscrasias; corticosteroid or radiation therapy; gamma globulin disorders; active, untreated tuberculosis; fever. Use cautiously in hypersensitivity to neomycin, chickens, ducks, eggs, or feathers. Defer in acute illness and after administration of human immune serum globulin, blood, or plasma.
• Stress importance of avoiding pregnancy for 3 months after immunization.

If necessary, provide contraceptive information.
• Store in refrigerator and protect from light. Solution may be used if red, pink, or yellow, but must be clear.
• Use only diluent supplied. Discard 8 hours after reconstituting.
• Obtain history of allergies, especially to ducks and rabbits, and past reaction to immunization.
• Inject into outer aspect of upper arm. Don't inject I.V.
• Keep epinephrine 1:1,000 available.

smallpox vaccine
Dryvax

INDICATIONS & DOSAGE
Immunization—
Adults and children: deposit drop of vaccine onto cleansed site and make series of multiple pressures with sharp needle through drop. Use only for lab personnel working with virus.

SIDE EFFECTS
Systemic: encephalopathy, transverse myelitis, acute infection, polyneuritis, eczema vaccinatum, eye infection, rash, *anaphylaxis,* fever.
Local: necrosis, pustule (expected), infection.

INTERACTIONS
Immune serum globulin, whole blood, plasma: antibodies in serum may interfere with immune response. Don't use vaccine within 3 months of transfusion.
Methotrexate: may interfere with immune response. Don't use together.

NURSING CONSIDERATIONS
• Contraindicated in infants failing to thrive, wounds or burns, skin disorders, patients with direct contact with smallpox virus, immunosuppression, antimetabolite and radiation therapy. Weigh risks against benefits. Use cau-

tiously in hypersensitivity to eggs, chickens, or feathers, or to neomycin or other antibiotic preservatives in this vaccine (polymyxin B, streptomycin, chlortetracycline).
• Don't expose site to direct sunlight for several days or water for 2 hours. Don't cover site initially. In pustular stage, loose dressing may be applied. Warn against touching site: may spread lesion and cause secondary infection.
• Obtain history of allergies, especially to chickens or beef, antibiotics, and past reaction to immunization.
• Do not inject.
• Reconstituted solution may be kept for 3 months under refrigeration.
• Keep epinephrine 1:1,000 available.

staphylococcus toxoid

INDICATIONS & DOSAGE
Prophylaxis and treatment of recurrent boils, carbuncles, pustular acne (when combined with antibiotics)—
Adults and children: administer a graded series of I.M. or S.C. injections based on sensitivity testing results. Give injections q 2 to 7 days, utilizing two dilutions supplied.

SIDE EFFECTS
Systemic: hypersensitivity, *anaphylaxis.*

INTERACTIONS
None significant.

NURSING CONSIDERATIONS
• Use with antibiotics.
• Give test dose first.
• Obtain history of allergies and past reaction to immunization.
• Keep epinephrine 1:1,000 available.

Italicized side effects are common or life-threatening.

tetanus toxoid, adsorbed♦
Tet Tox Adsorbed
tetanus toxoid fluid
Tet Tox Fluid

INDICATIONS & DOSAGE
Primary immunization—
Adults and children: 0.5 ml (adsorbed) I.M. 4 to 6 weeks apart for 2 doses, then third dose 1 year after the second.
Primary immunization—
Adults and children: 0.5 ml (fluid) I.M. or S.C. 4 to 8 weeks apart, for 3 doses, then fourth dose of 0.5 ml 6 to 12 months after third dose.
Booster: 0.5 ml I.M. at 10-year intervals.

SIDE EFFECTS
Systemic: slight fever, chills, malaise, aches and pains, flushing, urticaria, pruritus, tachycardia, hypotension, *anaphylaxis.*
Local: erythema, induration, nodule.

INTERACTIONS
None significant.

NURSING CONSIDERATIONS
• Contraindicated in immunosuppression and immunoglobulin abnormalities. Defer in acute illness and polio outbreaks, except in emergencies.
• For prevention, not treatment, of tetanus infections.
• Determine date of last tetanus immunization.
• Don't use hot or cold compresses; may increase severity of local reaction.
• Obtain history of allergies and past reaction to immunization.
• Keep epinephrine 1:1,000 available.
• Adsorbed form produces longer duration of immunity. Fluid form provides quicker booster effect in patients actively immunized previously.

typhoid vaccine

INDICATIONS & DOSAGE
Primary immunization—
Adults, and children over 10 years: 0.5 ml S.C.; repeat in 4 weeks.
Booster: same dose as primary immunization q 3 years.
Children 6 months to 10 years: 0.25 ml S.C.; repeat in 4 weeks.
Booster: same dose as primary immunization q 3 years.

SIDE EFFECTS
Systemic: *fever,* malaise, headache, nausea, *anaphylaxis.*
Local: swelling, pain, inflammation.

INTERACTIONS
None significant.

NURSING CONSIDERATIONS
• Contraindicated in corticosteroid therapy. Defer in acute illness.
• Treat fever with antipyretics.
• Do not give intradermally.
• Obtain history of allergies and past reaction to immunization.
• Keep epinephrine 1:1,000 available.
• Store at 2° to 10° C. (35.6° to 50° F.).
• Shake thoroughly before withdrawal from vial.

typhus vaccine

INDICATIONS & DOSAGE
Immunization against louse-borne epidemic typhus—
Adults: 0.5 ml Lederle vaccine or 1 ml Lilly vaccine S.C.; repeat in 4 weeks.
Children under 10 years: 0.25 ml Lederle vaccine or 0.5 ml Lilly vaccine S.C.; repeat in 4 weeks.

SIDE EFFECTS
Systemic: fever, malaise, *anaphylaxis*.
Local: pain, induration, erythema.

INTERACTIONS
None significant.

NURSING CONSIDERATIONS
• Contraindicated in corticosteroid therapy and in egg hypersensitivity. Defer in acute illness.
• Use for classical epidemic typhus, not endemic forms.
• Obtain history of allergies, especially to eggs, and past reaction to immunization.
• Keep epinephrine 1:1,000 available.

---

yellow fever vaccine

INDICATIONS & DOSAGE
Primary vaccination—
Adults, and children over 6 months: 0.5 ml S.C. Booster: repeat 0.5 ml S.C. q 10 years.

SIDE EFFECTS
Systemic: fever, malaise, *anaphylaxis*.

INTERACTIONS
None significant.

NURSING CONSIDERATIONS
• Contraindicated in gamma globulin deficiency, immunosuppression, cancer, corticosteroid or radiation therapy, allergies to chickens or eggs, and in pregnancy and in infants under 6 months except in high-risk areas.
• Reconstitute with sodium chloride injection that contains no preservatives (preservatives decrease potency of vaccine).
• Must be kept frozen. Shake well before using. Use within 1 hour following reconstitution. Discard remainder.
• Obtain history of allergies, especially to eggs, and past reaction to immunization.
• Don't give within 1 month of other live virus vaccines.
• Keep epinephrine 1:1,000 available.

95

Antitoxins and antivenins

black widow spider antivenin
botulism antitoxin,
  bivalent equine
crotaline antivenin, polyvalent
diphtheria antitoxin, equine
Micrurus fulvius antivenin
tetanus antitoxin (TAT), equine

---

black widow spider antivenin
Antivenin (*Latrodectus mactans*) ♦

INDICATIONS & DOSAGE
Black widow spider bite—
Adults and children: 2.5 ml I.M. in deltoid. Second dose may be needed.

SIDE EFFECTS
Systemic: hypersensitivity, *anaphylaxis, neurotoxicity.*

INTERACTIONS
None significant.

NURSING CONSIDERATIONS
- If possible, hospitalize patient.
- Immobilize patient or splint bitten limb to prevent spread of venom.
- Test for sensitivity before giving.
- Epinephrine should be available in case of adverse reaction.
- Venom is neurotoxic and may cause respiratory paralysis and convulsions. Watch patient carefully for 2 to 3 days.
- Obtain accurate patient history of allergies, especially to horses, and past reaction to immunization.
- Earliest possible use of the antivenin is recommended for best results.

---

botulism antitoxin, bivalent equine

INDICATIONS & DOSAGE
Botulism—
Adults and children: 1 vial I.V. stat and q 4 hours, p.r.n., until patient's condition improves. Dilute antitoxin 1:10 in 5% or 10% dextrose in water or normal saline solution before giving. Give first 10 ml of dilution over 5 minutes; after 15 minutes, rate may be increased.

SIDE EFFECTS
Systemic: hypersensitivity, *anaphylaxis,* serum sickness (urticaria, pruritus, fever, malaise, arthralgia) may occur in 5 to 13 days.

INTERACTIONS
None significant.

NURSING CONSIDERATIONS
- Test for sensitivity before giving.
- Epinephrine should be available in case of adverse reaction. Bivalent antitoxin contains antibodies against types A and B *Clostridium botulinum.* Antitoxins against all other types available only from Center for Disease Control in Atlanta, Georgia.
- Obtain accurate patient history of allergies, especially to horses, and past reaction to immunization.
- Earliest possible use of the antitoxin is recommended for best results.

crotaline antivenin, polyvalent

INDICATIONS & DOSAGE
Crotalid (rattlesnake) bites—
Adults and children: initially, 10 to 50 ml or more I.M. or S.C., depending on severity of bite and patient's response. If large amount of venom, 70 to 100 ml I.V. directly into superficial vein. Subsequent doses based on patient's response; may give 10 ml q ½ to 2 hours, p.r.n. If bite is in extremity, inject part of initial dose at various sites around limb above swelling; don't inject in finger or toe. The smaller the patient, the larger the initial dose.

SIDE EFFECTS
Systemic: hypersensitivity, *anaphylaxis.*

INTERACTIONS
Antihistamines: enhanced toxicity of crotaline venoms. Don't use together.

NURSING CONSIDERATIONS
• Test for sensitivity before giving.
• Immobilize patient immediately. Splint bitten extremity.
• Epinephrine should be available in case of adverse reaction.
• Type and crossmatch as soon as possible since hemolysis from venom prevents accurate crossmatching.
• Early use of antivenin recommended for best results.
• Watch patient carefully for delayed allergic reaction or relapse.
• Because children have less resistance and less body fluid to dilute venom, they may need twice the adult dose.
• Obtain accurate patient history of allergies, especially to horses, and past reaction to immunization.
• Discard unused reconstituted drug.

diphtheria antitoxin, equine

INDICATIONS & DOSAGE
Diphtheria prevention—
Adults and children: 1,000 to 5,000 units I.M.
Diphtheria treatment—
Adults and children: 20,000 to 80,000 units or more slow I.V. Additional doses may be given in 24 hours. I.M. route may be used in mild cases.

SIDE EFFECTS
Systemic: hypersensitivity, *anaphylaxis,* serum sickness (urticaria, pruritus, fever, malaise, arthralgia) may occur in 7 to 12 days.

INTERACTIONS
None significant.

NURSING CONSIDERATIONS
• Test for sensitivity before giving.
• Epinephrine should be available in case of adverse reaction.
• Obtain accurate patient history of allergies, especially to horses, and past reaction to immunization.
• Therapy should be started immediately, without waiting for culture and sensitivity reports, if patient has clinical symptoms of diphtheria (sore throat, fever, tonsillar membrane).
• Refrigerate antitoxin at 35.6° to 50° F. (2° to 10° C.). May be warmed to 90° to 95° F. (32.2° to 35° C.), never higher.

Micrurus fulvius antivenin

INDICATIONS & DOSAGE
Eastern and Texas coral snake bite—
Adults and children: 3 to 5 vials slow I.V. through running I.V. of 0.9% normal saline solution. Give first 1 to 2 ml over 3 to 5 minutes, and watch for signs of allergic reaction. If

no signs develop, continue injection.
Up to 10 vials may be needed. Not effective for Sonoran or Arizona coral snake bites.

SIDE EFFECTS
Systemic: hypersensitivity, *anaphylaxis*.

INTERACTIONS
None significant.

NURSING CONSIDERATIONS
• Test for sensitivity before giving.
• Immobilize patient or splint bitten limb to prevent spread of venom.
• Hospitalize patient if possible.
• Early use of antivenin recommended for best results.
• Venom is neurotoxic and may cause respiratory paralysis. Watch patient carefully for 24 hours. Be ready to take supportive measures. Epinephrine should be available in case of adverse reaction.
• Obtain accurate patient history of allergies, especially to horses, and past reaction to immunization.

tetanus antitoxin (TAT), equine

INDICATIONS & DOSAGE
Tetanus prophylaxis—
Patients over 29.5 Kg: 3,000 to 5,000 units I.M. or S.C.
Patients under 29.5 Kg: 1,500 to 3,000 units I.M. or S.C.
Tetanus treatment—
All patients: 10,000 to 20,000 units injected into wound. Give additional 40,000 to 200,000 units I.V. Start tetanus toxoid at same time but at different site and with a different syringe.

SIDE EFFECTS
Local: pain, numbness, skin eruptions.
Systemic: joint pain, hypersensitivity, *anaphylaxis*.

INTERACTIONS
None significant.

NURSING CONSIDERATIONS
• Test for sensitivity before giving.
• Use only when tetanus immune globulin (human) not available.
• Obtain accurate patient history of allergies, especially to horses, and past reaction to immunization. If respiratory difficulty develops, give 0.4 ml of 1:1,000 solution epinephrine HCl.
• Preventive dose should be given to those who have had 2 or fewer injections of tetanus toxoid and who have tetanus-prone injuries more than 24 hours old.

96

Acidifiers and alkalinizers

Acidifiers:
ammonium chloride
dilute hydrochloric acid
Alkalinizers:
sodium bicarbonate
sodium lactate
tromethamine

---

ammonium chloride

INDICATIONS & DOSAGE
Metabolic alkalosis—
Adults and children: 4 mEq/Kg slow
I.V. or calculated by amount of chloride deficit. Infusion rate: 0.9 to
1.3 ml/min 2.14% solution. Do not
exceed 2 ml/min. Hypodermoclysis
has been used in infants and young
children. One half calculated volume
should be given and then patient reassessed.
*As an acidifying agent—*4 to 12 g P.O.
daily in divided doses.

SIDE EFFECTS
Side effects usually result from ammonia toxicity or too rapid I.V.
administration.
CNS: headache, confusion, progressive drowsiness, excitement alternating with coma, hyperventilation,
jerky respirations with apneic periods, *calcium-deficient tetany, twitching, hyperreflexia, EEG abnormalities.*
CV: bradycardia.
GI (with oral dose): *gastric irritation,
nausea, vomiting,* thirst, anorexia,
retching.

GU: glycosuria.
Metabolic: *acidosis, hyperchloremia,
hypokalemia,* hyperglycemia.
Skin: rash, pallor.
Local: pain at injection site.

INTERACTIONS
Spironolactone: systemic acidosis.
Use together cautiously.

NURSING CONSIDERATIONS
• Contraindicated in severe hepatic
or renal dysfunction. Use cautiously
in pulmonary insufficiency or cardiac
edema and in infants.
• Give after meals to decrease GI
side effects. Enteric-coated tablets
may also minimize GI symptoms but
are absorbed erratically.
• Pain of I.V. injection may be lessened by decreasing rate of infusion.
• Determine CO_2 combining power
and serum electrolytes before and during therapy.
• Monitor urine pH and output. Diuresis normal for first 2 days.
• Dilute concentrated solutions
(21.4%, 26.75%) to 2.14% before
giving.
• Monitor rate and depth of respirations frequently.
• Hypodermoclysis should be into
lateral aspect of thigh. Stop infusion
immediately if pain occurs.

---

dilute hydrochloric acid

INDICATIONS & DOSAGE
Metabolic alkalosis— pharmacy pre-

pares (0.1 normal HCl solution in sterile water) 100 mEq hydrogen and 100 mEq chloride/liter.

SIDE EFFECTS
None confirmed.

INTERACTIONS
None significant.

NURSING CONSIDERATIONS
• Not available commercially; prepared in pharmacy.
• Administer I.V. solution slowly through a central venous line.
• Monitor pH, blood gases, and electrolytes at 4- to 6-hour intervals.

---

sodium bicarbonate

INDICATIONS & DOSAGE
Cardiac arrest—
Adults and children: as a 7.5% or 8.4% solution, 1 to 3 mEq/Kg I.V. initially; may repeat in 10 minutes. Further doses based on blood gases. If blood gases unavailable, use 0.5 mEq/Kg q 10 minutes until spontaneous circulation returns.
Infants up to 2 years: 4.2% solution, I.V. infusion. Rate not to exceed 8 mEq/Kg/day.
Metabolic acidosis—
Adults and children: dose depends on blood CO_2 content, pH, and patient's clinical condition. Generally, 2 to 5 mEq/Kg I.V. infused over 4- to 8-hour period.
Systemic or urinary alkalinization—
Adults: 325 mg to 2 g P.O. q.i.d.

SIDE EFFECTS
GI: gastric distention, belching, flatulence.
GU: renal calculi or crystals.
Metabolic: with overdose: alkalosis, hypernatremia, hyperosmolarity.

INTERACTIONS
None significant.

NURSING CONSIDERATIONS
• No contraindications for use in life-threatening emergencies. Contraindicated in hypertension, in patients with tendency toward edema, in patients who are losing chlorides by vomiting or from continuous GI suction, in patients receiving diuretics known to produce hypochloremic alkalosis, and in patients on salt restriction or with renal disease.
• May be added to other I.V. fluids.
• Parenteral bicarbonate solutions will precipitate calcium salts. Do not mix in same infusion fluid. I.V. bolus injections should be given only through running I.V. lines free of calcium salts.
• To avoid risk of alkalosis, determine blood pH, PO_2, PCO_2, and electrolytes. Keep doctor informed of lab results.
• Tell patient not to take with milk. May cause hypercalcemia, alkalosis, and possibly renal calculi.
• Because sodium bicarbonate inactivates catecholamines such as epinephrine and levarterenol, do not mix with I.V. solutions of these agents.

---

sodium lactate

INDICATIONS & DOSAGE
Alkalinize urine—
Adults: 30 ml of a $1/_6$ molar solution/Kg of body weight given in divided doses over 24 hours.
Metabolic acidosis—
Adults: usually given as $1/_6$ molar injection (167 mEq lactate/liter). Dosage depends on degree of bicarbonate deficit.

SIDE EFFECTS
Metabolic: with overdose: alkalosis, hypernatremia, hyperosmolarity.

Unmarked trade names available in the United States only.
♦ Also available in Canada   ♦ ♦ Available in Canada only.

INTERACTIONS
None significant.

NURSING CONSIDERATIONS
• Contraindicated in respiratory alkalosis and in acidosis associated with congenital heart disease with persistent cyanosis.

---

tromethamine
THAM♦

INDICATIONS & DOSAGE
Metabolic acidosis (associated with cardiac bypass surgery or with cardiac arrest)—
Adults: dose depends on bicarbonate deficit. Calculate as follows: ml of 0.3 M tromethamine solution required = wt in Kg x bicarbonate deficit (mEq/L). Additional therapy based on serial determinations of existing bicarbonate deficit.
Children: calculate dose as above. Give slowly over 3 to 6 hours. Additional therapy based on degree of acidosis. Total 24-hour dose should not exceed 33 to 40 ml/Kg.

SIDE EFFECTS
CNS: respiratory depression.
Metabolic: hypoglycemia, hyperkalemia (with decreased urinary output).
Local: venospasm; intravenous thrombosis; inflammation, necrosis, and slough if extravasation occurs.

INTERACTIONS
None significant.

NURSING CONSIDERATIONS
• Contraindicated in anuria, uremia, chronic respiratory acidosis, pregnancy (except acute, life-threatening situations). Use cautiously in renal disease or poor urinary output. Monitor EKG and serum K^+ in these patients.
• To prevent blood pH from rising above normal, adjust dose carefully.
• Give slowly through large needle (18G to 20G) into largest antecubital vein or by indwelling catheter.
• Before, during, and after therapy, make the following determinations: blood pH; carbon dioxide tension; bicarbonate, glucose, and electrolyte levels.
• Mechanical ventilation should be available. Use when giving drug to patient with associated respiratory acidosis.
• Except in life-threatening situations, do not use longer than 1 day.
• If I.V. extravasates, infiltrate area with 1% procaine and hyaluronidase 150 units; may reduce vasospasm and dilute remaining drug in local area.
• Concentration of tromethamine should not exceed 0.3 M.

97

Uricosurics

probenecid
sulfinpyrazone

probenecid

Benemid♦, Benn, Benuryl♦♦,
Probalan, Probenimead, Robenecid,
SK-Probenecid

INDICATIONS & DOSAGE

Adjunct to penicillin or cephalosporin therapy—
Adults, and children over 50 Kg:
500 mg P.O. q.i.d.
Children 2 to 14 years (under 50 Kg): initially, 25 mg/Kg P.O., then 40 mg/Kg divided q.i.d.
Single-dose treatment of gonorrhea—
Adults: 3.5 g ampicillin P.O. with 1 g probenecid P.O. given together; or 1 g probenecid P.O. 30 minutes before dose of 4.8 million units of I.M. aqueous penicillin G procaine, injected at 2 different sites.
Treatment of hyperuricemia of gout, gouty arthritis—
Adults: 250 mg P.O. b.i.d. for first week, then 500 mg b.i.d., to maximum of 2 g daily. Maintenance: 500 mg daily for 6 months.

SIDE EFFECTS

Blood: *hemolytic anemia.*
CNS: headache, dizziness.
CV: hypotension.
GI: anorexia, nausea, vomiting, *gastric distress.*
GU: urinary frequency.
Skin: dermatitis, pruritus.
Other: flushing, sore gums, fever.

INTERACTIONS

Salicylates: inhibited uricosuric effect of probenecid, causing urate retention. Do not use together.

NURSING CONSIDERATIONS

• Contraindicated in blood dyscrasias; acute gout attack; penicillin therapy in presence of known renal impairment; gouty nephropathy; urinary tract stones or obstruction; azotemia, hyperuricemia secondary to cancer chemotherapy, radiation, or myeloproliferative neoplastic diseases. Use cautiously with peptic ulcer or renal impairment.
• Usually preferred over sulfinpyrazone because probenecid produces fewer, less severe GI and hematologic side effects.
• Contains no analgesic or anti-inflammatory agent, and is of no value during acute gout attacks.
• Suitable for long-term use; no cumulative effects or tolerance.
• Not effective with chronic renal insufficiency (glomerular filtration rate less than 30 ml/minute).
• Periodic BUN and renal function tests recommended in long-term therapy.
• May increase frequency, severity, and length of acute gout attacks during first 6 to 12 months of therapy. Prophylactic colchicine is given during first 3 to 6 months.
• Tell patient to avoid alcohol; increases urate level.
• Force fluids to maintain daily output of 2 to 3 liters minimum. Alkalin-

ize urine with sodium bicarbonate or other agent ordered by doctor.
● Give with milk, food, or antacids to minimize GI distress. Continued disturbances might indicate need to lower dose.
● Restrict foods high in purine: anchovies, liver, sardines, kidneys, sweetbreads, peas, lentils.
● Instruct patient and family that drug must be taken regularly as ordered or gout attacks may result. Tell him to visit doctor regularly so blood levels can be monitored and dosage can be adjusted if necessary.
● May have false positive glucose tests with Benedict's solution or Clinitest, but not with glucose oxidase method (Clinistix, Diastix, Tes-Tape).
● Decreases urinary excretion of 17-ketosteroids, PSP, BSP, aminohippuric acid, iodine-related organic acids, interfering with laboratory procedures.

---

sulfinpyrazone
Anturan♦◆, Anturane

INDICATIONS & DOSAGE

Inhibition of platelet aggregation, increase of platelet survival time in treatment of thromboembolic disorders, angina, myocardial infarction, transient cerebral ischemic attacks, peripheral arterial atherosclerosis—
Adults: 200 mg P.O. q.i.d.
Maintenance therapy of common gout: reduction, prevention of joint changes and tophi formation—
Adults: 100 to 200 mg P.O. b.i.d. first week, then 200 to 400 mg P.O. b.i.d. Maximum 800 mg daily.

SIDE EFFECTS

GI: *nausea, dyspepsia,* pain, blood loss, reactivation of peptic ulcers.
Skin: rash.

INTERACTIONS

Probenecid: inhibited renal excretion of sulfinpyrazone. Use together with caution.
Salicylates: inhibited uricosuric effect of sulfinpyrazone. Do not use together.

NURSING CONSIDERATIONS

● Contraindicated in hypersensitivity to pyrazole derivatives (including oxyphenbutazone, phenylbutazone); active peptic ulcer; during or within 2 weeks after gout attack; gouty nephropathy; urolithiasis or urinary obstruction; bone marrow depression; azotemia, hyperuricemia secondary to cancer chemotherapy, radiation, or myeloproliferative neoplastic diseases. Use cautiously with diminished hepatic or renal function.
● Use for treating thromboembolic conditions is investigational and is most often directed at prevention of recurrent myocardial infarction.
● Recommended for patients unresponsive to other uricosurics. Suitable for long-term use; no cumulative effects or tolerance.
● Contains no analgesic or antiinflammatory agent, and is of no value during acute gout attacks.
● Periodic BUN and renal function studies advised (long-term use).
● May increase frequency, severity, and length of acute gout attacks during first 6 to 12 months of therapy; prophylactic colchicine is given during first 3 to 6 months.
● Therapy, especially at start, may lead to renal colic and formation of uric acid stones. Until acid levels are normal (about 6 mg/100 ml), monitor intake and output closely.
● Force fluids to maintain daily output of 2 to 3 liters minimum. Alkalinize urine with sodium bicarbonate or other agent ordered by doctor.
● Give with milk, food, or antacids to minimize GI disturbances.
● Restrict foods high in purine: an-

Italicized side effects are common or life-threatening.

chovies, liver, sardines, kidneys, sweetbreads, peas, lentils.
• Instruct patient and family that drug must be taken regularly as ordered or gout attacks may result. Tell him to visit doctor regularly so blood levels can be monitored and dosage adjusted if necessary.

• Decreases urinary excretion of aminohippuric acid and PSP, interfering with laboratory procedures.
• Alkalinizing agents are used therapeutically to increase sulfinpyrazone activity, preventing urolithiasis.

Enzymes

bromelains
chymotrypsin
fibrinolysin and desoxyribonuclease
hyaluronidase
papain
streptokinase-streptodornase
trypsin

bromelains
Ananase

INDICATIONS & DOSAGE
Adjunct to reduce inflammation and edema, ease pain, and speed tissue repair of traumatic injuries (contusions, sprains, strains, dislocations), cellulitis, furunculosis, ulcerations—
Adults: initially, 100,000 units P.O. q.i.d., then 50,000 units t.i.d. or q.i.d. for maintenance.

SIDE EFFECTS
Blood: bleeding tendencies.
GI: mild diarrhea, nausea, vomiting.
GU: menorrhagia, metrorrhagia.
Other: fever, hypersensitivity reactions (rash, urticaria).

INTERACTIONS
Alkaline solutions, antacids: dissolved enteric coating of tablet. Do not use within 1 hour of bromelains.

NURSING CONSIDERATIONS
• Contraindicated in hypersensitivity to pineapple or pineapple products. Use cautiously with anticoagulant therapy and in patients with blood-clotting abnormalities, including hemophilia, hepatic or renal disease, and systemic infection.
• Obtain history of previous allergies. Watch for hypersensitivity reactions.
• Destruction of enteric coating may decrease effectiveness. Tablets must be swallowed whole; do not crush or break.
• Observe wound to monitor progress of therapy. Appearance of granulation tissue may indicate effectiveness. Notify doctor if inflammation or color of drainage indicates spread of infection.
• Protect from heat.

chymotrypsin
Avazyme

INDICATIONS & DOSAGE
Adjunct in general, rectal, oral, and dental surgery—
Adults: preoperatively, 2,500 units I.M.; then 2,500 units once or twice daily, as indicated.
Adjunct in treatment of respiratory conditions (asthma, bronchitis, rhinitis, sinusitis)—
Adults: 2,500 to 5,000 units I.M. once or twice weekly; more often if needed.
Children: ½ adult dose.
Chronic or recurrent inflammation (peptic ulcer, ulcerative colitis, phlebitis, thrombophlebitis, dermatologic conditions)—
Adults: 2,500 to 5,000 units I.M. once or twice weekly. Tablet containing 10,000 units may be given buc-

cally q.i.d. alone or in conjunction with I.M. therapy.
Relief of episiotomy symptoms—
Adults: 5,000 units I.M. repeated twice at 12-hour intervals. Tablet containing 20 mg (20,000 units) may be given P.O. q.i.d.
Pelvic inflammatory diseases—
Adults: 2,500 units daily for 7 days; repeat course if needed.

SIDE EFFECTS
Blood: increased bleeding tendency.
GI: nausea and vomiting, diarrhea with oral administration.
GU: hematuria, albuminuria, menorrhagia.
Local: pain, induration at injection site.
Other: chills, dizziness, fever, rapid dissolution of animal-origin sutures, *hypersensitivity (rash, urticaria, itching, anaphylaxis).*

INTERACTIONS
Alkaline solutions, antacids: dissolved enteric coating of tablet. Do not use within 1 hour of oral administration of chymotrypsin.

NURSING CONSIDERATIONS
• Contraindicated in hypersensitivity to trypsin or to sesame oil (injectable form), septicemia, severe generalized or localized infection, and blood coagulation disorders such as hemophilia. Use with caution in severe hepatic or renal disease.
• Parenteral administration: Do not give I.V. Test for sensitivity before giving. Inject deep into gluteal muscle; rotate sites. Watch for hypersensitivity reactions, including changes in blood pressure and pulse. Watch for pain, induration at injection site. Stop if reaction occurs.
• Avoid getting in eyes. If it does get into eyes, flood with water at once.
• Protect from heat.

fibrinolysin and desoxyribonuclease
Elase♦

INDICATIONS & DOSAGE
Debridement of inflammatory and infected lesions (surgical wounds, ulcerative lesions, second- and third-degree burns, circumcision, episiotomy, cervicitis, vaginitis, abscesses, fistulas and sinus tracts)—
Intravaginally: 5 ml ointment may be inserted using applicator supplied, once daily for vaginitis or cervicitis.
Topical use: apply ointment 30 units fibrinolysin, 20,000 units desoxyribonuclease/30 g at intervals as long as enzyme action is desired.
*Irrigating agent for infected wounds, empyema cavities, abscesses, otorhinolaryngologic wounds, subcutaneous hematomas—*dilution for irrigation depends on extent and severity of wound: 25 units fibrinolysin powder, 15,000 units desoxyribonuclease per 30 ml vial.

SIDE EFFECTS
Local: hyperemia with high doses.

INTERACTIONS
None significant.

NURSING CONSIDERATIONS
• Contraindicated for parenteral use.
• Dense, dry eschar must be removed surgically before enzymatic debridement. Enzyme must be in constant contact with substrate. Accumulated necrotic debris must be removed periodically.
• Clean wound with water or peroxide and dry gently; cover with thin layer of Elase. Cover with nonadhering dressing.
• Change dressing at least once a day. Flush away necrotic debris and reapply ointment.
• Solution as wet dressing: Mix 1 vial

Unmarked trade names available in the United States only.
♦ Also available in Canada   ♦ ♦ Available in Canada only.

of Elase powder with 10 to 50 ml saline solution; saturate strips of fine gauze with solution. Pack ulcerated area with Elase gauze. Allow gauze to dry in contact with ulcerated lesion for about 6 to 8 hours. Remove dried gauze and repeat 3 to 4 times daily.
• Solution as irrigant: Drain cavity and replace Elase every 6 to 10 hours to reduce amount of by-product accumulation and to minimize loss of enzyme activity. Although parenteral use is contraindicated, Elase is used as an irrigant in certain specific conditions.
• Prepare solution just before use. Discard after 24 hours.

hyaluronidase
Hyazyme, Wydase♦

INDICATIONS & DOSAGE
Adjunct to increase absorption and dispersion of other injected drugs—
Adults and children: 150 units to injection medium containing other medication.
Hypodermoclysis—
Adults, and children over 3 years: 150 units injected S.C. before clysis or injected into clysis tubing near needle for each 1,000 ml clysis solution.
Subcutaneous urography—
Adults and children: with patient prone, give 75 units S.C. over each scapula, followed by injection of contrast medium at same sites.

SIDE EFFECTS
Skin: rash, urticaria.
Local: irritation.

INTERACTIONS
Local anesthetics: increased potential for toxic local reaction. Use together cautiously.

NURSING CONSIDERATIONS
• Use with caution in blood-clotting abnormalities, severe hepatic or renal disease.
• Do not inject into acutely inflamed or cancerous areas.
• In hypodermoclysis, adjust dose, rate of injection, and type of solution to patient response.
• Administration precautions: Skin-test for sensitivity. Avoid injecting into diseased areas (may spread infection). Observe injection site for local reactions.
• Avoid getting solution in eyes. If it does get into eyes, flood with water at once.
• Protect from heat. Do not use cloudy or discolored solution.

papain
Panafil, Papase♦

INDICATIONS & DOSAGE
Prevention of inflammation and edema in surgical procedures—
Adults and children: 10,000 to 20,000 units P.O. or buccal 1 to 2 hours before surgery, then 20,000 units q.i.d. for up to 5 days.
Treatment of inflammation and burns, enzymatic debridement, promotion of normal healing and deodorization of surface lesions, particularly in local infection, necrosis, fibrinous or purulent debris, sloughing—
Adults and children: apply ointment 10% directly to lesion 1 to 2 times daily. Cover with gauze.

SIDE EFFECTS
Blood: increased bleeding tendencies.
GI: nausea, vomiting, diarrhea with oral administration.
Local: tenderness after buccal administration, occasional itching or stinging with first application of ointment.
Other: fever, hypersensitivity reactions (rash, urticaria, pruritus).

Italicized side effects are common or life-threatening.

INTERACTIONS
With topical use, detergents and anti-septics (benzalkonium chloride, hexa-chlorophene, iodine, hydrogen perox-ide): decreased enzymatic activity. Do not use together.

NURSING CONSIDERATIONS
• Contraindicated in hypersensitivity to papaya fruit. Oral administration contraindicated in anticoagulant therapy; blood-clotting abnormalities, including hemophilia; and systemic infections. Use cautiously in severe hepatic or renal disease.
• Instruct patient on proper route to be used. Oral tablets may be swallowed with water or chewed.
• Before treatment, thoroughly cleanse and irrigate wound area with sterile normal saline or water to remove antiseptics, detergents, and heavy metal antibacterials, which can decrease enzyme activity. Don't use hydrogen peroxide. Moisten area for optimal enzymatic activity. Apply ointment in thin layers to assure contact with necrotic tissue. Cover with gauze.
• Irrigate lesion with mild cleansing solution (not hydrogen peroxide) at each redressing.
• Observe wound to monitor progress of therapy. Appearance of granulation tissue may indicate effectiveness. Notify doctor if inflammation or color of drainage indicates spread of infection.
• Avoid getting ointment in eyes. If it does get into eyes, flood with water at once.
• Protect drug from heat.

---

streptokinase-streptodornase
Varidase♦

INDICATIONS & DOSAGE
Anti-inflammatory agent to relieve pain, swelling, tenderness, erythema; management of edema and localized

*extravasation of blood from infection, trauma, certain dental conditions—*dose, route of administration are determined by patient's response, location of lesion, ease of drainage or aspiration, size of cavity, and ability of cavity to expand. Higher doses than those stated may be advisable in severe cases.

Adults and children: 1 tablet P.O. containing 10,000 IU streptokinase (SK) and 2,500 IU streptodornase (SD) q.i.d. for 4 to 6 days; 0.5 ml I.M. of injectable solution (5,000 IU SK) b.i.d.

SIDE EFFECTS
GI: nausea, vomiting, diarrhea with oral administration.
Skin: rash, urticaria.

INTERACTIONS
None significant.

NURSING CONSIDERATIONS
• Contraindicated in active hemorrhage; decreased level of fibrinogen; acute cellulitis without suppuration; or risk of reopening preexisting bronchopleural fistulas, especially in active tuberculosis. Use oral and I.M. forms with caution in severe renal disease, depressed hepatic function or hepatic disease, or abnormalities of blood-clotting mechanism.
• Do not give I.V.
• If infection is present, consider concomitant antimicrobial therapy with compatible agent, such as tetracycline, penicillin, streptomycin.
• I.M. use: Add 2 ml sterile water for injection or sterile physiologic saline solution to 25,000-unit vial streptokinase-streptodornase (result is solution of 5,000 IU SK per 0.5 ml). Inject deep I.M., preferably into gluteal muscle. Store remaining solution for 2 weeks in refrigerator or 24 hours at room temperature.
• Avoid getting solution in eyes. If it

does get into eyes, flood with water at once.

• Protect from heat.

• Streptokinase and streptodornase are antigenic; antienzymes may develop following prolonged therapy or acute hemolytic streptococcal infections. High antienzyme titer apparently not harmful, but dosage may have to be increased to overcome its effect.

---

trypsin
Tryptar

INDICATIONS & DOSAGE

In general and oral surgical procedures to reduce inflammation, accelerate reabsorption of attendant edema, facilitate restoration of local tissue circulation; to reduce inflammation and edema of bronchial mucosa; as adjunct in treatment of phlebothrombosis, thrombophlebitis, iritis, iridocyclitis, chorioretinitis, cutaneous ulcerative conditions—
Adults: 50,000 to 100,000 units P.O. q.i.d.; or 12,500 units I.M. daily or for severe conditions b.i.d. for 1 to 2 days, then 12,500 units daily.
Solution for wet dressings:
10,000 units in each ml normal saline solution or water for injection. Apply new dressings when dry.
Ointment: 5,000 units/g once daily or b.i.d.
Inhalation: 125,000 units dissolved in 3 ml saline solution or water inhaled at least once daily.

SIDE EFFECTS

Blood: increased bleeding tendency.
CNS: dizziness, fainting.

EENT: rhinorrhea, sneezing, with aerosol inhalation.
GI: nausea, vomiting, diarrhea, abdominal pain.
GU: albuminuria, hematuria.
Skin: rash, pruritus, urticaria.
Local: pain and induration, local irritation.
Other: febrile reactions, angioneurotic edema, rapid dissolution of sutures of animal origins, *anaphylaxis.*

INTERACTIONS

With topical use, detergents and antiseptics (benzalkonium chloride, hexachlorophene, iodine, hydrogen peroxide): decreased enzymatic activity. Do not use together.

NURSING CONSIDERATIONS

• Contraindicated in history of allergic reactions to parenteral enzyme therapy. Use with extreme caution in severe hepatic or renal disease, abnormalities of blood-clotting mechanism.

• Test for possible hypersensitivity reactions before I.M. administration. Observe for 30 minutes after I.M. administration. Have epinephrine 1:1,000 available.

• Do not apply to actively bleeding areas, ocular lesions, or to ulcerated carcinomas.

• Do not give I.V.

• Enteric-coated tablets must be swallowed whole; do not crush or break.

• Give deep I.M. in gluteal muscle, alternating sites. Do not use I.M. route in infants or children.

• Follow nasal inhalation with water or saline spray. Have patient take several swallows of water to remove large droplets from oropharynx.

• Store in tight container. Protect from heat.

Oxytocics

carboprost tromethamine
dinoprost tromethamine
dinoprostone
ergonovine maleate
methylergonovine maleate
oxytocin citrate, buccal
oxytocin, synthetic injection
oxytocin, synthetic nasal
sodium chloride 20% solution

---

carboprost tromethamine
Prostin/M15

INDICATIONS & DOSAGE
Abort pregnancy between 13th and 20th weeks of gestation—initially, 250 mcg is administered deep in the muscle. Subsequent doses of 250 mcg should be administered at intervals of 1½ to 3½ hours, depending upon uterine response. Increments in dosage may be increased to 500 mcg if contractility is inadequate after several 250 mcg doses. Total dose should not exceed 12 mg.

SIDE EFFECTS
GI: *vomiting, diarrhea.*
Other: *fever.*

INTERACTIONS
None significant.

NURSING CONSIDERATIONS
• Contraindicated in those with pelvic inflammatory disease or active cardiac, pulmonary, renal, or hepatic disease. Use cautiously in patients with a history of asthma; hypertension; cardiovascular, renal, or hepatic disease; anemia; jaundice; diabetes; epilepsy.
• Intramuscular injection of this drug is technically less difficult and poses fewer potential risks inherent in other prostaglandin abortifacients.
• Carboprost can be used without concern that expulsion of vaginal suppositories may occur in the presence of profuse vaginal bleeding.
• Live birth may result.
• Should be used only in a hospital setting by trained personnel.

---

dinoprost tromethamine
Prostin F₂ Alpha

INDICATIONS & DOSAGE
Abort second trimester pregnancy— 1 ml amniotic fluid is withdrawn via transabdominal intra-amniotic catheter. If no blood is present in tap, 40 mg dinoprost is injected directly into amniotic sac. Initially, 5 mg is given very slowly (1 mg/minute), and patient watched for adverse reactions. Then, remainder is injected. If abortion not completed in 24 hours, another 10 to 40 mg may be given. Uterine activity may continue 10 to 30 minutes after drug is stopped.

SIDE EFFECTS
CNS: dizziness, fainting.
GI: *nausea, vomiting, diarrhea,* abdominal cramps, epigastric pain.
Other: bronchospasm, wheezing.

INTERACTIONS

Alcohol (I.V. infusions of 500 ml of 10% over 1 hour): inhibited uterine activity.

I.V. oxytocin: cervical perforation, especially in primigravida patients or in those with inadequately dilated cervices. Use with caution.

NURSING CONSIDERATIONS

• Contraindicated in those with pelvic inflammatory disease. Use with caution in cardiovascular, renal, or hypertensive disease; asthma; glaucoma; or epilepsy.
• Observe and record character and amount of vaginal bleeding.
• Live birth may result.
• Other measures may be needed if dinoprost fails to terminate pregnancy completely. Utilization of hypertonic saline should be delayed until uterine contractions stop.
• Monitor vital signs. Report rapid fall in blood pressure or hypertonic uterine contractions.
• Instruct patient to remain in prone position.
• After abortion, observe patient frequently for cervical injuries.
• Store at 2° to 8° C. (35.6° to 46.4° F.). Discard 24 months after manufacture date.
• Should be used only in hospital setting by trained personnel.

dinoprostone
Prostin E₂♦

INDICATIONS & DOSAGE

Abort second trimester pregnancy, evacuate uterus in cases of missed abortion, intrauterine fetal deaths up to 28 weeks of age, benign hydatidiform mole—insert 20 mg suppository high into posterior vaginal formix. Repeat q 3 to 5 hours until abortion is complete.

SIDE EFFECTS

CNS: *headache.*
CV: hypotension (in large doses).
GI: *nausea, vomiting, diarrhea.*
GU: vaginal pain, vaginitis.
Other: fever, shivering, chills.

INTERACTIONS
None significant.

NURSING CONSIDERATIONS

• Contraindicated in those with pelvic inflammatory disease or history of pelvic surgery, incisions, uterine fibroids, or cervical stenosis. Use with caution in asthma, epilepsy, anemia, diabetes, hypertension, hypotension, jaundice, or cardiovascular, renal, or hepatic disease.
• Live birth may result.
• Warm dinoprostone suppositories in their wrapping to room temperature.
• After insertion, patient should stay supine for 10 minutes.
• Store suppositories at temperature no higher than −20° C. (−4° F.).
• Should be used only when critical care facilities are readily available.
• Dinoprostone-induced fever is self-limiting and transient. Treat with water or alcohol sponging and increased fluid intake rather than with aspirin, which has not proved effective.
• Abortion should be complete within 30 hours.

ergonovine maleate
Ergotrate Maleate♦

INDICATIONS & DOSAGE

Prevent or treat postpartum and post-abortion hemorrhage due to uterine atony or subinvolution—0.2 mg I.M. q 2 to 4 hours, maximum 5 doses; or 0.2 mg I.V. (only for severe uterine bleeding or other life-threatening emergency) over 1 minute while blood pressure and uterine contractions are monitored. I.V. dose may be

---

Italicized side effects are common or life-threatening.

diluted to 5 ml with 0.9% sodium chloride injection. Following initial I.M. or I.V. dose, may give 0.2 to 0.4 mg P.O. q 6 to 12 hours for 2 to 7 days. Decrease dose if severe uterine cramping occurs.

SIDE EFFECTS
CNS: dizziness, headache.
CV: hypertension.
EENT: tinnitus.
GI: *nausea, vomiting*.
GU: uterine cramping.
Other: sweating, chest pain, dyspnea, hypersensitivity.

INTERACTIONS
Regional anesthetics, dopamine, I.V. oxytocin: excessive vasoconstriction. Use together cautiously.

NURSING CONSIDERATIONS
• Contraindicated for induction or augmentation of labor; before delivery of placenta; in threatened spontaneous abortion; in patients with allergy or sensitivity to ergot preparations. Use cautiously in hypertension, heart disease, venoatrial shunts, mitral valve stenosis, obliterative vascular disease, sepsis, or hepatic or renal impairment.
• Monitor blood pressure, pulse, uterine response, and report any sudden changes in vital signs or frequent periods of uterine relaxation, and character and amount of vaginal bleeding.
• Hypocalcemia may decrease patient response. If patient is not also taking digitalis, cautious administration of calcium gluconate I.V. may produce desired oxytocic action.
• Contractions begin 5 to 15 minutes after P.O. administration; immediately following I.V. injection. May continue 3 hours or more after P.O. or I.M. administration; 45 minutes after I.V. injection.
• Store in tightly closed, light-resistant container. Discard if discolored.

• Store I.V. solutions below 8° C. (46.4° F.). Daily stock may be kept at cool room temperature for 60 days.
• Keep patient warm.
• Have drug ready for immediate use if it is to be given postpartum.

---

methylergonovine maleate
Methergine

INDICATIONS & DOSAGE
Prevent and treat postpartum hemorrhage due to uterine atony or subinvolution—0.2 mg I.M. q 2 to 5 hours for maximum of 5 doses; or I.V. (excessive uterine bleeding or other emergencies) over 1 minute while blood pressure and uterine contractions are monitored. I.V. dose may be diluted to 5 ml with 0.9% sodium chloride injection. Following initial I.M. or I.V. dose, may give 0.2 to 0.4 mg P.O. q 6 to 12 hours for 2 to 7 days. Dose may be decreased if severe cramping occurs.

SIDE EFFECTS
CNS: dizziness, headache.
CV: hypertension, transient chest pain, dyspnea, palpitation.
EENT: tinnitus.
GI: *nausea, vomiting*.
Other: sweating, hypersensitivity.

INTERACTIONS
Regional anesthetics, dopamine, I.V. oxytocin: excessive vasoconstriction. Use together cautiously.

NURSING CONSIDERATIONS
• Contraindicated for induction of labor; before delivery of placenta; in patients with hypertension, toxemia, or sensitivity to ergot preparations; in threatened spontaneous abortion. Use with caution in sepsis, obliterative vascular disease, hepatic or renal disease, hypertension, heart disease,

venoatrial shunts, mitral valve stenosis.

• Monitor and record blood pressure, pulse, uterine response; and report any sudden change in vital signs or frequent periods of uterine relaxation and character and amount of vaginal bleeding.

• Contractions begin 5 to 15 minutes after P.O. administration; 2 to 5 minutes after I.M. injection; immediately following I.V. injection. May continue 3 hours or more after P.O. or I.M. administration; 45 minutes after I.V. injection.

• Store in tightly closed, light-resistant containers. Discard if discolored.

• Store below 8° C. (46.4° F.). Daily stock may be kept at room temperature for 60 to 90 days.

---

oxytocin citrate, buccal
Pitocin Citrate♦

INDICATIONS & DOSAGE
Induction of labor—1 tablet (200 U.S.P. units) in alternate cheeks until firm, regular uterine contractions, 40 to 60 seconds long, q 3 minutes, are achieved. Repeat q 30 minutes until 15 tablets (3,000 units) have been given over 24 hours, or until delivery is imminent or anesthestic is administered. Average dose to complete labor, 1,700 units; same number of tablets are used to maintain labor once induced.

SIDE EFFECTS
Maternal:
CV: hypertension; premature ventricular contractions; hypotension; increase in heart rate, venous return, cardiac output; *arrhythmias in large doses.*
GI: nausea, vomiting.
GU: uterine hypertonicity, spasm, tetanic contraction or rupture, postpartum hemorrhage.

Local: parabuccal irritation.
Fetal:
CV: bradycardia, cardiac arrhythmias.
Other: birth canal trauma, jaundice.

INTERACTIONS
Cyclopropane anesthesia: increased risk of hypotension or bradycardia. Use together cautiously.
Thiopental anesthesia: delayed induction time. Adjust dose.
Vasoconstrictors (vasopressors): severe hypertension if oxytocin is used within 3 to 4 hours of vasoconstrictor. Monitor patient closely.

NURSING CONSIDERATIONS
• Contraindicated in control and management of third stage of labor; to expel placenta; to control postpartum bleeding; in unconscious or postpartum patients; in management of inevitable, incomplete, or missed abortion, abruptio placentae, placenta previa, fetal distress, or other obstetrical emergencies. Use cautiously in prematurity, previous major cervical or uterine surgery (including cesarean section), grand multiparity, invasive cervical carcinoma, overdistention of uterus, history of uterine sepsis.

• In eclampsia, if delivery isn't imminent within 12 hours after oxytocin is started, cesarean section is recommended.

• Used to induce or reinforce labor only when pelvis is known to be adequate, when fetal maturity is assured, when fetal position is favorable and vaginal delivery is indicated.

• May be hazardous in patients with heart disease or in those receiving spinal or epidural anesthesia.

• Should be given only in hospital setting under qualified supervision.

• Buccal administration is more difficult to control than I.M. or I.V. route; can be given by different routes sequentially but never at same time.

• Monitor uterine contractions, heart rate, blood pressure, intrauterine pres-

---

Italicized side effects are common or life-threatening.

sure, and character and volume of blood loss.
- Monitor and record fetal heart beat.
- Patient may rinse mouth with cold water before tablet is placed in para-buccal space. For maximum buccal absorption, patient should avoid disturbing tablet. A tablet swallowed accidentally is not harmful, but the digestive process destroys its oxytocic action.
- Store at temperature lower than 25° C. (77° F.).

---

oxytocin, synthetic injection
Oxytocin♦, Pitocin♦,
Syntocinon♦, Uteracon

INDICATIONS & DOSAGE
Induction or stimulation of labor—initially, 1 ml (10 units) ampule in 1,000 ml 5% dextrose injection or 0.9% sodium chloride I.V. infused at 1 to 2 milliunits/minute. Increase rate at 15- to 30-minute intervals until normal contraction pattern is established. Maximum 1 to 2 ml (20 milliunits)/minute. Decrease rate when labor is firmly established.
Reduction of postpartum bleeding after expulsion of placenta—10 to 40 units added to 1,000 ml 5% dextrose in water or 0.9% sodium chloride infused at rate necessary to control bleeding.
Facilitate threatened abortion—10 to 40 units (1 to 4 ml) oxytocin added to 1,000 ml 5% dextrose in water, normal saline solution, or other nonhydrating solution; infused at rate necessary to control uterine atony.

SIDE EFFECTS
Maternal:
Blood: afibrinogenemia; may be related to increase in postpartum bleeding.
CNS: subarachnoid hemorrhage

resulting from hypertension; *convulsions or coma resulting from water intoxication.*
CV: hypotension; increased heart rate, systemic venous return, and cardiac output; arrhythmia.
GI: nausea, vomiting.
Other: hypersensitivity, tetanic contractions, abruptio placentae, impaired uterine blood flow, and increased uterine motility.
Fetal:
Blood: increased risk of hyperbilirubinemia.
CV: bradycardia, tachycardia, premature ventricular contractions, *anoxia, asphyxia.*

INTERACTIONS
Cyclopropane anesthesia: less pronounced bradycardia; more severe hypotension than occurs with oxytocin alone. Use together cautiously.
Thiopentol anesthesia: delayed induction reported. May require dosage adjustment.
*Vasoconstrictors:*severe hypertension if oxytocin is given within 3 to 4 hours of vasoconstrictor in patient receiving caudal block anesthesia. Monitor patient closely.

NURSING CONSIDERATIONS
- Contraindicated in cases of cephalopelvic disproportion or where delivery requires conversion, as in transverse lie; fetal distress, when delivery isn't imminent; severe toxemia; and other obstetrical emergencies. Use cautiously in history of cervical or uterine surgery, grand multiparity, uterine sepsis, traumatic delivery, or overdistended uterus, and in primipara over 35 years. Use with extreme caution during first and second stages of labor, since cervical laceration, uterine rupture, and maternal and fetal death are reported.
- Used to induce or reinforce labor only when pelvis is known to be adequate, when vaginal delivery is indi-

---

cated, when fetal maturity is assured, and when fetal position is favorable. Should be used only in hospital where critical care facilities and doctor are immediately available.
• Oxytocin should never be given simultaneously by more than one route.
• Incompatible with fibrinolysis, levarterenol bitartrate, prochlorperazine edisylate, protein hydrolysate, and warfarin sodium. Compatibility with other I.V. infusion fluids may be influenced by drug concentration, temperature, pH, and other factors. Rotate bottle gently to distribute drug in diluted solution.
• Monitor and record uterine contractions, heart rate, blood pressure, intrauterine pressure, fetal heart rate, and character and volume of blood loss.
• Store at temperature below 25° C. (77° F.), but do not freeze.
• Oxytocin may produce antidiuretic effect; monitor fluid intake/output.
• If contractions occur less than 2 minutes apart and if contractions above 50 mm Hg are recorded, or if contractions last 90 seconds or longer, stop infusion, turn patient on her side, and notify doctor.
• Oxygen administration may be necessary.
• Not recommended for I.M. use.

oxytocin, synthetic nasal

INDICATIONS & DOSAGE
To promote initial milk ejection; may be useful in relieving postpartum breast engorgement—1 spray or 3 drops into one or both nostrils 2 or 3 minutes before nursing or pumping breasts.

SIDE EFFECTS
None reported.

INTERACTIONS
None significant.

NURSING CONSIDERATIONS
• Instruct patient to clear nasal passages first. With patient's head in vertical position, hold squeeze bottle upright and eject solution into patient's nostril.
• Support patient's wish to breastfeed with quiet, nonstressful environment and encouragement.

sodium chloride 20% solution

INDICATIONS & DOSAGE
To induce fetal death and abortion in second trimester of pregnancy (beyond 16th week of gestation)—following transabdominal tap of amniotic sac, at least 1 ml fluid is withdrawn and examined. If no blood is found, 250 ml of amniotic fluid may be aspirated and 250 ml (maximum dose) of sodium chloride instilled over 20 to 30 minutes, while patient is observed for adverse reactions. Sodium chloride instillation may be repeated in 48 hours if membranes are still intact. I.V. infusion of oxytocin or intra-amniotic dinoprost tromethamine may be given to patients who fail to respond to second dose after oxytocic action of saline has ceased.

SIDE EFFECTS
Blood: mild, self-limiting disseminated intravascular coagulation; coagulation changes, including decreased platelet count, hematocrit, fibrinogen, and Factors V and VIII; increased plasma volume, fibrin levels and thrombin, PT and PTT times. Occur within first 12 to 24 hours.
CV: *pulmonary embolism*, pneumonia.
GU: *cortical necrosis of kidneys*, cervical laceration and perforation, cervico-vaginal fistula, and uterine rupture reported in primigravida patients

receiving concomitant I.V. oxytocin before cervix is adequately dilated.
Local: infection at injection site.
Other: fever, flushing.

INTERACTIONS

Indomethacin: may prolong abortion if used within 4 to 6 hours after intra-amniotic instillation of sodium chloride. Defer indomethacin dose.
Oxytocin: intense uterine contractions and increased risk of uterine rupture or cervical laceration. Don't use together.

NURSING CONSIDERATIONS

• Contraindicated in blood disorders or in actively contracting or hypertonic uterus. Use with extreme caution in heart disease, hypertension, epilepsy, renal impairment, uterine incision, or pelvic adhesions, or in history of pelvic surgery.

• Should be done only by doctors trained in amniocentesis when critical care facilities are immediately available.

• Monitor constantly for signs of accidental intravascular, endometrial, or intraperitoneal injection. Procedure usually painless. If patient complains of pain, burning, feeling of heat, thirst, severe headache, mental confusion, distress, tinnitus, numbness of fingertips, or anxiety, stop instillation at once. Inadvertent I.V. injection can cause hypernatremia, myometrial necrosis, with secondary vomiting, cerebral blood clots, cardiovascular collapse, and death.

• Patient should drink at least 2 liters of water on day of procedure to improve salt excretion.

• General anesthetics or sedatives should not be used during administration of hypertonic saline.

100

Spasmolytics

aminophylline
  or theophylline ethylenediamine
dyphylline
flavoxate hydrochloride
oxtriphylline
oxybutynin chloride
theophylline
theophylline sodium glycinate

---

aminophylline or theophylline ethylenediamine

Aminodur Dura-Tab, Aminophyl♦♦,
Aminophyllin, Corophyllin♦♦,
Lixaminol, Mini-Lix, Phyllocontin,
Somophyllin

INDICATIONS & DOSAGE

*For treatment of acute and chronic
bronchial asthma, bronchospasm;
also used for Cheyne-Stokes respiration, pulmonary vasodilator—*
Oral: **Adults:** 500 mg stat; then 250 to
500 mg q 6 to 8 hours.
Children: 7.5 mg/Kg stat; then 3 to
6 mg/Kg q 6 to 8 hours.
I.V.: inject very slowly, minimum
time of 4 to 5 minutes; do not exceed
25 mg/minute infusion rate.
Loading dose: 5.6 mg/Kg over
30 minutes.
Maintenance dose: **Adults:** 0.6 to 0.9
mg/Kg/hour I.V. by continuous infusion.
Children less than 9 years:
1mg/Kg/hour.
I.M.: **Adults:** 500 mg. Painful. Not
recommended.
Rectal: **Adults:** 500 mg suppository
or by retention enema q 6 to 8 hours.

SIDE EFFECTS

CNS: *restlessness, dizziness,* headache, *insomnia,* light-headedness,
convulsions.
CV: *palpitations, sinus tachycardia,*
extrasystoles, flushing, marked hypotension, increase in respiratory rate.
GI: *nausea, vomiting, anorexia,* bitter
aftertaste, dyspepsia, heavy feeling in
stomach.
Skin: urticaria.
Local: *rectal suppositories may cause
irritation.*

INTERACTIONS

Alkali-sensitive drugs: reduced activity. Do not add to I.V. fluids containing aminophylline.
Propranolol and nadolol: antagonism. Propranolol and nadolol may
cause bronchospasm in sensitive patients. Use together cautiously.
Troleandomycin, erythromycin: decreased hepatic clearance of theophylline; elevated theophylline levels.
Monitor for signs of toxicity.
Barbiturates: enhanced metabolism
and decreased theophylline blood levels. Monitor for decreased aminophylline effect.

NURSING CONSIDERATIONS

• Contraindicated in hypersensitivity
to xanthine compounds (caffeine,
theobromine); preexisting cardiac arrhythmias, especially tachyarrhythmias. Use cautiously in young children; in elderly patients with congestive heart failure or other cardiac or
circulatory impairment, cor pulmonale, hepatic disease; in patients with

active peptic ulcer, since it may increase volume and acidity of gastric secretions; and in hyperthyroidism or diabetes mellitus.
- Individuals metabolize xanthines at different rates. Adjust dose by monitoring response, tolerance, pulmonary function, and theophylline plasma levels: therapeutic level = 10 to 20 mcg/ml; toxicity seen over 20 mcg/ml.
- Plasma clearance may be decreased in patients with congestive heart failure, hepatic dysfunction, or pulmonary edema. Smokers show accelerated clearance. Dose adjustments necessary.
- Monitor vital signs; measure and record intake/output. Expected clinical effects include improvement in quality of pulse and respiration.
- Warn elderly patient of dizziness, common side effect at start of therapy.
- GI symptoms may be relieved by taking oral drug with full glass of water at meals, although food in stomach delays absorption. Enteric-coated tablets may also delay and impair absorption. No evidence that antacids reduce GI side effects.
- Suppositories slowly and erratically absorbed; retention enemas may be absorbed more rapidly. Rectally administered preparations can be given when patient cannot take drug orally. Schedule following evacuation, if possible; may be retained better if given before meal. Advise patient to remain recumbent 15 to 20 minutes following insertion.
- Question patient closely about other drugs used. Warn that over-the-counter remedies may contain ephedrine in combination with theophylline salts; excessive CNS stimulation may result. Tell him to check with doctor before taking *any* other medications.
- Before giving loading dose, check that patient has not had recent theophylline therapy.
- Supply instructions for home care and dosage schedule. Some patients

may require round-the-clock dosage schedule.

---

dyphylline
Airet, Air-Tabs, Brophylline, Coeurophylline♦♦, Dilin♦, Dilor, Dyflex, Dylline, Emfabid, Lufyllin, Neothylline, Protophylline♦♦

INDICATIONS & DOSAGE
For relief of acute and chronic bronchial asthma and reversible bronchospasm associated with chronic bronchitis and emphysema—
Adults: 200 to 800 mg P.O. q 6 hours; or 250 to 500 mg I.M. injected slowly at 6-hour intervals.
Children over 6 years: 4 to 7 mg/Kg P.O. daily, in divided doses.

SIDE EFFECTS
CNS: *restlessness, dizziness,* headache, *insomnia,* light-headedness, *convulsions.*
CV: *palpitations, sinus tachycardia,* extrasystoles, flushing, marked hypotension, increase in respiratory rate.
GI: *nausea, vomiting, anorexia,* bitter aftertaste, dyspepsia, heavy feeling in stomach.
Skin: urticaria.

INTERACTIONS
None significant.

NURSING CONSIDERATIONS
- Contraindicated in hypersensitivity to xanthine compounds (caffeine, theobromine); preexisting cardiac arrythmias, especially tachycardias. Use cautiously in young children; in elderly patients with congestive heart failure, any impaired cardiac or circulatory function, cor pulmonale, renal or hepatic disease; in patients with peptic ulcer, hyperthyroidism, or diabetes mellitus.
- I.V. use not recommended.
- Dyphylline is metabolized faster

than theophylline; dosage intervals may have to be decreased to ensure continual therapeutic effect. Higher daily doses may be needed.
• Dose should be decreased in renal insufficiency.
• Monitor vital signs; measure and record intake/output. Expected clinical effects include improvement in quality of pulse and respiration.
• Warn elderly patient of dizziness, a common side effect.
• Gastric irritation may be relieved by taking oral drug after meals; no evidence that antacids reduce this side effect. May produce less gastric discomfort than theophylline.
• Discard dyphylline ampule if precipitate is present. Protect from light.
• Question patient closely about other drugs used. Warn that over-the-counter remedies may contain ephedrine in combination with theophylline salts; excessive CNS stimulation may result. Tell him to check with doctor before taking *any* other medications.
• Supply instructions for home care and dosage schedule.

---

flavoxate hydrochloride
Urispas

INDICATIONS & DOSAGE
Symptomatic relief of dysuria, frequency, urgency, nocturia, incontinence, and suprapubic pain associated with urologic disorders—
Adults, and children over 12 years: 100 to 200 mg P.O. q.i.d.

SIDE EFFECTS
CNS: *mental confusion* (especially in elderly), nervousness, dizziness, headache, drowsiness, difficulty with concentration.
CV: tachycardia, palpitations.
EENT: *dry mouth and throat, blurred vision,* disturbed eye accommodation.

GI: abdominal pain, constipation (with high doses), nausea, vomiting.
Skin: urticaria, dermatoses.
Other: fever.

INTERACTIONS
None significant.

NURSING CONSIDERATIONS
• Contraindicated in pyloric or duodenal obstruction, obstructive intestinal lesions or ileus, achalasia, GI hemorrhage, obstructive uropathies of lower urinary tract.
• Check history for other drug use before giving drugs with anticholinergic side effects.
• Warn about possible drowsiness, mental confusion, and blurred vision.
• Tell patient to report adverse effects or lack of response to drug.

---

oxtriphylline
Choledyl♦, Theophylline Choline♦♦

INDICATIONS & DOSAGE
To relieve acute bronchial asthma and reversible bronchospasm associated with chronic bronchitis and emphysema—
Adults, and children over 12 years: 200 mg P.O. q 6 hours.
Children 2 to 12 years: 4 mg/Kg P.O. q 6 hours. Increase as needed to maintain therapeutic levels of theophylline (10 to 20 mcg/ml).

SIDE EFFECTS
CNS: *restlessness, dizziness,* headache, *insomnia,* light-headedness, *convulsions.*
CV: *palpitations, sinus tachycardia,* extrasystoles, flushing, marked hypotension, increase in respiratory rate.
GI: *nausea, vomiting, anorexia,* bitter aftertaste, dyspepsia, heavy feeling in stomach.
Skin: urticaria.

INTERACTIONS
Erythromycin, troleandomycin: decreased hepatic clearance of theophylline; increased plasma level. Monitor for signs of toxicity.
Barbiturates: enhanced metabolism and decreased theophylline blood levels. Monitor for decreased effect.
Propranolol and nadolol: antagonism. May cause bronchospasms in sensitive patients. Use together cautiously.

NURSING CONSIDERATIONS
• Contraindicated in hypersensitivity to xanthines (caffeine, theobromine); preexisting cardiac arrhythmias, especially tachyarrhythmias.
• Tell patient to report GI distress, palpitations, irritability, restlessness, nervousness, or insomnia; may indicate excessive CNS stimulation.
• Administer drug after meals and at bedtime.
• Store at 15° to 30° C. (59° to 86° F.). Protect elixir from light, tablets from moisture.
• Equivalent to 80% anhydrous theophylline.
• Monitor therapy carefully.
• Combination products that contain ephedrine not recommended; excessive CNS stimulation may result.

---

oxybutynin chloride
Ditropan

INDICATIONS & DOSAGE
Antispasmodic for neurogenic bladder—
Adults: 5 mg P.O. b.i.d. to t.i.d. to maximum of 5 mg q.i.d.
Children over 5 years: 5 mg P.O. b.i.d. to maximum of 5 mg t.i.d.

SIDE EFFECTS
CNS: *drowsiness,* dizziness, insomnia, *dry mouth,* flushing.
CV: *palpitations, tachycardia.*

EENT: *transient blurred vision,* mydriasis, cycloplegia.
GI: nausea, vomiting, *constipation,* bloated feeling.
GU: impotence, suppression of lactation, *urinary hesitance or retention.*
Skin: urticaria, severe allergic reactions in patients sensitive to anticholinergics.
Other: decreased sweating, fever.

INTERACTIONS
None significant.

NURSING CONSIDERATIONS
• Contraindicated in myasthenia gravis, GI obstruction, adynamic ileus, megacolon, severe or ulcerative colitis; in elderly or debilitated patients with intestinal atony; and in patients with obstructive uropathy. Use cautiously in elderly patients; in patients with autonomic neuropathy, reflux esophagitis, or hepatic or renal disease.
• May aggravate symptoms of hyperthyroidism, coronary artery disease, congestive heart failure, cardiac arrhythmias, tachycardia, hypertension, or prostatic hypertrophy.
• Therapy should be stopped periodically to determine whether patient can get along without it. Minimizes tendency toward tolerance.
• Rapid onset of action, peaks at 3 to 4 hours, lasts 6 to 10 hours.
• Neurogenic bladder should be confirmed by cystometry before oxybutynin is given. Evaluate patient response to therapy periodically by cystometry.
• Rule out partial intestinal obstruction in patients with diarrhea, especially those with colostomy or ileostomy, before giving oxybutynin.
• If urinary tract infection is present, patient should receive antibiotics concomitantly.
• Warn patient that drug may impair alertness or vision.
• Since oxybutynin suppresses sweat-

ing, its use during very hot weather may precipitate fever or heat stroke.
• Store in tightly closed containers at 15° to 30° C. (59° to 86° F.).

---

theophylline
Accurbron, Adophyllin, Aerolate, Aqualin, Asthmophylline♦♦, Bronkodyl, Elixicon, Elixophyllin♦, Labid, Lanophyllin, Liquophylline, Norophylline, Optiphyllin, Oralphyllin, Physpan, Quibron BID, Slo-Phyllin, Somophyllin♦, Theo-dur, Theo-Lix, Theo II, Theobid, Theocap, Theoclear, Theolair♦, Theolixir♦, Theolline, Theon, Theophyl♦, Theo-Span, Theostat, Theotal, Theovent
theophylline sodium glycinate
Acet-Am♦♦, Panophylline Forte, Synophylate, Theocyne♦♦, Theo-tort

INDICATIONS & DOSAGE
Prophylaxis and symptomatic relief of bronchial asthma, bronchospasm of chronic bronchitis and emphysema—
Adults: 100 to 200 mg P.O. q 6 hours; or 250 to 500 mg rectally q 8 to 12 hours.
Children: 50 to 100 mg P.O. q 6 hours, not to exceed 10 to 12 mg/Kg/24 hours, in divided doses q 8 to 12 hours.
Oral timed-release form given q 8 to 12 hours.
Symptomatic relief of bronchial asthma, pulmonary emphysema, and chronic bronchitis—
Adults: 330 to 660 mg (sodium glycinate) P.O. q 6 to 8 hours, after meals.
Children over 12 years: 220 to 330 mg (sodium glycinate) P.O. q 6 to 8 hours.
Children 6 to 12 years: 330 mg (sodium glycinate) P.O. q 6 to 8 hours.
Children 3 to 6 years: 110 to 165 mg (sodium glycinate) P.O. q 6 to 8 hours.
Children 1 to 3 years: 55 to 110 mg

(sodium glycinate) P.O. q 6 to 8 hours.

SIDE EFFECTS
CNS: *restlessness, dizziness,* headache, *insomnia,* light-headedness, *convulsions.*
CV: *palpitations, sinus tachycardia,* extrasystoles, flushing, marked hypotension, increase in respiratory rate.
GI: *nausea, vomiting, anorexia,* bitter aftertaste, dyspepsia, heavy feeling in stomach.
Skin: urticaria.

INTERACTIONS
Erythromycin, troleandomycin: decreased hepatic clearance of theophylline; increased plasma levels. Monitor for signs of toxicity.
Barbiturates: enhanced metabolism and decreased theophylline blood levels. Monitor for decreased effect.
Propranolol and nadolol: antagonism. May cause bronchospasms in sensitive patients. Use together cautiously.

NURSING CONSIDERATIONS
• Contraindicated in hypersensitivity to xanthine compounds (caffeine, theobromine); preexisting cardiac arrhythmias, especially tachyarrhythmias. Use cautiously in young children; in elderly patients with congestive heart failure or other circulatory impairment, cor pulmonale, renal or hepatic disease; and in patients with peptic ulcer, hyperthyroidism, or diabetes mellitus.
• Individuals metabolize xanthines at different rates; determine dose by monitoring response, tolerance, pulmonary function, and theophylline plasma levels: therapeutic level = 10 to 20 mcg/ml.
• Monitor vital signs; measure and record intake/output. Expected clinical effects include improvement in quality of pulse and respiration.

Italicized side effects are common or life-threatening.

• Warn elderly patients of dizziness, common side effect at start of therapy.
• GI symptoms may be relieved by taking oral drug with full glass of water after meals, although food in stomach delays absorption.
• Question patient closely about other drugs used. Warn that over-the-counter remedies may contain ephedrine in combination with theophylline salts; excessive CNS stimulation may result. Tell him to check with doctor before taking *any* other medications.

• Supply instructions for home care and dosage schedule.
• Decrease daily dosage in congestive heart failure, hepatic disease, or in elderly patients, since metabolism and excretion may be decreased. Monitor carefully, using serum levels, observation, examination, and interview. Give drug around the clock, using sustained-release product at bedtime.
• Be careful not to confuse sustained-release dosage forms with standard-release dosage forms.

101

Heavy metal antagonists

deferoxamine mesylate
dimercaprol
edetate calcium disodium
edetate disodium
D-penicillamine

---

deferoxamine mesylate
Desferal♦

INDICATIONS & DOSAGE
Acute iron intoxication—
Adults and children: 1 g I.M. or I.V. followed by 500 mg I.M. or I.V. for 2 doses, q 4 hours; then 500 mg I.M. or I.V. q 4 to 12 hours. Infusion rate shouldn't exceed 15 mg/Kg/hour.
Chronic iron overload and in patients requiring multiple transfusions—
Adults and children: 500 mg to 1 g I.M. daily and 2 g slow I.V. infusion in separate solution along with each unit blood transfused. Maximum dose 6 g daily. I.V. infusion rate shouldn't exceed 15 mg/Kg/hour.
S.C.: 1 to 2 g administered q 8 to 24 hours.

SIDE EFFECTS
Local: pain and induration at injection site. *After rapid I.V. administration: erythema, urticaria, hypotension.*
With long-term use: sensitivity reaction (cutaneous wheal formation, pruritus, rash, *anaphylaxis), diarrhea, leg cramps, fever, tachycardia, blurred vision, dysuria, abdominal discomfort.*

INTERACTIONS
None significant.

NURSING CONSIDERATIONS
• Contraindicated in severe renal disease or anuria. Use cautiously in impaired renal function.
• Monitor intake/output carefully.
• I.M. route preferred.
• Use I.V. only when patient has cardiovascular collapse or shock. For I.V. use, dissolve as for I.M. use; dilute in normal saline, 5% dextrose in water, or lactated Ringer's solution.
• If giving I.V., change to I.M. as soon as possible.
• For reconstitution, add 2 ml sterile water for injection to each ampule. Make sure drug is completely dissolved. Reconstituted solution good for 1 week at room temperature. Protect from light.
• Urine may be colored red.

---

dimercaprol
BAL in Oil♦

INDICATIONS & DOSAGE
Adults and children:
Severe arsenic or gold poisoning—
3 mg/Kg deep I.M. q 4 hours for 2 days, then q.i.d. on 3rd day, then b.i.d. for 10 days.
Mild arsenic or gold poisoning—
2.5 mg/Kg deep I.M. q.i.d. for 2 days, then b.i.d. on 3rd day, then once daily for 10 days.
*Mercury poisoning—*5 mg/Kg deep

I.M. initially, then 2.5 mg/Kg daily or b.i.d. for 10 days.

Acute lead encephalopathy or lead level more than 100 mcg/ml—
4 mg/Kg deep I.M. injection, then q 4 hours with edetate calcium disodium (12.5 mg/Kg I.M.). Use separate sites. Maximum dose 5 mg/Kg per dose.

SIDE EFFECTS

CNS: pain or tightness in throat, chest, or hands; headache; paresthesias; muscle pain or weakness.
CV: *transient increase in blood pressure, returns to normal in 2 hours; tachycardia.*
EENT: blepharal spasm, conjunctivitis, lacrimation, rhinorrhea, excessive salivation.
GI: halitosis; nausea; vomiting; burning sensation in lips, mouth, and throat.
GU: renal damage if alkaline urine not maintained.
Metabolic: decreased iodine uptake.
Local: sterile abscess, pain at injection site.
Other: fever (especially in children), sweating, pain in teeth.

INTERACTIONS

^{131}I uptake thyroid tests decreased: don't schedule patient for this test during course of dimercaprol therapy.
Iron: formed toxic metal complex; concurrent therapy contraindicated.

NURSING CONSIDERATIONS

• Contraindicated in hepatic dysfunction (except postarsenical jaundice), acute renal insufficiency.
• Don't use for iron, cadmium, or selenium toxicity. Complex formed is highly toxic, even fatal.
• Ephedrine or antihistamine may prevent or relieve mild side effects.
• Ineffective in arsine gas poisoning.
• Solution with slight sediment usable.

• Keep urine alkaline to prevent renal damage. Oral NaHCO$_3$ may be ordered.
• Don't give I.V.; give by deep I.M. route only.

---

edetate calcium disodium
Calcium Disodium Versenate♦,
Calcium EDTA

INDICATIONS & DOSAGE

Lead poisoning—
Adults: 1 g/250 to 500 ml 5% dextrose in water or 0.9% normal saline solution I.V. over 1 to 2 hours daily or q 12 hours for 3 to 5 days; repeat after 2 days if indicated. Maximum dose 50 mg/Kg daily.
Children: 35 mg/Kg I.M. daily divided q 8 to 12 hours. Maximum dose 50 mg/Kg daily.
Acute lead encephalopathy or lead levels more than 100 mcg/ml—
Adults and children: 12.5 mg/Kg with dimercaprol 4 mg/Kg deep I.M. after initial dose of dimercaprol 4 mg deep I.M. Use separate sites. After first dose, reduce to 3 mg/Kg for 2 to 7 days.

SIDE EFFECTS

CNS: headache, paresthesias, numbness.
CV: cardiac arrhythmias, hypotension.
GI: anorexia, nausea, vomiting.
GU: *proteinuria, hematuria; nephrotoxicity with renal tubular necrosis leading to fatal nephrosis in excessive dose.*
Other: arthralgia, myalgia, hypercalcemia.
4 to 8 hours after infusion: sudden fever and chills, fatigue, excessive thirst, sneezing, nasal congestion.

INTERACTIONS
None significant.

NURSING CONSIDERATIONS

- Contraindicated in severe renal disease or anuria.
- I.V. use contraindicated in lead encephalopathy; may increase intracranial pressure. Use I.M. route instead.
- Force fluids in all patients except those with lead encephalopathy.
- Monitor intake/output, urinalysis, BUN, and EKGs.
- To avoid toxicity, use with dimercaprol.
- Oral form available but use discouraged because of poor GI absorption; often used ineffectively as prophylaxis against lead exposure; can even increase lead absorption from GI tract.
- Procaine HCl may be added to I.M. solutions to minimize pain. Watch for local reactions.
- Avoid rapid I.V. infusions. I.M. route preferred.

edetate disodium
Disodium EDTA, Disotate, Endrate, Sodium Versenate

INDICATIONS & DOSAGE
Hypercalcemic crisis—
Adults and children: 15 to 50 mg/Kg slow I.V. infusion. Dilute in 500 ml 5% dextrose in water or 0.9% normal saline solution. Give over 3 to 4 hours. Maximum adult dose 3 g/day. Maximum children's dose 70 mg/Kg/day.

SIDE EFFECTS
CNS: circumoral paresthesias, numbness, headache, malaise, fatigue, muscle pain or weakness.
CV: hypertension, thrombophlebitis.
GI: nausea, vomiting, diarrhea, anorexia, abdominal cramps.
GU: in excessive doses—nephrotoxicity with urgency, nocturia, dysuria, polyuria, proteinuria, renal insufficiency and failure, tubular necrosis.

Metabolic: *severe hypocalcemia,* decreased magnesium.
Local: pain at site of infusion, erythema, dermatitis.

INTERACTIONS
None significant.

NURSING CONSIDERATIONS
- Contraindicated in anuria, known or suspected hypocalcemia, or significant renal disease; active or healed tubercular lesions; history of seizures or intracranial lesions; generalized arteriosclerosis associated with aging. Use cautiously in limited cardiac reserve, incipient congestive heart failure, hypokalemia, diabetes.
- Avoid rapid I.V. infusion; profound hypocalcemia may occur.
- Monitor EKG and test renal function frequently.
- Obtain serum calcium levels after each dose.
- Keep I.V. calcium available.
- Keep patient in bed for 15 minutes after infusion to avoid postural hypotension.
- Don't use to treat lead toxicity; use edetate calcium disodium instead.
- Edetate disodium not currently drug of choice for treatment of hypercalcemia; other treatments are safer and more effective.

D-penicillamine
Cuprimine♦, Depen

INDICATIONS & DOSAGE
Wilson's disease—
Adults: 250 mg P.O. q.i.d. before meals. Adjust dose to achieve urinary copper excretion of 0.5 to 1 mg daily.
Children: 20 mg/Kg daily P.O. divided q.i.d. before meals. Adjust dose to achieve urinary copper excretion of 0.5 to 1 mg daily.
Cystinuria—
Adults: 250 mg P.O. q.i.d. before

Italicized side effects are common or life-threatening.

meals. Adjust dose to achieve urinary cystine excretion of less than 100 mg daily when renal calculi present, or 100 to 200 mg daily when no calculi present. Maximum adult dose is 5 g daily.

Children: 30 mg/Kg daily P.O. divided q.i.d. before meals. Adjust dose to achieve urinary cystine excretion of less than 100 mg daily when renal calculi present, or 100 to 200 mg daily when no calculi present.

Rheumatoid arthritis—

Adults: 250 mg P.O. daily initially, with increases of 250 mg q 2 to 3 months if necessary. Maximum dose 1 g daily.

SIDE EFFECTS

Blood: *leukopenia, eosinophilia, thrombocytopenia, monocytosis, granulocytopenia,* elevated sedimentation rate, lupus erythematosus-like syndrome.

EENT: tinnitus.

GU: *nephrotic syndrome, glomerulonephritis.*

Hepatic: hepatotoxicity.

Metabolic: *decreased pyridoxine (may cause optic neuritis),* decreased zinc and mercury.

Skin: friability, especially at pressure spots; wrinkling; erythema; urticaria; ecchymoses.

Other: reversible taste impairment, especially of salts and sweets; hair loss. *About ⅓ of patients develop allergic reactions (rash, pruritus, fever), arthralgia, lymphadenopathy.* With long-term use, myasthenia gravis syndrome.

INTERACTIONS

Oral iron: decreased effectiveness of D-penicillamine. If used together, give at least 2 hours apart.

NURSING CONSIDERATIONS

• Contraindicated in pregnant women with cystinuria. Use cautiously in penicillin allergy; cross sensitivity may occur.

• Report to doctor if fever or other allergic reactions occur.

• Patient should receive pyridoxine daily.

• Handle patients carefully to avoid skin damage.

• Dose should be given on empty stomach.

• Patient should drink large amounts of fluid, especially at night.

• Tell patient that therapeutic effect may be delayed up to 3 months.

• Monitor CBC, renal and hepatic function.

102

Gold compounds

aurothioglucose
gold sodium thiomalate

---

aurothioglucose
Solganal
gold sodium thiomalate
Myochrysine♦

INDICATIONS & DOSAGE
Rheumatoid arthritis—
Adults: initially, 10 mg (aurothioglucose) I.M., followed by 25 mg for second and third doses at weekly intervals. Then, 50 mg weekly until 1 g has been given. If improvement occurs without toxicity, continue 25 to 50 mg at 3- to 4-week intervals indefinitely.
Children 6 to 12 years: ¼ usual adult dose. Alternatively, 1 mg/Kg I.M. once weekly for 20 weeks.

Rheumatoid arthritis—
Adults: initially, 10 mg (gold sodium thiomalate) I.M., followed by 25 mg in 1 week. Then, 50 mg weekly until 14 to 20 doses have been given. If improvement occurs without toxicity, continue 50 mg q 2 weeks for 4 doses; then, 50 mg q 3 weeks for 4 doses; then, 50 mg q month indefinitely. If relapse occurs during maintenance therapy, resume injections at weekly intervals.
Children: 1 mg/Kg I.M. per week for 20 weeks. If good response occurs, may be given q 3 to 4 weeks indefinitely.

SIDE EFFECTS
Adverse reactions to gold are considered severe and potentially life-threatening. Report any side effect to the doctor at once.
Blood: *thrombocytopenia* (with or without purpura), *aplastic anemia, agranulocytosis,* leukopenia, eosinophilia.
CV: bradycardia.
EENT: corneal gold deposition.
GU: *albuminuria, proteinuria, nephrotic syndrome,* nephritis, acute tubular necrosis.
Hepatic: hepatitis, jaundice.
Skin: *rash and dermatitis in 20%. (If drug is not stopped, may lead to fatal exfoliative dermatitis.)*
Other: *anaphylaxis,* angioneurotic edema, metallic taste, stomatitis.

INTERACTIONS
None significant.

NURSING CONSIDERATIONS
• Contraindicated in severe uncontrollable diabetes, renal disease, hepatic dysfunction, marked hypertension, heart failure, systemic lupus erythematosus, Sjögren's syndrome. Use cautiously with other drugs that cause blood dyscrasias.
• Indicated only in active rheumatoid arthritis that has not responded adequately to salicylates, penicillamine, rest, and physical therapy.
• Should be administered only under constant supervision of a doctor who is thoroughly familiar with its toxicities and benefits.

• Most side effects are readily reversible if drug is stopped immediately.
• Administer all gold compounds intramuscularly, preferably intragluteally.
• Observe patient for 30 minutes after administration because of possibility of anaphylactic reaction.
• Reassure patient that benefits of therapy may not appear for 6 to 8 weeks.
• Aurothioglucose is a suspension. Immerse vial in warm water and shake vigorously before injecting.

• When giving gold sodium thiomalate, advise patient to lie down and to remain recumbent for 10 minutes following injection.
• Complete blood counts should be performed at 2- to 4-week intervals.
• If side effects are mild, some rheumatologists resume gold therapy after 2 to 3 weeks' rest.
• Dimercaprol (BAL) should be kept on hand to treat acute toxicity.

103

Diagnostic skin tests

histoplasmin
Old Tuberculin
tuberculin purified protein
    derivative, Mantoux

---

histoplasmin♦

INDICATIONS & DOSAGE
Suspected histoplasmosis—
Adults and children: 0.1 ml of 1:100
dilution intradermally on inner forearm. Use tuberculin syringe with 26-
or 27-gauge, ⅜-inch needle.

SIDE EFFECTS
Local: urticaria, ulceration or necrosis in highly sensitive patients.
Other: shortness of breath, sweating,
anaphylaxis.

INTERACTIONS
None significant.

NURSING CONSIDERATIONS
• Read test at 24 to 48 hours. Indura-
tion of 5 mm or more is positive.
• Reaction may be depressed in mal-
nutrition or in immunosuppression.
• Cross-reaction may occur with
other fungi (e.g., *Candida albicans,*
Blastomyces dermatitides).
• Obtain accurate history of allergies
and past reactions to skin tests.
• Keep epinephrine 1:1,000 available.
• Cold packs or topical corticoste-
roids may relieve pain and itching if
severe local reaction occurs.

Old Tuberculin
Old Tuberculin Test♦; Tuberculin,
Mono-Vacc Test; Old Tuberculin Tine
Test

INDICATIONS & DOSAGE
Diagnosis of tuberculosis—
Adults and children: 10 tuberculin
units (0.1 ml of 1:1,000) Old Tuberculin intradermally on inner forearm.
In suspected tuberculosis, use 1 tuberculin unit first. Use tuberculin syringe
with 26- or 27-gauge, ⅜-inch needle.
Multiple-puncture test: cleanse skin
thoroughly with alcohol; make skin
taut on inner forearm; press points
firmly into selected site.

SIDE EFFECTS
Local: hypersensitivity (vesiculation,
ulceration, necrosis).
Other: *anaphylaxis.*

INTERACTIONS
None significant.

NURSING CONSIDERATIONS
• Contraindicated in known tuberculin positive reactors.
• False-positive reaction can occur in
sensitive patients.
• Reaction may be depressed in malnutrition or in immunosuppression.
• Read test in 48 to 72 hours. Induration of 10 mm or more is positive; 5 to
9 mm, doubtful; less than 5, negative.
• Multiple-puncture test: 1 to 2 mm
induration is positive.
• Old Tuberculin Tine Test equals

5 tuberculin units purified protein derivatives.
- Obtain accurate history of allergies, especially to acacia (contained in tine test as stabilizer), and past reactions to skin tests.
- Keep epinephrine 1:1,000 available.
- S.C. injection invalidates test results. Bleb must form on skin upon injection.
- Corticosteroids and other immunosuppressants may suppress skin test reaction.
- Cold packs or topical corticosteroids may relieve pain and itching if severe local reaction occurs.

tuberculin purified protein derivative, Mantoux
Aplisol, Aplitest, Sclavo test-PPD, Sterneedle, Tuberculin PPD-Heaf, Tuberculin PPD-Stabilized, Tubersol

INDICATIONS & DOSAGE
Diagnosis of tuberculosis—
Adults and children: 5 tuberculin units (0.1 ml) intradermally on inner forearm. Suspected sensitivity dose is 1 tuberculin unit. Patients failing to react to 5 tuberculin units should be tested with 250 tuberculin units. First strength equals 1 tuberculin unit/0.1 ml; intermediate strength, 5 tuberculin units/0.1 ml. Second strength equals 250 tuberculin units/0.1 ml.
Use tuberculin syringe with 26- or 27-gauge, 3/8-inch needle.
Multiple-puncture test: cleanse skin thoroughly with alcohol; make skin taut on inner forearm; press points firmly into selected site.

SIDE EFFECTS
Local: pain, pruritus, ulceration, necrosis.
Other: *anaphylaxis.*

INTERACTIONS
None significant.

NURSING CONSIDERATIONS
- Contraindicated in known tuberculin-positive reactors; severe reactions may occur. Use cautiously with active tuberculosis.
- Read test in 48 to 72 hours. Induration of 10 mm or more is positive; 5 to 9 mm, doubtful; less than 5 mm, negative.
- Multiple-puncture test: vesiculation is positive reaction; induration of less than 2 mm without vesiculation is negative.
- 1 tuberculin unit may give false-negative test; 250 tuberculin units may give false-positive test.
- Obtain accurate history of allergies and past reactions to skin tests.
- Reaction may be depressed in malnutrition, immunosuppression, or viral infections (up to 4 weeks postinfection).
- Antigen adsorbed by plastic. Use at once after drawing into plastic syringe.
- Keep epinephrine 1:1,000 available.
- S.C. injection invalidates test results. Bleb must form on skin upon injection.
- Cold packs or topical corticosteroids may relieve pain and itching if severe local reaction occurs.
- Never give initial test with second test strength (250 tuberculin units).
- A tine test is available for rapid screening (multiple-puncture test).
- Corticosteroids and other immunosuppressants may suppress skin test reaction.

104

Uncategorized drugs

adenosine phosphate
allopurinol
amantadine hydrochloride
bromocriptine mesylate
clomiphene citrate
colchicine
cromolyn sodium
diazoxide, oral
dimethyl sulfoxide 50% (DMSO)
disulfiram
lactulose
levodopa
levodopa-carbidopa
methoxsalen
metyrosine
pralidoxime chloride
ritodrine hydrochloride

---

adenosine phosphate
Adenocrest, Adenyl, Cobalasine,
My-B-Den

INDICATIONS & DOSAGE
*To relieve edema, pruritus, dermatitis,
and erythema of varicose veins; symptomatic treatment of bursitis, tendon-
itis, intractable pruritus—*
Adults: 20 to 100 mg I.M. (extended-
release) daily for 3 or 4 days, reduced
to same dosage every other day. Depending on patient response, reduce
dose to 20 mg once or twice weekly;
or 20 mg I.M. daily to t.i.d. (simple
aqueous solution); or every hour for
5 doses for first 3 days, followed by
20 mg daily as needed; or 100 mg in
aqueous solution injected as single
dose daily for 3 days, followed by

100 mg on alternate days thereafter as
needed.
*Sublingual dose to supplement I.M.
injection—*
Adults: 20 mg sublingually q hour,
5 to 7 doses per day for 4 to 7 days.
Maintenance dose: 40 to 100 mg daily
sublingually, adjusted to patient
response.

SIDE EFFECTS
CNS: dizziness.
CV: *palpitations, hypotension,
dyspnea.*
GI: epigastric discomfort, nausea.
Skin: erythema, flushing.
Other: *anaphylaxis.*

INTERACTIONS
None significant.

NURSING CONSIDERATIONS
• Contraindicated in myocardial infarction and cerebral hemorrhage.
Use cautiously in patients with history
of allergy. Obtain accurate history of
allergies before giving first dose.
• Anaphylactic reactions have occurred following use of gelatin I.M.
solution. Discontinue if patient complains of dyspnea or tightness in
chest.
• Don't give I.V.
• Place sublingual tablets under
tongue. Warn patient not to mix with
food or water, or to swallow exces-
sively until dissolved.
• I.M. extended-release in gelatin
vehicle: warm solution before using.
Inject into gluteal muscle, using 22G
to 20G needle, 1 to 1½ inches long.

allopurinol
Lopurin, Zyloprim♦

INDICATIONS & DOSAGE

Gout, primary or secondary to hyper-uricemia; secondary to diseases such as acute or chronic leukemia, polycy-themia vera, multiple myeloma, and psoriasis—
Dosage varies with severity of disease; can be given as single dose or divided, but doses larger than 300 mg should be divided.
Adults: mild gout, 200 to 300 mg P.O. daily; severe gout with large tophi, 400 to 600 mg P.O. daily. Same dose for maintenance in secondary hyperuricemia.
Hyperuricemia secondary to malignancies—
Children 6 to 10 years: 300 mg P.O. daily.
Children under 6 years: 150 mg P.O. daily.
Impaired renal function—
Adults: 200 mg daily if creatinine clearance is 10 to 20 ml/minute; 100 mg daily if creatinine is less than 10 ml/minute; 100 mg more than 24 hours apart if clearance is less than 3 ml/minute.
To prevent acute gouty attacks—
Adults: 100 mg daily; increase at weekly intervals by 100 mg without exceeding maximum (800 mg), until serum uric acid level falls to 6 mg/100 ml or less.
To prevent uric acid nephropathy during cancer chemotherapy—
Adults: 600 to 800 mg P.O. daily for 2 to 3 days, with high fluid intake.

SIDE EFFECTS

Blood: *agranulocytosis,* anemia, *aplastic anemia.*
CNS: drowsiness.
EENT: cataracts, retinopathy.
GI: nausea, vomiting, diarrhea, abdominal pain.
Skin: *rash, usually maculopapular; exfoliative,* urticarial, and purpuric lesions; erythema multiforme; severe furunculosis of nose; ichthyosis, *toxic epidermal necrolysis.*
Other: altered liver function tests.

INTERACTIONS

Uricosuric agents: additive effect; may be used to therapeutic advantage.

NURSING CONSIDERATIONS

• Contraindicated in hypersensitive individuals or those with idiopathic hemochromatosis; and in patients who have developed reactions to it. Use cautiously in hepatic or renal disease.
• Obtain accurate patient history; note possible allergies with other drug use before first dose.
• Discontinue at first sign of skin rash, which may precede severe hypersensitivity reaction, or any other adverse reaction. Warn patient to report all side effects immediately.
• Monitor intake/output; daily urinary output of at least 2 liters and maintenance of neutral or slightly alkaline urine are desirable.
• Periodically check CBC, hepatic and renal function, especially at start of therapy.
• Acute gouty attacks may occur in first 6 weeks of therapy; concurrent use of colchicine may be prescribed prophylactically.
• Minimize GI side effects by giving with meals or immediately after.
• Evaluate effectiveness, using serum uric acid levels. Goal is to lower serum level to 6 mg/100 ml, usually within 7 to 10 days; to gradually reduce size of tophi, with no new deposits within 6 months; and to relieve joint pain and increase mobility.
• Allopurinol may predispose patient to ampicillin-induced skin rash.

amantadine hydrochloride
Symmetrel ♦

INDICATIONS & DOSAGE
To treat drug-induced extrapyramidal reactions—
Adults: 100 mg P.O. b.i.d., up to 300 mg daily in divided doses. Patients may benefit from as much as 400 mg daily, but doses over 200 mg must be closely supervised.
To treat idiopathic parkinsonism, parkinsonian syndrome—
Adults: 100 mg P.O. b.i.d.; in patients who are seriously ill or receiving other antiparkinsonism drugs, 100 mg daily for at least 1 week, then 100 mg b.i.d., p.r.n.

SIDE EFFECTS
CNS: depression, fatigue, confusion, *dizziness,* psychosis, hallucinations, anxiety, irritability, *ataxia, insomnia,* weakness, headache.
CV: peripheral edema, *orthostatic hypotension,* congestive heart failure.
GI: anorexia, nausea, constipation, vomiting, dry mouth.
GU: urinary retention.
Skin: *livedo reticularis,* dermatitis.

INTERACTIONS
None significant.

NURSING CONSIDERATIONS
• Use cautiously in epilepsy or seizures, with congestive heart failure, renal impairment, peripheral edema, hepatic disease, eczematoid dermatitis, uncontrolled psychosis, or severe psychoneurosis.
• Don't stop abruptly, since this might precipitate a parkinsonian crisis; taper off gradually.
• Warn elderly patients about orthostatic hypotension. Suggest they change position slowly, dangle legs before getting up, and lie down if they feel faint or dizzy. Advise elderly males to sit down to urinate, especially at night.
• Last daily dose should be given as early as possible to avoid insomnia.
• Warn that drug may produce dizziness, blurred vision, impaired coordination; activities requiring mental alertness should be resumed gradually.
• Advise patient to report decrease in drug's effectiveness to doctor.

bromocriptine mesylate
Parlodel ♦

INDICATIONS & DOSAGE
To treat amenorrhea and galactorrhea associated with hyperprolactinemia —
2.5 mg P.O. b.i.d. or t.i.d. with meals for 14 days; and for no more than 6 months.
Prevention of postpartum lactation—
2.5 mg b.i.d. with meals for 14 days. Treatment may be extended for up to 21 days, if necessary.

SIDE EFFECTS
CNS: *dizziness,* headache, fatigue, nervousness.
EENT: nasal congestion, tinnitus, blurred vision.
GI: *nausea,* vomiting, abdominal cramps, constipation, diarrhea.

INTERACTIONS
None significant.

NURSING CONSIDERATIONS
• Contraindicated in hypersensitivity to ergot derivatives.
• Patient should be examined carefully for pituitary tumor (Forbes-Albright syndrome).
• May lead to early postpartum conception. Test for pregnancy every 4 weeks or whenever period is missed once menses are reinitiated.
• Advise patient to use contraceptive

Italicized side effects are common or life-threatening.

methods other than oral contraceptive during treatment.
• "First-dose phenomenon" occurs in 1% of patients. Sensitive patients may collapse for 15 to 60 minutes but can usually tolerate subsequent treatment without ill effects.
• Should be given with meals.
• Has been used investigationally in management of parkinsonism.

clomiphene citrate
Clomid♦

INDICATIONS & DOSAGE
To induce ovulation—50 to 100 mg P.O. daily for 5 days, starting any time; or 50 to 100 mg P.O. daily starting on day 5 of menstrual cycle (first day of menstrual flow is day 1). Repeat until conception occurs or until 3 courses of therapy are completed.

SIDE EFFECTS
CNS: headache, restlessness, insomnia, dizziness, light-headedness, depression, fatigue, tension.
CV: hypertension.
EENT: blurred vision, diplopia, scotomata, photophobia (signs of impending visual toxicity).
GI: nausea, vomiting, bloating, distention, increased appetite, weight gain.
GU: urinary frequency and polyuria; ovarian enlargement and cyst formation, which regress spontaneously when drug is stopped.
Metabolic: hyperglycemia.
Skin: urticaria, rash, dermatitis.
Other: *hot flashes,* reversible alopecia, *breast discomfort.*

INTERACTIONS
None significant.

NURSING CONSIDERATIONS
• Contraindicated in thrombophlebitis, thromboembolic disorders, or his-

tory of these conditions; cancer of breast or reproductive organs; undiagnosed abnormal genital bleeding; ovarian cyst; hepatic disease or dysfunction. Use cautiously in hypertension, mental depression, migraines, seizures, diabetes mellitus, or gonadotropin sensitivity. Report development or worsening of these conditions to doctor. May require stopping drug.
• Patient with visual disturbances should report symptoms to doctor at once.
• Tell patient possibility of multiple births exists with this drug. Risk increases with higher doses.

colchicine
Colchicine, Novocolchine♦ ♦

INDICATIONS & DOSAGE
To prevent acute attacks of gout as prophylactic or maintenance therapy—
Adults: 0.5 or 0.6 mg P.O. daily; or 1 to 1.8 mg P.O. daily for more severe cases.
To prevent attacks of gout in patients undergoing surgery—
Adults: 0.5 to 0.6 mg P.O. t.i.d. 3 days before and 3 days after surgery.
To treat acute gout, acute gouty arthritis—
Adults: initially, 1 to 1.2 mg P.O., then 0.5 or 0.6 mg q hour, or 1 to 1.2 mg q 2 hours until pain is relieved or until nausea, vomiting, or diarrhea ensues. Or 2 mg I.V. followed by 2 mg I.V. in 12 hours if necessary. Total I.V. dose over 24 hours not to exceed 4 mg.
Note: Give I.V. by slow I.V. push over 2 to 5 minutes. Avoid extravasation. Don't dilute colchicine injection with 0.9% sodium chloride or 5% dextrose injection, or any other fluid that might change pH of colchicine solution. If lower concentration of colchi-

cine injection needed, dilute with sterile water for injection. However, if diluted solution becomes turbid, don't inject.

SIDE EFFECTS
Blood: *aplastic anemia and agranulocytosis with prolonged use;* nonthrombocytopenic purpura.
CNS: peripheral neuritis.
GI: *nausea, vomiting, abdominal pain, diarrhea.*
Skin: urticaria, dermatitis.
Local: severe local irritation if extravasation occurs.
Other: alopecia.

INTERACTIONS
None significant.

NURSING CONSIDERATIONS
• Use cautiously in hepatic dysfunction, heart disease, renal disease, GI disorders, and in aged or debilitated patients.
• Reduce dosage if weakness, anorexia, nausea, vomiting, or diarrhea appears. First sign of acute overdosage may be GI symptoms, followed by vascular damage, muscle weakness, ascending paralysis. Delirium and convulsions may occur without patient losing consciousness.
• Do not administer I.M. or S.C.; severe local irritation occurs.
• As maintenance therapy, give with meals to reduce GI effects. May be used with uricosuric agents.
• Baseline lab studies including CBC should precede therapy and be repeated periodically.
• Monitor fluid intake/output. Keep output at 2,000 ml daily.
• Store in tightly closed, light-resistant container.
• Change needle before making direct I.V. injection.

cromolyn sodium
Intal♦, Rynacrom♦♦

INDICATIONS & DOSAGE
Adjunct in treatment of severe perennial bronchial asthma—
Adults, and children over 5 years: contents of 20 mg capsule inhaled q.i.d. at regular intervals.

SIDE EFFECTS
CNS: dizziness, headache.
EENT: *irritation of the throat and trachea, cough, bronchospasm following inhalation of dry powder; esophagitis;* nasal congestion; pharyngeal irritation; wheezing.
GI: nausea.
GU: dysuria, urinary frequency.
Skin: rash, urticaria.
Other: joint swelling and pain, lacrimation, swollen parotid gland, angioedema.

INTERACTIONS
None significant.

NURSING CONSIDERATIONS
• Contraindicated in acute asthma attacks and status asthmaticus.
• Not to be taken orally; insert capsule into inhaler provided; follow manufacturer's directions.
• Watch for recurrence of asthmatic symptoms when dosage is decreased, especially when corticosteroids are also used.
• Use only when acute episode has been controlled, airway is cleared, and patient is able to inhale.
• Patient considered for cromolyn therapy should have pulmonary function tests to show significant bronchodilator-reversible component to his airway obstruction.
• Teach correct use of inhaler: exhale completely before placing mouthpiece between lips, then inhale deeply and rapidly with steady, even breath; re-

move inhaler from mouth, hold breath a few seconds, and exhale. Repeat until all powder has been inhaled.
• Store capsules at room temperature in tightly closed containers; protect from moisture and temperatures higher than 40° C. (104° F.).
• Instruct patient to avoid excessive handling of capsule.
• Esophagitis may be relieved by antacids or a glass of milk.

---

diazoxide, oral
Proglycem

INDICATIONS & DOSAGE
Management of hypoglycemia due to a variety of conditions resulting in hyperinsulinism—
Adults and children: 3 to 8 mg/Kg/day P.O., divided into 3 equal doses q 8 hours.
Infants and newborns: 8 to 15 mg/Kg/day P.O., divided into 2 or 3 equal doses q 8 to 12 hours.

SIDE EFFECTS
Blood: *leukopenia, thrombocytopenia.*
CV: *cardiac arrhythmias.*
EENT: diplopia.
GI: nausea, vomiting.
Metabolic: sodium and fluid retention, ketoacidosis and hyperosmolar nonketotic coma, hyperuricemia.
Other: *severe hypertrichosis (hair growth) in 25% of adults and higher percentage of children.*

INTERACTIONS
Thiazide diuretics: may potentiate hyperglycemic, hyperuricemic, and hypotensive effects. Monitor appropriate lab values.

NURSING CONSIDERATIONS
• Contraindicated in thiazide hypersensitivity and functional hypoglycemia.

• Oral diazoxide does not significantly lower blood pressure.
• A nondiuretic congener of thiazide diuretics.
• Most important use is in management of hypoglycemia due to hyperinsulinism in infants and children.
• Monitor urine regularly for glucose and ketones; report any abnormalities to doctor.
• If not effective after 2 or 3 weeks, drug should be stopped.
• Hair growth on arms and forehead is a common side effect that will subside when drug treatment is completed. Reassure patient.
• Available in capsules and oral suspension.

---

dimethyl sulfoxide 50% (DMSO)
Rimso-50

INDICATIONS & DOSAGE
Symptomatic relief of interstitial cystitis—
Adults: instill 50 ml directly into bladder with catheter or syringe; allow to remain for 15 minutes. Repeat every 2 weeks until maximum symptomatic relief is obtained. Thereafter, time intervals between therapy may be increased.

SIDE EFFECTS
Other: *garlic-like taste in mouth,* hypersensitivity.

INTERACTIONS
None significant.

NURSING CONSIDERATIONS
• Chronic use of DMSO has been associated with ophthalmic changes. Eyes should be examined periodically.
• After retention of Rimso-50 for 15 minutes, it's expelled by spontaneous voiding.
• Administration of oral analgesics

Unmarked trade names available in the United States only.
♦ Also available in Canada   ♦ ♦ Available in Canada only.

before instillation can reduce bladder spasm in sensitive patients.
• Lidocaine jelly or similar local anesthetic should be applied to urethra before insertion of catheter to avoid spasm.
• Not for I.M. or I.V. injection.
• Used investigationally as a treatment for arthritis.

---

disulfiram
Antabuse♦, Cronetal, Ro-Sulfiram

INDICATIONS & DOSAGE
Adjunct in management of chronic alcoholism—
Adults: maximum of 500 mg q morning for 1 to 2 weeks. Can be taken in evening if drowsiness occurs. Maintenance: 125 to 500 mg daily (average dose 250 mg) until permanent self-control is established. Treatment may continue for months or years.

SIDE EFFECTS
CNS: drowsiness, headache, fatigue, neuritis.
EENT: optic neuritis.
GI: metallic or garlic-like aftertaste.
GU: impotence.
Skin: acneiform or allergic dermatitis.
Other: "disulfiram reaction," which may include flushing, throbbing headache, dyspnea, nausea, vomiting, sweating, thirst, chest pain, palpitations, hyperventilation, hypotension, syncope, anxiety, weakness, blurred vision, confusion.

INTERACTIONS
Isoniazid (INH): ataxia or marked change in behavior. Avoid use.
Metronidazole (Flagyl): psychotic reaction. Do not use together.
Paraldehyde: toxic levels of the acetaldehyde. Do not use together.

NURSING CONSIDERATIONS
• Contraindicated in alcohol intoxication, psychoses, myocardial disease, coronary occlusion, or those receiving metronidazole, paraldehyde, alcohol, or alcohol-containing preparations. Use cautiously in diabetes mellitus, hypothyroidism, epilepsy, cerebral damage, nephritis, hepatic cirrhosis or insufficiency, abnormal EEG, multiple drug dependence.
• Used only under close medical and nursing supervision. Patient should clearly understand consequences of disulfiram therapy and give permission. Drug should be used only in patients who are cooperative, well motivated, and are receiving supportive psychiatric therapy.
• Complete physical exam and lab studies, including CBC, SMA-12, and transaminase, should precede therapy and be repeated regularly.
• If compliance is questionable, crush tablets and mix with juice or other liquid; observe patient.
• Warn patient to avoid all sources of alcohol: sauces, cough syrups. Even external application of liniments, shaving lotion, back-rub preparations may precipitate disulfiram reaction. Tell him that alcohol reaction may occur as long as 2 weeks after single dose of disulfiram; the longer patient remains on drug, the more sensitive he will become to alcohol.
• Patient should wear a bracelet or carry a card supplied by drug manufacturer identifying him as disulfiram user.
Note: Mild reactions may occur in sensitive patients with blood alcohol level of 5 to 10 mg/100 ml; symptoms are fully developed at 50 mg/100 ml; unconsciousness usually occurs at 125 to 150 mg/100 ml level. Reaction may last ½ hour to several hours, or as long as alcohol remains in blood.
Caution: Warn patient to ingest no alcohol or alcohol-containing products

---

for at least 12 hours before administering.

lactulose
Cephulac♦, Chronulac♦

INDICATIONS & DOSAGE
To prevent and treat portal-systemic encephalopathy, including hepatic precoma and coma in patients with severe hepatic disease—
Adults: initially, 20 to 30 g P.O. (30 to 45 ml) t.i.d. or q.i.d., until 2 or 3 soft stools are produced daily. Usual dose is 60 to 100 g daily in divided doses. Can also be given by retention enema in at least 100 ml of fluid.
Treatment of constipation—
Adults: 15 to 30 ml P.O. daily.

SIDE EFFECTS
GI: abdominal cramps, belching, diarrhea, gaseous distention, flatulence.

INTERACTIONS
None significant.

NURSING CONSIDERATIONS
• Contraindicated in patients who need low-galactose diet. Use cautiously in diabetes mellitus.
• Reduce dosage if diarrhea occurs. Replace fluid loss.
• If desired, minimize drug's sweet taste by diluting with water or fruit juice or giving with food.
• Store at room temperature, preferably below 30° C. (86° F.). Don't freeze.

levodopa
Bendopa, Bio Dopa, Dopar, Larodopa♦, Levopa♦, Parda, Rio-Dopa

INDICATIONS & DOSAGE
*Treatment of idiopathic parkinsonism and parkinsonian syndrome resulting from lethargica encephalitis; carbon monoxide and chronic manganese intoxication; and cerebral arteriosclerosis—*administered orally with food in dosages carefully adjusted to individual requirements, tolerance, response.
Adults: initially, 0.5 to 1 g P.O. daily, given b.i.d., t.i.d., or q.i.d. with food; increase by no more than 0.75 g daily q 3 to 7 days, until usual maximum of 8 g is reached. Larger dose requires close supervision.

SIDE EFFECTS
Blood: hemolytic anemia, leukopenia.
CNS: *choreiform, dystonic, dyskinetic movements; involuntary grimacing, head movements, myoclonic body jerks, ataxia, tremors, muscle twitching; bradykinetic episodes; psychiatric disturbances, memory loss, nervousness, anxiety, disturbing dreams, euphoria, malaise, fatigue; severe depression, suicidal tendencies, dementia, delirium, hallucinations (may necessitate reduction or withdrawal of drug).*
CV: *orthostatic hypotension,* cardiac irregularities, flushing, hypertension, phlebitis.
EENT: blepharospasm, blurred vision, diplopia, mydriasis or miosis, widening of palpebral fissures, activation of latent Horner's syndrome, oculogyric crises, nasal discharge.
GI: *nausea, vomiting, anorexia;* weight loss may occur at start of therapy; constipation; flatulence; diarrhea; epigastric pain; hiccups; sialorrhea; dry mouth; bitter taste.
GU: urinary frequency, retention, incontinence; darkened urine; excessive and inappropriate sexual behavior; priapism.
Hepatic: hepatotoxicity.
Other: dark perspiration, hyperventilation.

INTERACTIONS

Anticholinergic drugs, tricyclic antidepressants, benzodiazepines, clonidine, papaverine, phenothiazines and other antipsychotics, phenytoin: watch for decreased levodopa effect. *Pyridoxine:* reduced efficacy of levodopa. Examine vitamin preparations for content of vitamin B₆ (pyridoxine). *Antacids, propranolol:* may increase levodopa effect. Use together cautiously.

NURSING CONSIDERATIONS

• Contraindicated in narrow-angle glaucoma, melanoma or undiagnosed skin lesions. Use cautiously in cardiovascular, renal, hepatic, pulmonary disorders; in those with peptic ulcer, psychiatric illness, myocardial infarction with residual arrhythmias; and in patients with bronchial asthma, emphysema, and endocrine disease.
• Carefully monitor patients also receiving antihypertensive medication, hypoglycemic agents. Stop MAO inhibitors at least 2 weeks before therapy is begun.
• Adjust dosage according to patient's response and tolerance. Observe and monitor vital signs, especially while adjusting dose. Report significant changes.
• Instruct patient to report adverse reactions and therapeutic effects.
• Warn of possible dizziness and orthostatic hypotension, especially at start of therapy. Patient should change position slowly and dangle legs before getting out of bed. Elastic stockings may control this side effect in some patients.
• Muscle twitching and blepharospasm (twitching of eyelids) may be an early sign of drug overdosage; report immediately.
• Patients on long-term use should be tested regularly for diabetes and acromegaly; repeat blood tests, liver and kidney function studies periodically.
• Multivitamin preparations, fortified cereals, and certain over-the-counter medications may contain pyridoxine (vitamin B₆), which can reverse the effects of levodopa.
• If therapy is interrupted for long period, drug should be adjusted gradually to previous level.
• Therapeutic response usually occurs following each dose and disappears within 5 hours but varies considerably.
• Patient who must undergo surgery should continue levodopa as long as oral intake is permitted, generally 6 to 24 hours before surgery. Drug should be resumed as soon as patient is able to take oral medication.
• Protect from heat, light, moisture. If preparation darkens, it has lost potency and should be discarded.
• Coombs' test occasionally becomes positive during extended use. Expect uric acid elevations with colorimetric method, but not with uricase method.
• Alkaline phosphatase, SGOT, SGPT, LDH, bilirubin, BUN, and PBI show transient elevations in patients receiving levodopa; WBC, hemoglobin, and hematocrit show occasional reduction.
• Combination of levodopa-carbidopa usually reduces amount of levodopa needed by 75%, thereby reducing incidence of side effects.

---

levodopa-carbidopa
(combination)
Sinemet♦

INDICATIONS & DOSAGE

Treatment of idiopathic Parkinson's disease, postencephalitic parkinsonism, and symptomatic parkinsonism; carbon monoxide and manganese intoxication—
Adults: 3 to 6 tablets of 25 mg carbidopa/250 mg levodopa daily given in divided doses. Do not exceed 8 tablets of 25 mg carbidopa/250 mg levodopa

---

Italicized side effects are common or life-threatening.

a day. Optimum daily dosage must be determined by careful titration for each patient.

SIDE EFFECTS
Blood: hemolytic anemia.
CNS: *choreiform, dystonic, dyskinetic movements; involuntary grimacing, head movements, myoclonic body jerks, ataxia,* tremors, muscle twitching; bradykinetic episodes; psychiatric disturbances, memory loss, nervousness, anxiety, disturbing dreams, euphoria, malaise, fatigue; severe depression, suicidal tendencies, dementia, delirium, hallucinations (may necessitate reduction or withdrawal of drug).
CV: *orthostatic hypotension,* cardiac irregularities, flushing, hypertension, phlebitis.
EENT: blepharospasm, blurred vision, diplopia, mydriasis or miosis, widening of palpebral fissures, activation of latent Horner's syndrome, oculogyric crises, nasal discharge.
GI: nausea, vomiting, anorexia, weight loss may occur at start of therapy; constipation; flatulence; diarrhea; epigastric pain; hiccups; sialorrhea; dry mouth; bitter taste.
GU: urinary frequency, retention, incontinence; darkened urine; excessive and inappropriate sexual behavior; priapism.
Hepatic: hepatotoxicity.
Other: dark perspiration, hyperventilation.

INTERACTIONS
Papaverine, diazepam, clonidine, phenothiazines: may antagonize antiparkinson actions. Use together cautiously.

NURSING CONSIDERATIONS
• Contraindicated in narrow-angle glaucoma, melanoma or undiagnosed skin lesions. Use cautiously in cardiovascular, renal, hepatic, pulmonary disorders; in history of peptic ulcer, psychiatric illness, myocardial infarction with residual arrhythmias; and in bronchial asthma, emphysema, and endocrine disease.
• Carefully monitor patients also receiving antihypertensive medication, hypoglycemic agents. Discontinue MAO inhibitors at least 2 weeks before therapy is begun.
• Dosage is adjusted according to patient's response and tolerance to drug. Therapeutic and adverse reactions occur more rapidly with levodopa-carbidopa than with levodopa alone. Observe and monitor vital signs, especially while dosage is being adjusted; report significant changes.
• Instruct patient to report adverse reactions and therapeutic effects.
• Warn patient of possible dizziness and orthostatic hypotension, especially at start of therapy. Patient should change position slowly and dangle legs before getting out of bed. Elastic stockings may control this side effect in some patients.
• Muscle twitching and blepharospasm (twitching of eyelids) may be an early sign of drug overdosage; report immediately.
• Patients on long-term therapy should be tested regularly for diabetes and acromegaly; blood tests, liver and kidney function studies should be repeated periodically.
• If patient is being treated with levodopa, discontinue at least 8 hours before starting Sinemet.
• This combination drug usually reduces the amount of levodopa needed by 75%, thereby reducing the incidence of side effects.
• Pyridoxine (B_6) does not reverse the beneficial effects of Sinemet. Multivitamins can be taken without fear of losing control of symptoms.
• If therapy is interrupted temporarily, the usual daily dosage may be given as soon as patient resumes oral medication.
• Available as tablets with carbidopa-

levodopa in a 1 to 10 ratio (Sinemet 10/100 and Sinemet 25/250); also in a 1 to 4 ratio (Sinemet 25/100).
• Sinemet 25/100 may reduce many side effects seen with 1 to 10 ratio strengths.
• Carbidopa (Lodosyn) as a single agent is available from Merck, Sharp and Dohme upon doctor's request.

methoxsalen
Oxsoralen♦

INDICATIONS & DOSAGE
To induce repigmentation in vitiligo—
Adults, and children over 12 years: 20 mg P.O. daily, 2 to 4 hours before carefully timed exposure to ultraviolet light.

SIDE EFFECTS
CNS: nervousness, insomnia, depression.
GI: *discomfort, nausea, diarrhea.*
Skin: edema, erythema, painful blistering, burning, peeling.

INTERACTIONS
Photosensitizing agents: do not use together. May increase toxicity.

NURSING CONSIDERATIONS
• Contraindicated in hepatic insufficiency, porphyria, acute lupus erythematosus, hydromorphic and polymorphic light eruptions. Use with caution in familial history of sunlight allergy, GI diseases, or chronic infection.
• Regulate therapy carefully. Overdosage or overexposure to light can cause serious burning or blistering.
• Drug should be taken orally with meals or milk.
• During light exposure treatments, protect eyes and lips.
• Monthly liver function tests should be done on patients with vitiligo (especially at beginning of therapy).

metyrosine
Demser

INDICATIONS & DOSAGE
Preoperative preparation of patients with pheochromocytoma; management of such patients when surgery is contraindicated; chronic treatment of malignant pheochromocytoma—
Adults, and children over 12 years: 250 mg P.O. q.i.d. May be increased by 250 to 500 mg q day to a maximum of 4 g/day in divided doses. When used for preoperative preparation, optimally effective dosage should be given for at least 5 to 7 days.

SIDE EFFECTS
CNS: *sedation,* extrapyramidal symptoms such as speech difficulty and tremors, disorientation.
GI: *diarrhea,* nausea, vomiting, abdominal pain.
GU: *crystalluria,* hematuria.
Other: impotence, hypersensitivity.

INTERACTIONS
Phenothiazines and haloperidol: increased inhibition of catecholamine synthesis may result in extrapyramidal symptoms. Use cautiously.

NURSING CONSIDERATIONS
• During surgery, monitor blood pressure and EKG continuously. If a serious arrhythmia occurs during anesthesia and surgery, treatment with a beta-blocking drug or lidocaine may be necessary.
• Warn patient that sedation almost always occurs in those treated with metyrosine. Sedation usually subsides after several days' treatment.
• Instruct patient to increase daily fluid intake to prevent crystalluria. Daily urine volume should be 2,000 ml or more.
• Tell patient to notify doctor if any of the listed side effects occurs.

Italicized side effects are common or life-threatening.

- Insomnia may occur when metyrosine is stopped.
- If patient is not adequately controlled by metyrosine, an alpha-adrenergic blocking agent, such as phenoxybenzamine, should be added to the regimen.
- Available as 250-mg capsules.

pralidoxime chloride
Protopam♦

INDICATIONS & DOSAGE
Antidote for organophosphate poisoning—
Adults: I.V. infusion of 1 to 2 g in 100 ml saline over 15 to 30 minutes. If pulmonary edema is present, give drug by slow I.V. push over 5 minutes. Repeat in 1 hour if muscle weakness persists. Additional doses may be given cautiously. I.M. or S.C. injection can be used if I.V. is not feasible; or 1 to 3 g P.O. q 5 hours.
Children: 20 to 40 mg/Kg I.V.
To treat cholinergic crisis in myasthenia gravis—
Adults: 1 to 2 g I.V., followed by increments of 250 mg I.V. q 5 minutes.

SIDE EFFECTS
CNS: dizziness, headache, drowsiness, excitement, and manic behavior following recovery of consciousness.
CV: tachycardia.
EENT: blurred vision, diplopia, impaired accommodation, laryngospasm.
GI: nausea.
Other: muscular weakness, muscle rigidity, hyperventilation.

INTERACTIONS
None significant.

NURSING CONSIDERATIONS
- Contraindicated in poisoning with Sevin, a carbamate insecticide, since it increases drug's toxicity. Use with extreme caution in renal insufficiency or myasthenia gravis (overdosage may precipitate myasthenic crisis).
- Use in hospitalized patients only; have respiratory and other supportive measures available. Obtain accurate medical history and chronology of poisoning if possible. Give as soon as possible after poisoning.
- I.V. preparation should be given slowly, as dilute solution.
- Initial measures should include removal of secretions, maintenance of patent airway, artificial ventilation if needed.
- Drug relieves paralysis of respiratory muscles but is less effective in relieving depression of respiratory center.
- Atropine along with pralidoxime should be given I.V., 2 to 4 mg, if cyanosis is not present. If cyanosis is present, atropine should be given I.M. Give atropine every 5 to 10 minutes until signs of atropine toxicity appear; maintain atropinization for at least 48 hours.
- Dilute with sterile water without preservatives.
- Not effective against poisoning due to phosphorus, inorganic phosphates, or organophosphates with no anticholinesterase activity.
- Difficult to distinguish toxic effects produced by atropine, or organophosphate compounds, from pralidoxime. Observe patient for 48 to 72 hours if poison ingested. Delayed absorption may occur from lower bowel.

ritodrine hydrochloride
Yutopar

INDICATIONS & DOSAGE
Management of preterm labor—
Intravenous therapy: dilute 150 mg (3 ampuls) in 500 ml fluid yielding a final concentration of 0.3 mg/ml. Usual initial dose is 0.1 mg/minute, to

be gradually increased according to
the results by 0.05 mg/minute q 10
minutes until desired result obtained.
Effective dosage range usually lies between 0.15 and 0.35 mg/minute.
Oral maintenance: 1 tablet (10 mg)
may be given approximately 30 minutes before termination of intravenous
therapy. Usual dosage for first
24 hours of oral maintenance is 10
mg q 2 hours. Thereafter, usual dose
is 10 to 20 mg q 4 to 6 hours. Total
daily dose should not exceed 120 mg.

SIDE EFFECTS
Intravenous—
CNS: nervousness, anxiety, headache.
CV: *dose-related alterations in blood
pressure, palpitations,* EKG changes.
GI: nausea, vomiting.
Other: erythema.
Oral—
CNS: tremor.
CV: palpitations.
GI: nausea, vomiting.
Skin: rash.

INTERACTIONS
Corticosteroids: may produce pulmonary edema in mother. When these
drugs are used concomitantly, monitor
closely.

NURSING CONSIDERATIONS
• Contraindicated before 20th week
of pregnancy.
• Contraindicated in the following
conditions: antepartum hemorrhage,
eclampsia, intrauterine fetal death,
chorioamnionitis, maternal cardiac
disease, pulmonary hypertension, maternal hyperthyroidism, uncontrolled
maternal diabetes mellitus.
• Because cardiovascular responses
are common and more pronounced
during intravenous administration,
cardiovascular effects, including maternal pulse rate and blood pressure
and fetal heart rate, should be closely
monitored.
• Monitor amount of fluids administered intravenously, to avoid circulatory overload.
• Ritodrine decreases intensity and
frequency of uterine contractions.
• Don't use intravenous ritodrine if
solution is discolored or contains a
precipitate.

B

C

D

F

Gly-Trate, 151
Glytuss, 338
gold sodium thiomalate, 742
Golden Peacock, 657
Gonadex, 442
Gormel Cream, 649
Gravigen, 434
Gravol, 371
G-Recillin-T, 58
Grifulvin V, 23
Grisactin, 23
griseofulvin microsize, 23
griseofulvin ultramicrosize, 23
Grisovin-FP, 23
Grisowen, 23
Gris-PEG, 23
G-Sox, 92
G-Tussin, 338
Guaiatussin, 338
guaifenesin, 338
guanethidine sulfate, 132
Gustalac, 345
Gyne-Lotrimin, 598
Gynergen, 305
Gynovules, 12
Gyrocaps, 303

H

Halciderm, 620
halcinonide, 620
Haldol, 247
Haldrone, 409
Halog, 620
haloperidol, 247
haloprogin, 599
Halotestin, 415
Halotex, 599
hamamelis water, 632
Harmar, 184
Harmonyl, 131
Hartmann's solution. See Ringer's
    injection, lactated, 497
Hazel-Balm, 632
H-BIG, 696
HBP, 142
HC Cream, 621
Heb Cream Base, 645
Heb-Cort, 621
Hedulin, 509
Hematon, 501
Hematran, 503
Hemocyte, 501
Hemofil, 515
Henomint, 200, 216
Hepahydrin, 352
Hepalean, 507
heparin sodium, 507
hepatitis B immune globulin, human,
    696

Hep-B-Gammagee, 696
Heprinar, 507
Herisan Antibiotic, 601
Herplex, 555
Hespan, 492
hetacillin, 54
hetacillin potassium, 54
hetastarch, 492
Hetrazan, 16
Hexa-Betalin, 681
hexachlorophene, 637
Hexacrest, 681
Hexadrol, 402, 614
Hexadrol Phosphate, 402
hexafluorenium bromide, 318
Hexalet, 94
Hexamead-Ph, 637
Hexaphen, 290
Hexavibex, 681
hexobarbital, 195
hexocyclium methylsulfate, 383
Hibiclens Liquid, 636
Hibitane, 636
HI-COR-2.5, 621
Hip-Rex, 94, 94
Hiserpia, 144
Hispril, 330
Histalon, 326
Histantil, 332
Histaspan, 326
Histerone, 423
Histex, 326
histoplasmin, 744
Histrey, 326
Hiwolfia, 142
HMS Liquifilm Ophthalmic, 562
Homatrocel Ophthalmic, 572
homatropine hydrobromide, 572
homatropine methylbromide, 384
Homo-Tet, 698
Honvol, 429
H.P. Acthar Gel, 462
HQC Kit, 657
Humafac Koate, 515
human growth hormone. See
    somatropin, 464
Humatin, 14
Humorsol, 565
Hurricaine, 626
Hu-Tet, 698
hyaluronidase, 722
Hyasorb, 58
Hyazyme, 722
Hycodan, 339
Hycort, 621
Hycortole, 621
Hydeltrasol Ophthalmic, 562
Hydeltra-TBA, 410
Hydextran, 503
hydralazine hydrochloride, 133
Hydralyn, 133

iodinated glycerol, 340
iodine, 458, 637, 688
iodine solution, 637
iodine tincture, 637
iodochlorhydroxyquin, 600
Ionamin, 274
Ionax Foam, 635
Ionax Scrub, 635
Iosel 250, 659
ipecac syrup, 372
Ircon, 501
iron dextran, 503
Irospan, 503
I-Sedrin Plain, 591
Ismelin, 132
Iso-Autohaler, 296
Isobec, 188
Iso-Bid, 149
Isocaine, 666
isocarboxazid, 225
Iso-D, 149
Isodine, 640
isoetharine hydrochloride 1%, 295
isoetharine mesylate, 295
Isofedrol, 591
isoflurophate, 567
isoniazid (INH), 35
isophane insulin suspension (NPH),
    447
Isophrin, 593
isopropamide iodide, 385
isopropyl alcohol 99%, 634
isopropyl aqueous alcohol 75%,
    634
isopropyl rubbing alcohol 70%, 634
isoproterenol hydrochloride, 296
isoproterenol sulfate, 296
Isopto Alkaline, 580
Isopto Atropine, 570
Isopto Carbachol, 564
Isopto Carpine, 569
Isopto Cetamide Ophthalmic, 557
Isopto Eserine, 568
Isopto Fenicol, 552
Isopto Frin, 576
Isopto Homatropine, 572
Isopto Hyoscine, 574
Isopto Plain, 580
Isopto Tears, 580
Isordil, 149
Isosorb, 149
isosorbide dinitrate, 149
Isotamine, 35
Isotrate, 149
Isovex, 148
isoxsuprine hydrochloride, 150
Isuprel, 296
Ivadantin, 96
Ivocort, 621

J

Jactatest, 424
Janimine, 225
Jayne's P-W Vermifuge, 17
J-Dantin, 96
Jecto Sal, 172
J-Liberty, 232
J-Pav, 153
J-Sul, 92

K

K Tab, 494
K-10, 494
Kabikinase, 521
Kafocin, 68
Kalinate Elixir, 495
Kalmm, 236
kanamycin sulfate, 43
Kantrex, 43
Kaochlor 10%, 494
Kaochlor S-F 10%, 494
kaolin and pectin mixtures, 356
Kaon, 494
Kaon Liquid, 495
Kaon Tablets, 495
Kaon-Cl, 494
Kaon-Cl 20%, 494
Kaoparin, 356
Kaopectate, 356
Kapectin, 356
Ka-Pen, 58
Kappadione, 685
Kardonyl, 277
Karidium, 688
Kasof, 363
Kato Powder, 494
Kavrin, 153
Kaybovite, 678
KayCiel, 494
Kayexalate, 499
Kaytrate, 154
K-Cillin, 58
Keflex, 68
Keflin Neutral, 70
Kefzol, 65
Kelex, 501
Kell-E, 685
Kemadrin, 289
Kenacort, 412
Kenalog, 412, 625
Kenalog in Orabase, 594
Kenazide, 479
Keotin, 356
Keralyt, 653
Ketaject, 672
Ketalar, 672

M

oxychlorosene sodium, 638
oxycodone hydrochloride, 182
Oxy-Kesso-Tetra, 79
Oxylone, 618
oxymetazoline hydrochloride, 592
oxymetholone, 420
oxymorphone hydrochloride, 183
oxyphenbutazone, 168
oxyphencyclimine hydrochloride,
    390
oxyphenonium bromide, 391
Oxytetrachlor, 79
oxytetracycline hydrochloride, 79,
    587
Oxytocin, 729
oxytocin citrate, buccal, 728
oxytocin, synthetic injection, 729
oxytocin, synthetic nasal, 730

P

P-50, 58
PABA, 647
Pabagel, 647
Pabanol, 647
Pagitane Hydrochloride, 287
Palafer, 501
Palmiron, 501
Palocillin, 58
Paltet 250, 80
Pamelor, 226
Pamine, 389
Pamovin, 19
Panafil, 722
Pancrease, 354
pancreatin, 353
pancrelipase, 354
pancuronium bromide, 319
Panectyl, 332
Panheprin, 507
Panmycin, 80
Panophylline Forte, 736
Panoxyl, 656
Panteric Double Strength, 353
Panthoderm Cream, 644
Panthoderm Lotion, 644
Panwarfin, 512
Papacon, 153
papain, 722
Papalease, 153
Papase, 722
papaverine hydrochloride, 153
Papital T.R., 153
PapKaps-150, 153
para-aminobenzoic acid, 647
para-aminosalicylic acid, 36
Paracort, 411
Paradione, 215
Paraflex, 310
Paral, 198, 214

paraldehyde, 198, 214
Paralgin, 160
paramethadione, 215
paramethasone acetate, 409
Parasal Sodium, 36
Para-thor-mone, 469
parathyroid hormone, 469
Parcillin, 58
Parda, 753
Paredrine, 573
Paregoric, 358
Parest, 196
Parest 400, 196
Parfuran, 96
Pargel, 356
Pargesic 65, 184
pargyline hydrochloride, 138
Parlodel, 748
Par-Mag, 349
Parmine, 274
Parnate, 229
Paroidin, 469
paromomycin sulfate, 14
Partrex, 80
PAS, 36
Pasdium, 36
Pathilon, 393
Pathocil, 53
P-A-V, 153
Pavabid, 153
Pavacap, 153
Pavacen, 153
Pavaclor, 153
Pavacron, 153
Pavadel, 153
Pavadur, 153
Pavadyl, 153
Pavakey S.A., 153
Pava-lyn, 153
Pava-Par, 153
Pava-Rx, 153
Pavaspan, 148
Pavasule, 153
Pavatime, 153
Pavatran T.D., 153
Pava-Wol, 153
Paveril Phosphate, 147
Paverolan, 153
Pavex, 153
Pavulon, 319
Pax-400, 236
Paxel, 234
PB, 216
PBR, 216
PBR 12, 200
PBZ-SR, 333
Peacock's Bromides, 207
Pecto-Kalin, 356
Pectokay, 356
Pediaflor, 688
Pediamycin, 102

R

R

S

U

NOTES

NOTES